Differential Diagnosis of Tumors *and* Tumor-like Lesions of Bones and Joints

Differential Diagnosis of Tumors *and* Tumor-like Lesions of Bones and Joints

Adam Greenspan, M.D.
Professor of Radiology and Orthopedic Surgery
University of California, Davis School of Medicine
Chief, Musculoskeletal Radiology
Department of Diagnostic Radiology
University of California, Davis Medical Center
Sacramento, California

and

Wolfgang Remagen, M.D.
Professor Emeritus of General and Special Pathology
Institute of Pathology, University of Basel
Former Head of Swiss Bone Tumor Reference Center
Basel, Switzerland

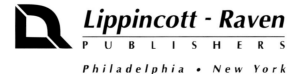

Lippincott - Raven
P U B L I S H E R S

Philadelphia • New York

Acquisitions Editor: James D. Ryan
Developmental Editor: Michelle M. LaPlante
Manufacturing Manager: Dennis Teston
Production Manager: Lawrence Bernstein
Production Editor: Janice G. Lochansky
Cover Designer: Karen Quigley
Indexer: Susan Thomas
Compositor: Maryland Composition Inc.
Printer: Worzalla

Printed in the United States of America

9 8 7 6 5 4 3 2 1

Library of Congress Cataloging-in-Publication Data

Greenspan, Adam.
    Differential diagnosis of tumors and tumor-like lesions of bones and joints /
Adam Greenspan and Wolfgang Remagen. — 1st ed.
        p.   cm.
    Includes bibliographical references and index.
    ISBN 0-397-51710-6
    1. Bones—Tumors—Diagnosis.   2. Joints—Tumors—Diagnosis.
3. Diagnosis, Differential.   I. Remagen, Wolfgang. II. Title.
    [DNLM: 1. Bone Neoplasms—diagnosis.   2. Joint Diseases—diagnosis.
3. Diagnosis, Differential.   WE 258 G815d 1997]
RC280.B6G74   1997
616.99′271075—dc21
DNLM/DLC
for Library of Congress   97-37501
                                                              CIP

To my wife Barbara, and to my children Luddy, Samantha, and Michael, with love.
—A.G.

To my wife Karin for her patience, understanding and encouragement.
—W.R.

Contents

Preface

Differential Diagnosis of Tumors and Tumor-like Lesions of Bones and Joints was written to facilitate the complex process of differential diagnosis of bone and joint lesions that confronts the radiologist and the pathologist. The book was designed to provide a single, concise source of recognition for the majority of bone and joint lesions with emphasis on radiologic and histopathologic approaches. Because the differential diagnosis of a given tumor deemed by the radiologist may be different from that deemed by the pathologist, the diagnostic approach is discussed separately from radiologic and pathologic points-of-view. The text gives an overview of the diversity of the radiologic and histopathologic appearance of benign and malignant bone lesions and lesions situated in or around the joint; typical and atypical features are discussed.

Each chapter provides information concerning clinical presentation of the lesion, imaging techniques and radiologic features, histopathology, and radiologic and pathologic differential diagnosis. The chapters are richly illustrated with roentgenograms, CT and MR images, photomicrographs (in color), and schematic drawings. Important diagnostic features are provided in concise tables, and the summary of differential diagnosis is included at the end of each section in the form of a schematic drawing. This drawing also depicts the less likely differential possibilities that are not discussed in the text. All major tumors and tumor-like lesions are accompanied by line drawings of a skeleton depicting the specific distribution of a given lesion. Detailed and up-to-date references are provided at the end of each chapter.

The histopathologic material, with a few exceptions, was obtained from the Swiss Bone Tumor Reference Center at the Institute of Pathology, University of Basel, Switzerland.

This text has been written with the radiologist and the pathologist in mind as the intended audience, although we believe that the orthopedic oncologist and other physicians may find it useful as well.

A.G.
W.R.

Acknowledgments

We would like to acknowledge the guidance and help in preparation of this text from our many friends at Lippincott–Raven Publishers; in particular, Editor-in-Chief James D. Ryan, Developmental Editor Michelle M. LaPlante, Creative Director Diana Andrews, Cover Designer Karen Quigley, and Associate Production Editor Janice Lochansky.

Special thanks to: Sharon Rule for her initial meticulous editing; Deborah Ann Hoang and Carol Harris for their invaluable secretarial assistance; Gernot Jundt, M.D., lecturer in pathology and now head of the Tumor Reference Center, for his patience and help during the long period of preparation of the manuscript; and Petra Huber at the Tumor Reference Center for unending assistance with finding cases, histopathologic slides, x-ray films, and literature.

CHAPTER 1

Radiologic and Pathologic Approach to Bone Tumors

RADIOLOGY
  Plain Film Radiography
    Site of the Lesion
    Borders of the Lesion
    Type of Bone Destruction
    Periosteal Response

    Type of Matrix
    Soft Tissue Mass
    Benign vs. Malignant Nature
  Scintigraphy, CT, and MRI
PATHOLOGY

INTRODUCTION

The ideal therapeutic goals for managing patients with primary or metastatic lesions can be incorporated into a triad of important factors: (a) do not overtreat a benign bone tumor; (b) do not undertreat a malignant bone tumor; and (c) do not take an incorrect biopsy approach to the lesion, as this may suggest a need for radical rather than more conservative surgery (61,67,79). Achieving these goals depends on close cooperation among the radiologist, the pathologist, and the tumor surgeon.

Several factors make precise diagnosis of osseous tumors difficult. Although radiographic features have a high correlation with malignancy, benignity, and sometimes even an exact histologic diagnosis, radiographic determination of these characteristics is based on statistical probabilities. Moreover, errors in the radiologic interpretation may occur. These can usually be ascribed to failure to recognize a specific pathologic finding or to misinterpretation of normal structures as pathologic. Regardless of how persuasive a radiologist's clinical assessment of the biologic potential of a lesion may be to a pathologist colleague, any lesion, no matter how radiologically typical it appears, may represent an entirely different entity on histologic examination (35). A confident radiologic diagnosis may not outweigh the microscopic appearance of the lesion.

Both the radiologist and the pathologist play important roles by providing the diagnosis and/or differential diagnosis of a bone tumor, thus aiding the clinician in the complex process of patient management. Before a final diagnosis or differential diagnosis is made, clinical information, radiologic imaging, and pathologic material should be carefully studied and correlated. The radiologist has the significant advantage of being able to view the three-dimensional extent of a bone tumor, whereas the pathologist can view only a small biopsy specimen of the lesion selected by the surgeon (67), which may not reflect the histology of the entire lesion. Obviously, viewing the entire resected specimen enhances the final pathologic evaluation. Many years ago, Ewing commented that "the gross anatomy (as revealed in radiographs) is often a safer guide to a correct clinical conception of the disease than the variable and uncertain nature of a small piece of tissue" (22). It is important to emphasize that the differential diagnosis contemplated by the radiologist may be identical to or different from that contemplated by the pathologist. For example, a radiologist who is evaluating a lesion that looks like an aneurysmal bone cyst must include in the differential diagnosis the possibility of telangiectatic osteosarcoma. Likewise, the pathologist who is looking at the histologic sections of the same lesion must also consider the possibility of telangiectatic osteosarcoma because both lesions have several histopathologic similarities. On the other hand, in the radiologic evaluation of a purely lytic lesion at the articular end of a long bone, that looks like a giant cell tumor plasmacytoma might enter into the differential diagnosis, whereas for a pathologist examining the same lesion (which in fact *is* a giant cell tumor), the differential diagnosis will obviously include other lesions that may contain giant-cells. However, the pathologist would not consider plasmacytoma as one of the differential possibilities because of the completely different histologic pattern of this tumor.

For teaching purposes, the diagnostic approach to bone tu-

1

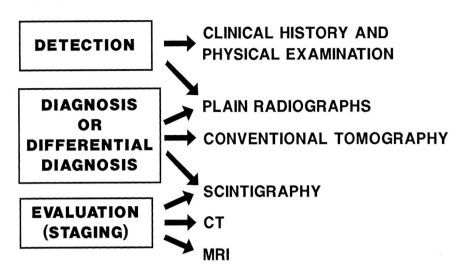

FIG. 1. Imaging of musculoskeletal neoplasms can be considered from three aspects: detection, diagnosis (or differential diagnosis), and evaluation.

mors will be discussed separately from the radiologic and the pathologic point of view.

RADIOLOGY

In general, the imaging of musculoskeletal neoplasms can be considered from three standpoints: detection, diagnosis and differential diagnosis, and evaluation (staging) (Fig. 1). Detection of a bone tumor does not always require the expertise of a radiologist. The clinical history and the physical examination are often sufficient to raise the suspicion of a tumor, although plain radiography is the most common means of revealing one. Bone scintigraphy can also pinpoint lesions, but its findings are nonspecific.

Despite the dramatic advances in imaging technology that have occurred in recent decades, especially the introduction of cross-sectional imaging modalities such as computed tomography (CT) and magnetic resonance imaging (MRI), plain radiography remains the single most important modality for establishing a diagnosis (34) and serves as the basis for differential diagnosis (17,60,69). It yields the most useful information about the location and morphology of a lesion, particularly concerning the type of bone destruction, calcifications, ossifications, and periosteal reaction. Conventional tomography also continues to be a useful diagnostic tool, particularly on those occasions when questions arise regarding cortical destruction, periosteal reaction, or mineralization of the tumor matrix. It can also detect occult pathologic fracture (1). Scintigraphy is only occasionally helpful in making a specific diagnosis but can be valuable in distinguishing, for example, multiple myeloma from similar-appearing metastases (63) or for distinguishing a benign or malignant sclerotic tumor from a bone island (36).

The imaging advances of the past decade have been most profoundly felt in the evaluation (staging) of bone tumors (20,51,72). The multiplanar capabilities and unsurpassed soft tissue contrast offered by CT (11,59) and MRI (2,3) have rendered these modalities indispensable in tumor staging (15,25,29,73). They have enabled radiologists to deter-

mine tumor size, location, and configuration more accurately than ever before and have facilitated demonstration of intra- and extramedullary extension of tumors and the relationship of tumors to individual muscles, muscle compartments, fascial planes, and neurovascular bundles, as well as to neighboring joints and organs (93,4,5). MRI, in fact, affords more accurate anatomic staging than any other imaging method (9,10,14). Nevertheless, it is not helpful in differentiating benign from malignant tumors, despite attempts to identify signal intensity patterns, the appearance of tumor margins, the presence of edema, and neurovascular bundle involvement as markers for this essential determination (40,46).

A number of pulse sequences can be used to evaluate musculoskeletal tumors (32). These include spin-echo (SE) sequences, inversion recovery (IR) sequences, short time inversion-recovery (STIR) sequences, gradient echo (GRE) sequences, and fast T2 or fat-suppression T2-weighted sequences (3,19,31,80). SE sequences are the most effective for identification and staging of most skeletal tumors (2,110). The signal intensity for normal tissues is predictable using these sequences. On T1-weighted images, fat and bone marrow have a high signal intensity that changes to intermediate intensity on T2 weighting. Muscles have intermediate signal intensity on both T1 and T2 sequences. Cortical bone and fibrocartilage have low signal on both sequences. Fluid has intermediate signal on T1-weighted and high signal intensity on T2-weighted images (Table 1). Most bone tumors have increased T1 and T2 relaxation times compared with normal tissue and therefore are imaged as areas of low or intermediate signal intensity on T1-weighted SE sequences and high signal intensity on T2-weighted sequences (3,30,110). T1-weighted SE sequences enhance tumor contrast with bone marrow and fatty tissue, whereas T2-weighted images enhance tumor contrast with muscle and accentuate peritumoral edema (66).

Several investigators have stressed the advantage of contrast enhancement of MR images using intravenous injection of gadopentate dimeglumine (gadolinium diethylenetri-aminepentaacetic acid, or Gd-DTPA) (38,90). This param-

TABLE 1. *MRI signal intensities of various tissues*

Tissue	Image	
	T1-weighted	T2-weighted
Hematoma	High	High
Fat, fatty marrow	High	Intermediate
Muscle, nerves, hyaline cartilage	Intermediate	Intermediate
Cortical bone, tendons, ligaments, fibrocartilage, scar tissue, air	Low	Low
Hyaline cartilage	Intermediate	Intermediate
Red (hematopoietic) marrow	Low	Intermediate
Fluid	Intermediate	High
Tumors (generally)	Intermediate-to-low	High
Lipoma	High	Intermediate
Hemangioma	Intermediate (slightly higher than muscle)	High

agnetic contrast enhancement on conventional T1-weighted sequences decreases the T1 relaxation time in tumor tissue causing the lesion to be of higher signal intensity (hence making the demarcation of the tumor more obvious). In particular, enhancement was found to give better delineation of tumor in richly vascularized parts, in compressed tissue immediately surrounding the tumor, and in atrophic but richly vascularized muscle (77). Both static and dynamic Gd-DTPA studies show significant promise for evaluation of musculoskeletal tumors (21,48,105). Areas that demonstrate contrast enhancement on T1 weighting are typically more vascular, whereas those without enhancement usually represent necrotic tissue (21). In addition, utilization of a chemical shift or fat suppression technique is even more effective (65) because the fat signal becomes markedly suppressed, whereas the abnormal contrast-enhanced tumor displays a high signal intensity (64,100,101). This combination improves the interface between tumor and peritumoral edema, the interface between tumor and reactive zone, and the interface between tumor and adjacent muscle (91,100,101).

Other techniques also play roles in evaluation of bone tumors. These include scintigraphic techniques using technetium (Tc-99), gallium citrate (Ga-67), and indium (In-111)–labeled white blood cells, as well as single photon emission computed tomography (SPECT), among others (4,5,21,24,45,63,93). Because these imaging methods use radiopharmaceutical labeling, they can provide information about the pathophysiologic function of bone and surrounding soft tissues, as well as the size and location of a lesion (62). Bone scintigraphy is a highly sensitive method for detecting bone neoplasms, but its specificity is low. In addition, radioisotope techniques are less accurate than CT and MRI for defining intraosseous tumor extension (12).

Plain Film Radiography

Plain films continue to provide a wealth of information whose implications can be helpful in the precise diagnosis of

a bone tumor (34,47,70,95,107). However, plain radiography does not provide a diagnosis in every case (44). Some types of tumor can be diagnosed with certainty by their radiographic appearance alone; other types can be diagnosed only with various degrees of probability; and still others may have an appearance compatible with that of more than one type of tumor and therefore allow only a differential diagnosis to be made (68,82). The information yielded by plain films includes (Fig. 2):

Topography of the lesion (location in the skeleton and in the individual bone)
Borders of the lesion (the so-called zone of transition)
Type of bone destruction
Type of periosteal response to the lesion (periosteal reaction)
Type of matrix of the lesion (composition of the tumor tissue), and
Nature and extent of soft tissue involvement

Patient age and determination of whether a lesion is solitary or multiple are the starting approaches in the diagnosis of bone tumors (Fig. 3). The age of the patient is the single most important item of clinical data that can be used in conjunction with the radiographic findings to establish a diagnosis (49). Certain tumors occur almost exclusively in a specific age group (Fig. 4). For example, aneurysmal bone cyst, chondromyxoid fibroma, and chondroblastoma rarely occur in individuals >20 years of age. Conversely, giant cell tumor of bone almost invariably arises after growth plate closure, and metastatic lesions, myeloma, and conventional chondrosarcoma are rarely encountered in patients <40 years of age (52,55). Some bone tumors associated with specific age groups may have different radiographic presentations and appear in atypical locations, when they arise outside of their usual age population. Simple bone cysts, for example, are found almost exclusively in the long bones (proximal humerus, proximal femur) before skeletal maturity. After skeletal maturity they may arise in the pelvis, scapula, or calcaneus, among other sites, and may exhibit unconventional radiographic features with progressing age (71).

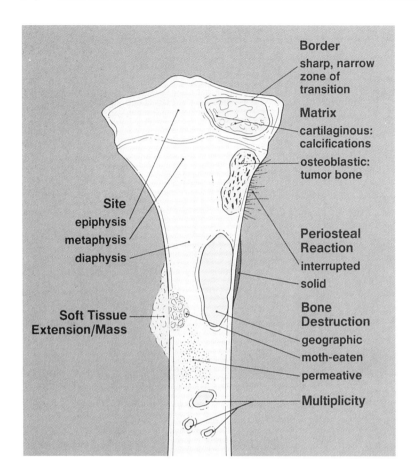

FIG. 2. Radiographic features of tumors and tumor-like lesions of bone.

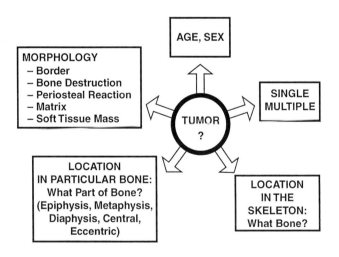

FIG. 3. Analytic approach to evaluation of the bone neoplasm must include patient age, multiplicity of a lesion, location in the skeleton and in the particular bone, and radiographic morphology.

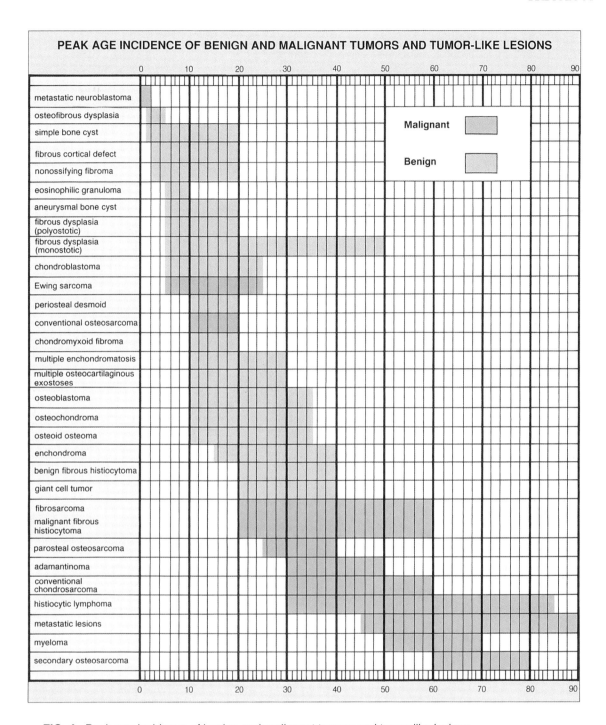

FIG. 4. Peak age incidence of benign and malignant tumors and tumor-like lesions.

Determining the number of lesions also has important implications. Benign lesions tend to involve multiple sites, as in polyostotic fibrous dysplasia, enchondromatosis, multiple osteocartilaginous exostoses, Langerhans-cell granuloma, hemangiomatosis, and fibromatosis. In contrast, primary malignancies, such as osteosarcoma, Ewing sarcoma, fibrosarcoma, and malignant fibrous histiocytoma, rarely present as multifocal disease. Multiple malignant lesions usu-ally indicate metastatic disease, multiple myeloma, or lymphoma.

Site of the Lesion

Some tumors have a predilection for specific bones or specific sites in bone (Table 2 and Fig. 5). This location is de-

TABLE 2. *Predilection of tumors for specific sites in the skeleton*

	A. Skeletal predilection of benign osseous neoplasms and tumor-like lesions	B. Skeletal predilection of malignant osseous neoplasms
Axial skeleton	*Skull and facial bones:* Osteoma, osteoblastoma, Langerhans-cell granuloma, fibrous dysplasia, solitary hemangioma, osteoporosis circumscripta (lytic phase of Paget disease)	*Skull and facial bones:* Mesenchymal chondrosarcoma, chordoma, multiple myeloma, metastatic neuroblastoma, metastatic carcinoma
	Jaw: Giant cell reparative granuloma, myxoma, ossifying fibroma, desmoplastic fibroma	*Mandible:* Osteosarcoma
	Spine: Aneurysmal bone cyst, osteoblastoma, Langerhans-cell granuloma, hemangioma	*Spine:* Chordoma, myeloma, metastases
Appendicular skeleton	*Long tubular bones:* Osteoid osteoma, simple bone cyst, aneurysmal bone cyst, osteochondroma, enchondroma, periosteal chondroma, chondroblastoma, chondromyxoid fibroma, nonossifying fibroma, giant cell tumor, osteofibrous dysplasia, desmoplastic fibroma, intraosseous ganglion	*Long tubular bones:* Osteosarcoma (all variants), adamantinoma, malignant fibrous histiocytoma, angiosarcoma, fibrosarcoma, primary lymphoma, chondrosarcoma
	Hands and feet: Giant cell reparative granuloma, florid reactive periostitis, enchondroma, glomus tumor, epidermoid cyst, subungual exostosis, bizarre parosteal osteochondromatous lesion	*Hands and feet:* None
Specific predilections	Simple bone cyst—proximal humerus, proximal femur	Adamantinoma—tibia, fibula
	Osteofibrous dysplasia—tibia, fibula (anterior cortex)	Parosteal osteosarcoma—distal femur (posterior cortex)
	Osteoid osteoma—femur, tibia	Periosteal osteosarcoma—tibia
	Chondromyxoid fibroma— tibia, metaphyses	Clear cell chondrosarcoma— proximal femur and humerus
	Chondroblastoma—epiphyses	Chordoma—sacrum, clivus, C2
	Giant cell tumor—articular ends of femur, tibia, radius	Multiple myeloma—pelvis, spine, skull

Modified from Fechner, RE, Mills, SE. *Tumors of the bones and joints,* 3rd ed., Vol. 8. Armed Forces Institute of Pathology, 1993;1–16.

termined by the laws of field behavior and developmental anatomy of the affected bone, a concept first popularized by Johnson (42,67). Parosteal osteosarcoma, for example, arises with very rare exceptions in the posterior aspect of the distal femur, a feature so characteristic that it alone can suggest the diagnosis (Fig. 6). The same can be said of chondroblastoma, which has a strong preference for the epiphysis of long bones before skeletal maturity (Fig. 7). Adamantinoma and osteofibrous dysplasia have a specific predilection for the tibia (Fig. 8; **see also Figs. 4-34, 4-35, and 7-52**). A lesion's location can also exclude certain entities from the differential diagnosis. Giant-cell tumor, for example, should not be considered if the lesion does not affect the articular end of a bone because very few of these tumors are found anywhere else.

Equally important in the evaluation of a lesion's site is its location in relation to the central axis of the bone (Fig. 9). This is particularly true when the lesion is located in a long tubular bone, such as humerus, radius, femur, or tibia (37). For example, simple bone cyst, enchondroma, or a focus of fibrous dysplasia always appears centrally located (**see Figs. 3-6B, 3-9, 3-8, 4-19, 7-15, and 7-16**). In contrast, eccentric location is characteristically observed in aneurysmal bone cyst, chondromyxoid fibroma, and nonossifying fibroma (**see Figs. 3-70, 3-71, 4-2B, 4-3, 4-4, 7-25, and 7-28**).

Borders of the Lesion

The borders or margins of a lesion are crucial factors in determining the growth rate of a lesion and hence whether it is benign or malignant (58). Three types of lesion margins are encountered: (a) a margin with sharp demarcation by sclerosis between the peripheral aspect of the tumor and the adjacent host bone (IA margin); (b) a margin with sharp demarcation without sclerosis around the periphery of the lesion (IB margin); and (c) a margin with an ill-defined region (either the entire circumference or only a portion of it) at the interface between lesion and host bone (IC margin) (Fig. 10). Slow-growing lesions are marked by sharply outlined,

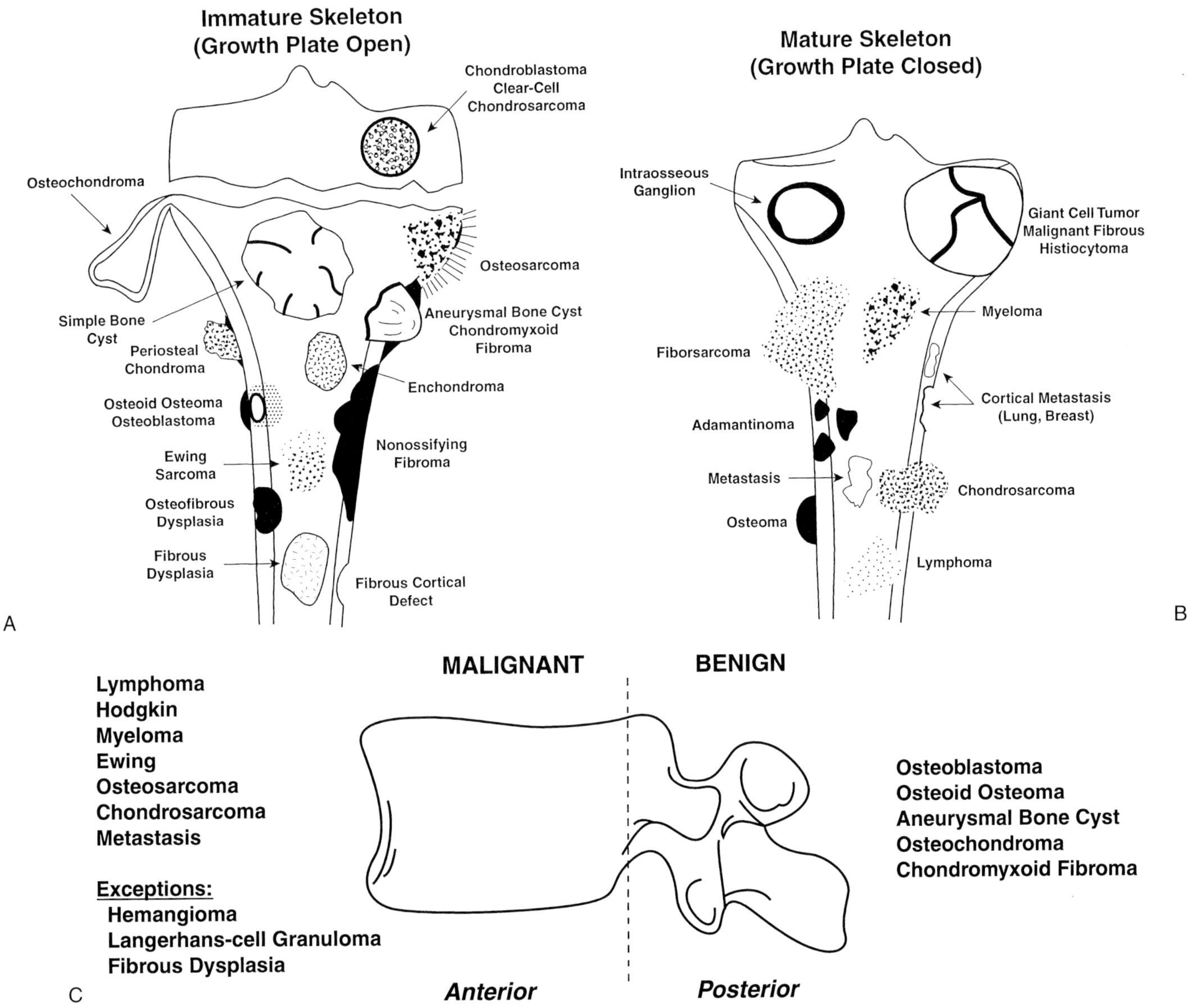

Immature Skeleton (Growth Plate Open)

Chondroblastoma
Clear-Cell
Chondrosarcoma

Osteochondroma

Osteosarcoma

Simple Bone
Cyst

Periosteal
Chondroma

Aneurysmal Bone Cyst
Chondromyxoid
Fibroma

Enchondroma

Osteoid Osteoma
Osteoblastoma

Ewing
Sarcoma

Nonossifying
Fibroma

Osteofibrous
Dysplasia

Fibrous
Dysplasia

Fibrous Cortical
Defect

A

Mature Skeleton (Growth Plate Closed)

Intraosseous
Ganglion

Giant Cell Tumor
Malignant Fibrous
Histiocytoma

Myeloma

Fiborsarcoma

Cortical Metastasis
(Lung, Breast)

Adamantinoma

Chondrosarcoma

Metastasis

Osteoma

Lymphoma

B

MALIGNANT   **BENIGN**

Lymphoma
Hodgkin
Myeloma
Ewing
Osteosarcoma
Chondrosarcoma
Metastasis

Osteoblastoma
Osteoid Osteoma
Aneurysmal Bone Cyst
Osteochondroma
Chondromyxoid Fibroma

Exceptions:
Hemangioma
Langerhans-cell Granuloma
Fibrous Dysplasia

C

Anterior   *Posterior*

FIG. 5. Site of the lesion. **A:** Distribution of various lesions in a long tubular bone in a growing skeleton (growth plate is open). **B:** Distribution of various lesions in a long tubular bone after skeletal maturity (growth plate is closed). **C:** Distribution of various lesions in a vertebra. Malignant lesions are seen predominantly in its anterior part (body), whereas benign lesions predominate in its posterior elements.

sclerotic borders, and this narrow zone of transition usually indicates that a tumor is benign (67). Benign lesions such as nonossifying fibroma, simple bone cyst, and chondromyxoid fibroma almost invariably exhibit sclerosis at their borders. Indistinct borders (a wide zone of transition), on the other hand, are typical of malignant or aggressive lesions. Primary malignancies such as fibrosarcoma, malignant fibrous histiocytoma, lymphoma, multiple myeloma (or solitary plasmacytoma), and metastases from primary tumors of the kidney, thyroid, and gastrointestinal tract usually lack a sclerotic border, as does the giant-cell tumor of bone. Radio- or chemotherapy of malignant bone tumors can alter their appearance, causing them to exhibit sclerosis and a narrow zone of transition.

The more well-defined the margin (e.g., IA, IB), the slower the biologic activity, and therefore the more likely that the lesion is benign. Conversely, the less well-defined the margin (IC), the greater the biologic activity, and therefore the more likely that the lesion is malignant (65).

Type of Bone Destruction

Destruction of bone represents not only a direct effect of tumor cells but also reflects a complex mechanism in which

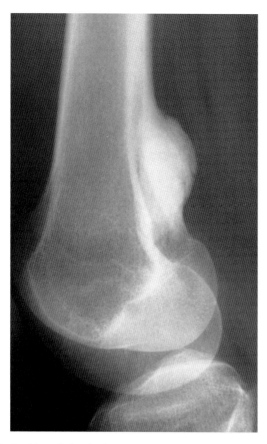

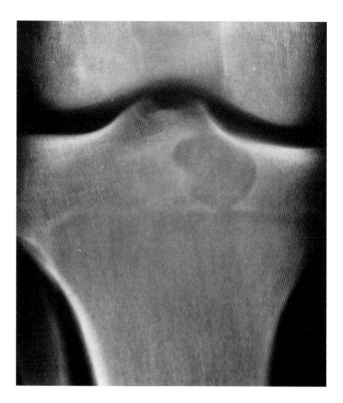

FIG. 7. Site of the lesion. Chondroblastoma has a predilection for the epiphysis of a long bone.

FIG. 6. Site of the lesion. Parosteal osteosarcoma has a predilection for the posterior aspect of the distal femur.

normal osteoclasts of the host bone respond to pressure generated by the enlarging mass and by active hyperemia associated with the tumor (68). Cortical bone is destroyed less rapidly than trabecular bone. However, loss of cortical bone appears earlier on radiography because its density is highly homogeneous compared with that of trabecular bone. In the latter, greater amounts of bone must be destroyed (about 70% loss of mineral content) before the loss becomes radiographically evident (68). Like the borders of a lesion, the type of bone destruction caused by a tumor indicates its growth rate. Bone destruction can be described as geographic (type I), moth-eaten (type II), and permeative (type III) (52,54) (Fig. 11). Although none of these features are pathognomonic for any specific neoplasm, the type of destruction may suggest a benign or a malignant process. Geographic bone destruction is characterized by a uniformly destroyed area usually within sharply defined borders. It typifies slow-growing, benign lesions, such as simple bone cyst, enchondroma, chondromyxoid fibroma, or giant cell tumor. On the other hand, moth-eaten (i.e., characterized by multiple, small, often clustered lytic areas) and permeative (i.e., characterized by ill-defined, very small oval radiolucencies or lucent streaks) types of bone destruction mark rapidly growing, infiltrating tumors, such as myeloma, lymphoma, fibrosarcoma, or Ewing sarcoma. However, some

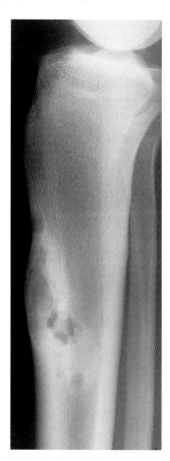

FIG. 8. Site of the lesion. Tibia is a common site for adamantinoma.

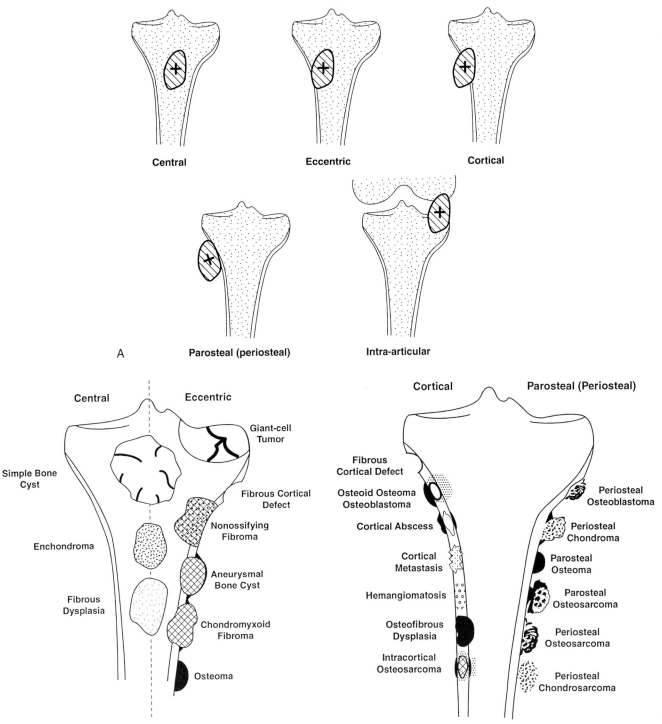

FIG. 9. Site of the lesion. **A:** Location of the epicenter of the lesion usually determines the site of its origin, whether medullary, cortical, periosteal, soft tissue, or in the joint. **B:** Eccentric vs. central location of the similar-appearing lesions is helpful in differential diagnosis. **C:** Cortical and parosteal (periosteal) lesions.

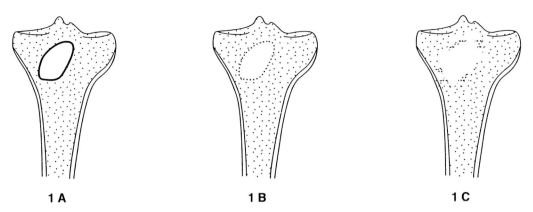

1 A   **1 B**   **1 C**

FIG. 10. Borders of the lesion determine its growth rate. *1A*, sharp sclerotic; *1B*, sharp lytic; *1C*, ill-defined. (Modified from Madewell JE, Ragsdale BD, Sweet DE. Radiologic and pathologic analysis of solitary bone lesions. Part I. Internal margins. *Radiol Clin North Am* 1981;19:715–748.)

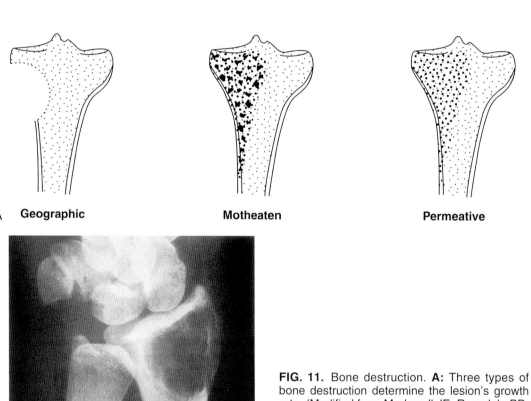

A   **Geographic**   **Motheaten**   **Permeative**

B

FIG. 11. Bone destruction. **A:** Three types of bone destruction determine the lesion's growth rate. (Modified from Madewell JE, Ragsdale BD, Sweet DE. Radiologic and pathologic analysis of solitary bone lesions. Part I. Internal margins. *Radiol Clin North Am* 1981;19:715–748.) **B:** The geographic type of bone destruction is characterized by a uniformly affected area within sharply defined borders, in this case a giant cell tumor.

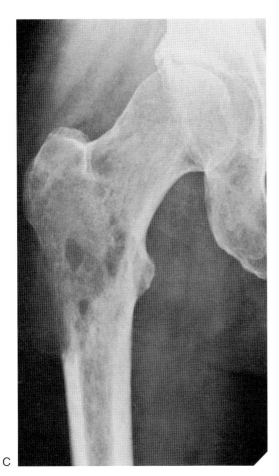
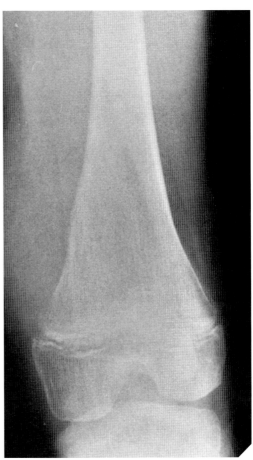

C

D

FIG. 11. *Continued.* **C:** The moth-eaten bone destruction is characteristic of rapidly growing infiltrating lesions, in this case myeloma. **D:** The permeative type of bone destruction is characteristic of round cell tumors, in this case Ewing sarcoma. Note the almost imperceptible destruction of the metaphysis of the femur by a tumor that has infiltrated the medullary cavity and cortex and extended into the surrounding soft tissues, forming a large mass.

non-neoplastic lesions may demonstrate this aggressive pattern. For example, osteomyelitis can exhibit both type II (moth-eaten) and type III (permeative) patterns of destruction (67). Similarly, hyperparathyroidism can cause a permeative pattern (58). The distinction between a moth-eaten and a permeative pattern of destruction may be subtle; often the two patterns coexist in the same lesion.

Periosteal Response

Like the pattern of bone destruction, the pattern of periosteal reaction is an indicator of the biologic activity of a lesion (106). Bone neoplasms elicit periosteal reactions that can be categorized as uninterrupted (continuous) or interrupted (discontinuous) (81) (Fig. 12 and Table 3). Any widening and irregularity of bone contour may represent periosteal activity. The solid periosteal reaction represents a single solid layer or multiple closely apposed and fused layers of new bone attached to the outer surface of the cortex (81) (Fig. 13). The resulting pattern is often referred to as cortical thickening (23). Although no single periosteal response is unique for a given lesion, an uninterrupted periosteal reaction indicates a long-standing (slow-growing), usually indolent, benign process. There are several types of solid periosteal reaction: a solid buttress, such as is frequently seen accompanying aneurysmal bone cyst and chondromyxoid fibroma; a solid smooth or elliptical layer, such as is seen in osteoid osteoma and osteoblastoma; an undulating type, most frequently seen in long-standing varicosities, pulmonary osteoarthropathy, chronic lymphedema, periostitis, and, rarely, with neoplasms (81); and a single lamellar reaction, such as accompanies osteomyelitis, Langerhans-cell granuloma, and stress fracture. An interrupted periosteal response, on the other hand, is commonly seen in malignant primary tumors and less commonly in some metastatic lesions and highly aggressive nonmalignant processes. In these tumors, the periosteal reaction may appear in a sun-

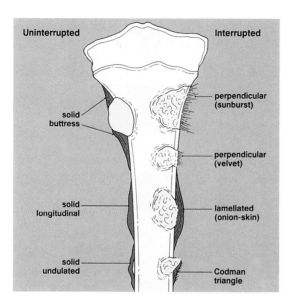

FIG. 12. Types of periosteal reaction. An uninterrupted periosteal reaction usually indicates a benign process, whereas an interrupted reaction indicates a malignant or aggressive nonmalignant process.

burst ("hair-on-end") (Fig. 14A) or onion-skin (lamellated) pattern (Fig. 14B, C). When the tumor breaks through the cortex and destroys the newly formed lamellated bone, the remnants of the latter on both ends of the break-through area may remain as a triangular structure known as a Codman triangle (Fig. 14D, E).

Type of Matrix

The matrix represents the intercellular material produced by mesenchymal cells and includes osteoid, bone, chondroid, myxoid, and collagen material (99). Assessment of the type of matrix allows differentiation of some similar-appearing lesions and, in particular, the tumor matrix provides a useful means of differentiating osteoblastic from chondroblastic processes. Although it should be kept in mind that tumor bone is often radiographically indistinguishable from reparative new bone deposited secondary to bone destruction by a reactive sclerosis or callus formation, the presence of irregular, not fully mineralized bone matrix within or adjacent to an area of bone destruction strongly suggests osteosarcoma (Fig. 15). Similarly, cottony or cloud-like densities within the medullary cavity and in the adjacent soft tissues are likely to represent tumor bone and hence osteosarcoma.

Calcifications in the tumor matrix, on the other hand, point to a chondroblastic process. These calcifications typically appear punctate (stippled), irregularly shaped (flocculent), or curvilinear (annular or comma-shaped, rings and arcs). In benign or well-differentiated malignant tumors they may reflect the process of endochondral ossification (99) (Fig. 16A). Differential diagnosis of stippled, flocculent, or ring-and-arc calcifications includes enchondroma (Fig. 16B), chondroblastoma, and chondrosarcoma (Fig. 16C). Sometimes it is difficult to distinguish osseous matrix from cartilaginous matrix. The former usually appears radiographically more organized and structural (trabecular), whereas the latter is more amorphous, with frequently distinguished characteristic calcifications (described above).

TABLE 3. *Examples of nonneoplastic and neoplastic processes categorized by type of periosteal reaction*

Uninterrupted Periosteal Reaction	
Benign tumors and tumor-like lesions	*Non-neoplastic conditions*
Osteoid osteoma	Osteomyelitis
Osteoblastoma	Langerhans-cell granuloma
Aneurysmal bone cyst	Healing fracture
Chondromyxoid fibroma	Juxtacortical myositis ossificans
Periosteal chondroma	Hypertrophic pulmonary osteoarthropathy
Chondroblastoma	Hemophilia (subperiosteal bleeding)
	Varicose veins and peripheral vascular
Malignant tumors	insufficiency
Chondrosarcoma (rare)	Caffey disease
	Thyroid acropachy
	Treated scurvy
	Pachydermoperiostosis
	Gaucher disease

Interrupted Periosteal Reaction	
Malignant tumors	*Non-neoplastic conditions*
Osteosarcoma	Osteomyelitis (occasionally)
Ewing sarcoma	Langerhans cell granuloma (occasionally)
Chondrosarcoma	Subperiosteal hemorrhage (occasionally)
Lymphoma (rare)	
Fibrosarcoma (rare)	
MFH (rare)	
Metastatic carcinoma	

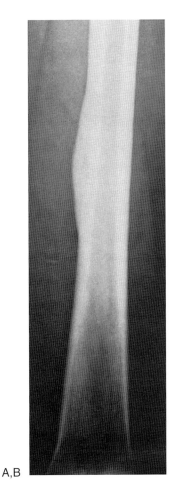
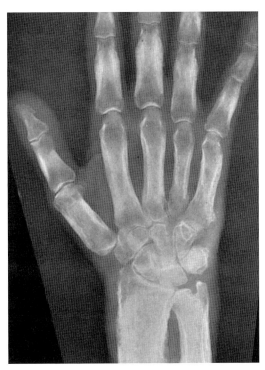

A,B

FIG. 13. Solid type of periosteal reaction. **A:** An uninterrupted solid periosteal reaction is characteristic of benign lesions, in this case a cortical osteoid osteoma. **B:** An uninterrupted periosteal reaction typifies changes of hypertrophic pulmonary osteoarthropathy as seen here in the distal radius and ulna and bones of the hand in a patient with carcinoma of the lung.

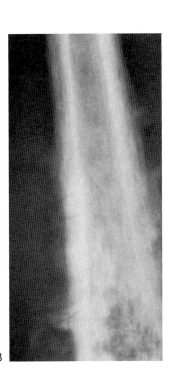
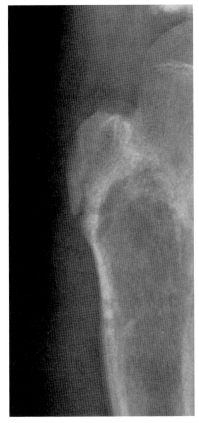

A,B

FIG. 14. Interrupted type of periosteal reaction. **A:** Highly aggressive and malignant lesions may present radiographically with a sunburst pattern of periosteal reaction, as seen in this case of osteosarcoma. **B:** Another pattern of interrupted periosteal reaction is the lamellated or onion-skin type as seen here in Ewing sarcoma involving the proximal femur.

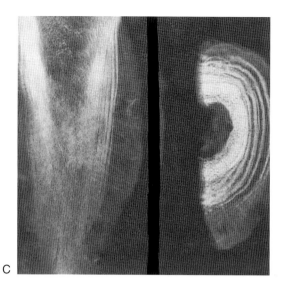

FIG. 14. *(cont.)* C: Radiographs of the slab sections (coronal at left and transverse at right) of the resected specimen from Ewing sarcoma demonstrate lamellated type in more detail. **D:** Codman triangle also reflects an aggressive, usually malignant type of periosteal response. **E:** Schematic representation of periosteal reactive bone formation. (a) Tumor (*red dashes*) growing against endosteal border of the cortex blocks vascular supply and provokes reactive hyperemia of periosteum with secondary formation of a single layer of bone. (b) With progressive destruction of cortical bone additional layers of periosteal bone form lamellated ("onion-peel") appearance. (c) After the rapidly growing tumor has destroyed cortex and newly formed periosteal bone, remnants of the latter at the tumor border form Codman triangle. (d) Slowly growing tumor leaves time to form perpendicular reactive periosteal bone (spiculae, sunburst appearance).

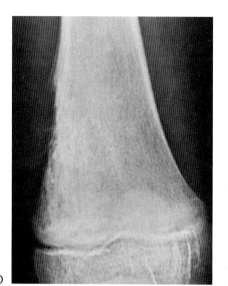

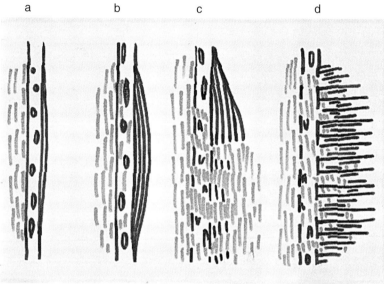

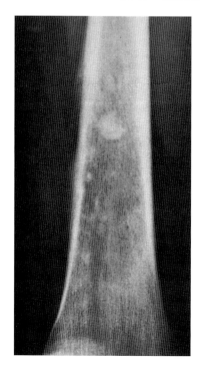

FIG. 15. Types of matrix: osteoblastic. The matrix of a typical osteoblastic lesion, in this case an osteosarcoma, is characterized by the presence of fluffy, cotton-like densities within the medullary cavity of the distal femur.

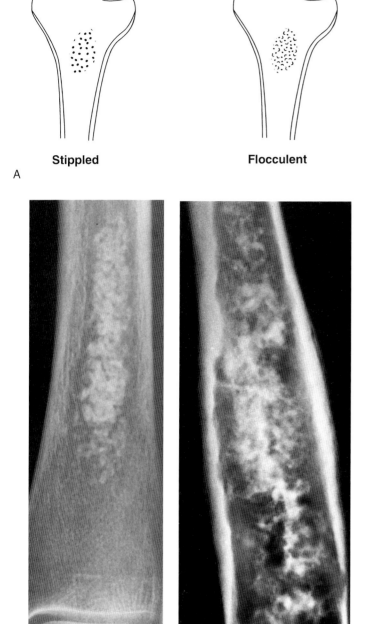

Stippled   Flocculent   Rings and Arcs
("o"'s and "c"'s)

A

B,C

FIG. 16. Types of matrix: chondroid. **A:** Schematic representation of various appearances of chondroid matrix calcifications. (Modified from Sweet DE, Madewell JE, Ragsdale BD. Radiologic and pathologic analysis of solitary bone lesions. Part III. Matrix patterns. *Radiol Clin North Am* 1981;19:785–814.). **B:** Enchondroma displays a typical chondroid matrix. **C:** Chondrosarcoma with characteristic chondroid matrix.

TABLE 4. *Tumors and pseudotumors that may present as radiolucent lesions*

A. Solid	B. Cystic
Osteoblastic (osteoid osteoma, osteoblastoma, telangiectatic osteosarcoma)	Simple bone cyst
Cartilaginous (enchondroma, chondroblastoma, chondromyxoid fibroma, chondrosarcoma)	Aneurysmal bone cyst
Fibrous and histiocytic (nonossifying fibroma, fibrous dysplasia, osteofibrous dysplasia, desmoplastic fibroma, fibrosarcoma, malignant fibrous histiocytoma)	Various bone cysts (synovial, degenerative)
Intraosseous lipoma	Brown tumor of hyperparathyroidism
Lymphoma	Vascular lesions
Myeloma (plasmacytoma)	Hydatid cyst
Ewing sarcoma	Hemophilic pseudotumor
Metastatic (from lung, breast, gastrointestinal tract, kidney, thyroid)	Intraosseous ganglion
Giant cell tumor	Bone abscess
Langerhans cell granuloma	
Paget disease (osteolytic phase—osteoporosis circumscripta)	

A completely radiolucent lesion may be either fibrous or cartilaginous in origin, although hollow structures produced by tumor-like lesions, such as simple bone cysts or intraosseous ganglion, can also present as radiolucent areas (Table 4).

Soft Tissue Mass

With few exceptions—giant-cell tumor, aneurysmal bone cyst, and desmoplastic fibroma among the more common examples—benign bone tumors usually do not have an associated soft tissue mass, which is an invariable feature of many advanced malignant and aggressive lesions (Fig. 17). Nevertheless, it is important to note that some nonneoplastic conditions also manifest with a soft tissue component, e.g., osteomyelitis. In such cases, however, the associated mass is usually poorly defined and the fatty tissue layers appear obliterated. This is in sharp contrast to the soft tissue extensions typical of malignant processes, in which a defined mass extends through the destroyed cortex but the tissue planes are usually intact.

A bone lesion associated with a soft tissue mass should prompt the question of which came first. Is the soft tissue lesion an extension of a primary bone tumor, or is it a primary tumor invading bone? Some clues may help to answer this question, but these observations are by no means absolute (Fig. 18). A large soft tissue mass with a smaller bone lesion usually indicates secondary bone involvement. That said, it is worth noting that Ewing sarcoma and less commonly malignant tumors may exhibit a large soft tissue mass accompanying a small primary bone malignancy. Another clue to help determine the primary malignancy may be found in the periosteal response. Primary soft tissue tumors adjacent to bone usually destroy the neighboring periosteum without

eliciting a periosteal response. Primary bone malignancies, however, typically prompt a periosteal reaction when they grow into the cortex and extend into adjacent soft tissues (34,67,81).

Benign vs. Malignant Nature

Although it is sometimes very difficult to establish a lesion as benign or malignant by plain radiography alone, the clusters of features that can be gathered from plain films can help in favoring one designation over the other (Fig. 19). Benign tumors usually have well-defined sclerotic borders and exhibit a geographic type of bone destruction; the periosteal reaction is solid and uninterrupted, and there is no soft tissue mass. In contrast, malignant lesions often exhibit poorly defined borders with a wide zone of transition; bone destruction appears in a moth-eaten or permeative pattern, and the periosteum shows an interrupted, sunburst, or onion-skin re-

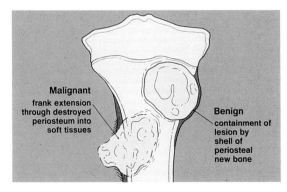

Fig. 17. Radiographic features of soft tissue extension characterizing malignant or aggressive bone lesions and benign processes.

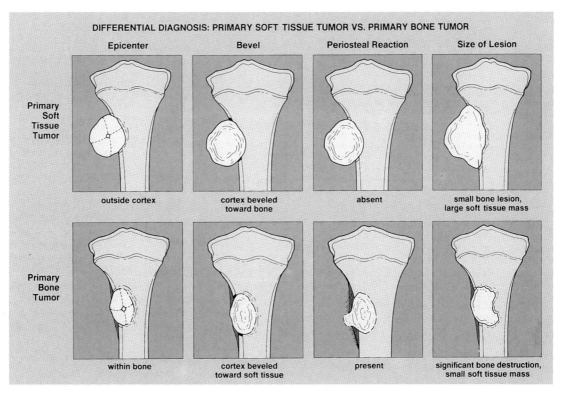

FIG. 18. Certain radiographic features of bone and soft tissue lesions may help differentiate a primary soft tissue tumor invading the bone from a primary bone tumor invading soft tissues. (From Greenspan A. *Orthopedic radiology,* 2nd ed. Philadelphia: Lippincott-Raven, 1992.)

action with an adjacent soft tissue mass. It should be kept in mind, however, that some benign lesions may also exhibit aggressive features (Table 5).

Scintigraphy, CT, and MRI

An essential factor in the evaluation of a bone lesion is intra- and extraosseous extension. Although plain radiography

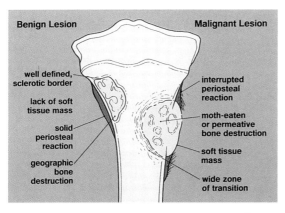

FIG. 19. Radiographic features that may help differentiate benign from malignant lesions.

and conventional tomography can yield significant information about tumor extension, bone scintigraphy, CT, and MRI are indispensable techniques for evaluating whether a tumor has spread beyond its site of origin (6,27,39,76,78,83,84,97). Radionuclide bone imaging better demonstrates the extent of intramedullary involvement by tumor than plain films or conventional tomograms, but it tends to show a larger than actual area of extension because the radiopharmaceutical also localizes to areas of hyperemia and edema adjacent to the tumor (7). Therefore, bone scans are not adequate for evaluating the exact level of intramedullary invasion. However, scintigraphy has no competitor (except for MRI) for identifying additional remote skeletal lesions, so-called skip lesions, and intraosseous metastases (24).

Scintigraphy and MRI or CT are truly complementary examinations that provide quite different staging information for the patient who presents with a bone tumor that requires biopsy (85,86,87). The main role of scintigraphy is not so much for local staging as for evaluating the remainder of the skeleton. Although scintigraphy provides information on the intraosseous extent of disease, it cannot entirely be relied on for local extent of the lesion [because of the augmented uptake that has been described in osteosarcomas (12,41)], its inability to match MRI in differentiating normal from abnormal marrow, and its inability to adequately demonstrate extracompartmental disease. Increased uptake of radionuclides is highly nonspecific. Any pathologic process in bone that

TABLE 5. *Benign lesions with aggressive features*

Lesion	Radiographic presentation	Lesion	Radiographic presentation
Osteoblastoma (aggressive)	Bone destruction and soft tissue extension similar to osteosarcoma	Osteomyelitis	Bone destruction, aggressive periosteal reaction. Occasionally, features resembling osteosarcoma, Ewing sarcoma, or lymphoma
Desmoplastic fibroma	Expansive, destructive lesion, frequently trabeculated	Langerhans-cell granuloma	Bone destruction, aggressive periosteal reaction. Occasionally, features resembling Ewing sarcoma
Periosteal desmoid	Irregular cortical outline, mimics osteosarcoma or Ewing sarcoma	Pseudtumor of hemophilia	Bone destruction, periosteal reaction occasionally mimics malignant tumor
Giant-cell tumor	Occasionally, aggressive features such as osteolytic bone destruction, cortical penetration, and soft tissue extension	Myositis ossificans	Features of parosteal or periosteal osteosarcoma, soft tissue osteosarcoma, or liposarcoma
Aneurysmal bone cyst	Soft tissue extension, occasionally mimicking malignant tumor	Brown tumor of hyperparathyroidism	Lytic bone lesion, resembling malignant tumor

leads to new bone formation (reactive or tumor bone), increased blood flow, or bone turnover, will show increased radionuclide uptake (26). Therefore, a bone scan is usually not reliable for identifying the specific type of tumor or for differentiating malignant from benign processes. Despite these factors, scintigraphy is still an important technique for evaluation of solitary bone tumors. Because scintigraphy is the most sensitive examination for evaluation of the entire skeleton, it should always be performed to determine whether skeletal involvement is solitary or multiple. Metastases are the most common malignant tumors of bone and can frequently present as a solitary abnormality. In the pediatric age group, as in adults, metastases may mimic solitary tumors of bone. Metastatic neuroblastoma and leukemia may resemble true solitary lesions such as Ewing sarcoma, Langerhans-cell granuloma, and acute osteomyelitis. Because synchronous and delayed skeletal metastases may occur, scintigraphy is recommended at initial presentation and in follow-up of patients after extirpation of primary Ewing tumor (28). Scintigraphy can suggest the presence or absence of disseminated skeletal disease. In the proper clinical setting its appearance can be quite specific for the diagnosis of osteoid osteoma (88).

Both CT and MRI are highly accurate for determining the presence of soft tissue invasion by a tumor (48,74,96,102,109). MRI provides valuable information regarding the intraosseous and extraosseous extent of neoplasms. Its primary advantages include the provision of soft tissue contrast superior to that of CT, its multiplanar imaging ability (sagittal, coronal, axial, and oblique), its lack of beam-hardening artifacts from cortical bone, and its superior ability to characterize certain tissues (3,110). For characterization of soft tissue masses, MRI has distinct advantages

over CT (13). Coronal plane MR images, in particular, are often superior to axial CT scans in providing details of extra- and intramedullary tumor extent and its relationship to surrounding structures. Combining axial and coronal plane imaging has also been helpful in assessing important vascular structures adjacent to tumors. In addition, MRI offers better visualization of tissue planes surrounding a lesion and can evaluate neurovascular involvement without the use of intravenous contrast. Particularly in tumors of the extremities, the ability of MRI to demarcate normal from abnormal tissue more sharply than CT can reliably delineate the spatial boundaries of tumor masses, encasement and displacement of major neurovascular bundles, and the extent of joint involvement (1,50). T1-weighted SE images enhance tumor contrast with bone, bone marrow, and fatty tissue. T2-weighted SE or T2-weighted gradient echo images, on the other hand, enhance tumor contrast with muscle and accentuate peritumor edema (75,94,98,104).

In several respects, however, CT unquestionably rivals MRI. MR images do not clearly depict calcifications in the tumor matrix or allow it to be characterized as readily as CT. In fact, large amounts of calcification and ossification have occasionally gone almost undetected by MRI (98). In addition, MRI demonstration of cortical destruction and periosteal reaction is less satisfactory than that of CT or even of plain films and tomography (33,94). Although neither technique is usually suitable for establishing the precise nature of a bone tumor (except perhaps the characteristic MRI features of intraosseous lipoma and hemangioma), much faith has been placed in MRI in particular as a method capable of distinguishing benign from malignant lesions (21,40,46,56). An overlap between the classic characteristics of benign and malignant tumor is often observed (57). Moreover, some malignant bone tumors can appear misleadingly benign on MR images and, conversely, some benign lesions may exhibit a misleadingly malignant appearance. Attempts to formulate precise criteria for correlating MRI findings with histologic diagnosis have been largely unsuccessful (98). Tissue characterization on the basis of MRI signal intensities is still unreliable. Because of the wide spectrum of bone tumor composition and their differing histologic patterns, as well as in tumors of similar histologic diagnosis, signal intensities of histologically different tumors may overlap or there may be variability of signal intensity in histologically similar tumors. MRI is sensitive for delineating the extent of disease but unfortunately is relatively nonspecific (94).

PATHOLOGY

The task of categorizing an osseous lesion as benign or malignant is even more complex for the pathologist than for the radiologist. In bone tumor pathology, more than 65 entities must be differentiated, most of them representing a very low incidence. In fact, primary malignant bone tumors comprise only 1% of all malignancies, and about half of these represent multiple myeloma. Accordingly, the diagnostic density, even in a large institution, may not be sufficient to ensure diagnostic security. Therefore, an opinion from a bone tumor reference center should be obtained in all doubtful cases. For the pathologist, it is mandatory to consider all the radiologic criteria (see above), together with the data supplied by the clinician. Ideally, the pathologist should also consult with both the radiologist and the orthopedic surgeon. Although it may be obvious to a clinician that a child with a rock-hard, tender, 15-cm swelling of the femur almost undoubtedly has a tumor, a 4-mm sampling of tissue from the same lesion, unaccompanied by a history and radiologic studies, is fraught with diagnostic risk (35). Without consideration of all available correlative measurements before an attempt is made to interpret histologic sections, there is no assurance that a biopsy specimen is representative of the lesion or, in fact, that the actual abnormality has been sampled. This is particularly true for chondroblastic tumors, in which benign tissue may be dispersed within the malignant portion of a tumor, and vice versa.

After results of the necessary clinical correlation studies have been considered, the histologic diagnosis is rendered. The tumor cells and their arrangement, and the intercellular matrix produced, are compared with the appearance of radiographs and other imaging studies to verify adequate and representative sampling. The histologic patterns are then compared and matched with similar or identical histologic patterns of known examples of bone tumors (103). For daily diagnostic requirements, the standard hematoxylin and eosin (H&E) stain after decalcification is usually sufficient (Fig. 20). Only for some histochemical and immunocytochemical methods does previous decalcification represent an obstacle.

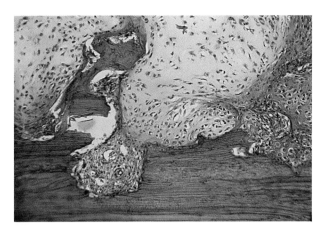

FIG. 20. Hematoxylin and eosin stain. The cortex of the femur (*bottom*) shows large resorption lacunae (*center and right*) with cartilaginous tumor tissue (chondrosarcoma) invading the bone. Some osteoclasts that created the excavations are still visible (*center*). The cartilage stains pink, the bone stains red (hematoxylin and eosin, original magnification ×100).

The method introduced some 20 years ago of embedding the bone specimen in plastic and cutting it without prior decalcification, which is necessary for histomorphometric purposes, does not substantially contribute to bone tumor diagnostics. Among the special stains available is van Gieson stain, which is more commonly used in Europe. This stain helps to identify the presence and amount of collagen in bone and other connective tissues by staining it intensely red (Fig. 21). Giemsa stain should be used in the differentiation of small, blue, round cell tumors, particularly the lymphomas (Fig. 22). It also intensely stains the arrest lines in the bone matrix, thus making apposition and reconstruction processes clearer than in an H&E preparation. We have found it useful in the differentiation of bone and cartilage when both tissues are intermingled because of the metachromatic properties of

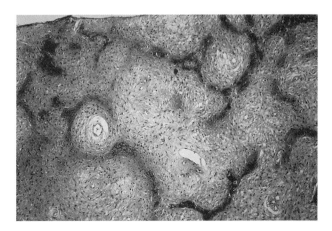

FIG. 21. Van Gieson stain. Chinese characters-like bone trabeculae typical of fibrous dysplasia show no evidence of osteoblastic rimming. Collagen fibers stain intensely red (van Gieson, original magnification ×50).

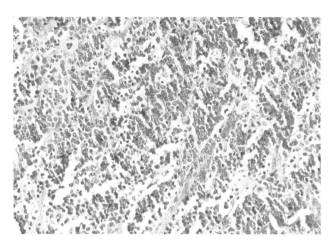

FIG. 22. Giemsa stain. In Burkitt lymphoma the large clear cells become more evident with this staining. The small cells contain large nuclei which stain intensely (Giemsa, original magnification ×50).

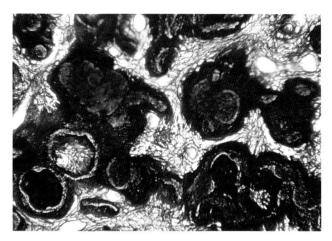

FIG. 24. Gomori stain. With this stain, the densely arranged reticulin fibers in the trabeculae of fibrous dysplasia and in the near surroundings appear in black. (Gomori stain, original magnification ×10).

the hyaline cartilage matrix. This staining technique helps to differentiate fibrocartilage because of its much lower metachromatic properties. The Alcian blue stain can be useful in a similar manner (Fig. 23). Reticulin fibers are usually stained with Gomori stain, which is helpful in the differentiation against collagen fibers (Fig. 24). We prefer the variation of this stain described by Novotny, in which the fibers stand out more clearly (Fig. 25). Another helpful tool is enzyme histochemistry, in particular the demonstration of alkaline phosphatase as marker for osteoblasts (Fig. 26A) and acid phosphatase as marker for osteoclasts (Fig. 26B).

A more recent method is immunohistochemistry, more properly called immunocytochemistry (18), which consists of the demonstration of markers on the surface and on the inner structures of cells by immunologic methods (89) (Fig. 27). For example, the application of leukocyte common anti-

gen and neuron-specific stains, as well as the ultrastructural identification of neurosecretory granules, can assist in distinguishing malignant lymphoma and neuroblastoma from Ewing sarcoma (16). However, it must be stated here that the expectations that center around electron microscopy have been disappointing to a certain extent, mostly because at the electron microscopic level most cells more or less resemble each other (43). There are, however, some exceptions as in the above-mentioned examples, in which electron microscopy is useful for practical diagnostic purposes (Fig. 28). These will be mentioned in the corresponding chapters. It should be remembered that immunocytochemistry is a rapidly expanding field. New markers are described almost every month. They are first considered to be and announced as "specific" for some tumors. With increasing experience they become only "characteristic" of, and are eventually

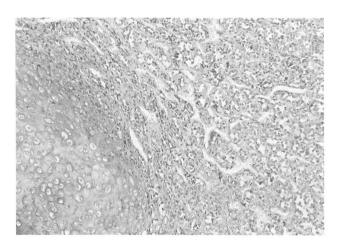

FIG. 23. Alcian blue stain. In mesenchymal chondrosarcoma stained with this method, the chondroblastic areas are light blue, and the spindle cell areas do not stain (Alcian blue, original magnification ×25).

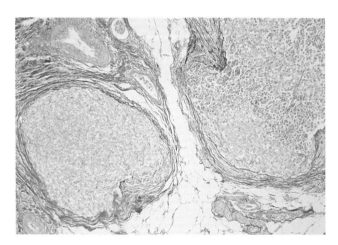

FIG. 25. Novotny stain. In this preparation from Ewing sarcoma, reticulin fibers that stain black are absent within tumor cell areas, thus excluding diagnosis of malignant lymphoma and small cell osteosarcoma (Novotny stain, original magnification ×12).

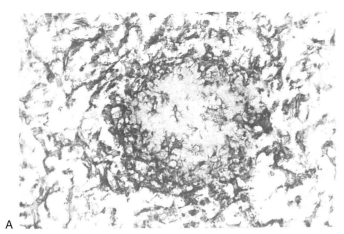
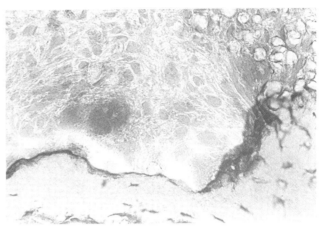

A

B

FIG. 26. Enzyme histochemistry. **A:** Alkaline phosphatase. A small round bone trabecula (*center*) is surrounded by typical for fibrous dysplasia stroma. All cells, in the stroma as well as the osteoblasts at the bone border and osteocytes within the bone, are more or less positive, indicating their bone-forming capability (alkaline phosphatase, original magnification ×50). **B:** Acid phosphatase. In fibrous dysplasia, with reaction for acid phosphatase an osteoclast with four nuclei (*left center*) shows intense activity. The surrounding mononuclear cells show a weak, finely granulated activity. The bone trabecula (*bottom*) shows negative reaction to acid phosphatase marker (acid phosphatase, original magnification ×500).

found in a number of different entities. Therefore, we shall restrict ourselves to adding some tables with patterns of markers that are useful for differentiation.

Despite the use of the above studies, a small percentage of bone tumors are not easily categorized. The pathologist must then attempt to assess the biologic potential of the neoplasm, even if it cannot be given a specific name. In such cases, the classic signs of nuclear pleomorphism and hyperchromaticity, mitotic rate and the presence of atypical mitoses, and the identification of spontaneous necrosis are sought to help distinguish benign from malignant lesions. However, it must be kept in mind that in Ewing sarcoma, for example, the tumor with the highest grade of malignancy, mitoses are almost never found in the histologic preparation. This is probably

because in a tumor with a high growth rate mitoses take place so rapidly as to be completed before the tumor tissue, after its excision, has been subjected to fixation. Observation of the interface area of the tumor with normal bone may reveal subtle infiltration of intertrabecular marrow spaces or Haversian canals by tumor cells and thus point to malignancy. Finally, more recent techniques, such as flow cytometry for analysis of nuclear DNA content (108), are used increasingly in difficult diagnostic assessments (Fig. 29). Thus far, however, these measurements do not allow unequivocal differentiation between malignant and benign forms of tumors derived from the same stem tissue, e.g., in cartilage tumors, because there is a considerable degree of overlapping (Dr. Gernot Jundt, Basel Switzerland).

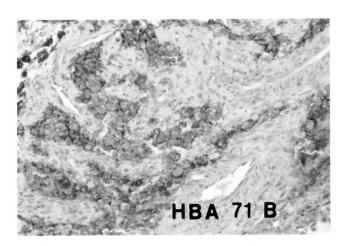

FIG. 27. Immunohistochemistry method. In Ewing sarcoma, most of the tumor cells are positive with the immunohistochemical marker HBA 71 (original magnification ×50).

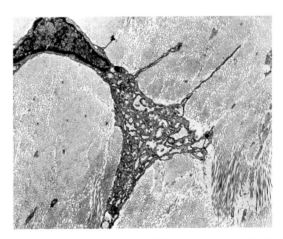

FIG. 28. Electron microscopy of fibrous cortical defect. Cell extension (*middle*) containing numerous organelles and the somewhat distorted nucleus (*upper left corner*) is surrounded by stroma with densely arranged immature fibrils. Only few mature-looking collagen fibrils are seen (*lower right corner*).

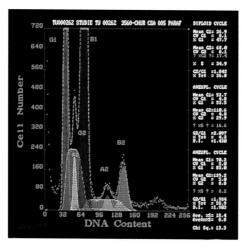

FIG. 29. Flow cytometry. Flow cytometry histogram of chondrocytes of chondrosarcoma grade 2 presents multiploid DNA pattern.

In the final analysis, only close cooperation among the radiologist, the pathologist, and the orthopedic surgeon in the review of history, radiographic studies, and biopsy materials may lead to an accurate diagnosis of a bone lesion. In most cases, careful analysis of all of these variables makes it possible to identify the various benign and malignant tumors and tumor-like conditions.

REFERENCES

1. Aisen AM, Martel W, Braunstein EM, McMillin KI. MRI and CT evaluation of primary bone and soft tissue tumors. *Am J Roentgenol* 1986;146:749–756.
2. Berquist TH. Magnetic resonance imaging of musculoskeletal neoplasms. *Clin Orthop* 1989;244:101–118.
3. Berquist TH. Magnetic resonance imaging of primary skeletal neoplasms. *Radiol Clin North Am* 1993;31:411–424.
4. Bloem JL, Bluemm RG, Taminiau AHM, van Oosterom AT, Stolk J, Doornbos J. Magnetic resonance imaging of primary malignant bone tumors. *RadioGraphics* 1987;7:425–445.
5. Bloem JL. Radiological staging of primary malignant musculoskeletal tumors. A correlative study of CT, MRI, ^{99m}Tc scintigraphy and angiography. The Hague: A. Jongbloed, 1988.
6. Bloem JL, Reiser MF, Vanel D. Magnetic resonance contrast agents in evaluation of the musculoskeletal system. *Magn Res Q* 1990; 6:136–163.
7. Bloem JL, Taminiau AHM, Eulderink F, Hermans J, Pauwels EKJ. Radiologic staging of primary bone sarcoma: MR imaging, scintigraphy, angiography, and CT correlated with pathologic examination. *Radiology* 1988;169:805–810.
8. Bloem JL, Van der Woude HJ, Giernaerdt M, Hogentorn PC, Taminiau AHM, Hermans J. Does magnetic resonance imaging make a difference for patients with musculoskeletal *sarcoma? Br J Radiol* 1997; 70:327–337.
9. Bohndorf K, Reiser M, Lochner B. Magnetic resonance imaging of primary tumors and tumor-like lesions of bone. *Skeletal Radiol* 1986; 15:511–517.
10. Boyko OB, Cory DA, Cohen MD, Provisor A, Mirkin D, DeRosa GP. MR imaging of osteogenic and Ewing's sarcoma. *Am J Roentgenol* 1987;148:317–322.
11. Brown KT, Kattapuram SV, Rosenthal DI. Computed tomography analysis of bone tumors: patterns of cortical destruction and soft tissue extension. *Skeletal Radiol* 1986;15:448–451.
12. Chew FS, Hudson TM. Radionuclide bone scanning of osteosarcoma: falsely extended uptake patterns. *Am J Roentgenol* 1982;139:49–54.
13. Coffre C, Vanel D, Contesso G, Kalifa C, Dubousset J, Genin J, Masselot J. Problems and pitfalls in the use of computed tomography for the local evaluation of long bone osteosarcoma. Report on 30 cases. *Skeletal Radiol* 1985;13:147–153.
14. Cohen EK, Kressel HY, Frank TS, Fallon M, Burk DL Jr., Dalinka MK, Schiebler ML. Hyaline cartilage-origin bone and soft-tissue neoplasms: MR appearance and histologic correlation. *Radiology* 1988; 167:477–481.
15. Cohen MD, Weetman RM, Provisor AJ, Grosfeld JL, West KW, Cory DA, Smith JA, McGuire W. Efficacy of magnetic resonance imaging in 139 children with tumors. *Arch Surg* 1986;121:522–529.
16. Cote RJ, Taylor CR. Immunohistochemistry and related marking techniques. In: Damjanov I, Linder J, eds. *Anderson's pathology*, 10th ed. St. Louis: Mosby, 1996;136–175.
17. Davies MA, Wellings RM. Imaging of bone tumors. *Curr Opin Radiol* 1992;4:32–38.
18. Domagala W, Osborn M. Immunocytochemistry. In: Koss LG, Woyke S, Olszewski W, eds. *Aspiration biopsy. Cytologic interpretation and histologic bases*, 2nd ed. New York: Igaku-Shoin, 1992; 55–108.
19. Dwyer AJ, Frank JA, Sank VJ, Reinig JW, Hickey AM, Doppman JL. Short-TI inversion-recovery pulse sequence: analysis and initial experience in cancer imaging. *Radiology* 1988;169:827–836.
20. Enneking WF. Staging of musculoskeletal neoplasms. *Skeletal Radiol* 1985;13:183–194.
21. Erlemann R, Reiser MF, Peters PE, Vasallo P, Nommensen B, Kusnierz-Glaz CR, Ritter J, Roessner A. Musculoskeletal neoplasms: static and dynamic Gd-DPTA-enhanced MR imaging. *Radiology* 1989;171: 767–773.
22. Ewing J. A review and classification of bone sarcomas. *Arch Surg* 1922;4:485–533.
23. Fechner RE, Mills SE. *Tumors of the bones and joints*. Washington, DC: Armed Forces Institute of Pathology, 1993;1–16.
24. Frank JA, Ling A, Patronas NJ, Carrasquillo JA, Horvath K, Hickey AM, Dwyer AJ. Detection of malignant bone tumors: MR imaging vs. scintigraphy. *Am J Roentgenol* 1990;155:1043–1048.
25. Frouge C, Vanel D, Coffre C, Couanet D, Contesso G, Sarrazin D. The role of magnetic resonance imaging in the evaluation of Ewing sarcoma. *Skeletal Radiol* 1988;17:387–392.
26. Galasko CS. The pathological basis for skeletal scintigraphy. *J Bone J Surg* 1975;57B:353–359.
27. Gillespy T III, Manfrini M, Ruggieri P, Spanier SS, Pettersson H, Springield DS. Staging of intraosseous extent of osteosarcoma: correlation of pre-operative CT and MR imaging with pathologic macroslides. *Radiology* 1988;167:765–767.
28. Gold RH, Bassett LW. Radionuclide evaluation of skeletal metastases: practical considerations. *Skeletal Radiol* 1986;15:1–9.
29. Golfieri R, Baddeley H, Pringle JS, Leung AWL, Greco A, Souhami R. MR imaging in primary bone tumors: therapeutic implications. *Eur J Radiol* 1991;12:201–207.
30. Golfieri R, Baddeley H, Pringle JS, Leung AW, Greco A, Souhami R, Kemp H. Primary bone tumors. MR morphologic appearance correlated with pathologic examinations. *Acta Radiol* 1991;32:290–298.
31. Golfieri R, Baddeley H, Pringle JS, Souhami R. The role of the STIR sequence in magnetic resonance imaging examination of bone tumors. *Br J Radiol* 1990;63:251–256.
32. Graif M, Pennock JM, Pringle J, Sweetman DR, Jelliffe AJ, Bydder GM, Young IR. Magnetic resonance imaging: comparison of four pulse sequences in assessing primary bone tumors. *Skeletal Radiol* 1989;18:439–444.
33. Greenfield GB, Warren DL, Clark RA. MR imaging of periosteal and cortical changes of bone. *RadioGraphics* 1991;11:611–623.
34. Greenspan A. Pragmatic approach to bone tumors. *Semin Orthop* 1991;6:125–133.
35. Greenspan A, Klein MJ. Radiology and pathology of bone tumors. In: Lewis MM, ed. *Musculoskeletal oncology. A multidisciplinary approach*. Philadelphia: WB Saunders, 1992;13–72.
36. Greenspan A, Stadalnik RC. Bone island: scintigraphic findings and their clinical application. *Can Assoc Radiol J* 1995;46:368–379.
37. Greenspan A, Stadalnik RC. Central versus eccentric lesions of long tubular bone. *Semin Nucl Med* 1996;26:201–206.
38. Hanna SL, Langston JW, Gronemeyer SA, Fletcher BD. Subtraction technique for contrast-enhanced MR images of musculoskeletal tumors. *Magn Reson Imag* 1990;8:213–215.

39. Hanna SL, Fletcher BD, Parham DM, Bugg MR. Muscle edema in musculoskeletal tumors: MR imaging charactristics and clinical significance. *J Magn Reson Imag* 1991;1:441–449.
40. Hayes CW, Conway WF, Sundaram M. Misleading aggressive MR imaging appearance of some benign musculoskeletal lesions. *RadioGraphics* 1992;12:1119–1134.
41. Hudson TM. *Radiologic-pathologic correlation of musculoskeletal lesions.* Baltimore: Williams and Wilkins, 1987.
42. Johnson LC. A general theory of bone tumors. *Bull NY Acad Med* 1953;29:164–171.
43. Joy DC, Pawley JB. High-resolution scanning electron microscopy. *Ultramicroscopy* 1992;47:80–100.
44. Jurik AG, Möller SH, Mosekilde L. Chronic sclerosing osteomyelitis of the iliac bone: Etiological possibilities. *Skeletal Radiol* 1988;17:114–118.
45. Kloiber R. Scintigraphy of bone tumors. In: *Current Concepts of Diagnosis and Treatment of Bone and Soft Tissue Tumors.* New York: Springer-Verlag, 1984;55–60.
46. Kransdorf M, Jelinek J, Moser RP Jr., Utz JA, Brower AC, Hudson TM, Berrey BH. Soft-tissue masses: diagnosis using MR imaging. *Am J Roentgenol* 1989;153:541–547.
47. Kricun ME. Radiographic evaluation of solitary bone lesions. *Orthop Clin North Am* 1983;14:39–64.
48. Lang P, Honda G. Roberts T, *et al.* Musculoskeletal neoplasm: perineoplastic edema versus tumor on dynamic postcontrast MR images with spatial mapping of instantaneous enhancement rates. *Radiology* 1995;197:831–839.
49. Larsson SE, Lorentzon R. The incidence of malignant primary bone tumors in relation to age, sex and site. A study of osteogenic sarcoma, chondrosarcoma, and Ewing's sarcoma diagnosed in Sweden from 1958–1968. *J Bone Joint Surg* 1974;56B:534–540.
50. Lee JK, Yao L, Wirth CR. MR imaging of solitary osteochondromas: Report of eight cases. *Am J Roentgenol* 1987;149–557.
51. Lewis MM, Sissons HA, Norman A, Greenspan A. Benign and malignant cartilage tumors. In: Griffin PP, ed. *Instructional course lectures.* Chicago: American Academy of Orthopaedic Surgeons, 1987; 87–114.
52. Lodwick GS. A systematic approach to the roentgen diagnosis of bone tumors. In: *M.D. Anderson Hospital and Tumor Institute— Clinical conference on cancer: tumors of bone and soft tissue.* Chicago: Year Book, 1965;49–68.
53. Lodwick GS. Solitary malignant tumors of bone: the application of predictor variables in diagnosis. *Semin Roentgenol* 1966;1:293–313.
54. Lodwick GS, Wilson AJ, Farrell C, Virtama P, Dittrich F. Determining growth rates of focal lesions of bone from radiographs. *Radiology* 1980;134:577–583.
55. Lodwick GS, Wilson AJ, Farrell C, Virtama P, Smeltzer FM, Dittrich F. Estimating rate of growth in bone lesions. Observer performance and error. *Radiology* 1980;134:585–590.
56. Ma LD, Frassica FJ, McCarthy EF, Bluenke DA, Zerhouni EA. Benign and malignant musculoskeletal masses: MR imaging differentiation with rim-to-center differential enhancement ratios. *Radiology* 1997; 202: 739–744.
57. Ma LD, Frassica FJ, Scott WW Jr, Fishman EK, Zerhouni EA. Differentiation of benign and malignant musculoskeletal tumors: potential pitfalls with MR imaging. *RadioGraphics* 1995;15:349–366.
58. Madewell JE, Ragsdale BD, Sweet DE. Radiologic and pathologic analysis of solitary bone lesions. Part I: Internal margins. *Radiol Clin North Am* 1981;19:715–748.
59. Magid D. Two-dimensional and three-dimensional computed tomographic imaging in musculoskeletal tumors. *Radiol Clin North Am* 1993;31:425–447.
60. Manaster BJ, Ensign MF. The role of imaging in musculoskeletal tumors. *Semin US CT MR* 1989;10:498–517.
61. Mankin HJ, Lange TA, Spanier SS. The hazards of biopsy in patients with malignant primary bone and soft-tissue tumors. *J Bone Joint Surg* 1982;64:1121–1127.
62. McCook BM, Sandler MP, Powers TA, Weaver GR, Nance EP Jr. Correlative bone imaging. In: *Nuclear medicine annual.* New York: Raven Press, 1989;143–171.
63. McNeil BJ. Value of bone scanning in neoplastic disease. *Semin Nucl Med* 1984;14:277–286.
64. Mirowitz SA. Fast scanning and fat-suppression MR imaging of musculoskeletal disorders. *Am J Roentgenol* 1993;161:1147–1157.
65. Mirowitz SA, Apicella P, Reinus WR, Hammerman AM. MR imaging of bone marrow lesions: relative conspicuousness on T1-weighted, fat-suppressed T2-weighted, and STIR images. *Am J Roentgenol* 1994;162:215–221.
66. Moore SG, Bisset GS, Siegel MJ, Donaldson JS. Pediatric musculoskeletal MR imaging. *Radiology* 1991;179:345–360.
67. Moser RP, Madewell JE. An approach to primary bone tumors. *Radiol Clin North Am* 1987;25:1049–1093.
68. Mulder JD, Kroon HM, Schütte HE, Taconis WK. *Radiologic atlas of bone tumors.* Amsterdam: Elsevier, Amsterdam;9–46.
69. Murphy WA Jr. Imaging bone tumros in the 1990s. *Cancer* 1991;67: 1169–1176.
70. Nelson SW. Some fundamentals in the radiologic differential diagnosis of solitary bone lesions. *Semin Roentgenol* 1966;1:244–267.
71. Norman A, Schiffman M. Simple bone cyst: factors of age dependency. *Radiology* 1977;124:779–782.
72. Olson P, Everson LI, Griffith HJ. Staging of musculoskeletal tumors. *Radiol Clin North Am* 1994;32:151–162.
73. Panicek DM, Gatsonis C, Rosenthal DI, Seeger LL, Huvos AG, Moore SG, Cavdry DJ, Palmer WE, McNeil BJ. CT and MR imaging in the local staging of primary malignant musculoskeletal neoplasms: report of the Radiology Diagnostic Oncology Group. *Radiology* 1997; 202:237–246.
74. Petasnick JP, Turner DA, Charters JR, Gitelis S, Zacharias CE. Soft-tissue masses of the locomotor system: comparison of MR imaging with CT. *Radiology* 1986;160:125–133.
75. Pettersson H, Eliasson J, Egund N, Rooser B, Willen H, Rydholm A, Berg NO, Holtas S. Gadolinium-DTPA enhancement of soft tissue tumors in magnetic resonance imaging —preliminary clinical experience in five patients. *Skeletal Radiol* 1988;14:319–323.
76. Pettersson H, Gillespie T III, Hamlin DJ, Enneking WF, Springfield DS, Andrew ER, Spanier S, Slone R. Primary musculoskeletal tumors: examination with MR imaging compared with conventional modalities. *Radiology* 1987;164:237–241.
77. Pettersson H, Slone RM, Spanier S, Gillespie T III, Fitzsimmons JR, Scott KN. Musculoskeletal tumors: T1 and T2 relaxation times. *Radiology* 1988;167:783–785.
78. Pettersson H, Spanier S, Fitzsimmons JR, Slone R, Scott KN. MR imaging relaxation measurements in musculoskeletal tumors and surrounding tissue. *Radiology* 1985;157(P):109.
79. Pettersson H, Springfield DS, Enneking WF. *Radiologic management of musculoskeletal tumors.* New York: Springer-Verlag, 1987;9–13.
80. Pui MH, Chang SK. Comparison of inversion recovery fast spin-echo (FSE) with T2-weighted fat-saturated FSE and T1-weighted MR imaging in bone marrow lesion detection. *Skeletal Radiol* 1996;25: 149–152.
81. Ragsdale BD, Madewell JE, Sweet DE. Radiologic and pathologic analysis of solitary bone lesions. Part II: Periosteal reactions. *Radiol Clin North Am* 1981;19:749–783.
82. Reinus WR, Wilson AJ. Quantitative analysis of solitary lesions of bone. *Invest Radiol* 1995;30:427–432.
83. Reiser M, Rupp N, Biehl T. MR in diagnosis of bone tumors. *Eur J Radiol* 1985;5:1–7.
84. Richardson ML, Kilcoyne RF, Gillespie T III, Genant HK. Magnetic resonance imaging of musculoskeletal neoplasms. *Radiol Clin North Am* 1987;24:259–267.
85. Rosenthal DI. Computed tomography of orthopedic neoplasms. *Orthop Clin North Am* 1985;16:461–470.
86. Rossleigh MA, Smith J, Yeh SD. Scintigraphic features of primary sacral tumors. *J Nucl Med* 1986;27:627–630.
87. Rotte KH, Schmidt-Peter P, Kriedemann E. CT-evaluation of osseous tumors. *Eur J Radiol* 1986;6:5–8.
88. Schajowicz F. *Tumors and tumorlike lesions of bone. Pathology, radiology, and treatment,* 2nd ed. Berlin: Springer-Verlag, 1994;1–21.
89. Schulz A, Jundt G, Berghauser KH, Gehron-Robey P, Termine JD. Immunohistochemical study of osteonectin in various types of osteosarcoma. *Am J Pathol* 1988;132:233–238.
90. Seeger LL, Widoff BE, Bassett LW, Rosen G, Eckardt JJ. Preoperative evaluation of osteosarcoma: value of gadopentetate dimeglumine-enhanced MR imaging. *Am J Roentgenol* 1991;157:347–351.
91. Sepponen RE, Sipponen JT, Tanttu JI. A method for chemical shift imaging: demonstration of bone marrow involvement with proton chemical shift imaging. *J Comput Assist Tomogr* 1984;8:585–587.
92. Shuman WP, Patten RM, Baron RL, Liddell RM, Conrad EU, Richardson ML. Comparison of STIR and spin-echo MR imaging at 1.5T in 45 suspected extremity tumors: lesion conspicuity and extent. *Radiology* 1991;179:247–252.

93. Steinbach LS. MRI of musculoskeletal tumors. Contemporary *Diagn Radiol* 1989;12:1–6.

94. Sundaram M, McDonald DJ. Magnetic resonance imaging in the evaluation of the solitary tumor of bone. *Radiology* 1990;2:697–702.

95. Sundaram M, McDonald DJ. The solitary tumor or tumor-like lesion of bone. *Top Magn Reson Imag* 1989;1:17–29.

96. Sundaram M, McGuire MH. Computed tomography or magnetic resonance imaging for evaluating the solitary tumor or tumor-like lesion of bone. *Skeletal Radiol* 1988;17:393–401.

97. Sundaram M, McGuire MH, Herbold DR, Wolverson MK, Heiberg E. Magnetic resonance imaging in planning limb-salvage surgery for primary malignant tumors of bone. *J Bone Joint Surg* 1986; 68A:809–819.

98. Sundaram M, McLeod R. MR imaging of tumor and tumorlike lesions of bone and soft tissue. *Am J Roentgenol* 1990;155:817–824.

99. Sweet DE, Madewell JE, Ragsdale BD. Radiologic and pathologic analysis of solitary bone lesions. Part III: Matrix patterns. *Radiol Clin North Am* 1981;19:785–814.

100. Szumowski J, Eisen JK, Vinitski S, Haake PW, Plewes DB. Hybrid methods of chemical shift-imaging. *Magn Reson Med* 1989; 9:379–388.

101. Szumowski J, Plewes D. Fat suppression in the time domain in fast MR imaging. *J Magn Reson Med* 1988;8:345–354.

102. Tehranzadeh J, Mnaymneh W, Ghavam C, Morillo G, Murphy BJ. Comparison of CT and MR imaging in musculoskeletal neoplasms. *J Comput Assist Tomogr* 1989;13:466–472.

103. Thomas C. *Sandritter histopathology. Textbook and color atlas,* 8th ed., Toronto: BC Decker, 1989;305–309.

104. Vanel D, Verstraele KL, Shagero LG. Primary tumors of the musculoskeletal system. *Radiol Clin North Am* 1997; 35: 213–237.

105. Verstraete KL, De Deene Y, Roels H, Dierick A, Uyttendaele D, Kunnen M. Benign and malignant musculoskeletal lesions: dynamic contrast-enhanced MR imaging—parametric first-pass images depict tissue vascularization and perfusion. *Radiology* 1994;192:835–843.

106. Volberg FM Jr, Whalen JP, Krook L, Winchester P. Lamellated periosteal reactions: a radiologic and histologic investigation. *Am J Roentgenol* 1977;128:85–87.

107. Watt I. Radiology in the diagnosis and management of bone tumours. Review article. *J Bone Joint Surg* 1985;67B:520–529.

108. Weinberg DS, Carey JL. Flow and imaging cytometry. In: Damjanov I, Linder J, eds. *Anderson's pathology,* 10th ed. St. Louis: CV Mosby, 1996;258–280.

109. Wetzel LH, Levine E. Murphcy MD. A comparison of MR imaging and CT in the evaluation of musculoskeletal masses. *RadioGraphics* 1987;7:851–874.

110. Zimmer WD, Berquist TH, McLeod RA, Sim FH, Pritchard DJ, Shives TC, Wold LE, May GR. Bone tumors: magnetic resonance imaging versus computed tomography. *Radiology* 1985;155:709–718.

CHAPTER 2

Bone-Forming Tumors

BENIGN LESIONS	Intracortical osteosarcoma
Osteoma	Gnathic osteosarcoma
Osteoid Osteoma	Multicentric (multifocal) osteosarcoma
Osteoblastoma	**Juxtacortical Osteosarcoma**
MALIGNANT LESIONS	Parosteal osteosarcoma
Osteosarcomas	Periosteal osteosarcoma
Conventional (medullary) osteosarcoma	High-grade surface osteosarcoma and dedifferentiated
Small-cell osteosarcoma	parosteal osteosarcoma
Fibrohistiocytic osteosarcoma	**Secondary Osteosarcomas**
Telangiectatic osteosarcoma	Paget sarcoma
Giant cell-rich osteosarcoma	Postirradiation osteosarcoma
Low-grade (well-differentiated) central osteosarcoma	**Soft-tissue (extraskeletal) osteosarcoma**

INTRODUCTION

Whether benign or malignant, bone-forming neoplasms are characterized by the formation of osteoid or mature bone directly by the tumor cells (23,24). Only one malignant tumor, osteosarcoma, is capable of doing this. The other bone-forming tumors are benign: osteoma, osteoid osteoma, and osteoblastoma.

BENIGN LESIONS

Osteoma

Osteoma is a benign, slow-growing lesion consisting of well-differentiated mature bone tissue with a predominantly laminar structure, commonly arising in the frontal and ethmoid sinuses (approximately 75% of cases) (37). It may also occur on the surface of the outer table of the calvaria ("ivory exostosis"), the bones of the jaw (41), and, rarely, on the surface of the flat bones and the long and short tubular bones (2,26,28,32,44,45) (Fig. 1). Extracranial parosteal osteomas compose only 0.03% of biopsied primary bone lesions (30). Exceptionally osteoma can exhibit endosteal extension (20).

Clinical Presentation

Osteomas have been reported in patients from 10 to 79 years of age, with most in the fourth and fifth decades (11,41). Males and females are equally affected. The signs and symptoms associated with osteoma vary depending on the size of the lesion and its location (33). Small lesions are usually asymptomatic and incidental findings. Large paranasal sinus tumors in particular may produce a variety of manifestations. Attached to the sinus wall and covered by the sinus mucoperiosteum (34), they often block the nasal ducts, causing mucoceles, sinusitis, nasal discharge, headache, and pain. At times a patient may lose the sense of smell (34). Occasionally, paranasal osteomas exhibit more dramatic features such as orbital or intracranial invasion (37). Tumors near the orbit can produce exophthalmos, double vision, and pressure on the optic nerve that may result in loss of vision. At other sites, they can erode the wall of the cranial fossa, perforate the dura, and compress the frontal lobe. Paranasal osteomas are usually discovered in the third and fourth decades, and the finding is most often incidental. One retrospective study involving 16,000 patients found a frequency of 0.4% for these tumors (9). They occur twice as frequently in males as in females and are believed to have a growth peak at the time of maximum skeletal development; they are only occasionally found before puberty (42).

Osteomas seldom develop in the long and short tubular bones (1,3,16,44) and are extremely rare in the flat bones (5,29,43). Tumors at these sites are known as parosteal osteomas. Like osteomas elsewhere, they are usually asymptomatic. Most parosteal lesions measure 1 to 4 cm in diame-

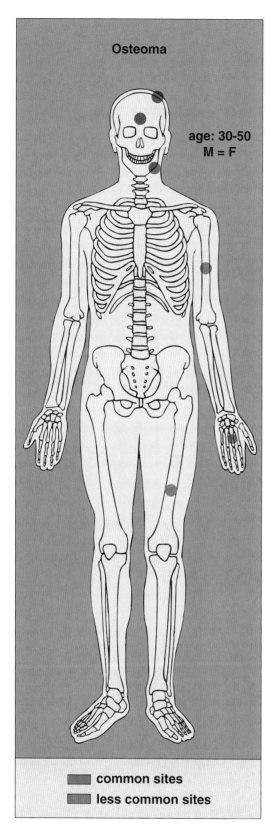

Osteoma

age: 30-50
M = F

common sites
less common sites

FIG. 1. Osteoma: skeletal sites of predilection, peak age range, and male-to-female ratio.

ter, rarely reaching the dimensions reported by Baum et al. (16.5 × 4.2 cm) and Mirra et al. (6 × 5 × 5 cm) (1,29). Many long bone lesions are multiple.

It is worth noting the association of osteomas with Gardner syndrome, an autosomal-dominant disorder frequently seen in Mormons in Utah (8,14). In addition to bone lesions, the syndrome is marked by multiple cutaneous and subcutaneous lesions (e.g., sebaceous cysts, skin fibromas, and desmoid tumors) and intestinal, particularly colonic, polyposis (13). The bone tumors may precede the appearance of the intestinal polyps, which have a marked propensity to carcinomatous change (6,13). Osteomas have also been reported in association with tuberous sclerosis (29). Finally, osteomas of the soft tissues (so-called osseous choristomas) are rare occurrences that have been described in the thigh and the intraoral soft parts (10,25,40).

Imaging

Plain film radiography is the basis for the diagnosis of osteoma. Radiographs typically show a dense, ivory-like sclerotic mass with sharply demarcated borders attached to the bone (Fig. 2). Conventional tomography (Fig. 3) and computed tomography (CT) (Fig. 4) are effective in demonstrating lack of cortical invasion (45), which not infrequently is a feature of parosteal osteosarcoma, or lack of cortical and medullar continuity with a host bone, a feature of osteochondroma (see "Differential Diagnosis" below). Magnetic resonance imaging (MRI) shows low signal intensity on both T1 and T2 sequences, consistent with cortical bone (45).

Histopathology

Histologically, two types of osteoma may be encountered: cancellous and compact (46). Most investigators consider the former to be the forerunner of the latter. The cancellous (or trabecular, or spongy) osteoma reveals a cancellous, trabecular architecture. Trabeculae are thin with fatty marrow present in the intertrabecular spaces (21) (Fig. 5A). They usually contain more woven bone and show evidence of active bone formation with transformation to lamellar bone (35). Woven bone consists of a more or less mature matrix with a plait of collagen fibers; it contains roundish osteocyte lacunae in high numbers per space unit. Lamellar bone is composed of narrow parallel layers of mature matrix with densely packed collagen fibers; it contains spindle-shaped osteocyte lacunae in smaller numbers than woven bone. Compact osteoma, on the other hand, consists of dense, compact, mature lamellar bone (Figs. 5B, C) (7). No Haversian systems are present and only occasionally marrow spaces are visible. A compact osteoma usually exhibits empty osteocyte lacunae in varying numbers, probably as a result of increased distance between the small marrow spaces and the cells that interferes with cell nourishment by diffusion.

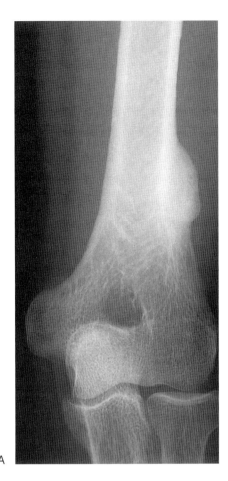

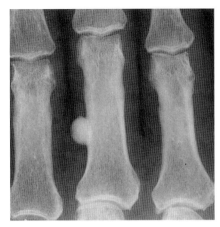

A

B

FIG. 2. Osteoma. A: An anteroposterior radiograph of the humerus shows sclerotic, ivory-like mass attached to the cortex. (Reprinted with permission from Greenspan A. Benign bone-forming lesions: osteoma, osteoid osteoma, and osteoblastoma. *Skeletal Radiol* 1993;22: 485–500.) B: A small osteoma of the proximal phalanx of the middle finger.

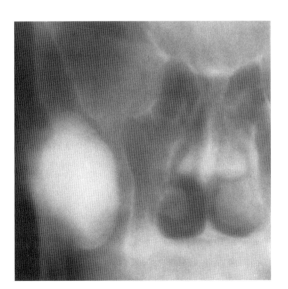

FIG. 3. Osteoma: conventional tomography. Conventional tomogram shows a large osteoma arising from the coronoid process of the right mandible. The tumor abuts the floor of the orbit and maxillary sinus, but there is no evidence of invasion in the adjacent structures. (Reprinted with permission from Greenspan A. Benign bone-forming lesions: osteoma, osteoid osteoma, and osteoblastoma. *Skeletal Radiol* 1993;22: 485–500.)

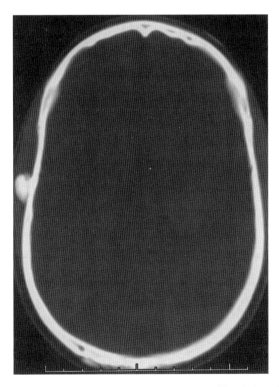

FIG. 4. Osteoma: computed tomography. CT of the skull shows a small osteoma attached to the outer table.

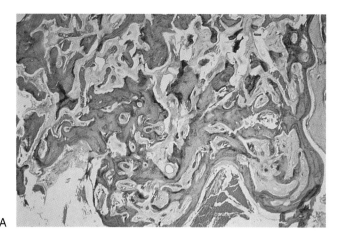

A

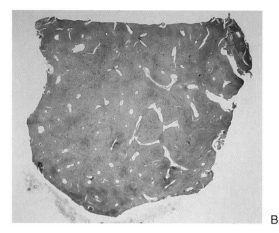

B

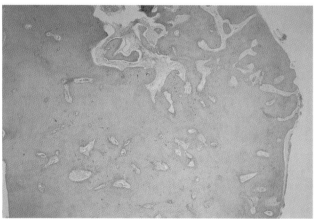

C

FIG. 5. Histopathology of osteoma. **A:** Cancellous osteoma. Irregularly formed bone trabeculae, consisting mostly of lamellar bone, enclose highly vascular fibrous marrow tissue (Giemsa, original magnification ×25). **B:** Compact osteoma. Dense, compact, mostly lamellar bone surrounds narrow marrow spaces. The surface is rather smooth (Giemsa, original magnification ×2.5). **C:** Compact osteoma. At higher magnification, the newly formed mature lamellar bone surrounding the marrow spaces appears in a darker red (hematoxylin and eosin, original magnification ×12).

DIFFERENTIAL DIAGNOSIS

Radiology

The radiologic differential diagnosis of solitary osteoma should include parosteal osteosarcoma, sessile osteochondroma, juxtacortical myositis ossificans, periosteal osteoblastoma, ossified parosteal lipoma, and focus of melorheostosis (Fig. 6 and Table 1) (17). Among these, *parosteal osteosarcoma* is the most important entity that needs to be excluded, and that may be a difficult task radiographically because both lesions appear as ivory-like masses attached to the bone's surface (Fig. 7) (19). The keys to recognizing osteoma, however, are its usually exquisitely smooth borders and well-circumscribed, intensely homogeneous sclerotic appearance on plain radiographs. Parosteal osteosarcoma, in contrast, may show a zone of decreased density at the periphery and usually appears less dense and homogeneous than osteoma (47).

Sessile osteochondroma can usually be identified by its characteristic radiographic features: the cortex of the lesion merges without interruption with the cortex of the host bone, and the cancellous portion is continuous with the host medullary cavity of the adjacent metaphysis or diaphysis (Fig. 8).

A well-matured focus of *juxtacortical myositis ossificans* may occasionally mimic osteoma. The radiographic hallmark of myositis ossificans is the so-called zonal phenomenon, characterized by a radiolucent area in the center of the lesion that indicates immature bone formation and a dense zone of mature ossification at the periphery. Often a thin radiolucent cleft separates the ossific mass from the adjacent cortex (Fig. 9A). Occasionally, however, a lesion (frequently, but not always, a mature one) may adhere to and fuse with the cortex, thus mimicking parosteal osteoma (Fig. 9B). In these instances CT may demonstrate the classic zonal phenomenon of the lesion (Fig. 9C).

Periosteal osteoblastoma, an extremely rare bone-producing lesion (27,39), appears radiographically as a round-to-ovoid juxtacortical mass (15). Its less intense and less homogeneous density (Fig. 10) distinguishes it from osteoma.

Ossified parosteal (or periosteal) lipoma is a rare neoplasm, which in the majority of cases measures 5 to 7 cm at its greatest dimension (12,36,48). Pain is an unusual symptom; most patients give a history of a slow-growing, painless mass that has been present for many years (22). Consistent with fatty tumors generally, lobulation is the chief radiographic feature of the mass, which contains low-density fat in contrast to the surrounding muscle tissue that it displaces (Fig. 11) (31).

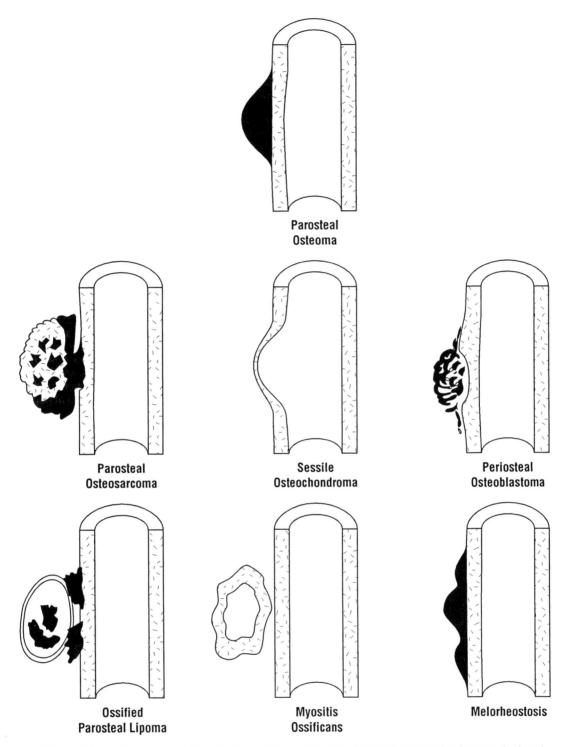

FIG. 6. Schematic representation of differential possibilities of similarly appearing juxtacortical and cortical lesions.

TABLE 1. *Differential diagnosis of parosteal osteoma*

Condition (lesions)	Radiologic features	Pathologic features
Parosteal osteoma	Ivory-like, homogeneously dense sclerotic mass, with sharply demarcated borders, intimately attached to cortex. No cleft between lesion and adjacent cortex.	Mature lamellar bone (either consisting of concentric rings of compact bone, or parallel plates of cancellous bone), lack of active fibrous stoma.
Parosteal osteosarcoma	Ivory-like, frequently lobulated sclerotic mass, homo- or heterogeneous in density with more radiolucent areas at periphery. Incomplete cleft between lesion and adjacent cortex occasionally present.	Streamers of woven to woven-lamellar bone with heavily collagenized stroma. Moderately cellular foci with nuclei exhibiting slight pleomorphism.
Sessile osteochondroma	Cortex of host bone merges without interruption with cortex of lesion and respective cancellous portions of adjacent bone and osteochondroma communicate.	Cartilaginous cap composed of hyaline cartilage arranged similarly to growth plate. Beneath zone of endochondral ossification with vascular invasion and replacement of calcified cartilage by newly formed bone. Intertrabecular spaces may contain fatty or hematopoietic marrow.
Juxtacortical myositis ossificans	Zonal phenomenon: radiolucent area in center of lesion and dense zone of mature ossification at periphery. Frequently thin radiolucent cleft separates ossific mass from adjacent cortex.	Trabecular bone and fibrous marrow. Histologic zonal phenomenon: immature bone in the center with proliferating osteoblasts, fibroblasts, and areas of hemorrhage and necrosis; mature bone at the periphery.
Periosteal osteoblastoma	Round or ovoid heterogeneous in density mass attached to cortex.	Trabeculae of woven bone, numerous dilated capillaries, exuberant in number osteoblasts, osteoclasts, and fibroblasts.
Ossified parosteal (periosteal) lipoma	Lobulated mass containing irregular ossifications and radiolucent area of fat. Hyperostosis of adjacent cortex occasionally present.	Formation of mature bone within adipose tissue. Occasionally foci of necrosis and calcifications.
Melorheostosis (monostotic)	Cortical thickening resembling wax dripping down one side of a candle. Commonly extends to the joint.	Thickened cortical bone containing irregularly arranged Haversian canals surrounded by cellular fibrous tissue. Osteoblastic activity usually present.

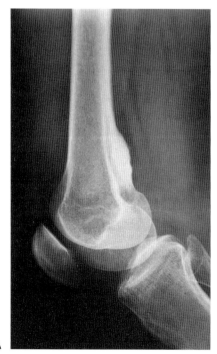 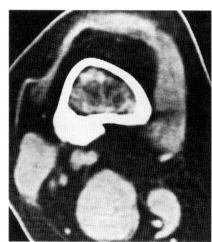

A   B

FIG. 7. Parosteal osteosarcoma. An ossific mass is attached to the posterior cortex of the distal femur.

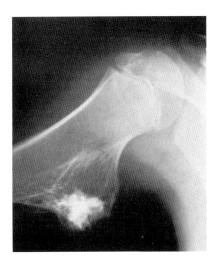

FIG. 8. Sessile osteochondroma. The radiographic hallmarks include uninterrupted cortical and medullary continuity between the lesion and the host bone (humerus).

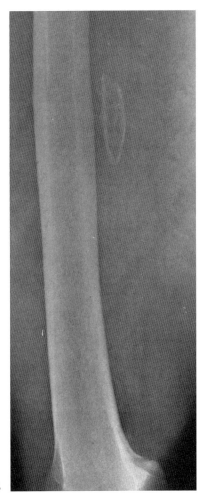

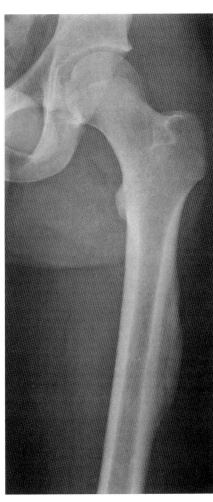

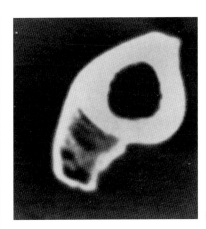

C

A,B

FIG. 9. Juxtacortical myositis ossificans. **A:** The radiographic hallmarks of the lesion include zonal phenomenon: a radiolucent area in the center of the lesion, which indicates immature bone formation, and a dense zone of mature ossification at the periphery. Note also a thin, radiolucent cleft separating the lesion from the adjacent cortex. **B:** A focus of mature post-traumatic myositis ossificans is tightly adherent to the cortex of the left femur. The radiolucent cleft that usually separates the lesion from the cortex is absent. **C:** In another patient with a post-traumatic focus of myositis ossificans that was firmly attached to the cortex, the CT section shows classic zonal phenomenon.

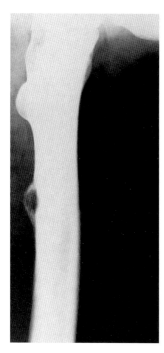

FIG. 10. Periosteal osteoblastoma. Lateral radiograph of the femur shows a juxtacortical lesion with radiolucent center and more dense periosteal shell.

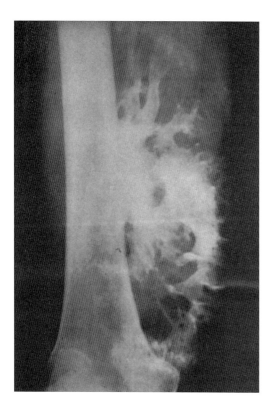

FIG. 11. Ossified parosteal lipoma. A large ossific mass is attached to the medial cortex of the right femur. The radiolucent character of the fatty tissue (distal part of the tumor) is apparent. (Reprinted with permission from Greenfield GB, Arrington JA. *Imaging of bone tumors.* 1995, Fig. 4.19).

Melorheostosis is a rare form of mixed sclerosing dysplasia that on radiography appears as a long segment of cortical thickening (flowing hyperostosis), often resembling wax dripping down one side of a candle (4,18). A typical focus of monostotic melorheostosis usually exhibits both parosteal and endosteal involvement and the lesion commonly extends into the articular end of the bone (Fig. 12), features rarely present in a parosteal osteoma.

Pathology

The difficulty in distinguishing between parosteal osteosarcoma and osteoma may extend to the histopathology. Conventional *parosteal osteosarcoma* is characterized by streamers of bone that appear woven to woven-lamellar and are produced by low-grade anaplastic, sometimes polar, cells of a fibroblastic stroma (29). Moderately cellular foci of stroma are noted, and nuclei may exhibit slight pleomorphism. Some lesions may exhibit a fairly cellular stroma containing neoplastic osteoid and bone, which clearly indicates malignancy. The heavily collagenous stroma of parosteal osteosarcoma is the key feature that distinguishes it from parosteal osteoma (Fig. 13) (46). In contrast, the presence of mature bone and the absence of an active fibrous stroma are the distinctive features of parosteal osteoma (1).

The microscopic features of *sessile osteochondroma* are similar to its radiographic appearance and are likewise diagnostic, with merging of the cortices and imperceptible blending of the spongiosa of the lesion and the host bone (Fig. 14). In addition, the spongiosa of sessile osteochondroma frequently contains remnants of calcified cartilage that was not

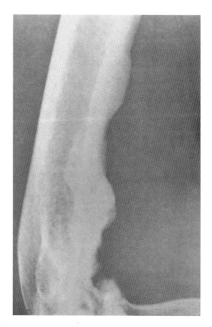

FIG. 12. Forme fruste of melorheostosis. Lateral radiograph of the elbow shows a flowing hyperostosis of the anterior cortex of the distal humerus. Note the extension of the lesion into the joint.

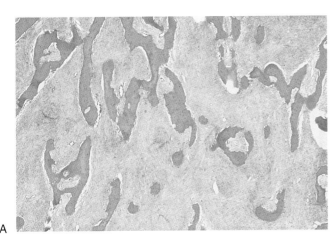
A

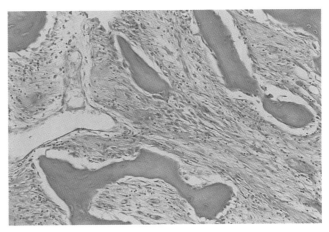
B

FIG. 13. Histopathology of parosteal osteosarcoma. **A:** A low-power photomicrograph shows the typical appearance of a heavily collagenized, fibrous matrix with irregular trabeculae of bone (hematoxylin and eosin, original magnification ×4). **B:** A higher power photomicrograph shows the cellular fibrous stroma with islands of bone tissue (hematoxylin and eosin, original magnification ×25). (Reprinted from Bullough PG. *Atlas of orthopedic pathology,* 2nd ed. New York: Gower, 1992;16.15.)

completely replaced by bone during the growth phase of the lesion (29), a finding not present in osteoma. A cartilaginous cap of variable thickness on the surface of the osteochondroma is a common finding. Because a sessile-type lesion may lose this cap by ossification in late adulthood, it may be confused with osteoma; however, the latter is always attached to the intact cortex.

The remaining entities that may create difficulties in the differential diagnosis for the radiologist can easily be excluded by histopathologic characteristics. For example, microscopic examination of *myositis ossificans circumscripta* reveals a correlative histologic zonal phenomenon. In contrast to osteoma, the lesion consists of trabecular bone and marrow fat, not solid cortical bone (Fig. 15).

Small trabeculae of woven bone, numerous dilated capillaries, and exuberant hyperplasia of osteoblasts, osteoclasts,

and, occasionally, fibroblasts are characteristic histopathologic findings of *periosteal osteoblastoma* (30) (Fig. 16). A thin shell of newly formed periosteal bone may cover the lesion (38).

Histologically, *ossified parosteal lipoma* can easily be distinguished from osteoma because it usually exhibits the typical features of lipoma, composed of adipose lobulated tumor tissue with mature fat cells and formation of woven bone trabeculae, and, at later stages, formation of lamellar bone with or without foci of necrosis and calcification (38).

Also, *melorheostosis* can easily be distinguished histologically from an osteoma. The former is characterized by thickened trabeculae containing irregularly arranged Haversian canals surrounded by cellular fibrous tissue (Fig. 17). Osteoblastic activity is usually present (4). This is in contrast to the thin trabeculae of the cancellous osteoma and the dense lamellar bone of the compact variant of this lesion.

The radiologic and pathologic differential diagnosis of parosteal osteoma are depicted in Fig. 18 and Table 1.

Osteoid Osteoma

Osteoid osteoma is a relatively common (4% of all primary bone tumors excluding myeloma) lesion of bone, characterized by a nidus of osteoid tissue, that is usually less than 1 cm in diameter (58). The nidus, consisting of cellular, highly vascularized tissue that contains osteoid, can be entirely radiolucent or it may have a sclerotic center. In many instances the nidus is surrounded by a zone of reactive bone formation (60,73).

Clinical Presentation

Patients with osteoid osteoma almost invariably present with a complaint of nocturnal pain that may be / severe

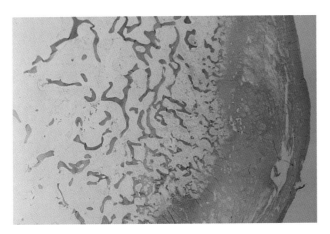

FIG. 14. Histopathology of sessile osteochondroma. Low-power magnification of a sessile lesion shows a hyaline cartilage cap covered with perichondrium. Endochondral ossification has occurred under the cartilage (hematoxylin and eosin, original magnification ×6). (Courtesy of Dr. M. Klein, New York, NY.)

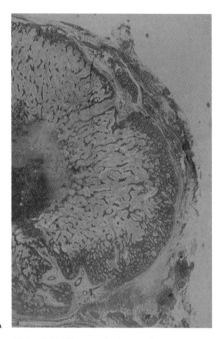
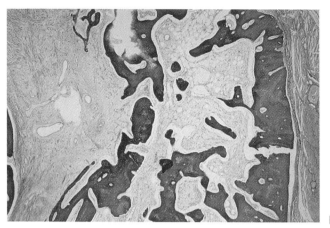

A

B

FIG. 15. Histopathology of myositis ossificans. **A:** Low-power photomicrograph shows the fibrous cellular center (darkly stained) (zone 1) surrounded by layers of more mature bone (zone 2). At the periphery of the lesion (zone 3), mature bone formation is present (hematoxylin and eosin, original magnification ×1.5). (Courtesy of Dr. A. Norman, Valhalla, NY.) **B:** At slightly higher magnification, mature lamellar bone borders the connective tissue and muscle (*right*). Toward the center of the lesion (*left*), less mature bone, consisting mainly of woven bone, borders almost boneless fibrous tissue (van Gieson, original magnification ×6).

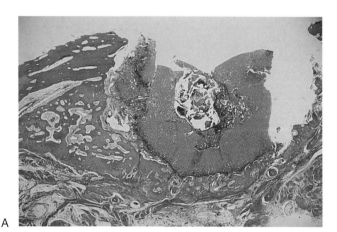
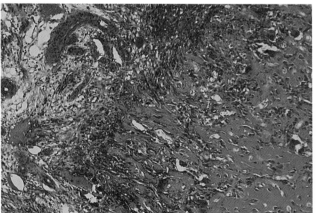

A

B

FIG. 16. Histopathology of periosteal osteoblastoma (here with secondary aneurysmal bone cyst). **A:** A ring-shaped plate of dense woven bone, almost without marrow spaces, indicating long-standing existence of tumor, with more cancellous bone at the border. The tumor lies at the outer surface of cortical bone. Some blood-filled spaces of ABC in the center (hematoxylin and eosin, original magnification ×6). **B:** At higher magnification, the periphery of the tumor shows densely arranged trabeculae of woven bone, bordered by osteoblasts and osteoclasts within the fibrous tissue of the bone marrow (hematoxylin and eosin, original magnification ×25).

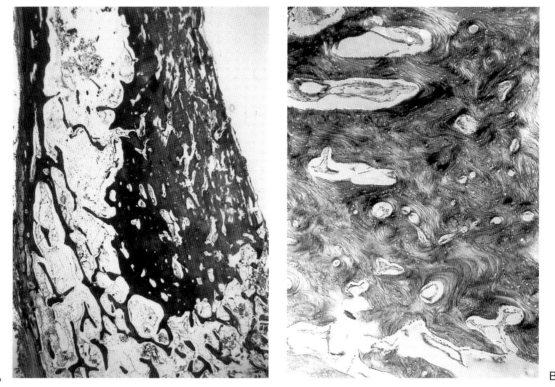

FIG. 17. Histopathology of melorheostosis. **A:** A low-power photomicrograph reveals extensive asymmetric sclerosis of the cortex, with encroachment on the endosteal surface, representing periosteal and endosteal bone formation (hematoxylin and eosin, original magnification ×9). **B:** Higher magnification of the abnormal cortex reveals that the new bone is largely lamellar in architecture, reflecting slow modeling (hematoxylin and eosin, polarized light, original magnification ×50). (A and B—courtesy of Michael J. Klein, M.D., New York, NY.)

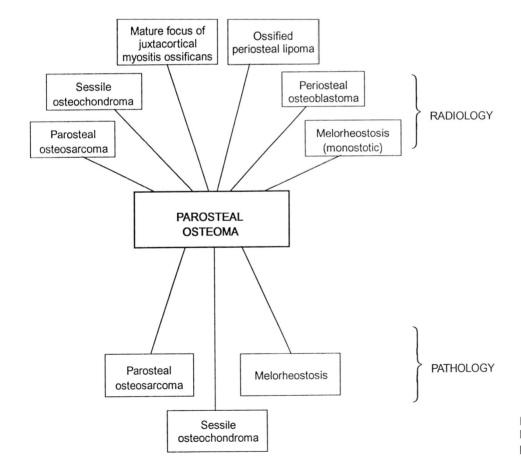

FIG. 18. Radiologic and pathologic differential diagnosis of parosteal osteoma.

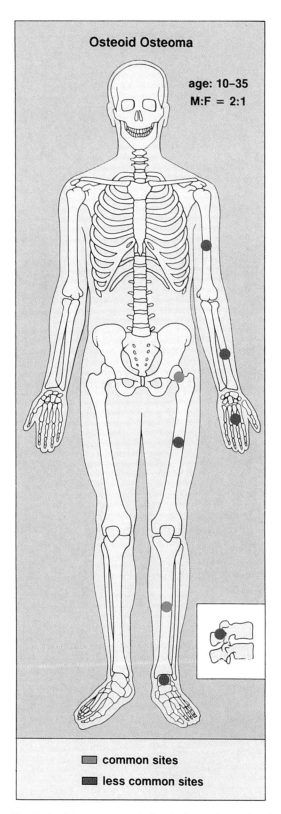

FIG. 19. Osteoid osteoma: skeletal sites of predilection, peak age range, and male-to-female ratio.

enough to cause awakening (59). Salicylates, such as aspirin, are remarkably effective in relieving the pain, usually in less than half an hour. This classical presentation is typical in >75% of patients and provides an important clue to the diagnosis (92). Local swelling and point tenderness are present in some patients (49,53). There may be also neurologic signs and symptoms, which can include muscle atrophy, a decrease in deep tendon reflex responses, and variable degrees of sensory loss (93). In most cases, osteoid osteoma arises in the age range of 10 to 35 years (55,77). There is a marked predominance in males, with a number of studies reporting a male/female ratio of 2:1 to 4:1 (Fig. 19) (30,58,61,72,73, 75–77).

Osteoid osteoma can arise in virtually any bone. The long bones are preferentially affected (approximately 65% of the lesions occur in the long bones), particularly the femur and tibia [over 53% of all osteoid osteomas are located in these bones with the proximal femur being most frequently affected (56)], in which the lesions usually occur near the end of the shaft. Less commonly affected sites are the phalanges of hands and feet (21%), the vertebrae (9%), and the humerus (78).

Depending on its location in the particular part of the bone, the lesion can be classified as cortical, medullary (cancellous), or subperiosteal. Osteoid osteomas can be further subclassified as extra- or intracapsular (intra-articular) (60,77).

Intraarticular osteoid osteomas preferentially affect the hip (93). However, lesions in the elbow, foot, wrist, knee, and vertebral facet joints have also been reported (62,65). These tumors are usually characterized by nonspecific symptoms that are indicative of an inflammatory synovitis (50,88). Sclerosis may be lacking and the periosteal reaction is absent. On physical examination, a joint effusion and synovitis may be identified (50,57). Intracapsular lesions may also cause a precocious appearance of arthritis. This can provide an important diagnostic clue in cases when the history is typical of osteoid osteoma but the nidus has not been confirmed by radiography (83). If a lesion is located near the growth plate, particularly in a young child, it may cause accelerated bone growth.

Osteoid osteoma involves the axial skeleton in 10% of cases (74,75,79,81). Osteoid osteoma of the spine most commonly involves the lumbar segment (59%). Less frequently affected are the cervical (27%), thoracic (12%), and sacral (2%) vertebrae (30,63,76,77,86). In patients with lesions of the neural arch painful scoliosis often occurs (frequently as a result of a spasm), the concavity of the curvature being toward the side of the lesion (74).

Imaging

The probability of identifying osteoid osteoma by conventional radiography is dependent on the location of the lesion. Cortical lesions are usually characterized by a radiolucent nidus (representing the tumor itself) with a surrounding area of reactive sclerosis. A periosteal reaction may or may not be identified (Fig. 20A). An intramedullary nidus is less easily identified on plain radiography because very little or no reactive sclerosis is present (Fig. 20B). Occasionally, the nidus may exhibit a focus of central calcification (sclerotic center). The nidus of a subperiosteal lesion may be visualized either as a central radiolucent or sclerotic focus, with or without reactive sclerosis (Fig. 20C) or as a shaggy, crescent-like focus of periosteal reaction (76). The radiographic presentation of intracapsular lesions is frequently characterized by periarticular osteoporosis and in some instances by premature osteoarthritis (Fig. 20D) (83).

In some instances conventional tomography is used to evaluate osteoid osteoma, with better visualization of the nidus than can be obtained with plain radiography (Fig. 21). It can also assist in confirming or excluding the presence of a sinus tract and is therefore useful when the differential diagnosis includes a possible bone abscess.

Skeletal scintigraphy is a highly sensitive method for detecting the nidus of osteoid osteoma (80,95). This modality can be particularly helpful in cases for which the symptoms are atypical and the initial radiographs appear normal (90). The use of a three-phase radionuclide bone scan has also been suggested (76). This technique can be especially valu-

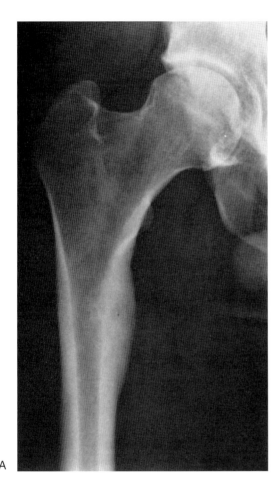

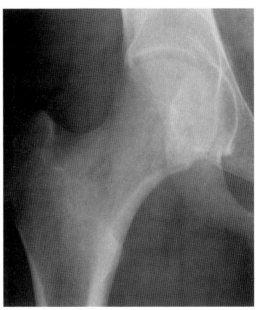

FIG. 20. Osteoid osteoma. **A:** Cortical lesion. A radiolucent nidus is surrounded laterally by reactive sclerosis and medially by a solid periosteal reaction. **B:** Intramedullary lesion. An intramedullary nidus shows no evidence of reactive sclerosis. **C:** Subperiosteal lesion. A sclerotic, subperiosteal nidus on the surface of talar bone shows minimal periosteal reaction without reactive sclerosis.

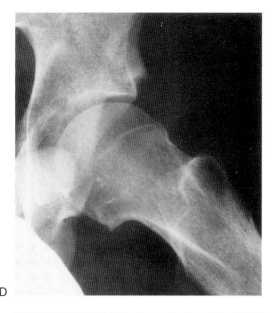

D

FIG. 20. *Continued.* **D:** Intracapsular lesion. A faintly discernible radiolucent nidus is present in the left femoral neck without evident perilesional sclerosis. Periarticular osteoporosis and early osteoarthritic changes (osteophytes) are the presumptive features of osteoid osteoma in this 14-year-old boy. **E:** Intracapsular lesion. Anteroposterior radiograph of the right hip in a 28-year-old man reveals osteoid osteoma in the medial femoral neck. **F:** Tomography of the same hip clearly shows osteoarthritic changes: collar osteophyte and slight narrowing of the weight-bearing segment of the hip joint.

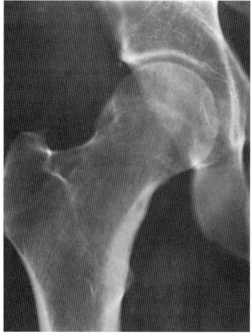

E

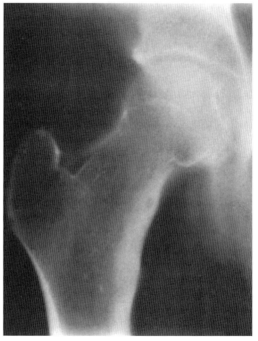

F

able when intraarticular or intramedullary lesions are not clearly visualized by conventional radiography. Radionuclide tracer activity can be observed on both immediate and delayed images (Fig. 22). Osteoid osteoma is characterized by an interesting scintigraphic feature, the so-called double-density sign. This phenomenon is believed to be related to increased vascularity of the nidus (69,70). In agreement with the appearance of the lesion on plain radiography, the double-density sign is seen as a small focus of increased activity associated with the nidus; this focus is surrounded by a larger area of less intense activity, related to the reactive sclerosis that surrounds the nidus (Fig. 23). Identification of the double-density sign can help to differentiate an osteoid osteoma from a bone abscess.

As the definite study for diagnosis of osteoid osteoma, computed tomography (CT) is recommended. Not only can CT identify the lesion, but it can also accurately determine its extent, thus enabling exact measurement of the size and location of the nidus (Fig. 24) (63,65,71). The nidus usually appears as a well-defined area of low attenuation, which is surrounded by a variably sized region of high attenuation reactive sclerosis. To delineate the lesion, thin (preferably 2-mm) contiguous sections are most appropriate (Fig. 25). CT is particularly useful to define lesions that arise in the axial skeleton, whose complex anatomy is less clear on routine radiography and conventional tomography (Fig. 26) (89).

The suitability of magnetic resonance imaging (MRI) for detection of osteoid osteoma remains unclear and published

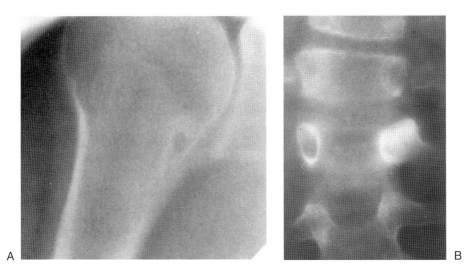

A   B

FIG. 21. Osteoid osteoma: conventional tomography. **A:** A trispiral tomogram reveals a radiolucent nidus of osteoid osteoma in the proximal humerus, which had not been apparent on plain radiography. **B:** A trispiral tomogram of the thoracolumbar junction demonstrates a nidus of osteoid osteoma with perilesional sclerosis in the left pedicle of L1.

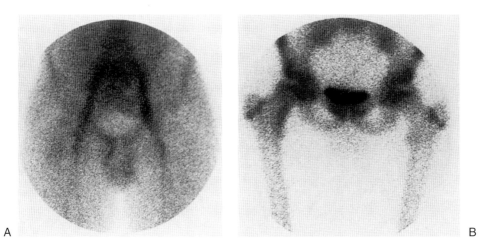

A   B

FIG. 22. Osteoid osteoma: scintigraphy. **A:** In the first phase of a three-phase radionuclide bone scan, 1 min after intravenous injection of 15 mCi (555 MBq) technetium-99m-labeled MDP, there is increased activity in the iliac and femoral vessels. Discrete activity in the area of the medial femoral neck is related to the nidus. **B:** In the third phase, 2 hr after injection, there is accumulation of a bone-seeking tracer in the femoral neck lesion. (Reprinted with permission from Greenspan A. Benign bone forming lesions: osteoma, osteoid osteoma, and osteoblastoma. *Skeletal Radiol* 1993;22:490.)

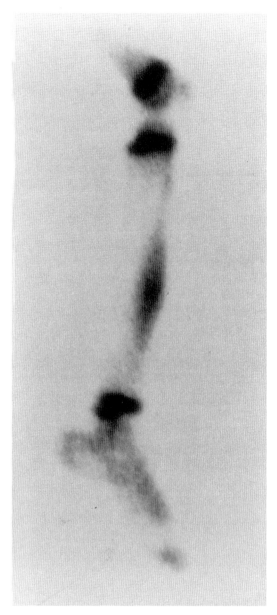

FIG. 23. Osteoid osteoma: scintigraphy. Scintigraphy of tibial osteoid osteoma shows a characteristic "double-density" sign: increased uptake in the center (related to the nidus of osteoid osteoma) and a less intensely active area at the periphery (denoting reactive sclerosis).

reports have had mixed results (94,97,99). Goldman et al. (65) reported on four cases of intracapsular osteoid osteoma of the femoral neck, in which the lesions were evaluated with bone scintigraphy, CT, and MRI. Although in all cases abnormal findings were apparent in the MR images, the nidi could not be identified prospectively. On the basis of MRI findings of secondary bone marrow edema or synovitis, several incorrect diagnoses were made, which included Ewing sarcoma, osteonecrosis, stress fracture, and juvenile arthritis. In these cases, it is noteworthy that the correct diagnoses

were made only after review of the radiographs and thin-section CT studies. Another report by Woods et al. (96) involved three patients with a highly unusual association of osteoid osteoma with a reactive soft tissue mass. In these cases, MRI studies might have led to confusion of osteoid osteoma with osteomyelitis or a malignant tumor. Moreover, in each case the nidus displayed different signal characteristics. In one case the intensity of signal was generally low on all pulse sequences but mild enhancement was seen after administration of gadolinium. In another case, the signal was of intermediate intensity and administration of gadolinium revealed inhomogeneous enhancement of the nidus. For the third case in which plain films showed the nidus to be intracortical, MRI could not identify the nidus distinctly.

However, some reports do suggest the effectiveness of MRI for demonstrating the nidus of osteoid osteoma (Figs. 27 and 28) (52,64,87,98). Bell et al. (54) clearly demonstrated an intracortical nidus on MRI that had not been seen on scintigraphy, angiography, or CT scans.

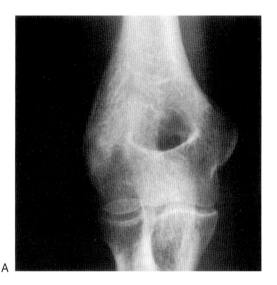

A

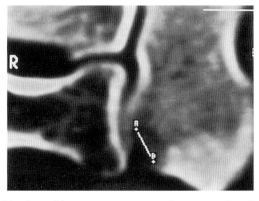

B

FIG. 24. Osteoid osteoma: computed tomography. **A:** Anteroposterior radiograph of the left elbow of a 31-year-old man with the typical clinical symptoms of osteoid osteoma shows periarticular osteoporosis. There is the suggestion of a lesion in the capitellum. **B:** A coronal CT section unequivocally demonstrates a subarticular nidus, measuring 6.5 mm.

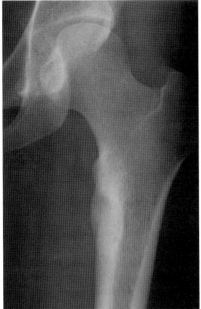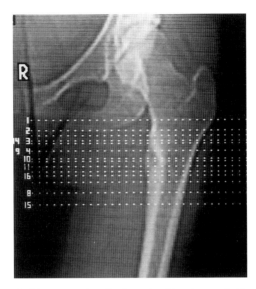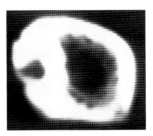

A, B   C

FIG. 25. Osteoid osteoma: computed tomography. **A:** An osteoid osteoma in the medial femoral cortex in an 18-year-old woman. **B:** Two-millimeter-thin CT sections through the lesion were obtained. **C:** The low-attenuation nidus of osteoid osteoma is surrounded by a high-attenuation zone of reactive sclerosis.

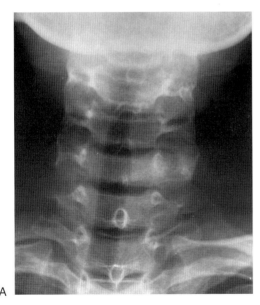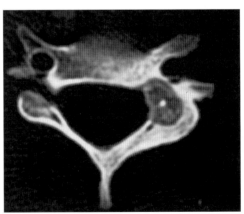

A   B

FIG. 26. Osteoid osteoma: computed tomography. **A:** A plain radiograph of the cervical spine does not clearly demonstrate the suspected lesion of osteoid osteoma. **B:** A CT section through C6 shows a low-attenuation nidus with a sclerotic center, located in the left pedicle and extending into the lamina. (Reprinted with permission from Greenspan A. Benign bone forming lesions: osteoma, osteoid osteoma, and osteoblastoma. *Skeletal Radiol* 1993;22:492.)

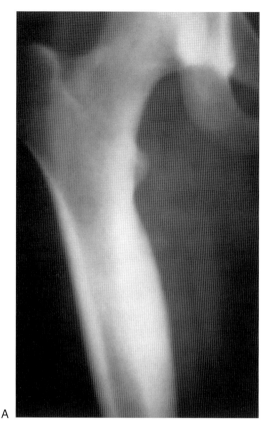

A

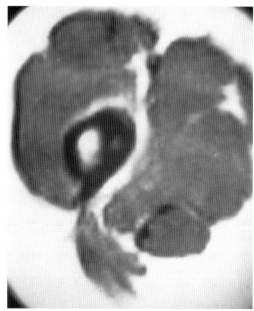

B

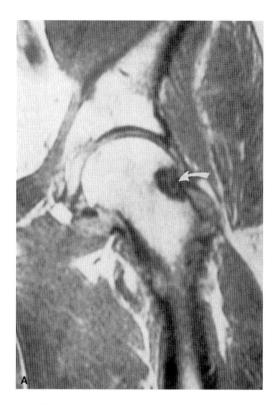

A

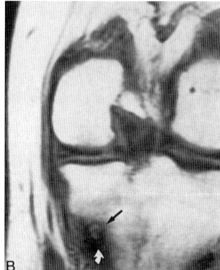

B

FIG. 27. Osteoid osteoma: magnetic resonance imaging. **A:** A plain radiograph shows a sclerotic area localized to the medial aspect of proximal femoral shaft. The nidus is not apparent. **B:** Axial T1-weighted MRI clearly demonstrates the high-intensity nidus within a low-intensity sclerotic cortex. (Courtesy of Lynne S. Steinbach, M.D., San Francisco, California. Reprinted with permission from Greenspan A. Benign bone forming lesions: osteoma, osteoid osteoma, and osteoblastoma. *Skeletal Radiol* 1993;22:492.)

FIG. 28. Osteoid osteoma: MRI. **A:** Coronal T1-weighted (SE; TR 600, TE 20) MRI shows an osteoid osteoma in the lateral aspect of the neck of the left femur. (Reprinted with permission from Stoller DW. *Magnetic resonance imaging in orthopedics and sports medicine,* 2nd ed. Philadelphia: JB Lippincott, 1993;1234.) **B:** Coronal T1-weighted (SE; TR 600, TE 20) MRI shows an osteoid osteoma in the medial cortex of the left tibia. (Reprinted with permission from Stoller SW. *Magnetic resonance imaging in orthopedics and sports medicine,* 2nd ed. Philadelphia: JB Lippincott, 1993;1236.)

Histopathology

In lesions of osteoid osteoma, the nidus is small, well circumscribed, and self-limited. It is composed of osteoid tissue or mineralized immature woven bone (Figs. 29A–C). The osteoid matrix and bone form small and irregular trabeculae, with a thickness ranging from thin and delicate to broad and sclerotic (76). The trabeculae are surrounded by a highly vascular fibrous stroma that exhibits prominent osteoblastic and osteoclastic activity (Fig. 29D). The sclerosis surrounding the lesion is composed of dense bone that displays a variety of maturation patterns. From the ultrastructural viewpoint, the morphology of osteoblasts of osteoid osteoma is generally similar to that of normal osteoblasts. However, these osteoblasts possess irregular, indented nuclei (indicative of high metabolic activity), glycogen particles, an abundance of fine intracytoplasmic fibers, and occasional iron-containing lysosomes (91). Moreover, some of these osteoblasts possess atypical mitochondria with a lobulated or "honeycomb" appearance. The areas of mineralized matrix exhibit the morphology of coarse woven bone. In two of the cases reported by Steiner, the osteoid contained, in addition to collagen, fine granular material, probably representing polysaccharides. It is noteworthy that Steiner observed no nerve fibers in any of the studied material (91), although recent observations (Jundt 1994, unpublished data) suggest the presence of such structures in the nidus of osteoid osteoma.

Differential Diagnosis

Radiology

Even when a cortical lesion exhibits the classic radiographic appearance of osteoid osteoma, the differential diag-

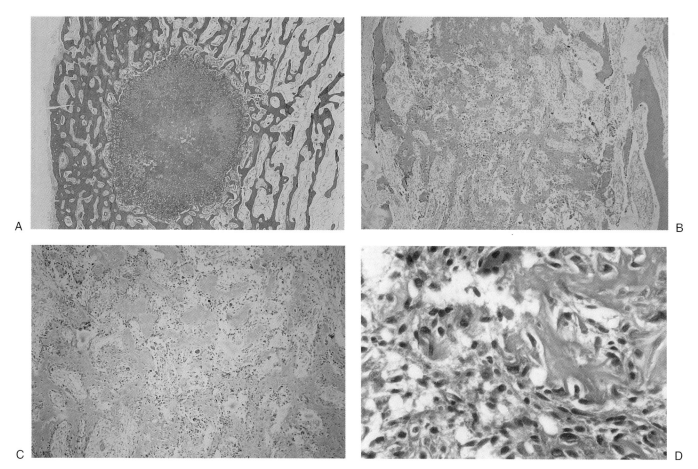

FIG. 29. Histopathology of osteoid osteoma. **A:** Low-power magnification shows a well-demarcated nidus composed of osteoid and trabeculae of immature woven bone (red, *center*), surrounded by a narrow, cell-rich outer zone (blue). At the periphery of the nidus, bone shows partial sclerosis (*left half*) (hematoxylin and eosin, original magnification ×6). **B:** Low-power magnification shows the nidus to be composed of irregular woven bone trabeculae with dense osteoblastic rimming. From the left and right the nidus is clearly delineated by the adjacent bone (Giemsa, original magnification ×12). **C:** At higher magnification, osteoblastic rimming of woven bone trabeculae is conspicuous. In addition, some osteoclasts are also present (Giemsa, original magnification ×50). **D:** High-power photomicrograph (hematoxylin and eosin, original magnification ×156) of the nidus shows interconnecting small trabeculae distributed within a fibrovascular stroma. Note the prominent osteoblastic activity. (**D**–Courtesy of Dr. KK Unni, Rochester, Minnesota.)

nosis must consider a cortical stress fracture, a focus of infection, and intracortical osteosarcoma. In *stress fracture*, the radiolucency is usually more linear than that of osteoid osteoma, running perpendicular to or at an angle to the cortex rather than parallel to it (Fig. 30). A *cortical bone abscess* may have a similar radiographic appearance to that of osteoid osteoma, but it can usually be differentiated by a linear, serpentine tract that extends away from the abscess cavity (Fig. 31). In some instances, intracortical osteoid osteoma must be differentiated from *intracortical osteosarcoma*, a rare bone-forming malignancy that arises solely within the cortex of bone and grossly involves neither the medullary cavity nor the soft tissues (79,85). On radiography, the latter tumor appears as a radiolucent focus within the cortex (femur or tibia), surrounded by zone of sclerosis. Occasionally, fluffy densities can be demonstrated in the radiolucent zone (81). The cortex at the site of the lesion may bulge slightly or may be thickened. The reported size of the lesion varies from 1.0 to 4.2 cm (51).

In intramedullary lesions, the differential must consider a *bone abscess* (Brodie abscess) and, in a lesion with calcified nidus, a bone island (enostosis). A *medullary bone abscess* exhibits a central radiolucency very similar to that of osteoid osteoma, but, similarly to the cortical focus of infection, it can usually be differentiated by the serpentine tract that ex-

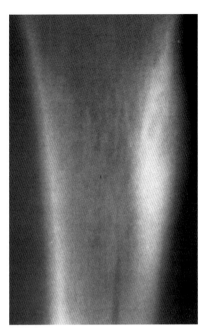

FIG. 31. Osteoid osteoma: differential diagnosis (bone abscess). A lateral tomogram of the tibia shows a radiolucent, serpentine tract of a cortical bone abscess that was originally diagnosed as osteoid osteoma.

tends from the abscess cavity toward the nearest growth plate (Figs. 32 and 33). *45* is characterized on radiography by the lesion's brush-like borders, which blend with surrounding trabeculae in a pattern likened to "thorny radiation" or "pseudopodia" (66,67) (Fig. 34). In addition, bone islands

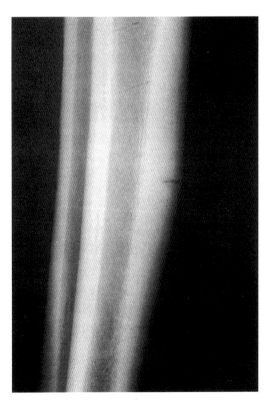

FIG. 30. Osteoid osteoma: differential diagnosis (stress fracture). A lateral radiograph of the tibia shows a cortical stress fracture. Note the perpendicular direction of radiolucency to the long axis of the tibial cortex.

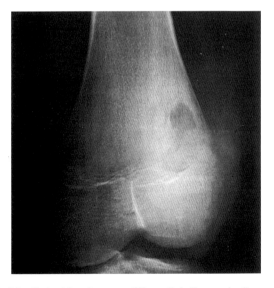

FIG. 32. Osteoid osteoma: differential diagnosis (bone abscess). In a medullary bone abscess, seen here at the junction of the distal femoral diaphysis and metaphysis, a serpentine tract extends from an abscess cavity towards the growth plate.

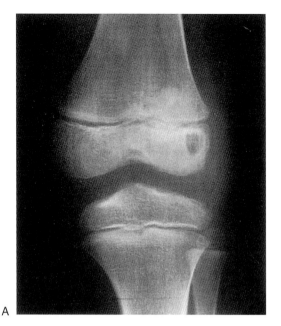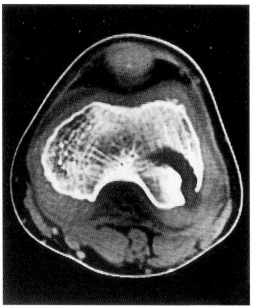

A   B

FIG. 33. Osteoid osteoma: differential diagnosis (bone abscess). **A:** A 7-year-old boy experienced intermittent pain in the left knee for 3 weeks; the pain was worse at night and was promptly relieved by salicylate. On the basis of clinical history and plain radiography showing a round radiolucency in the epiphysis with mild perilesional sclerosis, osteoid osteoma was considered in the differential diagnosis. **B:** CT section through the lesion reveals cortical disruption and the serpentine configuration of the radiolucent tract that extends into the articular cartilage. This is characteristic of bone abscess.

usually exhibit no increased activity on radionuclide bone scan (68) (Fig. 35).

A schematic representation of differential possibilities of cortical and medullary osteoid osteoma is depicted in Fig. 36.

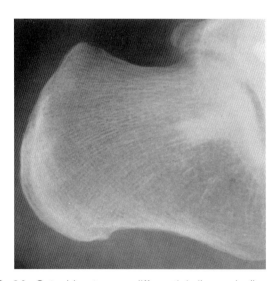

FIG. 34. Osteoid osteoma: differential diagnosis (bone island). A bone island in the os calcis exhibits characteristic features: a homogeneously dense, sclerotic focus in the cancellous bone with distinctive radiating bony streaks ("thorny radiation") that blend with the trabeculae of the host bone, creating a feathered, or brush-like, border.

Pathology

Histopathologic differential diagnosis of osteoid osteoma should include primarily osteoblastoma and osteosarcoma because the histologic appearances of stress fractures, Brodie abscesses, and bone islands are unmistakably characteristic and do not create identification problems (Table 2).

Probably the most difficult task is to differentiate osteoid osteoma from *osteoblastoma*. In fact, some authorities (39) consider these entities to represent the same lesion in different stages of development because they show such remarkable histologic similarities. On the other hand, some investigators contend that osteoid production is usually greater in osteoblastoma than in osteoid osteoma and that the former lesion shows greater vascularity. Whereas in osteoid osteoma there seems to be a more organized structure with maturation of the nidus toward its periphery, in osteoblastoma the distribution of osteoid and trabecular bone has a less organized pattern: the whole lesion may be in the same stage of development (38). The difference in the size of the nidus (1.0 cm or less for osteoid osteoma and >2 cm for osteoblastoma) may be an artificial division because osteoblastoma in the early stage of development has to be smaller than 2 cm. In the spine that division may be even more artificial, since the lesions of osteoblastoma are often smaller than 2 cm. The presence of more or less marked perilesional sclerosis in osteoid osteoma may allow this rather arbitrary differentiation.

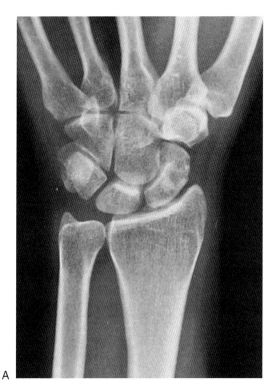
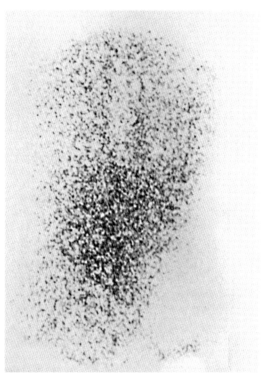

A   B

FIG. 35. Osteoid osteoma: differential diagnosis (bone island). A 32-year-old woman presented with nocturnal pain localized in the wrist area. **A:** A dorsovolar radiograph of the wrist shows a dense, round lesion in the scaphoid, and a diagnosis of osteoid osteoma was considered. **B:** Bone scan reveals normal uptake of the radiopharmaceutical tracer, ruling out osteoid osteoma, which is invariably associated with increased isotope uptake. The lesion proved to be a bone island. The pain was related not to the bone lesion but to tenosynovitis.

Histologic differentiation of osteoid osteoma from *osteosarcoma* (mainly from the intracortical variant) is less challenging. The latter tumor is rich in osteoid and woven bone, with minimal anaplasia due to so-called normalization of nuclei. Trapping of host cortical lamellar bone within the tumor, however, is an indicator of malignancy (81).

Differentiation of osteoid osteoma from a *bone island* is not difficult. The histopathologic features of bone island are characteristic: a dense, sclerotic focus of compact bone within the cancellous bone exhibits thickened peripheral trabeculae blending with the trabeculae of the spongiosa. In addition, the lesion shows mature compact lamellar bone with wide bands of parallel or concentric lamellae and marrow spaces having the appearance of Haversian canals (Fig. 37) (66, 67).

The radiologic and pathologic differential diagnosis of osteoid osteoma is depicted in Fig. 38 and Table 2.

Osteoblastoma

Osteoblastoma accounts for approximately 1% of all primary bone tumors and 3% of all benign bone tumors (114). Jaffe and Mayer are credited with identifying it as an entity in 1932 (116). Later it was described as "giant osteoid osteoma," underscoring its close histologic resemblance to oste-

oid osteoma and its larger size (105). The lesion is often >1.5 to 2 cm in diameter (115). Lichtenstein termed it an "osteogenic fibroma of bone," subsequently changing the name to "benign osteoblastoma" (26,27,119). The histologic similarities between osteoid osteoma and osteoblastoma are striking, and differentiation is often difficult if not impossible (102). Some authors subscribe to the concept that they represent different clinical expressions of the same pathologic process (39,108). In most of the world literature, however, osteoid osteoma and osteoblastoma are considered separate and distinct clinical entities, mainly because of their different clinical presentations and different radiologic characteristics. Their natural histories also differ: whereas osteoid osteoma tends toward regression, osteoblastoma tends toward progression and even malignant transformation (72) (although the possibility of the latter event remains controversial).

Clinical Presentation

Like osteoid osteoma, osteoblastomas are most often found in patients in the first to third decades with the peak incidence in the second decade; aggressive tumors are usually seen in an older age group (average age 33 years) (118,123). The male-to-female ratio appears to be approximately 2:1

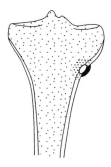

Cortical
Osteoid Osteoma

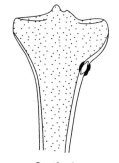

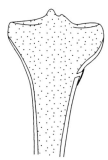

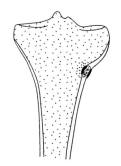

A

Cortical
Bone Abscess

Stress
Fracture

Intracortical
Osteosarcoma

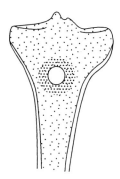

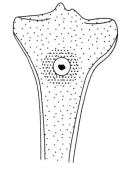

Medullary
Osteoid Osteoma

Medullary Osteoid Osteoma
with Sclerotic Center

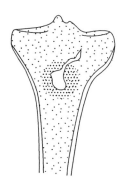

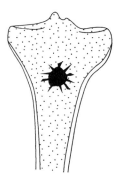

B

Brodie Abscess

Bone Island
(Enostosis)

FIG. 36. Schematic representation of differential possibilities of (**A**) cortical and (**B**) medullary osteoid osteoma.

TABLE 2. *Differential diagnosis of osteoid osteoma*

Condition (lesions)	Radiologic features	Pathologic features
Cortical osteoid osteoma	Radiolucent nidus, round or elliptical, surrounded by radiodense reactive sclerosis. Solid or laminated (but not interrupted) periosteal reaction. Scintigraphy invariably shows increased uptake of radiotracer. "Double-density" sign.	Nidus composed of osteoid tissue or mineralized immature bone. Osteoid matrix and bone form irregular islets and are surrounded by a richly vascular fibrous stroma. The islets have a trabecular structure, whose thickness ranges from thin and delicate to broad and sclerotic. The stroma shows prominent osteoblastic and osteoclastic activity. Perilesional sclerosis composed of dense bone exhibiting various maturation patterns.
Medullary osteoid osteoma	Radiolucent (or with central calcification) nidus, without or with only minimal perinidal sclerosis. Usually no or only minimal periosteal reaction. Scintigraphy—as above.	
Subperiosteal osteoid osteoma	Central radiolucent or sclerotic nidus with or without reactive sclerosis. Occasionally shaggy, crescent-like focus of periosteal reaction. Scintigraphy—increased uptake of radiotracer.	As above
Intracapsular (periarticular) osteoid osteoma	Periarticular osteoporosis. Premature onset of osteoarthritis. Nidus may or may not be visualized. Scintigraphy—as above.	
Osteoblastoma	See Table 3.	See Table 3.
Stress fracture (cortical)	Linear radiolucency runs perpendicular or at an angle to the cortex. Scintigraphy—increased uptake of radiotracer.	Features of bone repair: osteoid and cartilaginous callus, osteoblastic and osteoclastic activity.
Bone abscess (Brodie)	Irregular in outline radiolucency, usually with a sclerotic rim, associated with serpentine, linear tract. Predilection for metaphysis and the ends of tubular bones. Scintigraphy—increased uptake of radiotracer. MRI—on T1 WI a well-defined low-to-intermediate-signal lesion outlined by a low-intensity rim. On T2 WI a very bright homogeneous signal, outlined by a low-signal rim.	Necrotic tissue, giant cells, granulocytes, lymphocytes, plasma cells, and histiocytes.
Bone island (enostosis)	Homogeneously dense, sclerotic focus in cancellous bone with distinctive radiating streaks (thorny radiation) that blend with the trabeculae of the host bone. Scintigraphy—usually no increased uptake. MRI—low-intensity signal on T1 and T2 WI.	Focus of mature, compact bone with thickened peripheral trabeculae that blend with trabeculae of the spongiosa. Wide bands of parallel or concentric lamellae; marrow spaces resembling Haversian canals.
Intracortical osteosarcoma	Intracortical radiolucent focus surrounded by zone of sclerosis. Occasionally central "fluffy" densities. Cortex thickened or bulged. Scintigraphy—increased uptake of radiotracer.	Consistent with an osteoblastic osteosarcoma with focal evidence of chondroid and fibroblastic differentiation. Permeation of Haversian systems. "Trapping" of lamellar bone within the tumor.

(78,113). The long tubular bones are frequently affected, but the lesion shows a distinct predilection for the axial skeleton in general and the vertebral column in particular (11,30,103,118) (Fig. 39). Approximately 30% to 40% are localized in the spine (82), more or less equally in the cervical, thoracic, and lumbar segments, mainly in the posterior elements including the arch and spinous processes (122). In one series of 123 tumors, 39 (32%) were located in the spine and 23 (19%) in the jaw; the remaining 61 tumors were distributed throughout the appendicular skeleton with a predilection for the femur and tibia (123).

The clinical presentation of osteoblastoma is different from that of osteoid osteoma (100,114). Some patients are asymptomatic, and the lesion is found incidentally (120). Symptomatic patients in one study most often experienced a dull, localized pain, with a median duration of symptoms of 6 months before they presented for treatment. The pain very rarely interfered with sleep. Although the use of salicylates for pain relief is not mentioned in the study by Kroon and Schurmans (118), the pain of osteoblastoma does not appear to be as readily relieved by salicylates as the pain in osteoid osteoma. Tenderness at the tumor site is a consistent physi-

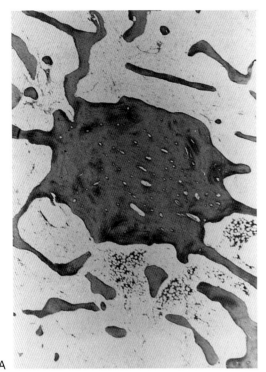

A

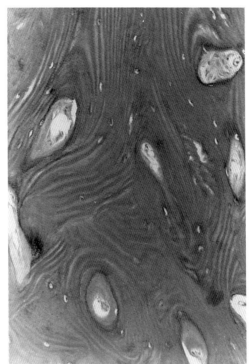

B

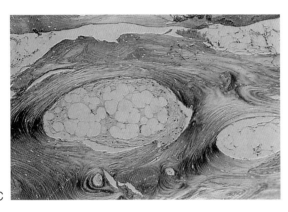

C

FIG. 37. Histopathology of bone island. **A:** A low-power photomicrograph demonstrates "pseudopodia" of the lesion. Note the multiple marrow spaces in the center, very similar to the Haversian system of nutrient canals (hematoxylin and eosin, original magnification ×16). (Reprinted with permission from Greenspan A. Sclerosing bone dysplasias—a target-site approach. *Skeletal Radiol* 1991;20:568.) **B:** A high-power photomicrograph reveals compact bone with wide bands of parallel lamellae and concentric rings (hematoxylin and eosin, original magnification ×90). **C:** Under polarized light, the mature configuration of bone island is well demonstrated (hematoxylin and eosin, polarized light, original magnification ×70). (Reprinted with permission from Greenspan A, Klein MJ. Giant bone island. *Skeletal Radiol* 1996;25:68.)

cal finding (122), and swelling may be present, particularly when the lesion is near the surface (118).

Patients with lumbar vertebral lesions will very commonly present with scoliosis. Scoliosis also commonly occurs in patients whose tumors arose in the ribs (107,110). Spinal lesions in particular may cause neurologic deficits ranging from muscle weakness to paraplegia.

Osteoblastomas rarely extend into the soft tissues and do not metastasize, although they do tend to recur locally.

Imaging

Plain film radiography is the basis for the diagnosis of osteoblastoma. In a review of the spectrum of osteoblastoma in 123 patients by McLeod et al (123), most tumors (75%) were either spherical or slightly oval, with the remainder being longitudinal; the tumor margin was well defined (83%). In half of the appendicular tumors, there was considerable reactive sclerosis; 13% of these tumors, however, had only a sclerotic rim, and 37% showed no surrounding sclerosis. The interior of the lesions was most often radiolucent (64%), whereas various degrees of ossification were present in the remaining cases. The authors speculated that lesions tend to be radiolucent when they are younger, ossifying as they mature. In the great majority of tumors, the cortex was either perfectly normal or intact, although expanded and thinned (75%); the cortical expansion was usually eccentric. Destruction or penetration of the cortex suggesting malignancy was present in a minority (20%) of tumors. The great majority of osteoblastomas showed periosteal new bone formation, which in some cases was extremely prominent. The periosteal reaction was predominantly benign and of the solid type (86%), whereas the remainder showed spiculation or multilamination, suggesting a more aggressive lesion.

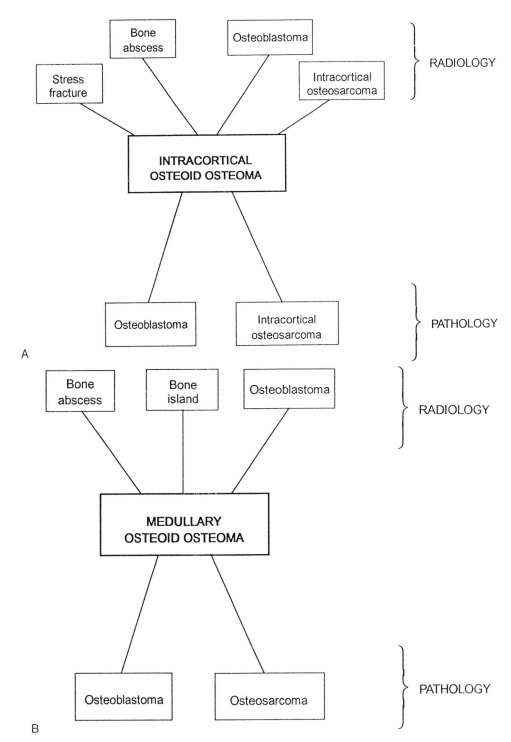

FIG. 38. A: Differential diagnosis of intracortical osteoid osteoma. **B:** Differential diagnosis of medullary osteoid osteoma.

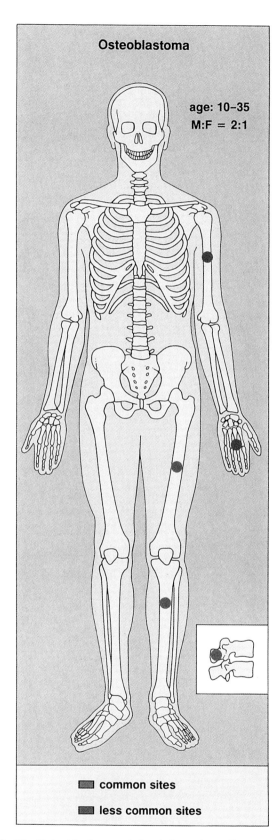

FIG. 39. Osteoblastoma: skeletal sites of predilection, peak age range, and male-to-female ratio.

Four distinctive types of osteoblastomas can be identified, based on the plain film findings (19). (a) The lesion may be almost identical radiographically to osteoid osteoma, although much larger (usually >2 cm in diameter). This type occasionally exhibits less reactive sclerosis than osteoid osteoma, but the periosteal reaction is more prominent (Fig. 40). In a review of the range of manifestations of osteoblastoma by Marsh et al. (122), the majority of tumors showed a shell of reactive bone separating the tumor from the surrounding normal bone. Osteoblastomas of the spongy bone of the spine, ilium, or talus exhibited less prominent reactive bone formation, and those arising in the cortex more pronounced reactive bone, than is seen in osteoid osteoma. (b) Osteoblastoma may also appear as a blow-out expansive lesion similar to an aneurysmal bone cyst, with small radiopacities in the center. This pattern is particularly common in tumors involving the spine (Fig. 41). (c) The tumor may occasionally appear as an aggressive lesion, simulating a

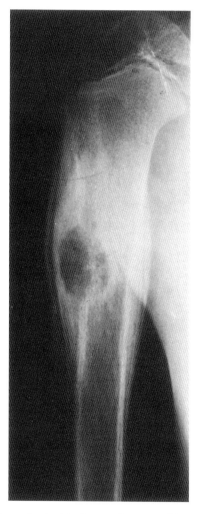

FIG. 40. Type of osteoblastoma: giant osteoid osteoma. The osteoblastoma of the proximal humerus in this 8-year-old boy appears similar to osteoid osteoma. However, the lesion is larger (2.5 cm in its largest dimension), and there is a more pronounced periosteal response.

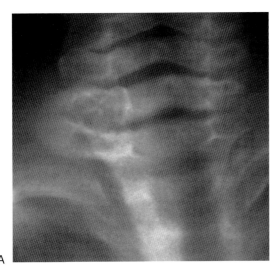
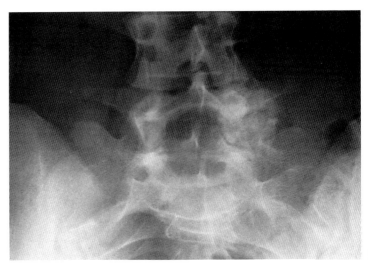

A
B

FIG. 41. Types of osteoblastoma: blow-out expansion. **A:** An expansive blow-out osteoblastoma with several small central opacities in the lamina of C6. **B:** A large osteoblastoma originating in the lamina and involving the pedicle, transverse process, and half of the vertebral body of L5, shows aneurysmal-like expansion with central radiopacities. (B—reprinted with permission from Greenspan A. Benign bone-forming lesions. *Skeletal Radiol* 1993;22:494.)

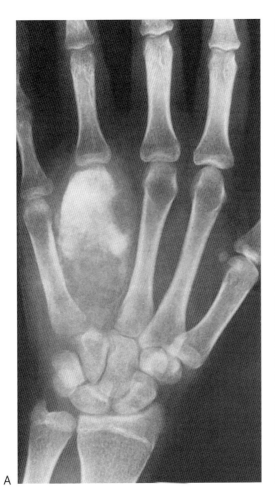
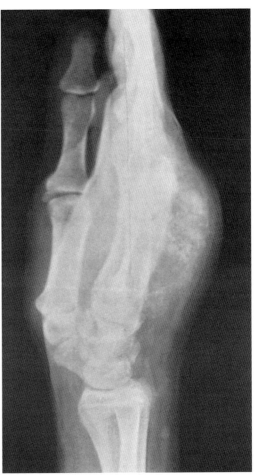

A
B

FIG. 42. Types of osteoblastoma: aggressive. **(A)** Dorsovolar and **(B)** lateral radiographs of the right hand show aggressive osteoblastoma. Note the destruction of the entire fourth metacarpal with massive bone formation. Although very similar in appearance to osteosarcoma, the lesion appears still to be contained by a shell of periosteal new bone.

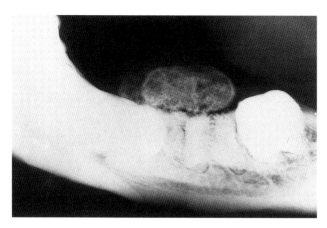

FIG. 43. Type of osteoblastoma: periosteal. Anteroposterior radiograph shows a juxtacortical lesion of the mandible.

malignant neoplasm (Fig. 42). Many of the so-called aggressive osteoblastomas belong to this group. (d) Exceptionally rare, osteoblastoma is juxtacortical (periosteal) in location, as described in 6 of 42 tumors reported by Schajowicz and Lemos (39) and in 2 of 20 tumors reported by Lichtenstein (27). These lesions generally lacked perifocal bone sclerosis and in addition, a thin shell of newly formed periosteal bone was noted covering the lesion (15, 30, 39) (Figs. 10 and 43).

Conventional tomography is often valuable for determining the extent of the tumor and whether and to what degree intralesional bone formation has occurred. It is particularly useful for spinal lesions, which may be difficult to interpret on routine radiographs. Tomography may also help gauge the size of the nidus, thus facilitating the distinction from osteoid osteoma (Fig. 44).

Skeletal scintigraphy invariably demonstrates intense fo-

cal accumulation of bone-seeking radiopharmaceutical agents (Fig. 45). Angiography is infrequently performed as part of the evaluation of osteoblastoma because of its questionable importance as a preoperative assessment tool (118).

Computed tomography, as in osteoid osteoma, is the most important imaging modality for facilitating the diagnosis of osteoblastoma and demonstrating its exact size and location (112) (Fig. 46). In addition, areas of calcifications and ossifications within the lesion (Fig. 47), as well as cortical destruction and soft tissue extension, are well delineated on CT sections (118). CT is particularly helpful in working up lesions of the spine (Fig. 48) (100).

Very few reports on the usefulness of MRI in the diagnosis and evaluation of osteoblastoma can be found in the literature (118). The strength of MRI would appear to be similar to those of CT, namely, defining the extent of bone and soft tissue involvement. Most osteoblastomas demonstrate signal intensity patterns on MR scans similar to those of the majority of bone neoplasms: spin-echo T1-weighted images show a low to intermediate intensity signal, whereas with T2-weighting signal intensity is intermediate to high. More sclerotic lesions are of low signal intensity on all pulse sequences (Fig. 49). MRI effectively reveals peritumoral edema in the adjacent marrow and in soft tissues. A recent report by Crim et al. (104) involving a 19-year-old man with osteoblastoma described an unusual "flare phenomenon" that caused a misleading appearance on MR scans, simulating a malignant process such as lymphoma or Ewing sarcoma. The phenomenon represented a widespread inflammatory response to the lesion that led to diffuse, reactive inflammatory infiltrates in two vertebrae, the adjacent ribs, and the paraspinal soft tissues. It is noteworthy that only CT-myelography was diagnostic in this case.

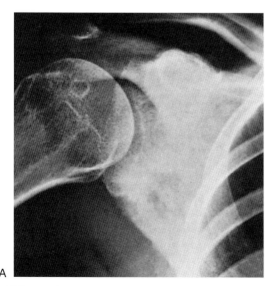
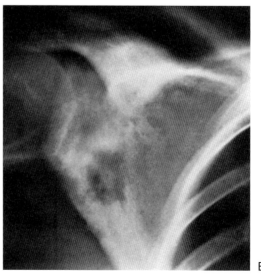

A

B

FIG. 44. Osteoblastoma: conventional tomography. **A:** A plain radiograph of the right scapula shows a faint radiolucent focus surrounded by a sclerotic area, accompanied by shaggy periosteal reaction at the axillary border. **B:** A conventional tomogram clearly demonstrates a radiolucent nidus with a sclerotic center resembling an osteoid osteoma. However, the size of this lesion (3 × 3 cm) marks it as an osteoblastoma, the diagnosis proven by excisional biopsy.

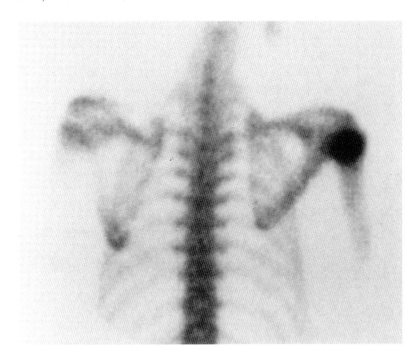

FIG. 45. Osteoblastoma: scintigraphy. A radionuclide bone scan, obtained after injection of 15 mCi (555 MBq) ^{99m}Tc-labeled MDP in a 15-year-old girl with osteoblastoma in the proximal humerus, reveals an increased uptake of tracer localized to the site of the lesion.

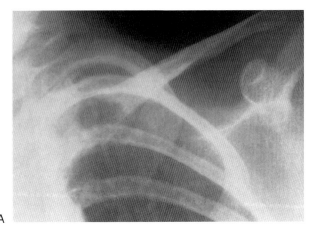

A

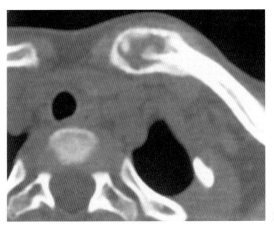

B

FIG. 46. Osteoblastoma: computed tomography. A: A plain radiograph of the left shoulder shows a radiolucent lesion in the sternal segment of the left clavicle in this 4-year-old girl. The exact location and the nature of this lesion are not clear. B: A CT section reveals the location and size of the lesion. Central ossifications are typical for osteoblastoma, the diagnosis confirmed on the histopathologic examination. (Courtesy of Dr. A. A. DeSmet, Madison, Wisconsin.)

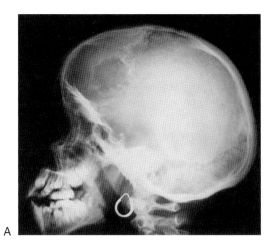
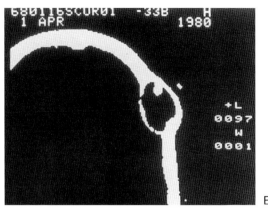

A

B

FIG. 47. Osteoblastoma: computed tomography. **A:** A lateral radiograph of the skull shows a well-defined lytic lesion in the frontal bone. **B:** A CT section shows, in addition, a focus of bone formation within the lesion, typical of osteoblastoma.

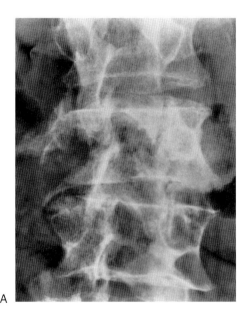
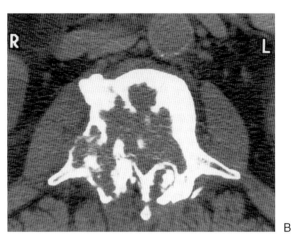

A

B

FIG. 48. Aggressive osteoblastoma. **A:** An anteroposterior radiograph of the lumbar spine shows a destructive lytic lesion affecting the right half of the vertebral body of L3 in a 65-year-old man who presented with insidious onset of pain in the lower back radiating to the right lower extremity. **B:** A CT section demonstrates focal areas of bone formation within the lesion and invasion of the cortex. Subsequent biopsy revealed an aggressive osteoblastoma. (Courtesy of Ibrahim F. Abdelwahab, M.D., New York, NY. Reprinted with permission from Greenspan A. Benign bone-forming lesions. *Skeletal Radiol* 1993; 22494.)

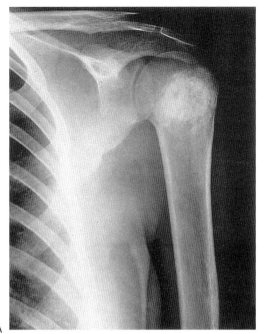

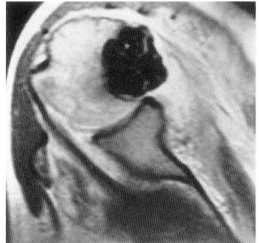

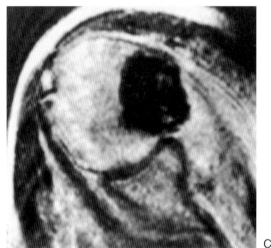

FIG. 49. Osteoblastoma: magnetic resonance imaging. **A:** A plain radiograph of the left proximal humerus (same patient as in Fig. 45) shows a large, sclerotic lesion, diagnosed on biopsy as osteoblastoma. **B:** Axial spin-echo, T1-weighted MRI demonstrates that the low-intensity lesion is located posteriorly. The cortex is destroyed and the tumor extends into the soft tissues. **C:** Axial spin-echo, T2-weighted MRI shows that the lesion remains of low signal intensity, indicating osteoblastic matrix.

Histopathology

Osteoblastoma is marked by a very active new formation of osteoid and immature bone trabeculae produced by compact masses of large osteoblasts (39). Osteoid production is generally greater in osteoblastoma than in osteoid osteoma, and the lesion shows greater vascularity (Fig. 50) (121). Furthermore, osteoblastoma exhibits a less organized pattern of osteoid and trabecular bone distribution than the nidus of osteoid osteoma, which invariably appears as a circumscribed, organized structure maturing toward its periphery; in effect, the lesion of osteoblastoma is at the same stage of development throughout (39). Occasionally, spindle-shaped hyperchromatic cells with uniform nuclei and irregular eosinophilic cytoplasm may be interdispersed among bony trabeculae (111). In contrast to most forms of osteosarcoma, osteoblastomas characteristically show variable numbers of osteoclasts at the surfaces of the bone trabeculae and seams of osteoblasts rimming the periphery of the lesion (Figs. 51A–C). In addition, they do not infiltrate or permeate the normal trabeculae at the interface with the lesion, as occurs

in osteosarcoma (30), but usually are separated from them by a narrow but distinct layer of bone-free fibrous tissue. Some atypical osteoblastomas may, however, closely resemble an osteosarcoma (Fig. 51D).

Aggressive osteoblastomas are characterized by "epithelioid" osteoblasts, twice the size of ordinary osteoblasts (109). The cells are rounded and have large nuclei containing one or more prominent nucleoli; their cytoplasm is usually abundant. Bone trabeculae are wider and more irregular than in conventional osteoblastoma, and cement lines are usually absent (Fig. 52) (117). Schajowicz and Lemos (128) described eight patients with "malignant" osteoblastoma whose tumors appear to be similar to aggressive osteoblastoma. They noted on microscopic examination more frequent atypical mitoses and increased numbers of osteoclast-like giant cells. In addition, there were bone spicules of regular shape (dark blue staining with hematoxylin), closely resembling those observed in osteosarcoma. A pseudomalignant variant of osteoblastoma contains bizarre multinucleated cells completely devoid of mitotic activity (123,125).

Della Rocca and Huvos recently stated that a clinically

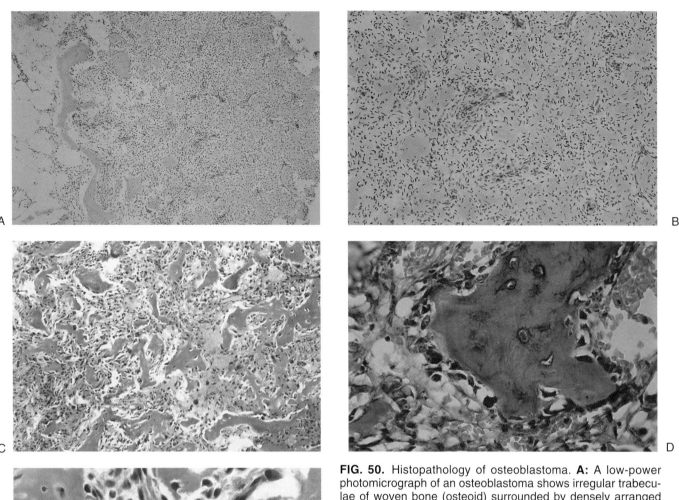

FIG. 50. Histopathology of osteoblastoma. **A:** A low-power photomicrograph of an osteoblastoma shows irregular trabeculae of woven bone (osteoid) surrounded by densely arranged osteoblasts (hematoxylin and eosin, original magnification ×12). **B:** At higher magnification, the dense osteoblastic rimming of the trabeculae is conspicuous. Some osteoclasts are also present (hematoxylin and eosin, original magnification ×25). **C:** Another photomicrograph of an osteoblastoma shows irregular trabeculae of woven bone haphazardly arranged within a vascular spindle cell stroma (hematoxylin and eosin, original magnification ×40). **D:** At high magnification, the bone trabecula is surrounded by osteoblasts containing large, dark nuclei. Many capillaries (one of which is dilated—upper right corner) filled with blood are also visible (Giemsa, original magnification ×100). **E:** A high-power photomicrograph reveals osteoblasts and osteoclasts on the surface of the immature small trabeculae (hematoxylin and eosin, original magnification ×152). (C and E—Courtesy of K. Krishnan Unni, M.B., B.S., Rochester, Minnesota. Reprinted with permission from Greenspan A. Benign bone-forming lesions. *Skeletal Radiol* 1993;22: 496.)

aggressive behavior is not correlated with histologic qualities but with the localization within the skeleton (106).

Differential Diagnosis

Radiology

To distinguish osteoblastoma from *osteoid osteoma* can be very difficult, if not impossible, on both radiologic and histologic grounds. Some authorities believe that because of

its striking histologic similarity to osteoid osteoma, osteoblastoma represents a variant of clinical expression of the same pathologic process. Both lesions are considered separate entities, however, because their clinical manifestations and skeletal distribution are distinct: osteoid osteoma is invariably accompanied by nocturnal pain promptly relieved by salicylates, whereas osteoblastoma is larger than osteoid osteoma and has a predilection for the axial skeleton. In addition, osteoid osteoma has a tendency to regress spontaneously, whereas osteoblastoma tends to progress and (al-

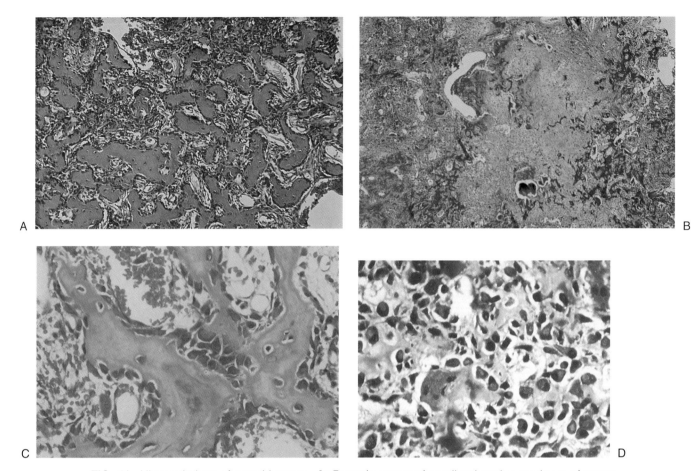

FIG. 51. Histopathology of osteoblastoma. **A:** Densely arranged small trabeculae made up of woven bone are surrounded by osteoblasts. In the narrow marrow spaces, some capillaries and giant cells of the osteoclast type are seen. These features, together with very regular appearing bone formation, militate against the diagnosis of osteosarcoma (hematoxylin and eosin, original magnification ×25). **B:** Osteoblastoma at the interface with normal (host) bone, unlike osteosarcoma, shows woven bone formation in plates (*middle*) and in delicate trabeculae (*right and left*), rimmed with densely arranged osteoblasts and giant cells of the osteoclast type (hematoxylin and eosin, original magnification ×50). **C:** At high magnification, the uniform-appearing osteoblasts line the newly formed trabeculae (hematoxylin and eosin, original magnification ×100). **D:** Atypical osteoblastoma with crowded, large epithelioid stromal cells and irregular foci of woven bone formation resembles an osteosarcoma (hematoxylin and eosin, original magnification ×400). (**D**—reprinted with permission from Bullough PG. *Atlas of orthopedic pathology with clinical and radiologic correlations,* 2nd ed. New York: Gower, 1992;16.4.)

though this is still a controversial speculation of some investigators) may undergo malignant transformation. The most useful differential factor is the size of a lesion: osteoblastoma usually measures 2 cm or more.

The differential diagnosis of osteoblastoma should also include *bone abscess* (Brodie abscess), *aneurysmal bone cyst*, and *osteosarcoma*. The same criteria distinguishing a bone abscess from osteoid osteoma apply in relation to osteoblastoma (see "Differential Diagnosis" under "Osteoid Osteoma"). The key to making the distinction is usually the serpentine track in bone abscess that extends toward the growth plate (**see Fig. 32**). At times the distinction between these two lesions may be difficult (Fig. 53A). Osteoblastoma located in a short tubular bone may be unmistakably diagnosed as *enchondroma* (Fig. 53B, C). Expansive osteoblastoma, particularly in spinal location, on plain film radiogra-

phy may occasionally mimic an aneurysmal bone cyst (**see Fig. 41**) or a giant cell tumor.

Aggressive osteoblastoma should be differentiated from *osteosarcoma* (101) (**see Fig. 42**). Cross-sectional imaging modalities such as CT and MRI are helpful in making the distinction by demonstrating the soft tissue component of osteosarcoma.

Intracortical osteosarcoma, because it may have a benign radiographic appearance, may mimic periosteal and intracortical osteoblastoma (124). The principal means for distinguishing these entities are histologic.

Pathology

Osteoblastoma may be confused with *osteoid osteoma*, unless clinical and radiologic factors are considered. Al-

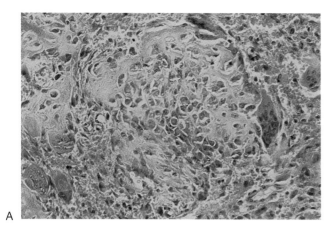
A

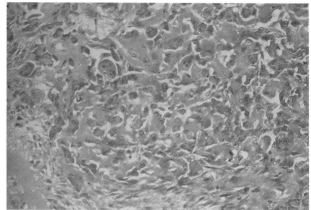
B

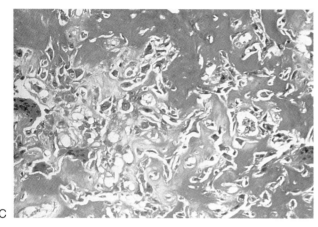
C

FIG. 52. Histopathology of aggressive osteoblastoma. A: Aggregates of large osteoblasts are producing osteoid and irregular bone trabeculae. Note the few scattered giant cells of the osteoclast type (hematoxylin and eosin, original magnification ×250). B: Large epithelioid-like osteoblasts surround an unorganized osteoid matrix (hematoxylin and eosin, original magnification ×300). C: In another area, dense and irregularly distributed islands of osteoid exhibit very few osteoblasts (hematoxylin and eosin, original magnification ×300).

though the nidus of osteoid osteoma is quite similar to that of osteoblastoma, some authorities postulate that there are minor microscopic differences (126,129): at the periphery of a nidus of osteoid osteoma a fibrovascular rim is often present, a feature only occasionally encountered in osteoblastoma. The latter tumor, on the other hand, often has a lobulated or multifocal outer margin (11). Moreover, the nidus of an osteoid osteoma often exhibits a distinct zonal pattern with central maturation to more mineralized woven bone.

Aneurysmal bone cyst can be easily distinguished from osteoblastoma. The former lesion consists of multiple blood-filled sinusoid spaces alternating with more solid areas. The solid tissue is composed of fibrous elements containing numerous giant cells and is richly vascular. The sinusoids have fibrous walls, often containing osteoid tissue or even lamellae of mature bone, though not in quantities seen in osteoblastoma (**see Figs. 7-31 to 7-33**). Furthermore, unlike in osteoblastoma, focal or diffuse collections of hemosiderin or reactive foam cells may be seen in the fibrous septae of aneurysmal bone cyst (127,130).

Giant-cell tumor characteristically demonstrates related dual populations of giant cells and mononuclear stromal cells. Giant cells are evenly distributed within the intervening spindle-celled stromal tissue without evidence of mineralization or osteoid formation.

Diagnosis of *osteosarcoma* should always be the differential possibility. Histopathologic examination can make the distinction (see "Histopathology"). Although in osteoblastoma a certain number of mitotic figures may be found, the lack of areas of necrosis and lack of cellular pleomorphism helps to distinguish this lesion from osteosarcoma (38).

Intracortical osteosarcoma exhibits distinctive characteristics. According to Mirra et al., the following histopathologic features are critical for diagnosis of intracortical osteosarcoma: (a) permeation of the Haversian systems with attenuation and trapping of cortical lamellar bone; (b) atypical mitoses or anaplasia; and (c) presence of tumor cartilage (124).

The radiologic and pathologic differential diagnoses of osteoblastoma are depicted in Fig. 54 and Table 3.

MALIGNANT LESIONS

Osteosarcomas

Osteosarcomas comprise a family of connective tissue tumors with various degrees of malignant potential. All of these tumors share the characteristic ability to produce bone or osteoid directly from neoplastic cells (224). Osteosarcomas constitute about 20% of all primary bone malignancies

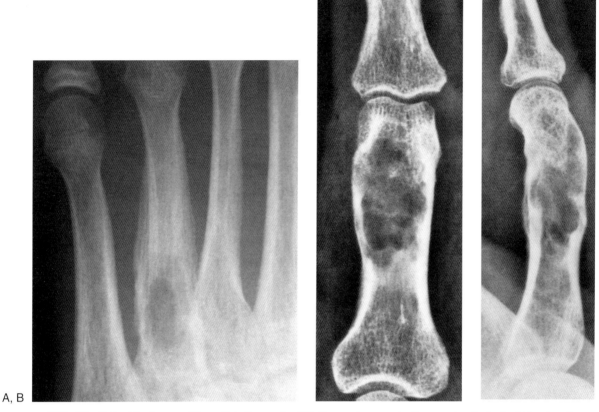

A, B

C

FIG. 53. Osteoblastoma: differential diagnosis. **(A)** Bone abscess in the proximal shaft of the fourth metatarsal in a 16-year-old boy was originally diagnosed as osteoblastoma. In another patient, dorso-volar **(B)** and lateral **(C)** radiographs of the small finger reveal a radiolucent lesion with scalloped borders in the middle phalanx, resembling an enchondroma. Small radiopacities in the center represent bone formation rather than chondroid matrix. The lesion proved to be an osteoblastoma.

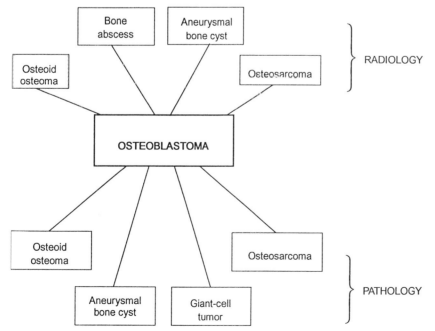

FIG. 54. Radiologic and pathologic differential diagnoses of osteoblastoma.

TABLE 3. *Differential diagnosis of osteoblastoma*

Condition (lesions)	Radiologic features	Pathologic features
Cortical and medullary osteoid-osteoma-like osteoblastoma (giant osteoid osteoma)	Radiolucent lesion, spherical or oval, with well-defined margins. Frequent perilesional sclerosis. Abundant periosteal reaction. Size of the nidus >2 cm.	Active formation of osteoid and immature bone trabeculae. Less organized pattern of osteoid and reticular bone distribution than seen in osteoid osteoma. Hypertrophic osteoblasts. Increased vascularity in the stroma. Occasionally spindle-shaped hyperchromatic cells with uniform nuclei and irregular eosinophilic cytoplasm interdispersed among bony trabeculae. Variable number of giant cells on the surface of bone trabeculae.
Aneurysmal bone cyst-like expansive osteoblastoma	Blow-out lesion, similar to aneurysmal bone cyst, but with central opacities.	
Aggressive osteoblastoma (simulating malignant neoplasm)	Ill-defined borders, destruction of the cortex; aggressive-looking periosteal reaction; occasionally soft tissue extension.	Large, "epithelioid" osteoblasts. Rounded cells with large nuclei containing one or more prominent nucleoli; abundant cytoplasm. Bone trabeculae wider and more irregular than in other types of osteoblastoma. Cement lines usually absent. Atypical mitoses. Bone spicules staining dark blue with hematoxylin-eosin.
Periosteal osteoblastoma	Round or ovoid heterogeneous in density mass attached to cortex.	Trabeculae of woven bone, numerous dilated capillaries, exuberant in number osteoblasts, osteoclasts, and occasionally fibroblasts.
Osteoid osteoma	See Table 2.	See Table 2.
Aneurysmal bone cyst	Blow-out, expansive lesion. In long bone buttress of periosteal reaction. Thin shell of reactive bone frequently covers the lesion, but may be absent in rapidly growing lesions. Soft tissue extension may be present.	Multiple blood-filled sinusoid spaces separated by fibrous septae displaying lamellae of primitive woven bone; may contain hemosiderin and reactive foam cells; solid areas composed of fibrous elements containing irregular bone trabeculae and giant cells, sometimes in great numbers.
Osteosarcoma	Permeative or moth-eaten bone destruction; wide zone of transition; tumor-bone cloud-like opacities; aggressive periosteal reaction; soft tissue mass.	Permeation of cortical bone; attenuation and "trapping" of lamellar bone; atypical mitoses or anaplasia; hyperchromatism and pleomorphism of cells and nuclei; tumor bone and tumor cartilage formed by malignant cells.

(199). The collection of large series of osteosarcomas has led to the identification of an increasing number of subtypes (242) (Fig. 55).

The vast majority of osteosarcomas are of unknown etiology and are therefore considered as idiopathic, or primary. A smaller number of tumors can be related to known factors that predispose to malignancy, such as Paget disease of bone, bone infarct, fibrous dysplasia, external ionizing irradiation, and ingestion of radioactive substances. These lesions are classified as secondary osteosarcomas (154).

All types of osteosarcomas can be further subclassified, according to their anatomic site, as either axial or appendicular (189). Furthermore, they can be classified, on the basis of their location in bone, as central (medullary), intracortical, or juxtacortical. A separate and very small group consists of primary osteosarcomas that originate in the soft tissues (so-called extraskeletal or soft tissue osteosarcomas). In general, central osteosarcomas are much more common than juxta-cortical tumors and tend to have a higher grade of malignancy (173, 174).

Clinical Presentation

The clinical presentation varies from case to case and is largely dependent on the type of osteosarcoma, its anatomic site, and the age of the patient (189). Pain and development of a soft tissue swelling or mass are the most common presenting symptoms. Rarely, a pathologic fracture is the first sign of malignancy (205). At first the pain may be slight and intermittent, but gradually it becomes more severe and constant (147). In juxtacortical tumors, the presence of a hard, slowly enlarging, painless mass is the most common clinical finding. Although pulmonary metastasis is the most usual and most significant complication in the majority of high-grade osteosarcomas, it is rare in osteosarcomas of the jaw and is a late complication in multicentric osteosarcomas.

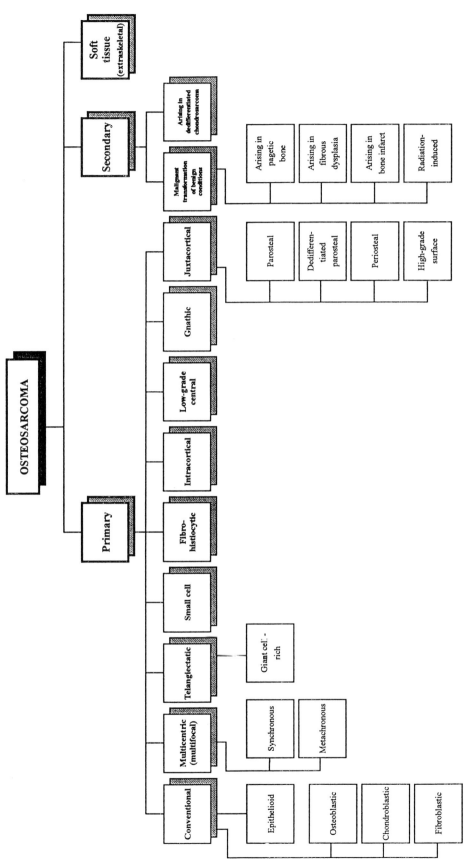

FIG. 55. Osteosarcoma and its subtypes.

Imaging

For diagnostic purposes, plain film radiography usually provides adequate information. The findings of bone destruction associated with sclerotic foci of tumor bone formation, an aggressive (sunburst-type, lamellated, or Codman triangle) periosteal reaction, and a soft tissue mass are highly suggestive of osteosarcoma. Conventional tomography may aid in delineating the osseous matrix and cortical destruction and in detection of occult pathologic fracture. Arteriography is usually reserved for mapping of the tumor and its vascular supply, and for identification of the area most suitable for an open biopsy. Radionuclide bone scan can assist in diagnosis of intraosseous metastases and skip lesions. CT and MRI are crucial for determining the intraosseous and extraosseous extension of a tumor (144,229,238, 258).

Histopathology

Like the imaging findings, the histopathologic features of osteosarcoma vary according to the particular subtype. The common characteristic of all subtypes, however, is the presence of tumor osteoid or tumor bone formed by the malignant cells.

Osteosarcomas can be graded on the basis of their cellularity, cytologic atypia (nuclear pleomorphism), and mitotic activity. In general, by Broder's system (145), the numerical grade (1 to 4) indicates the degree of malignancy (grade 1 indicating the least undifferentiated tumor and grade 4 the most undifferentiated tumor) (Table 4). For example, well-differentiated central osteosarcomas and parosteal osteosarcomas are regarded as grade 1, rarely grade 2 tumors; peri-

osteal osteosarcomas and gnathic osteosarcomas as grade 2, rarely grade 3; and conventional osteosarcomas as grade 3 or 4. Telangiectatic osteosarcomas, osteosarcomas developing in pagetic bone, postirradiation osteosarcomas, and multifocal osteosarcomas are usually grade 4 tumors. This grading has clinical, therapeutic, and prognostic importance (152, 238).

Primary Osteosarcomas

Conventional (Medullary) Osteosarcoma

Medullary osteosarcoma is the most common type of osteosarcoma, constituting approximately 85% of all forms of osteosarcoma (207). Formation of osteoid or bone by tumor cells is the criterion for the histologic diagnosis (151). The incidence of medullary osteosarcoma is greatest during the second decade of life, and males are affected slightly more often than females. The knee (distal femur, proximal tibia) is the most commonly affected site, followed by the proximal humerus (153) (Fig. 56). The metaphysis is more frequently affected than the diaphysis, and the growth plate usually serves as a barrier to tumor spread into the epiphysis, although invasion of the physis and involvement of the epiphysis and the joint have been reported (210,232). The most common complications of conventional osteosarcomas are pathologic fracture and development of pulmonary metastases.

Imaging

The distinctive radiologic features of conventional osteosarcoma, as demonstrated by plain film radiography, are medullary and cortical bone destruction, an aggressive periosteal reaction, a soft tissue mass, and the presence of tumor bone either within the destructive lesion or on its periphery, as well as within the soft tissue mass itself, often assuming a spiculated or sunburst pattern (154,193) (Fig. 57). In some instances the type of bone destruction is not so obvious (158,222), but patchy densities, representing tumor bone, and an aggressive periosteal reaction provide clues to the diagnosis (Fig. 58). The degree of radiopacity in the tumor reflects a combination of the amount of tumor bone production, calcified matrix, and osteoid. Tumors may present as purely sclerotic lesions, purely osteolytic lesions (157), but mostly a combination of both (Fig. 59). The borders are usually indistinct, with a wide zone of transition. The type of bone destruction is either moth-eaten or permeative, only rarely geographic. The most common periosteal reactions observed with this tumor are the sunburst type and the Codman triangle; the lamellated (onion-skin) type of periosteal

TABLE 4. *Histologic grading of osteosarcoma*[a]

Grade	Histologic features
1	Cellularity: slightly increased Cytologic atypia: minimal to slight Mitotic activity: low Osteoid matrix: regular
2	Cellularity: moderate Cytologic atypia: mild to moderate Mitotic activity: low to moderate Osteoid matrix: regular
3	Cellularity: increased Cytologic atypia: moderate to marked Mitotic activity: moderate to high Osteoid matrix: irregular
4	Cellularity: markedly increased Cytologic atypia: markedly pleomorphic cells Mitotic activity: high Osteoid matrix: irregular, abundant

[a] According to Unni KK, Dahlin DC. Grading of bone tumors. *Semin Diagn Pathol* 1984;1:165–172.

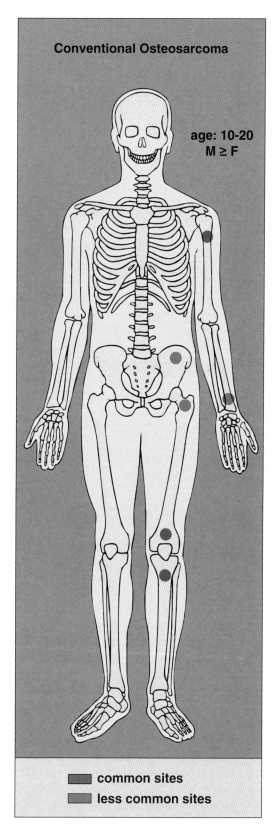

Conventional Osteosarcoma

age: 10-20
M ≥ F

■ common sites
■ less common sites

FIG. 56. Conventional osteosarcoma: skeletal sites of predilection, peak age range, and male-to-female ratio.

response is less common (Fig. 60). The presence of a soft tissue mass, which may contain sclerotic foci (tumor bone formation), is a common finding (Fig. 61).

Computed tomography is invaluable for evaluation of these tumors (228), particularly for determining the degree of tumor extension in the bone marrow. CT using Hounsfield units can accurately determine the attenuation coefficient of the medullary cavity (Fig. 62). The normal bone marrow has a fat density of −20 to −80 Hounsfield units. With tumor infiltration, this density is significantly increased (172).

Magnetic resonance imaging is equally if not more effective for evaluating intraosseous tumor extension and soft tissue involvement (144,214). On T1-weighted spin-echo images, the mineralized components of osteosarcoma display a low signal intensity, whereas the solid, nonmineralized portions of the tumor usually appear as areas of low to intermediate signal intensity. On T2-weighted spin-echo images and T2* gradient sequences, the mineralized portions of tumor display a low signal intensity, and nonmineralized areas and soft tissue mass are of high signal intensity (Figs. 63 and 64). Osteosclerotic tumors demonstrate a low signal intensity on both T1- and T2-weighted sequences (143). MRI may also effectively demonstrate the peritumoral edema, which will image as bright areas adjacent to the tumor on T2- or T2*-weighted sequences. In addition to staging both the extraosseous and intraosseous extent of the tumor, MRI can aid in the identification of various components within the tumor, such as cellular areas, and regions of necrosis and liquefaction. Cartilaginous components are particularly easy to identify by virtue of the septum-like enhancement seen on gadolinium-enhanced MR images (142).

Arteriography is rarely used, as it is primarily reserved for mapping of the vascular supply of the tumor, and sometimes for the identification of the areas most desirable for biopsy (Fig. 65).Scintigraphy will invariably show an increased uptake of the radiopharmaceutical tracer (Fig. 66). In addition, as indicated above, radionuclide bone scan can assist in the identification of intraosseous metastases (Fig. 67).

Histopathology

On the basis of the dominant histologic features, conventional osteosarcoma can be subdivided into three histologic subtypes: osteoblastic, chondroblastic, and fibroblastic (Fig. 68). As stated above, each of these is characterized by the formation of osteoid tissue or bone by the neoplastic cells. The specific appearance of osteosarcoma reflects its histologic grade. Microscopic examination usually reveals highly pleomorphic spindle-shaped and polyhedral tumor cells, producing different forms of osteoid (Fig. 69). Mitotic figures are commonly seen. Malignant giant cells may occasionally be found. Bone matrix formation may be subtle, displaying sporadic wisps in a lace-like pattern resembling a doily or a lotus root (174). The matrix sometimes takes the form of bulky deposits, which have been described as massive osteoid. Necrotic areas and hemorrhage may be present.

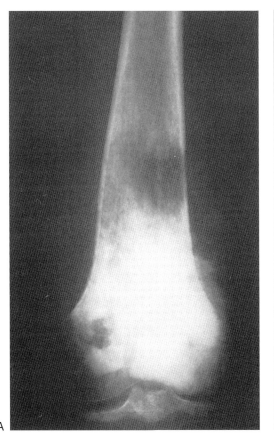
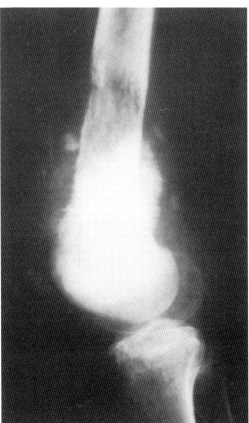

A

B

FIG. 57. Conventional osteosarcoma. Anteroposterior (**A**) and lateral (**B**) radiographs demonstrate the typical features of this tumor in the distal femur of a 19-year-old woman. Medullary and cortical bone destruction is present, in association with aggressive periosteal reaction of the velvet and sunburst types. A soft tissue mass contains tumor bone.

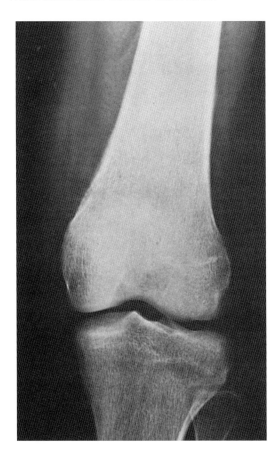

FIG. 58. Conventional osteosarcoma. Although no gross bone destruction is evident in the distal femur of this 16-year-old girl, the patchy densities in the medullary portion of the femur and the sunburst appearance of the periosteal response are clues to the diagnosis of osteosarcoma. Note also the presence of a Codman triangle.

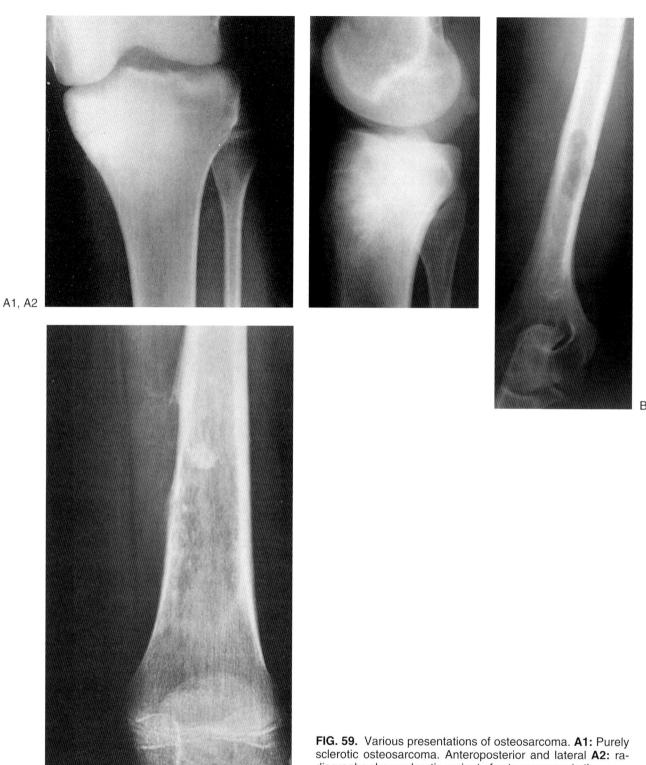

A1, A2

B

C

FIG. 59. Various presentations of osteosarcoma. **A1:** Purely sclerotic osteosarcoma. Anteroposterior and lateral **A2:** radiographs show sclerotic variant of osteosarcoma in the proximal tibia. **B:** Purely lytic osteosarcoma. An anteroposterior radiograph shows destructive lesion in the distal humerus, which proved to be a fibroblastic osteosarcoma. **C:** Mixed osteosarcoma. Areas of bone formation are present within a destructive lesion in the distal femur.

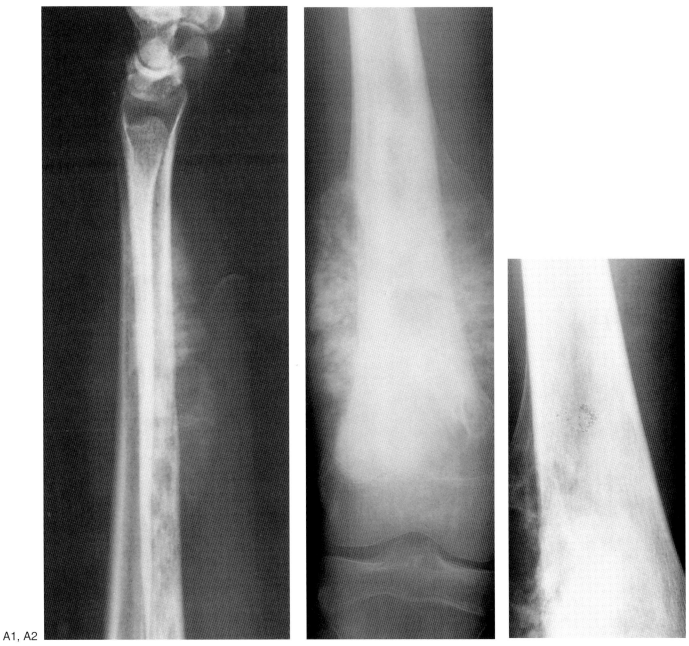

A1, A2

B

FIG. 60. Types of periosteal reaction in osteosarcoma. **A1, A2:** The sunburst type is the most common. **B:** A typical Codman triangle in osteosarcoma of the distal femur. *Continued on page 68.*

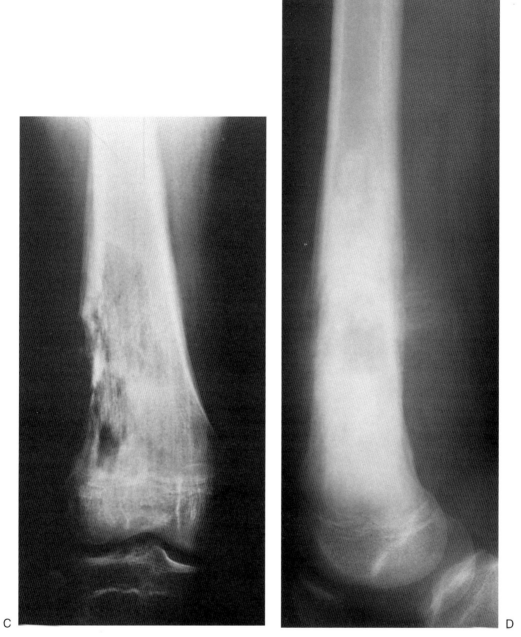

FIG. 60. *Continued.* **C:** The onion-skin or lamellated type of periosteal reaction. (From Greenspan A. *Orthopedic radiology,* 2nd ed. Philadelphia: Lippincott-Raven, 1992.) **D:** A combination of lamellated and sunburst periosteal reaction.

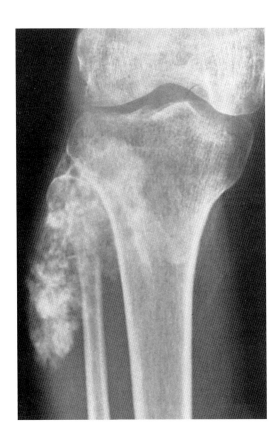

FIG. 61. Conventional osteosarcoma. A soft tissue mass containing tumor bone is a common finding in osteosarcoma, as seen in this 20-year-old man with a lesion in the right proximal fibula.

The intercellular material may be fibrous, cartilaginous, osteoid, or osseous, with various amounts of calcification (207). If osteoid deposition is plentiful, the tumor cells and their nuclei may become inconspicuous, a process referred to by Jaffe as normalization (184). In some instances, the tumor cells are so undifferentiated that cytologic study fails to clearly determine if they are mesenchymal or epithelial in origin, a variant of conventional osteosarcoma sometimes referred to as epithelioid osteosarcoma (150,156,190,242) (Fig. 70). This appearance may lead to an incorrect diagnosis of metastatic carcinoma. The diagnosis in such cases can usually be deduced on the basis of the patient's age, the production of obvious osteoblastic tumor matrix, the immunohistochemical demonstration of the mesenchymal character of the tumor, and a radiographic appearance typical of osteosarcoma (174). Occasionally, conventional osteosarcoma may exhibit large numbers of cytologically bland, reactive stromal giant cells that may obscure the underlying sarcomatous stroma (11). This variant is known as giant cell–rich osteosarcoma (see below).

Small-Cell Osteosarcoma

Originally described by Sim and associates (230), small cell osteosarcoma accounts for approximately 1% of all osteosarcomas. This subtype usually presents as a lucent lesion exhibiting permeative borders and a large soft tissue mass. Its appearance therefore mimics round cell tumors of bone, such as Ewing sarcoma. In some instances, small-cell osteo-

sarcoma presents as a sclerotic lesion that is indistinguishable from conventional osteosarcoma (163). The majority of tumors display an aggressive periosteal reaction (141). The distal femur, proximal humerus, and proximal tibia are preferred sites (137). Almost half of the patients are in their second decade at the time of clinical presentation (142).

On histopathologic study, these lesions usually exhibit loose aggregations of small round cells separated by collagenous bands of a fine eosinophilic matrix that resembles Ewing sarcoma (Fig. 71). (161) To blur the distinction further, this tumor may also exhibit a positive staining for glycogen, as described for Ewing sarcoma. However, the presence of ovoid nuclei and definite spindling of the tumor cells in some areas, and the often focal production of osteoid wisps or bone formation, should direct pathologists away from Ewing sarcoma and toward a confident diagnosis of small-cell osteosarcoma (174). The amount of cytoplasm varies considerably and is dependent on the degree of cellularity (137). In some instances, malignant cartilage can be detected.

Fibrohistiocytic Osteosarcoma

This variant, which resembles malignant fibrous histiocytoma (MFH), has recently been described in the literature (138). It can sometimes be confused with true MFH of bone because both of these tumors tend to arise at a greater age than conventional osteosarcoma, usually after the third decade. Both tend to involve the articular ends of long bones,

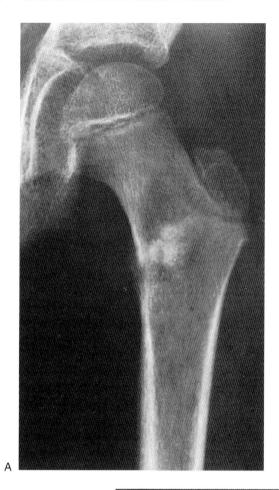
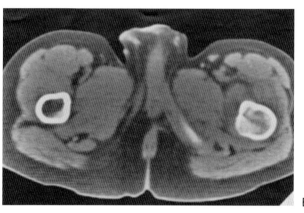
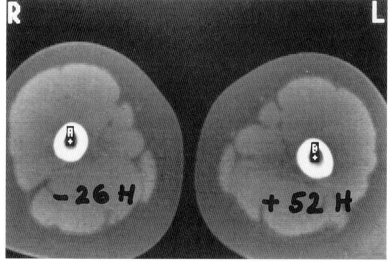

FIG. 62. Conventional osteosarcoma: computed tomography. (**A**) An anteroposterior radiograph of the left proximal femur of a 12-year-old boy demonstrates an osteolytic lesion in the intertrochanteric region, with a poorly defined margin and amorphous densities in the center, associated with a periosteal reaction medially. These features suggest osteosarcoma, which was confirmed on biopsy. Because a limb salvage procedure was contemplated, a CT scan was performed to determine the extent of marrow infiltration and the required level of bone resection. The most proximal section (**B**) shows obvious gross tumor involvement of the marrow cavity of the left femur. A more distal section (**C**) shows no gross marrow abnormality, but a positive Hounsfield value of 52 units indicates tumor involvement of the marrow, which was not shown on the standard radiographs. By comparison, the section of the right femur shows a normal Hounsfield value of −26 for bone marrow.

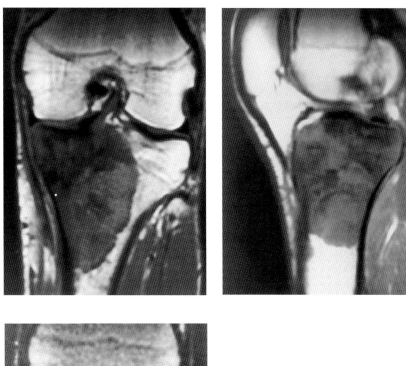

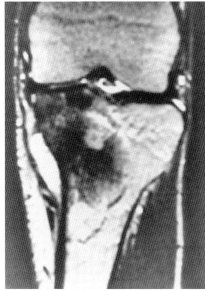

FIG. 63. Conventional osteosarcoma: magnetic resonance imaging. Coronal (**A1**) and sagittal (**A2**) spin-echo, T1-weighted MRI (TR 800, TE 20) in this 17-year-old boy with osteosarcoma of the left proximal tibia shows inhomogeneous appearance of a tumor. The mineralized parts of osteosarcoma display low signal intensity, whereas nonmineralized areas are of intermediate signal intensity. **B:** On spin-echo, T2-weighted MRI (TR 2000, TE 80), the sclerotic parts of the tumor remain of low signal intensity, whereas a nonmineralized part of the lesion (distally) shows high signal intensity. Likewise, the soft tissue extension of osteosarcoma displays high signal intensity.

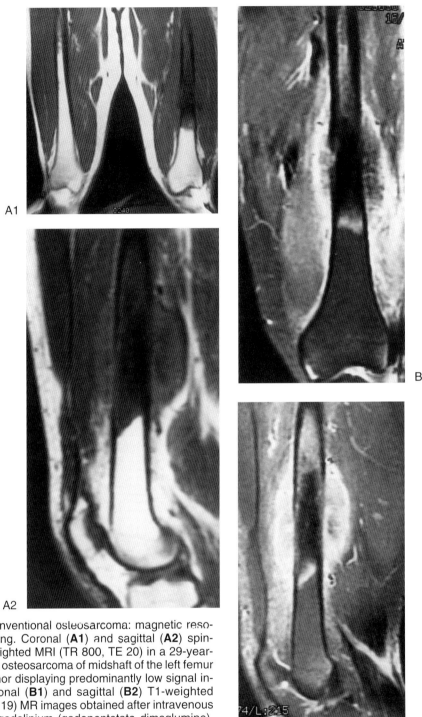

FIG. 64. Conventional osteosarcoma: magnetic resonance imaging. Coronal (**A1**) and sagittal (**A2**) spin-echo, T1-weighted MRI (TR 800, TE 20) in a 29-year-old man with osteosarcoma of midshaft of the left femur shows a tumor displaying predominantly low signal intensity. Coronal (**B1**) and sagittal (**B2**) T1-weighted (TR 650, TE 19) MR images obtained after intravenous injection of gadolinium (gadopentetate dimeglumine), using the fat suppression technique, show tumor enhancement in the medullary portion of bone and in the soft tissues. Heavily mineralized portions of tumor remain of low signal intensity.

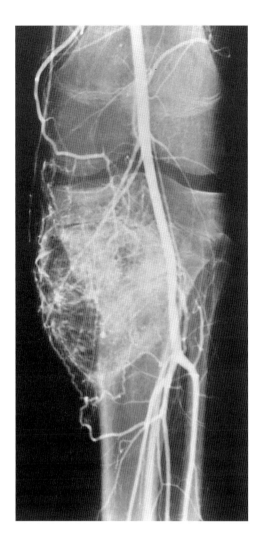

FIG. 65. Conventional osteosarcoma: angiography. Arteriography reveals increased vascularity of a tumor involving the left tibial metaphysis. Also noted are abnormal tumor vessels in the soft tissue mass. Biopsy is usually performed from the most viable (vascular) areas.

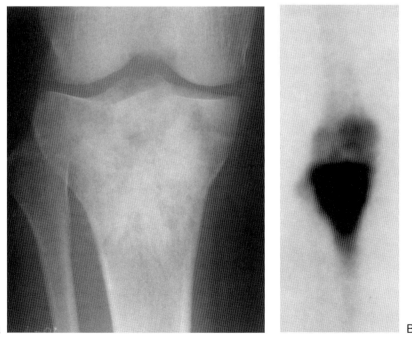

A   B

FIG. 66. Conventional osteosarcoma: scintigraphy. A: Anteroposterior radiograph shows a sclerotic variant of conventional osteosarcoma in the proximal tibia. B: After injection of 15 mCi (555 MBq) of ^{99m}Tc-labeled methylene diphosphonate (MDP), there is significantly increased uptake of the tracer in the tumor.

73

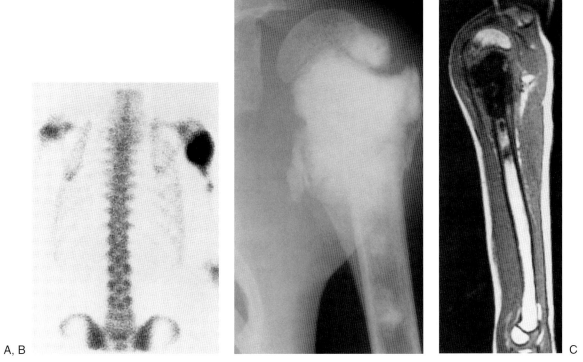

A, B

C

FIG. 67. Conventional osteosarcoma of the proximal humerus with intraosseous metastases ("skip lesions"). (**A**) Scintigraphy shows markedly increased uptake of the radiopharmaceutical agent in the proximal humerus, corresponding to the primary tumor. In addition two small foci of activity are seen distal to the main lesion. This finding, representing skip lesions, was confirmed by the plain radiography (**B**) and MRI (**C**).

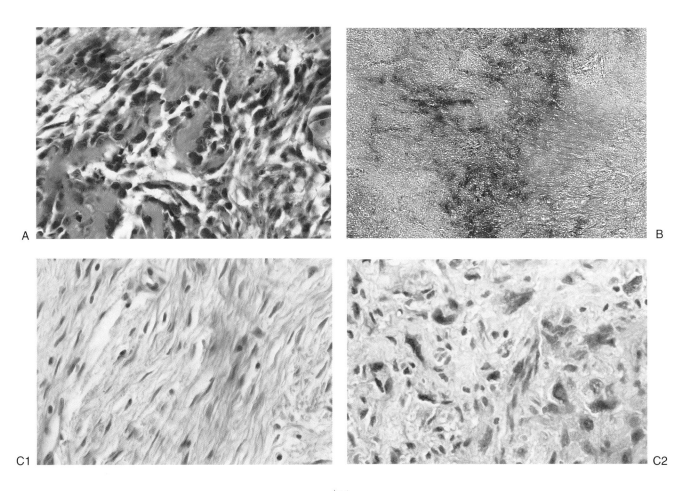

A

B

C1

C2

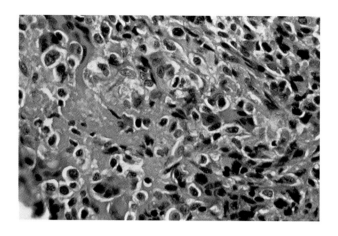

FIG. 69. Histopathology of conventional osteosarcoma. Markedly pleomorphic tumor cells are separated by lace-like osteoid (hematoxylin and eosin, original magnification ×400).

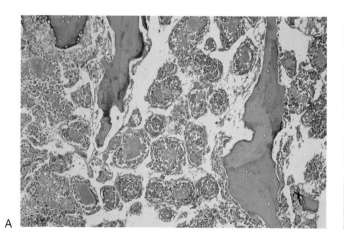

A

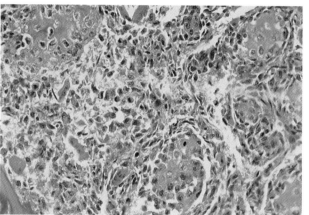

B

FIG. 70. Histopathology of epithelioid osteosarcoma. **A:** At low magnification, the tumor cells are arranged in a nesting pattern, resembling epithelial tumor (hematoxylin and eosin, original magnification ×63). **B:** At higher magnification there is evidence of osteoid formation by the tumor cells (hematoxylin and eosin, original magnification ×230). (Courtesy Dr. Michael J. Klein, New York, NY.)

FIG. 68. Histologic subtypes of osteosarcoma. **A:** Osteoblastic. Irregular woven bone trabeculae are rimmed by pleomorphic tumor osteoblasts with hyperchromatic nuclei (hematoxylin and eosin, original magnification ×100). **B:** Chondroblastic. The tumor consists mainly of cartilaginous tissue, with only scanty islands of tumor-osteoid (*upper right*) (Giemsa, original magnification ×12). **C:** Fibroblastic. (C1) Predominantly spindle fibroblast-like tumor cells with deeply stained nuclei are arranged in sheaths (hematoxylin and eosin, original magnification ×156). (C2) In another field, malignant cells produce osteoid (hematoxylin and eosin, original magnification ×150). (**C1**–Courtesy of Dr. L. Wold, Rochester, Minnesota.)

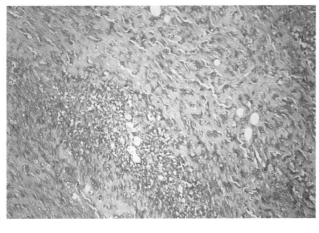

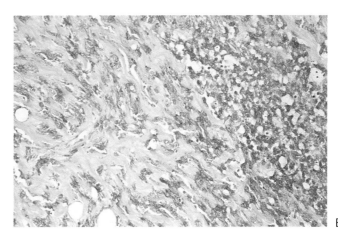

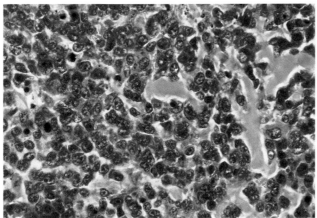

FIG. 71. Histopathology of small-cell osteosarcoma. **A:** Tumor tissue consisting of medium-sized round cells, with indistinct cytoplasm and slightly pleomorphic and hyperchromatic nuclei resembling those of Ewing sarcoma, form an abundant, primitive osteoid matrix (hematoxylin and eosin, original magnification ×25). **B:** At higher magnification, the resemblance of the matrix-free areas to a Ewing sarcoma (*upper right*) is even more obvious. The primitive osteoid is difficult to distinguish from hyalinized collagen (hematoxylin and eosin, original magnification ×50). **C:** At high magnification, malignant round cells are producing osteoid (hematoxylin and eosin, original magnification ×440).

and less periosteal reaction is typically present than in conventional osteosarcoma. Although on radiography both of these lesions tend to be radiolucent and thus do resemble giant cell tumor and fibrosarcoma, the MFH-like osteosarcoma usually exhibits areas of bone formation resembling cottonballs or cumulus clouds, whereas MFH does not (155). When such areas are identified on radiologic studies, a diligent search should be made for tumor bone in the resected specimen (189). Histologically, MFH-like osteosarcoma is characterized by pleomorphic spindle cells and giant cells, many of which have bizarre nuclei. This lesion therefore resembles giant cell–rich osteosarcoma. An inflammatory background is not unusual, and the storiform or spiral nebular arrangement, characteristic of MFH, although sometimes a dominant feature, may be less prominent or may be re-

placed by areas of large, pleomorphic cells arranged in diffuse sheets (138). As in all other subtypes of osteosarcoma, the distinction from other sarcomas depends on the demonstration of osteoid or bone formation by malignant cells in the very typical patterns seen in osteosarcomas (155, 221,252).

Telangiectatic Osteosarcoma

A very aggressive and unusual type of osteosarcoma, the telangiectatic variant affects males twice as often as females and occurs predominantly during the second and third decades (182). This variant, also called hemorrhagic osteosarcoma by Campanacci (148), accounts for <5% of osteo-

FIG. 72. Telangiectatic osteosarcoma. (**A**) A purely destructive lesion is seen in the femoral diaphysis of this 17-year-old girl. Note the velvet type of periosteal reaction. The sclerotic changes usually seen in conventional osteosarcoma are absent, and there is no radiographic evidence of tumor bone. (**B**) Lateral radiograph of the proximal tibia in a 21-year-old man shows a lytic lesion with relatively narrow zone of transition and no visible periosteal reaction. (**C**) Coronal and (**D**) sagittal T1-weighted (SE, TR 400, TE 10) MR images show the tumor to be predominantly of intermediate signal intensity with central areas of high signal. No definite soft tissue mass is demonstrated. (*Figure continues on page 78.*)

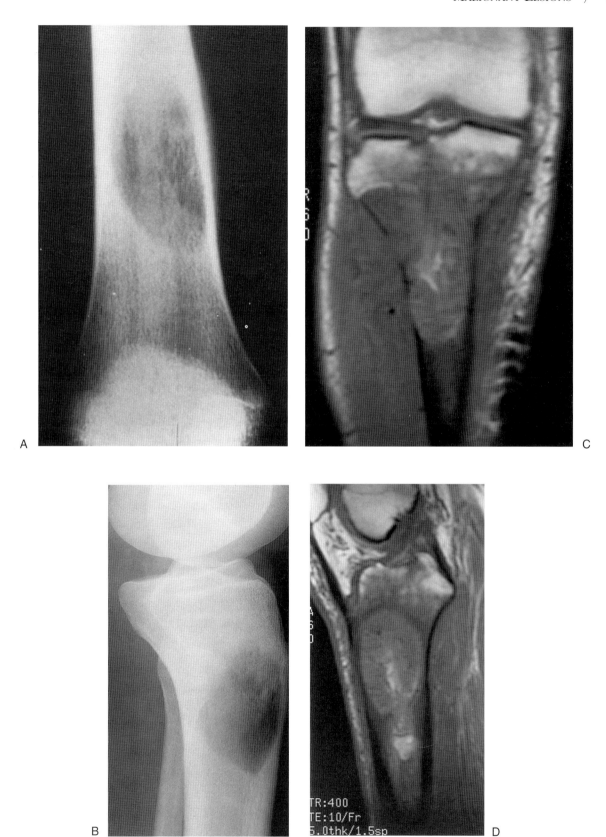

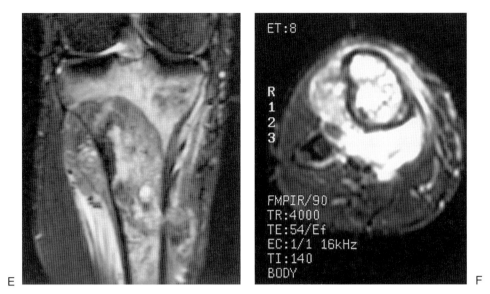

E   F

FIG. 72. *Continued.* (**E**) Coronal and (**F**) axial inversion recovery (FMPIR/90, TR 5000, TE 51 EF, TI 140) images show the extension of the tumor into the soft tissues and presence of peritumoral edema.

sarcomas (166,201). Most of these tumors arise in the femur or tibia (142). The tumor grossly resembles a bag of blood, characterized by blood-filled spaces, necrosis, and hemorrhage. These features account for its radiographic presentation as a purely lytic and destructive radiolucent lesion, almost devoid of sclerotic changes (Fig. 72A, B). A soft tissue mass may be present (Fig. 72E, F). An aggressive periosteal reaction (lamellar, sunburst, Codman triangle) is present in most patients, reflecting the malignant nature of this tumor (142) (Fig. 73). On radiography the lesion sometimes resembles an aneurysmal bone cyst. On MRI, it often exhibits areas of a high signal intensity on T1-weighted images, owing to the presence of methemoglobin (142) (see Fig. 72C, D). Fluid-fluid levels can occasionally be seen. These fluid-fluid levels indicate the presence of hemorrhage and are sometimes observed in other lesions that contain blood-filled cavities, such as aneurysmal bone cysts. Pathologic fracture is not uncommon in the case of large lesions (Fig. 74).

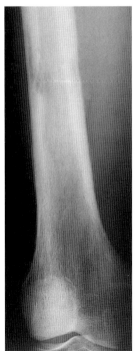
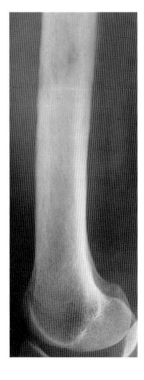

A,B

FIG. 73. Telangiectatic osteosarcoma. (**A**) Anteroposterior and (**B**) lateral radiographs show an ill-defined lesion that exhibits a permeative type of bone destruction in the middle portion of the right femur in a 41-year-old man. Note the velvet type of aggressive periosteal reaction.

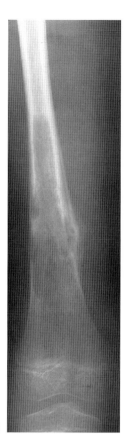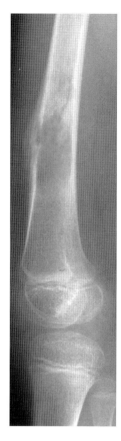

A,B

FIG. 74. Telangiectatic osteosarcoma. **A:** A predominantly lytic tumor associated with periosteal reaction is seen in the distal femoral diaphysis of this 6-year-old girl. **B:** On the lateral view, an oblique pathologic fracture is well demonstrated. (Courtesy of Dr. K. K. Unni, Rochester, Minnesota.)

Two histologic patterns may be observed. The tissue usually consists of blood-filled spaces divided by septa with few solid areas, a feature also shared by the major differential possibility, aneurysmal bone cyst (Fig. 75A, B, D). However, high-power microscopy of the cells lining the blood-filled spaces reveals significant pleomorphism, many mitotic figures, giant cells (benign and malignant), and focal osteoid production to a much greater extent than occurs in aneurysmal bone cysts (Fig. 75C). Some tumors exhibit only a minimal amount of osteoid production. However, according to Dahlin (7,154), if a tumor produces septa it should be classified as telangiectatic osteosarcoma, even in the absence of osteoid.

Giant Cell–Rich Osteosarcoma

This is a rare variant of osteosarcoma which appears as an undifferentiated sarcoma with an overabundance of osteoclasts (giant cells) and a paucity of tumor osteoid or tumor bone. It composes approximately 3% of all osteosarcomas and histologically is related to telangiectatic osteosarcoma and MFH-like osteosarcoma. Many of the classical radiologic features of osteosarcoma are absent, and differentiation from a benign lesion is sometimes difficult (140). In most cases the lytic lesion shows poorly defined borders. The typical location is the metaphysis or diaphysis of a long bone, usually the tibia or femur. A periosteal reaction is absent or scant, and a soft tissue mass is usually not present. The lesion has a striking histologic resemblance to giant cell tumor (Fig. 76). Tumor osteoid is usually scant and is therefore difficult to identify.

Low-Grade (Well-Differentiated) Central Osteosarcoma

This rare form of osteosarcoma, representing <2% of all osteosarcomas, usually affects patients older than those afflicted with conventional osteosarcoma (average age 28 years). Its sites of occurrence are similar, with a predilection for the femur and tibia (246). Unlike patients with conventional osteosarcoma, patients with this type of tumor often present with a long history of nonspecific aching, discomfort, or swelling over months or even years before the diagnosis is established. In many cases, the initial diagnosis on both a radiologic and a histologic basis is that of fibrous dysplasia. Although low-grade central osteosarcoma is occasionally indistinguishable on radiography from conventional osteosarcoma, more often the lesion appears benign, with a well-defined sclerotic rim (164). Expansion of the lesion is common, and the cortex is often thinned

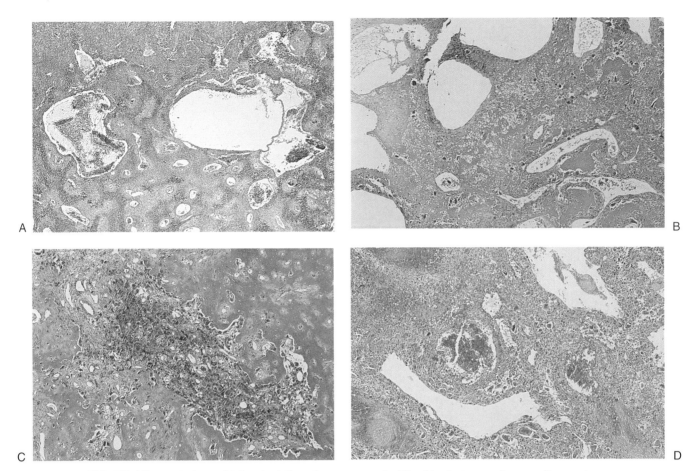

FIG. 75. Histopathology of telangiectatic osteosarcoma. **A:** Fibroblastic tumor stroma with scanty woven bone formation (red) and large, blood-filled capillary spaces (van Gieson, original magnification ×12). **B:** At higher magnification, a moderate amount of bone formation, characteristic of osteosarcoma, is clearly demonstrated. Large, blood-filled vascular spaces are typical of the telangiectatic variant (hematoxylin and eosin, original magnification ×25). **C:** Cellular areas of the tumor reveal bone formation by malignant cells (hematoxylin and eosin, original magnification ×25). **D:** In another section, there is almost complete lack of tumor bone formation, except for the areas in the upper left corner (van Gieson, original magnification ×25).

(Figs. 77 and 78). Periosteal reactions are rare, as is soft tissue extension of the tumor. This type of osteosarcoma is a slow-growing tumor and therefore has a better prognosis. Its radiographic presentation sometimes closely resembles that of fibrous dysplasia, giant cell tumor, desmoplastic fibroma, or even nonossifying fibroma (231).

The histologic diagnosis of low-grade osteosarcoma is extremely difficult. It may resemble fibrous dysplasia, desmoplastic fibroma, nonossifying fibroma, osteoblastoma, and chondromyoid fibroma (105), or nonspecific reactive lesions. Even the usual histology of low-grade parosteal osteosarcoma, with formation of mature-appearing bone trabeculae arranged in parallel arrays, has been reported (242). On microscopic examination, the tumor stroma consists of spindle cells arranged in interlacing bundles, which usually do not appear malignant (Fig. 79). The nuclei may exhibit some minimal atypia but the pleomorphism commonly observed in conventional osteosarcoma is absent. Mitotic fig-

ures are inconspicuous. Variable amounts of collagen and bone are produced, and the stromal cells may invade the marrow cavity and trabeculae of cancellous and cortical bone. The lesion may resemble desmoplastic fibroma at one end of the spectrum and fibrous dysplasia at the other, except that the bone spicules formed in this lesion are usually bulkier and lack the delicate, curvilinear shapes seen in fibrous dysplasia (189). Foci of atypical cartilage are only rarely observed. Giant cells may be present but are usually rare. As a consequence, a diagnosis is possible only with the aid of radiographic correlation.

Intracortical Osteosarcoma

This is one of the rarest forms of osteosarcoma. Only eight cases have thus far been reported (51,79,85,183,198,250), with an age range of 10 to 43 years (average 24 years) and a male predominance. The presenting symptom is pain, often

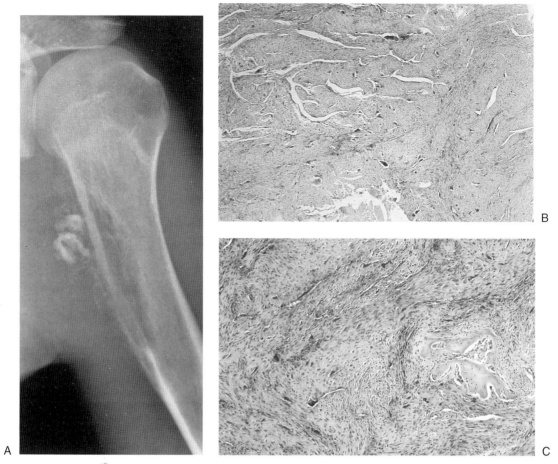

FIG. 76. Giant cell–rich osteosarcoma. **A:** An anteroposterior radiograph of the left proximal humerus shows a destructive lesion affecting the medullary portion of the bone, breaking through the medial cortex into the soft tissues. Bone formation is seen in the soft tissue mass. **B:** A low-power photomicrograph demonstrates fibrous tumor tissue of moderate cell density, containing numerous giant cells and branching vascular clefts (hematoxylin and eosin, original magnification ×12.5). **C:** At higher magnification bundles of spindle, clearly pleomorphous cells and giant cells, some of the tumor- and some of the osteoclast-type are seen. Tumor bone formation points to the diagnosis of osteosarcoma (hematoxylin and eosin, original magnification ×25).

associated with activity. In some patients, a history of previous trauma has been elicited. The tumor involves the cortex, without extension into the medullary portion of the bone or the soft tissues. The radiographic presentation is that of a radiolucent lesion with surrounding cortical sclerosis. The size of the lesion varies from 1.0 to 4.2 cm (51,194). In some instances the lesion mimics osteoid osteoma or intracortical osteoblastoma. Histologic studies show the tumor cells to be round or spindle-shaped, pleomorphic, with vesicular nuclei containing prominent nucleoli. Mitotic figures may be present. The bony matrix produced by malignant cells assumes a lace-like pattern with tumor osteoid.

Gnathic Osteosarcoma

Osteosarcoma arising in the maxilla or mandible is unlike osteosarcoma arising elsewhere in the skeleton because it occurs in older patients (fourth to sixth decades, with a mean age of 35 years) (195). It is usually a well-differentiated tumor with a low mitotic rate, possessing a predominantly cartilaginous component in a high percentage of cases (Fig. 80), and with less malignant potential and a better prognosis than for other forms of osteosarcoma (174).

Multicentric (Multifocal) Osteosarcoma

This very rare type of osteosarcoma (1.5% of all osteosarcomas), in which lesions develop simultaneously in multiple bones, is recognized at present as having two variants: synchronous and metachronous (168). A slight male predominance exists among patients of 18 years and younger, and a much greater (3:1) male predominance in patients of 19 years and older. The most commonly encountered sites in decreasing order of frequency are the distal end of the femur, proximal end of the tibia, proximal end of the femur, pelvis, and the proximal end of the humerus (153,180)

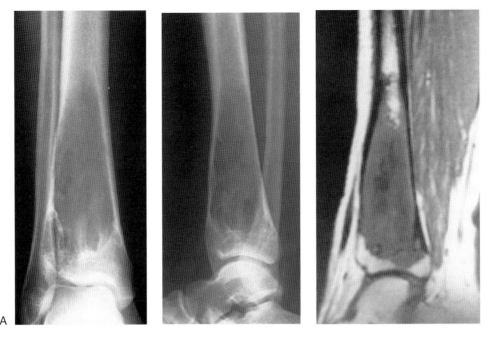

A   B, C

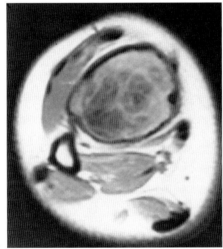

D

FIG. 77. Low-grade central osteosarcoma. (A) Anteroposterior and (B) lateral radiographs of the distal leg in an 18-year-old woman were originally interpreted as showing fibrous dysplasia of the distal tibia. Note a benign-appearing radiolucent lesion exhibiting a geographic type of bone destruction with a narrow zone of transition and no evidence of periosteal reaction. (C) Sagittal and (D) axial T1-weighted (SE, TR 600, TE 20) MRI demonstrates intermediate to low signal intensity of the lesion and lack of a soft tissue mass. (Courtesy of Dr. K. K. Unni, Rochester, Minnesota.)

(Figs. 81 and 82). Whether this type of osteosarcoma is truly a separate entity or whether it actually represents multiple bone metastases from a primary conventional osteosarcoma remains controversial (180). Because bone is a well-recognized site of metastasis for primary osteosarcoma, the possibility that a patient with multifocal involvement has a primary osteosarcoma with bone metastases should always be considered. When multiple bones are affected in the absence of pulmonary involvement, however, this situation probably indicates the independent development of multiple primary bone osteosarcomas. Amstutz (135) categorized multifocal osteosarcomas into three clinical patterns: type I are synchronous lesions occurring in younger patients; type II are low-grade synchronous lesions limited to the axial skeleton in adults; and type III are cases of metachronous lesions. Some of the patients in this group were believed to develop metastatic lesions from a solitary primary osteosarcoma.

Juxtacortical Osteosarcomas

The term juxtacortical is a general designation for a group of osteosarcomas that arise on the surface of a bone (187,196) (Fig. 83). In general, these lesions are much rarer and present a decade later than their intraosseous counterparts (234). The great majority of juxtacortical osteosarcomas are low-grade tumors (218), although there are moderately and highly malignant variants (179,185,247). Low-grade juxtacortical osteosarcoma is usually termed parosteal osteosarcoma. The lesion arises on the outside surface of the bone, virtually never provoking a periosteal reaction (212,239, 242). Histologically, the proliferating portion

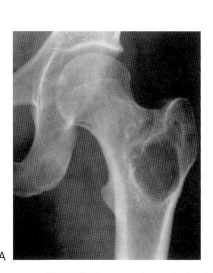
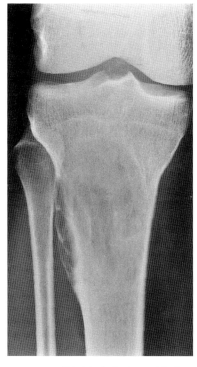
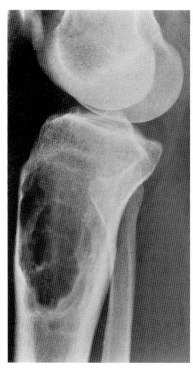

A

B, C

FIG. 78. Low-grade central osteosarcoma. (**A**) A lytic lesion with the geographic type of bone destruction and a narrow zone of sclerosis in the intertrochanteric region of the right femur has a benign appearance. (**B**) Anteroposterior and (**C**) lateral radiographs of another patient show a radiolucent lesion in the proximal tibial diaphysis, slightly expanding the lateral cortex.

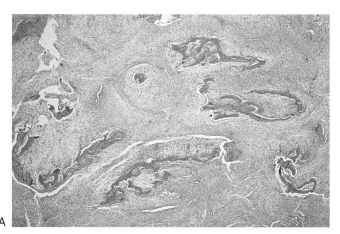

A

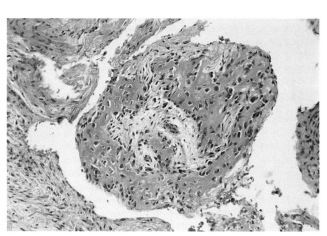

B

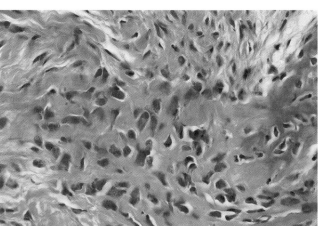

C

FIG. 79. Histopathology of a low-grade central osteosarcoma. **A:** The cellular stroma of medium density contains irregularly formed woven bone trabeculae, resembling fibrous dysplasia (hematoxylin and eosin, original magnification ×12). **B:** At higher magnification, benign-appearing spindle-cell tumor tissue is seen with formation of primitive woven bone pseudotrabeculae containing roundish osteocytes (*center*). Also present are large vascular spaces (hematoxylin and eosin, original magnification ×25). **C:** At high magnification, the malignant nature of the tumor is better appreciated. Densely packed, irregularly arranged osteoblastic cells with hyperchromatic nuclei are present in close approximation to the tumor bone revealing the malignant character of the tumor (hematoxylin and eosin, original magnification ×100).

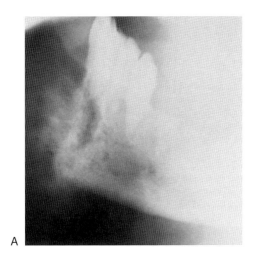

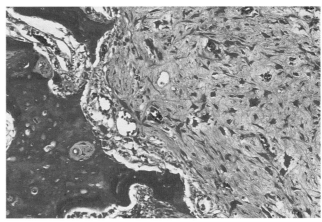

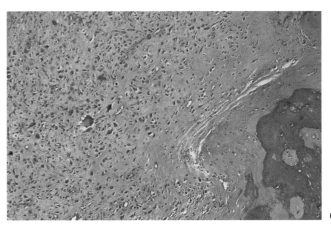

FIG. 80. Gnathic osteosarcoma. **A:** A radiograph of the mandible shows mixed sclerotic and lytic lesion destroying the cortex associated with a spiculated sunburst type of periosteal reaction. **B:** The tumor is composed of chondroblastic tissue growing into marrow spaces of tumor bone trabeculae (*left*) (hematoxylin and eosin, original magnification ×50). **C:** In other areas, purely cellular tissue with a moderate degree of pleomorphism of the cells and nuclei is present. Plate-like bone formation (*lower right*) confirms the diagnosis of osteosarcoma (hematoxylin and eosin, original magnification ×50). (Reprinted with permission from Prein J, Remagen W, Spiessl B, Uehlinger E. *Atlas of tumors of the facial skeleton.* Berlin: Springer-Verlag, 1986.)

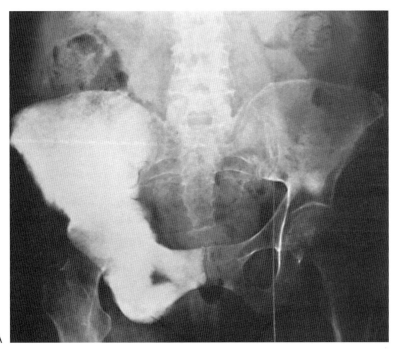

FIG. 81. Synchronous multicentric osteosarcoma involving right hemipelvis (**A**), proximal tibia

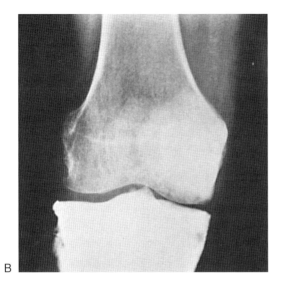

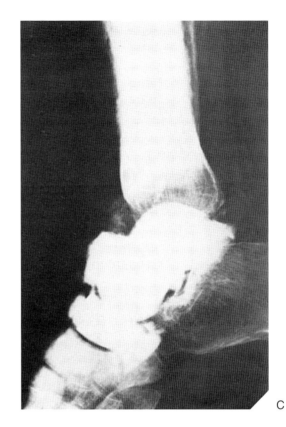

FIG. 81. (*Continued.*) (**B**), distal tibia and several bones of the right foot (**C**).

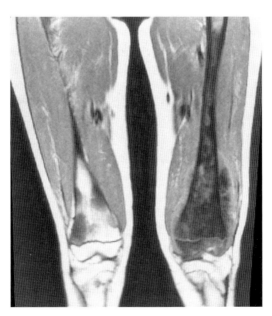

FIG. 82. Synchronous multicentric osteosarcoma: magnetic resonance imaging. In another patient, MRI shows involvement of the left femur and distal right femur.

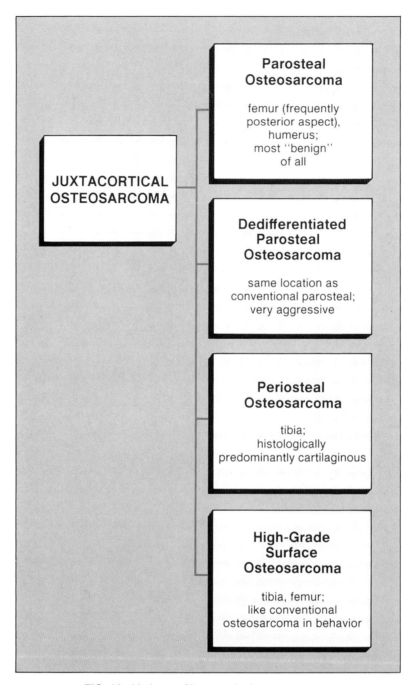

FIG. 83. Variants of juxtacortical osteosarcoma.

of the neoplasm consists of a fibrous stroma, considered to be derived from the outer fibrous periosteal layer. Dedifferentiated parosteal osteosarcoma is a high-grade variant of the former tumor (225,253). Periosteal osteosarcoma belongs to an intermediate grade of surface lesions (245). This lesion may cause periosteal response and usually consists mostly of cartilage (219). The lesion is believed to be derived from the inner, or cambium, layer of the periosteum. High-grade surface osteosarcoma is a lesion located on the periphery of a bone. It has a histology identical to that of conventional

medullary osteosarcoma and a similar metastatic potential (213,254,257).

Parosteal Osteosarcoma

This type of surface osteosarcoma, which accounts for about 5% of all osteosarcomas, is seen in patients in their third and fourth decades, and characteristically affects the posterior aspect of the distal femur (Fig. 84) (237). Other lo-

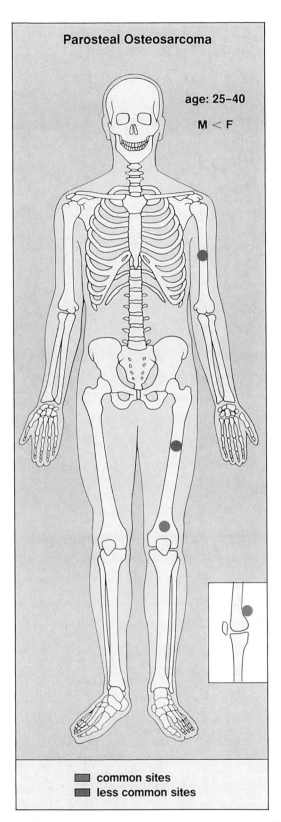

FIG. 84. Parosteal osteosarcoma: skeletal sites of predilection, peak age range, and male-to-female ratio.

cations include the tibia, the fibula, and the proximal portions of the femur and humerus (197). Rarely are other bones affected (188). Because the tumor is slow growing and usually involves only the surface of the bone, the prognosis is much better than for the other types of osteosarcoma.

On radiologic studies, the neoplasm presents as a dense oval or spherical mass attached to the surface of the cortical bone (Fig. 85). The surface is lobulated and may be less dense than the base of the tumor (Fig. 86). The mass appears sharply delineated from the peripheral soft tissues. The medullary cavity is usually spared unless the lesion is of long duration. A linear, translucent cleft usually forms an incomplete separation of the bulk of the tumor from the underlying cortex (Fig. 87). Larger lesions, however, tend to encircle the host bone (212). Although these features can be adequately demonstrated by conventional radiography, CT (Fig. 88) or MRI (Fig. 89) is often necessary to determine the extent of cortical penetration and intramedullary invasion by tumor (181).

The histology of this tumor is characterized by a high degree of structural differentiation and consists of immature (woven) bone in different stages of maturation to lamellar bone (226). The lamellar trabeculae, which predominate in most areas, are separated by a bland, well-differentiated fibrous stroma composed of spindle cells. The latter show minimal cytologic atypia, are minimally pleomorphic, and rarely exhibit mitotic activity (Fig. 90). Determining malignancy may present some difficulty, as the indolent nature of this tumor is also evidenced by lack of significant tumor hemorrhage or necrosis. Multiple sections are usually required to reveal regions of prominent osteoblastic activity around bony trabeculae (243).

Periosteal Osteosarcoma

This very rare type of osteosarcoma (accounting for 1% to 2% of all osteosarcomas) grows on the surface of a bone and is usually located in the midshaft of a long bone; it is most common in adolescence (176). Although the age range varies, most lesions occur during the second decade of life. There is a slight female preponderance, and the majority of lesions affect the tibia and femur.

The radiologic characteristics were defined by deSantos et al. (159). These include an inhomogeneous tumor matrix with calcified spiculations interspersed with areas of radiolucency representing uncalcified matrix; occasional periosteal reaction in the form of a Codman triangle (Fig. 91); thickening of the periosteal surface of the cortex at the base of the lesion, with sparing of the endosteal surface; extension of the tumor into the soft tissues; and sparing of the medullary cavity (Figs. 92 and 93).

By microscopy, these tumors are of low- or medium-grade malignancy and are composed mainly of lobulated chondroid tissue with moderate cellularity (Fig. 94). They

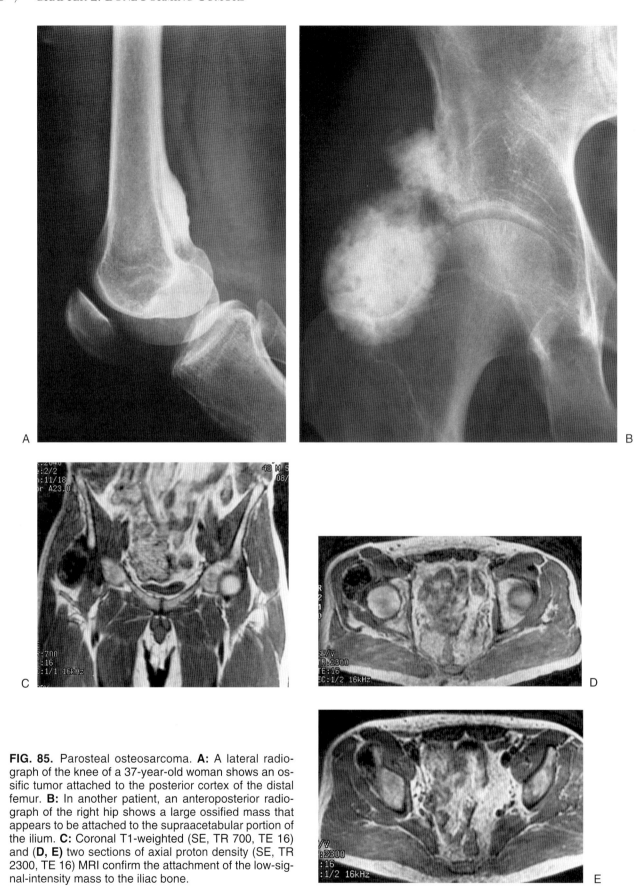

FIG. 85. Parosteal osteosarcoma. **A:** A lateral radiograph of the knee of a 37-year-old woman shows an ossific tumor attached to the posterior cortex of the distal femur. **B:** In another patient, an anteroposterior radiograph of the right hip shows a large ossified mass that appears to be attached to the supraacetabular portion of the ilium. **C:** Coronal T1-weighted (SE, TR 700, TE 16) and **(D, E)** two sections of axial proton density (SE, TR 2300, TE 16) MRI confirm the attachment of the low-signal-intensity mass to the iliac bone.

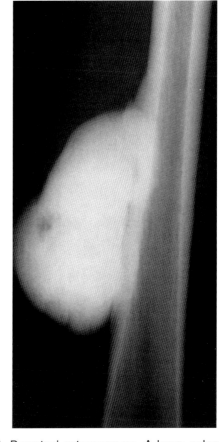

FIG. 86. Parosteal osteosarcoma. A sclerotic, lobulated mass is attached to the posterior cortex of distal femur. The periphery of the tumor is slightly less dense than the base.

FIG. 87. Parosteal osteosarcoma. A large, sclerotic tumor partially attached to the medial cortex of left femur displays inferiorly a radiolucent cleft.

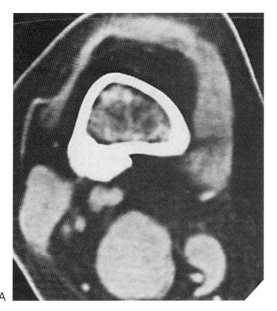

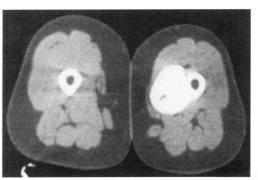

A

B

FIG. 88. Parosteal osteosarcoma: computed tomography. **A:** A contrast-enhanced CT section demonstrates that the medullary portion of the bone has not been invaded (same patient as in **Fig. 85A**). **B:** A CT section through the attached portion of the tumor (same patient as in **Fig. 86**) shows lack of invasion of the medullary cavity.

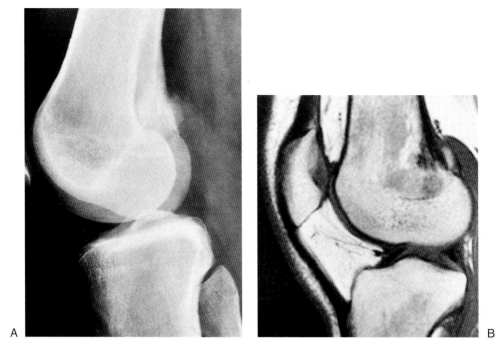

A   B

FIG. 89. Parosteal osteosarcoma: magnetic resonance imaging. **A:** A plain lateral radiograph shows a tumor involving the posterior aspect of the medial femoral condyle in this 22-year-old woman. It is not possible to determine whether the cortex has been violated. **B:** A sagittal MRI (SE;TR 517, TE 20) demonstrates invasion of the medullary cavity by that displays low signal intensity. (Reprinted with permission from Greenspan A. Osteosarcoma. *Contemp Diagn Radiol* 1993;16:1–6.)

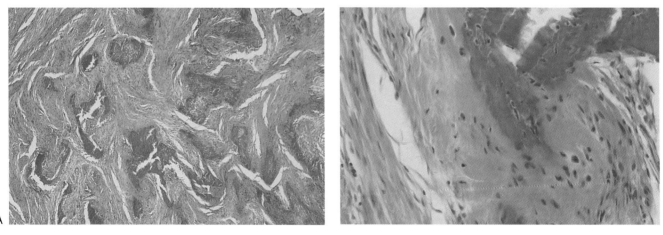

A   B

FIG. 90. Histopathology of parosteal osteosarcoma. **A:** A low-cellular, fibrous stroma of moderate density is arranged in bundles and contains bizarre-shaped trabeculae of woven bone, resembling fibrous dysplasia. The shape and arrangement of the trabeculae, however, are more irregular than in the latter condition (hematoxylin and eosin, original magnification ×12). **B:** At higher magnification, the irregular distribution of the cells, together with slight pleomorphism of their nuclei and indistinct merging of the bone with the connective tissue (*center*), points to the diagnosis of sarcoma rather than fibrous dysplasia (hematoxylin and eosin, original magnification ×100).

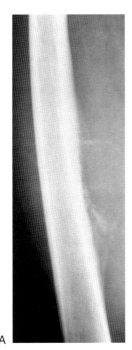

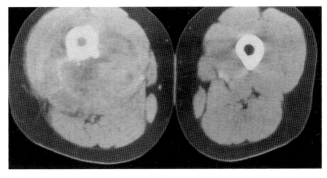

B

FIG. 91. Periosteal osteosarcoma. **A:** An anteroposterior radiograph of the right femur shows a surface lesion affecting the medial cortex, associated with a Codman triangle of periosteal reaction and a large soft tissue mass. **B:** CT shows the soft tissue component to better advantage. The medullary cavity was not involved by the tumor. However, an increase in attenuation value, as compared to the contralateral marrow cavity, indicates bone marrow edema.

A

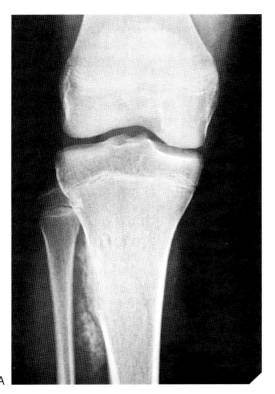

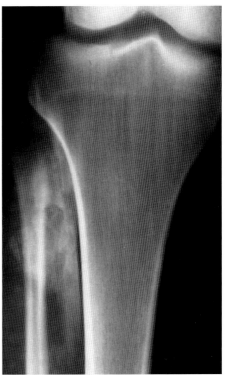

A

B

FIG. 92. Periosteal osteosarcoma. **A:** A frontal radiograph of the right knee of a 12-year-old girl with discomfort in the upper leg for 2 months shows poorly defined calcifications and ossifications in a mass attached to the surface of the lateral tibial cortex. **B:** An anteroposterior tomography shows the ossified mass partially separated from the lateral cortex of the tibia by a narrow radiolucent cleft, very similar to that seen in the juxtacortical myositis ossificans.

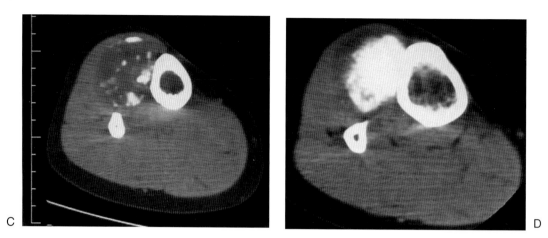

C

D

FIG. 92. (*Continued.*) **C:** A CT section obtained through the distal part of the lesion shows the extent of the soft tissue mass. Note low attenuation of the tumor with scattered high-attenuation ossifications. **D:** A CT section obtained through the proximal part of the lesion clearly demonstrates its attachment to the tibial cortex. The medullary cavity is not affected.

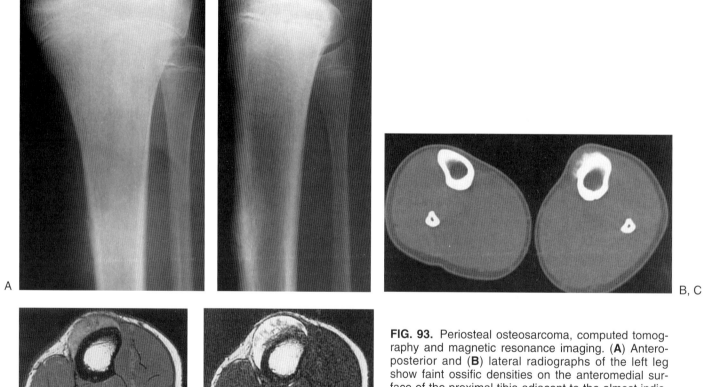

A

B, C

D, E

FIG. 93. Periosteal osteosarcoma, computed tomography and magnetic resonance imaging. (**A**) Anteroposterior and (**B**) lateral radiographs of the left leg show faint ossific densities on the anteromedial surface of the proximal tibia adjacent to the almost indistinct cortical destruction. An aggressive velvet type of periosteal reaction is evident. (**C**) A CT section through the tumor shows bone formation on the surface of the tibia and lack of invasion of the medullary cavity. (**D**) Axial SE T1-weighted MRI shows that tumor displays slightly higher signal than the muscles. (**E**) On axial T2-weighted image (TR 2000, TE 80) the mass becomes bright, except for the central areas at which bone formation displays low signal intensity.

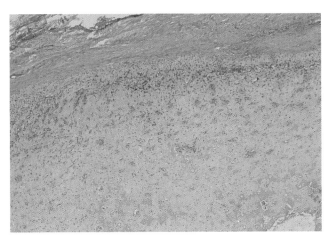

FIG. 94. Histopathology of periosteal osteosarcoma. The superficial part of the tumor consists of cellular cartilage with increasing cell density at the proliferation interface with covering fibrous tissue, indicating its malignant character (hematoxylin and eosin, original magnification ×25).

characteristically exhibit large amounts of cartilage matrix undergoing calcification or endochondral ossification, as well as small amounts of fine lace-like osteoid surrounding malignant cells (Fig. 95). The ultrastructural features consist of round or polyhedral chondroblast-like cells. The nuclei are rounded and have prominent nucleoli, and the nuclear envelope shows discrete indentations. The cytoplasm contains conspicuous rough endoplasmic reticulum, lakes of glycogen, and lipid vacuoles. The cytoplasmic membrane displays scanty, thin projections. The cells are surrounded by an abundant intercellular matrix of low electron density, with thin fibrils and granules (200). The prognosis for periosteal osteosarcoma is somewhat better than for conventional osteosarcoma but worse than for parosteal osteosarcoma (226).

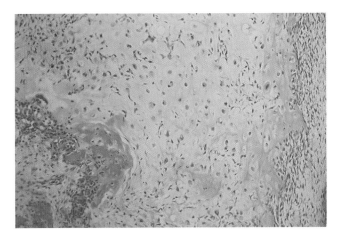

FIG. 95. Histopathology of periosteal osteosarcoma. A low-power photomicrograph shows predominantly cartilaginous matrix, which is a major component of the tumor. Areas of osteoid formation (*lower left corner*) confirm the diagnosis (hematoxylin and eosin, original magnification ×40).

High-Grade Surface Osteosarcoma and Dedifferentiated Parosteal Osteosarcoma

A small percentage of juxtacortical osteosarcomas are high-grade tumors and they carry the same prognosis as conventional osteosarcoma. The less common of these lesions, high-grade surface osteosarcoma, accounting for <1% of all osteosarcomas in a Mayo Clinic study (253), exhibits radiologic features similar to those of parosteal or periosteal osteosarcoma (Fig. 96) (178). Men are affected more frequently than women (M/F = 1.6:1). The most frequent site for this tumor is the femur (46%), followed by the humerus (16%) (213). It is histologically indistinct from conventional osteosarcoma (Fig. 97) and, like the latter, it has a high potential for distant metastases (254). Although intramedullary extension of the tumor is uncommon, the cortex may be involved and pathologic fractures may occur. Dedifferentiated parosteal osteosarcoma, the more common variant of the high-grade malignant surface osteosarcomas, usually arises as a conventional low-grade parosteal osteosarcoma (253). Then, either spontaneously (in which case both low- and high-grade components can be identified histologically) or secondarily (in recurrences of inadequately resected low-grade parosteal tumors), the lesion undergoes transformation to a high-grade malignancy (215). The latter situation is more common. Unni (242) cites a dedifferentiation rate of 20% in such recurrences. In radiographic and histologic studies, dedifferentiated parosteal osteosarcoma mimics the features of conventional parosteal osteosarcoma. There are, however, some characteristics of a high-grade sarcoma, such as radiographically identifiable cortical destruction and histologically identifiable pleomorphic tumor cells with hyperchromatic nuclei and a high mitotic rate. Cross-sectional imaging reveals medullary involvement in 22% of patients and adjacent soft tissue invasion in 46% (212) (Fig. 98). Hence, the prognosis is much worse than for parosteal osteosarcoma.

Secondary Osteosarcomas

The term "secondary" applied to osteosarcoma refers to a tumor that arises in association with a preexisting lesion of the bone, which may or may not be neoplastic. In contrast to primary osteosarcomas, secondary lesions predominantly affect an older population.

Paget Sarcoma

A large proportion of secondary sarcomas arise as a complication of Paget disease and characteristically develop in Pagetic bone (202, 206). Most cases of transformation to osteosarcoma occur in polyostotic Paget disease (227). Osteosarcoma can develop in any part of any bone affected by Paget disease (233), although the pelvic bones and femur are the preferential sites for this complication (202). The other

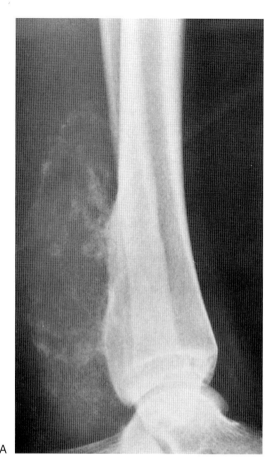

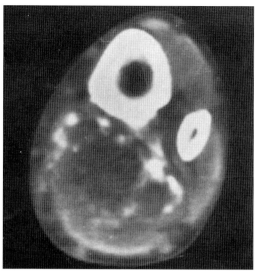

FIG. 96. High-grade surface osteosarcoma. **A:** A lateral radiograph of the distal leg shows a tumor arising from the surface of the posterior tibial cortex in a 24-year-old man. Poorly defined ossific foci are seen within a large soft tissue mass. Note the similarity of this tumor to periosteal osteosarcoma (compare with **Figs. 91A** and **92A**). **B:** A CT section demonstrates the extent of the lesion. Characteristically, the marrow cavity is not affected.

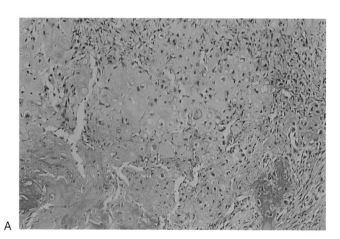

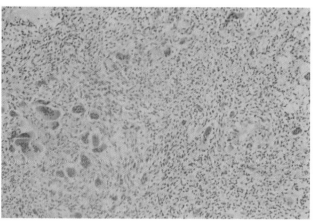

FIG. 97. Histopathology of high-grade surface osteosarcoma. **A:** High cellularity and marked pleomorphism of the stromal cells, together with foci of tumor osteoid formation, are characteristic of this tumor. The histologic appearance is indistinguishable from that of high-grade central osteosarcoma (hematoxylin and eosin, original magnification ×70). **B:** High cellularity of the tumor and areas containing several giant cells can be observed (hematoxylin and eosin, original magnification ×70). (Courtesy of Dr. G. Steiner, New York, NY.)

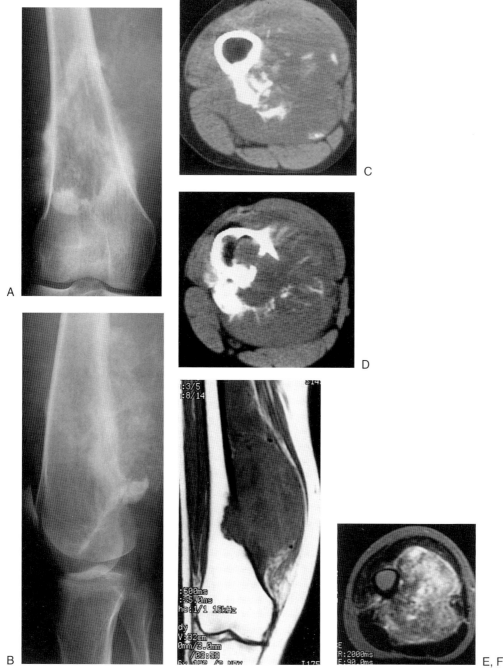

FIG. 98. Dedifferentiated parosteal osteosarcoma. A 24-year-old woman presented with pain and palpable mass above the popliteal fossa of 2 months duration. Three years prior to the current complaints a parosteal osteosarcoma had been resected from her distal femur. **A:** An anteroposterior radiograph of the distal femur shows an aggressive type of periosteal reaction and a large soft tissue mass with foci of bone formation. **B:** A lateral radiograph shows in addition the remnants of the previously resected parosteal osteosarcoma. **C:** The proximal CT section shows a surface tumor exhibiting bone formation and a large soft tissue mass with foci of tumor bone. At this level the bone marrow is not invaded. **D:** The more distal section reveals in addition the invasion of the medullary cavity, a feature not consistent with a conventional parosteal osteosarcoma. **E:** Coronal T1-weighted (SE, TR 600, TE 25) MRI demonstrates the extent of both intramedullary invasion and a soft tissue mass. **F:** Axial T2-weighted (SE, TR 2000, TE 90) MRI shows inhomogeneous signal of a large soft tissue mass. At the level of this section the bone marrow is not involved by a tumor.

sites commonly affected are the humerus and the tibia (216). Patients with advanced disease are at greater risk (206,227). The radiographic changes typically observed in malignant transformation of Paget disease include a destructive lesion in the affected bone, the presence of tumor bone in the lesion, pathologic fracture, and an associated soft tissue mass (235) (Figs. 99, 100, and 101). Periosteal reaction is only rarely encountered.

On microscopy, most Paget sarcomas are histologically conventional, high-grade osteoblastic intramedullary osteosarcomas (11) (Fig. 102). Other types of osteosarcoma, such as fibrohistiocytic, chondroblastic, and fibroblastic, are

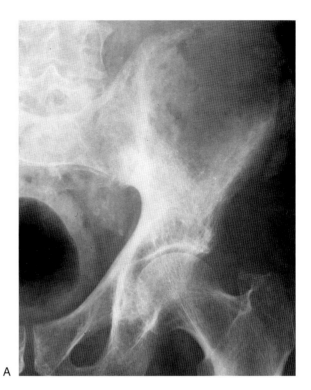

A

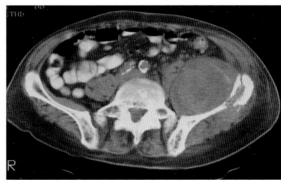

B

FIG. 100. Osteosarcoma complicating Paget disease. **A:** An anteroposterior radiograph of the left hip in a 73-year-old man with polyostotic Paget disease shows destructive lesion of the ilium associated with a pathologic fracture. A soft tissue mass containing tumor bone is seen inferiorly to the sacro-iliac joint. **B:** A CT section demonstrates to the better advantage the pathologic fracture and a large soft tissue mass with central necrosis, imaged as lower attenuation areas.

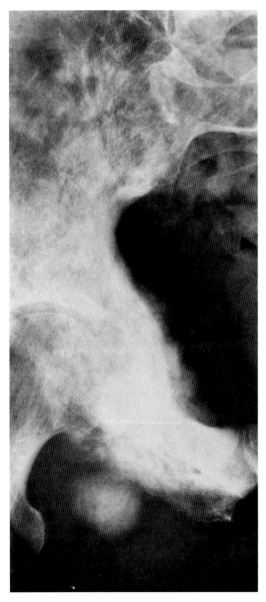

FIG. 99. Osteosarcoma complicating Paget disease. An anteroposterior radiograph of the right hip in a 66-year-old man who had extensive skeletal involvement by Paget disease shows destruction of the cortex of the ischial bone, associated with a soft tissue mass containing tumor bone.

also commonly observed. Osteosarcoma in these patients must be differentiated from metastases to Pagetic bone from primary carcinoma elsewhere in the body, most commonly the prostate, breast, or kidney (see below). Nevertheless, metastases are a most uncommon event in Paget disease, despite the increased vascularity of Pagetic bone (146).

Postirradiation Osteosarcoma

Radiation therapy for an unrelated previous condition also may give rise to secondary osteosarcoma (133). The thresh-

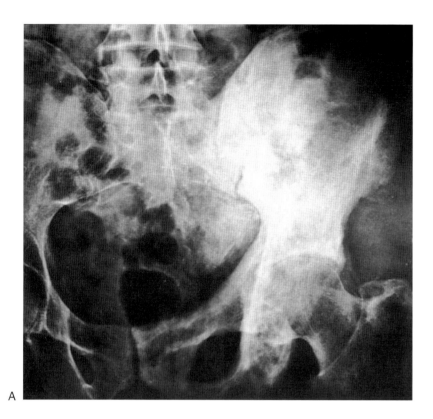

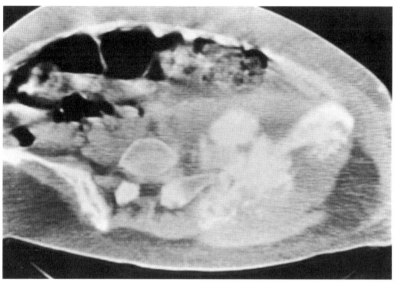

FIG. 101. Paget sarcoma. **A:** An anteroposterior radiograph of the pelvis of a 70-year-old woman shows extensive involvement of the left ilium, pubis, and ischium by Paget disease. There is also destruction of the cortex and a large soft tissue mass accompanied by bone formation, typical findings for osteosarcoma. **B:** A CT scan demonstrates the bone formation in the soft tissue mass more clearly.

old is approximately 800 to 1000 cGy, but usually a dose of at least 3000 cGy administered within 3 weeks is required (169). The latent period is between 4 and 42 years, with an average of 11 years (204). The criteria for diagnosis of post-irradiation sarcoma include the following (41): (a) the initial disease and the postirradiation sarcoma must not be of the same histologic type; (b) the site of the new tumor must be within the field of irradiation; and (c) at least 3 years must have elapsed since the previous radiation therapy (133,204).

Postirradiation osteosarcomas may develop either after radiation therapy for benign bone lesions, such as fibrous dysplasia (Fig. 103) and giant cell tumor, or after irradiation of malignant processes in the soft tissues, such as breast carcinoma and lymphoma. These tumors may also develop as a result of ingestion and intraosseous accumulation of radioisotopes, as has been described in painters of radium watch dials. Differentiation of radiation-induced sarcoma from osteonecrosis secondary to irradiation may be difficult. Progression and pain militate in favor of sarcoma. The double-line sign (parallel low- and high-signal-intensity lines)

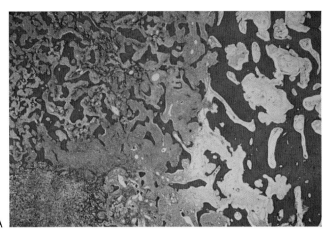

A

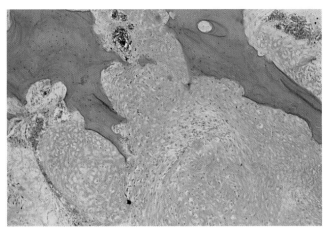

B

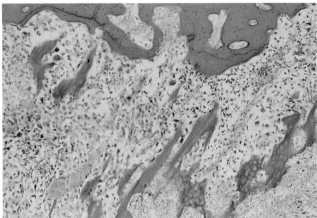

C

FIG. 102. Histopathology of Paget sarcoma. **A:** There is clear separation between deformed trabeculae pathognomonic for Paget disease (*right*) and osteosarcoma (*left*) (hematoxylin and eosin, original magnification ×15). **B:** Marrow spaces between the abnormal trabeculae typical of Paget disease are infiltrated by markedly pleomorphic tumor cells that form tumor osteoid (*lower left*) (van Gieson, original magnification ×25). **C:** Typical Pagetic bone exhibiting prominent cement lines (red, *upper half*) is surrounded by tumor osteoid (rose, *lower half*). Some dilated vessels (upper left) are also present (van Gieson, original magnification ×25).

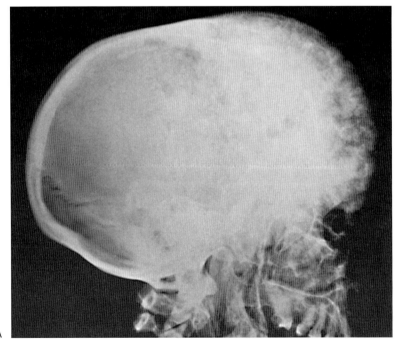

A

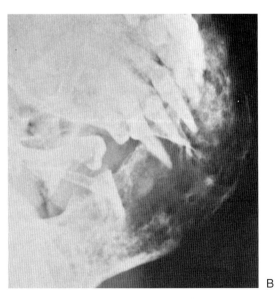

B

FIG. 103. Postirradiation osteosarcoma. **A:** Lateral radiograph of the skull of a 35-year-old woman with polyostotic fibrous dysplasia, who 11 years before this examination underwent radiation treatment of the mandible, shows predominant involvement of the frontal bones and the base of the skull. **B:** An oblique radiograph of the mandible shows an expansive lytic lesion in the body of the left mandible, with partial destruction of the cortex. Biopsy confirmed an osteosarcoma.

revealed with MRI indicates osteonecrosis. The presence of a soft tissue mass on MRI indicates the development of an osteosarcoma. The viability of the lesion can be confirmed with gadolinium-enhanced MRI (143).

The least commonly encountered instance in which a secondary osteosarcoma has been known to develop involves completely benign bone lesions, such as a medullary bone infarct (240) or fibrous dysplasia, without prior irradiation (244). Whatever its etiology, the histopathology of secondary osteosarcomas is identical to that of primary osteosarcomas, and the prognosis for these tumors is equally ominous.

Soft Tissue (Extraskeletal) Osteosarcoma

Osteosarcoma of the soft tissues (extraskeletal, extraosseous) is an uncommon malignant tumor of mesenchymal origin, with the capacity to form neoplastic osteoid, bone, and cartilage (139). Middle-aged and elderly individuals are most often affected, with a mean age at presentation of 54 years (149,236). This lesion is considerably less common than osteosarcoma of bone, accounting for only 4% of all osteosarcomas (132). The preferential sites for this neoplasm are in the lower extremities and buttocks (167,175, 191,220,256). The lesion may also develop in a variety of soft tissues such as breast, lung, thyroid, renal capsule, urinary bladder, and prostate, and even within the pelvic retroperitoneum. Occasionally, a soft tissue osteosarcoma arises after radiation therapy.

The most common clinical presentation is that of a slowly enlarging mass, with or without pain. The radiographic hallmarks include a soft tissue mass with scattered, amorphous calcifications and ossifications. The mass exhibits a disorganized arrangement of osteogenic elements in the center of the tumor (Figs. 104 and 105A). If the mass develops in close proximity to bone, it may invade the cortex.

CT usually reveals a heavily mineralized soft tissue mass, occasionally with areas of necrosis (162). This modality may demonstrate better than plain film radiography the pattern of central ossification or the reverse zoning phenomenon (217) (Fig. 105B, C). It also demonstrates a lack of attachment of the mass onto the bone. MRI usually reveals a mass with mixed low signal intensity on T1-weighted images (Fig. 105D) and mixed but predominantly high signal intensity on T2-weighted and inversion recovery sequences (Fig. 105 E–G) (248). MRI may also show a pseudocapsule of tumor (162).

The histopathology of soft tissue osteosarcoma is indistinguishable from that of a conventional osteosarcoma (Fig. 105H–J) (251).

Differential Diagnosis

Radiology

On the basis of the subtype of osteosarcoma and the radiographic appearance of different variants, several lesions should be considered in the differential diagnosis. As mentioned above, the radiologic differential possibilities do not always correspond to the histologic differential diagnosis,

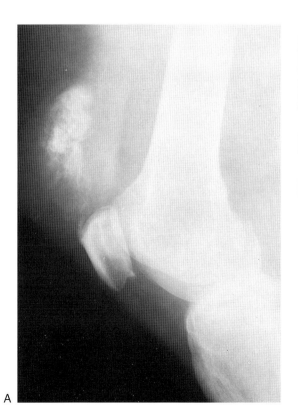
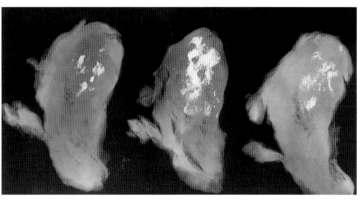

FIG. 104. Soft tissue osteosarcoma. **A:** A lateral radiograph of the right knee of a 51-year-old woman shows a poorly defined soft tissue mass situated above the patella merging with the quadriceps muscle. Approximately in the center of the lesion amorphous calcifications and ossifications are noted. The suprapatellar bursa appears unaffected. **B:** A radiograph of the specimen of the tumor depicted in A demonstrates foci of ossification in the center of the tumor, surrounded by the radiolucent zone at the periphery ("reverse zoning"). (Reprinted with permission from Greenspan A, et al. Skeletal Radiol 1987;16: 489–492.)

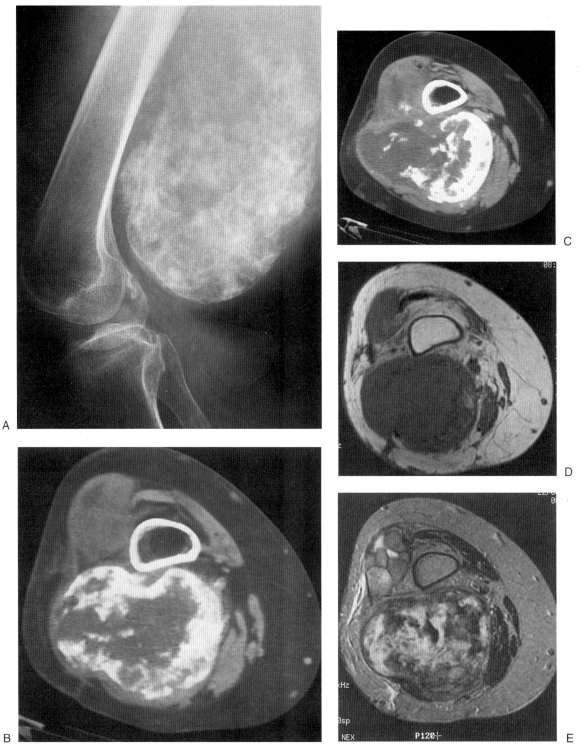

FIG.105. Soft tissue osteosarcoma. A 68-year-old woman presented with a progressively enlarging soft tissue mass in the popliteal region of the right knee. (**A**) A lateral radiograph shows a large soft tissue mass, sharply outlined in its distal extent, but poorly delineated at the proximal end. Calcifications and ossifications are present throughout the tumor. (**B**) One of the CT sections through the distal portion of the tumor shows predominantly peripheral mineralization of the mass, very similar to that of myositis ossificans. (**C**) The more proximal CT section clearly demonstrates reverse zoning, typical for soft tissue osteosarcoma. (**D**) Axial T1-weighted (SE, TR 700, TE 19) MRI shows the mass being of slightly inhomogeneous low-intensity signal. A smaller extension of the tumor is seen anterolaterally. (**E**) Axial fast spin-echo (FSE, TR 5200, TE 102 Ef) MRI reveals inhomogeneity of the tumor, displaying variation of signals, from high to intermediate intensity. *Continued.*

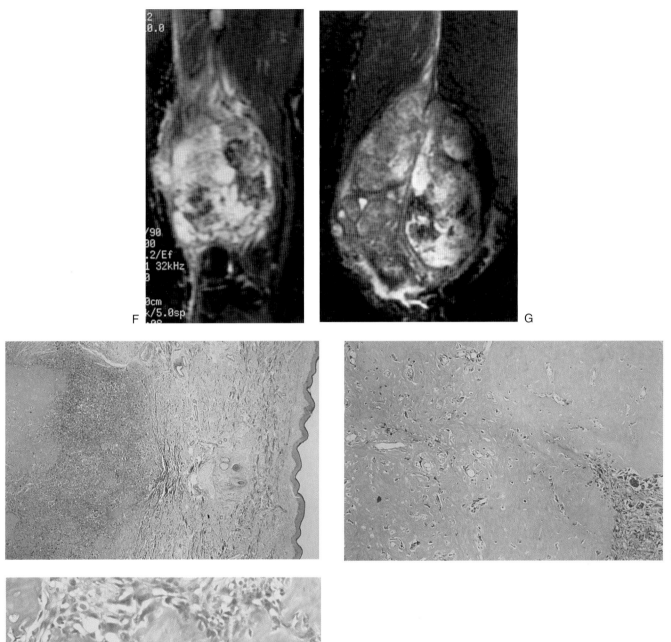

FIG. 105. *Continued.* (**F**) Coronal and (**G**) sagittal inversion recovery images further reveal the internal septa and inhomogeneous character of the tumor. (**H**) Histologic section shows cellular tumor tissue containing tumor bone beneath the skin (*right*) (Giemsa, original magnification ×6). (**I**) At higher magnification plates of tumor bone are surrounded by cellular areas containing numerous giant cells (Giemsa, original magnification ×25). (**J**) High-power magnification reveals osteoblastic differentiation of the tumor (hematoxylin and eosin, original magnification ×400).

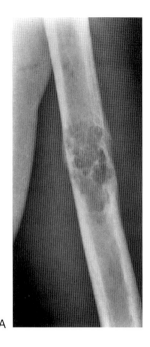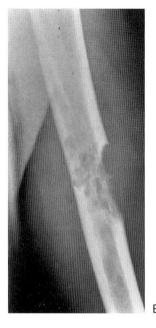

A
B

FIG. 106. Osteosarcoma resembling Ewing sarcoma. **(A)** An anteroposterior and **(B)** lateral radiographs of the midshaft of the left humerus in this 17-year-old boy show a lesion that exhibits moth-eaten pattern of bone destruction associated with Codman triangle of periosteal reaction and an adjacent soft tissue mass, similar to that of Ewing sarcoma. Histopathologic examination was consistent with grade 2 fibroblastic osteosarcoma.

and they may vary according to the subtype of osteosarcoma. In radiographic studies, the conventional medullary osteosarcoma should be differentiated mainly from *Ewing sarcoma* (Figs. 106 and 107). Ewing sarcoma usually affects the diaphysis of a long bone or the flat bones, such as the innominate bone and the scapula. The lesion is poorly defined and is characterized by a permeative or moth-eaten type of bone destruction (**see Fig. 5-14A and 5-16**). The periosteal

reaction is usually that of an aggressive, onion-skin (lamellated) type, although occasionally a sunburst type may be encountered. A soft tissue mass is almost invariably present, and at times there may be a disproportion between a small bony lesion and a large soft tissue mass (**see Fig. 5-15A, B and 5-16**). It is noteworthy that Ewing sarcoma is extremely rare in black subjects, a helpful point to remember in making the differential diagnosis. Osteosarcoma developing after skeletal maturity should be differentiated from *chondrosarcoma, fibrosarcoma,* and *malignant fibrous histiocytoma.* Osteosarcoma affecting an epiphysis must be differentiated from *clear-cell chondrosarcoma, chondroblastoma,* and *epiphyseal enchondroma* (241). The central low-grade osteosarcoma should be differentiated from *fibrous dysplasia.* This may be difficult because both lesions may show the same radiographic characteristics. The former lesion is expansive, the cortex is thinned, frequently without signs of invasion, and the medullary component may have a narrow zone of transition with a ground-glass appearance (231) (**see Figs. 77 and 78**). CT and MRI are not helpful in this respect. However, neither periosteal reaction nor cortical destruction is present in fibrous dysplasia. For telangiectatic osteosarcoma the differential diagnosis includes *fibrosarcoma, MFH, giant-cell tumor,* and *aneurysmal bone cyst.* Multicentric osteosarcoma must be differentiated from *metastatic*

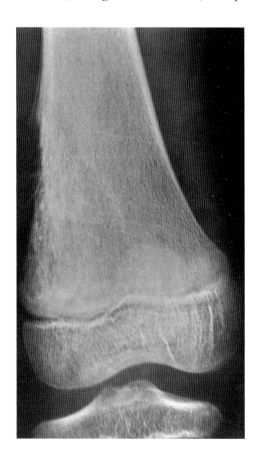

FIG. 107. Osteosarcoma resembling Ewing sarcoma. An anteroposterior radiograph of the distal femur of a 7-year-old girl shows a lesion in the metaphysis of the distal femur that exhibits a destructive, permeative, and moth-eaten pattern very similar to that seen in Ewing sarcoma. There is no evidence of significant bone formation. Aggressive periosteal reaction, in the form of Codman triangle, is present at the proximal extension of the tumor. Biopsy was consistent with a fibroblastic osteosarcoma.

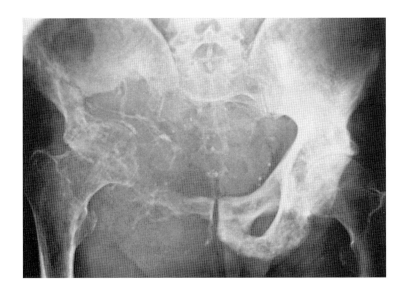

FIG. 108. Paget disease and lytic metastases. An anteroposterior radiograph of the pelvis of a 55-year-old woman with Paget disease shows extensive osteolytic destruction of the right ilium, ischium, and pubis secondary to metastatic renal cell carcinoma (hypernephroma). Note the characteristic features of Paget disease affecting the left hemipelvis. This metastatic lesion should not be mistaken for Paget sarcoma.

osteosarcoma or other *osteoblastic metastases*. Finally, parosteal osteosarcoma should be differentiated among others from *juxtacortical osteoma* (**see Fig. 2**), *soft tissue osteosarcoma* (**see Fig. 105A**), *sessile osteochondroma* (**see Fig. 3-38B**), *parosteal lipoma* with ossifications (see Fig. 11) and well-matured, *juxtacortical myositis ossificans* that became attached to the cortex (**see Fig. 9B**). The most common confusion in diagnosis involves the differentiation of this tumor from myositis ossificans (211) and sessile osteochondroma. Unlike parosteal osteosarcoma, *myositis ossificans* exhibits the distinctive radiologic features of a zonal phenomenon and a cleft that completely separates the ossific mass from the cortex (134,209) (**see Fig. 9A**). *Osteochondroma*, on the other hand, demonstrates uninterrupted cortical continuity and medullary communication between the lesion and the host bone (**see Fig. 8**), features that are not present in parosteal osteosarcoma. In addition, osteochondromas usually contain fatty or even hematopoietic marrow in their intertrabecular spaces, features that can be demonstrated with MRI.

Periosteal osteosarcoma may resemble *myositis ossificans*

and *periosteal chondrosarcoma* (255). Based only on radiologic examination differential diagnosis may be difficult. However, together with the young age of the patients, the radiologic presence of calcification and ossification in the base of the lesion (**see Figs. 91, 92, and 93**) and the histologic identification of at least some osteoid or bone formation by tumor cells are helpful in differentiating this tumor from periosteal chondrosarcoma (245).

Osteosarcoma developing in Pagetic bone must be differentiated from *bone metastases* such as from primaries in the breast, prostate, or kidney, localized either in an area of Pagetic bone or in unaffected bone (233). The metastatic foci may be either lytic (Fig. 108) or blastic (Fig. 109).

In the differential diagnosis of extraskeletal osteosarcoma the possibilities include myositis ossificans, synovial sarcoma, extraskeletal chondrosarcoma, liposarcoma of soft tissues with ossification, and pseudomalignant osseous tumor of soft tissue.

Myositis ossificans is a benign reactive lesion of the soft tissues, predominantly observed in adolescents and young adults (160). The zoning phenomenon represents the matu-

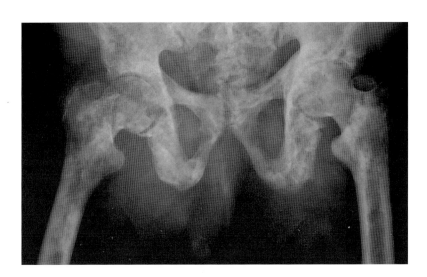

FIG. 109. Paget disease and blastic metastases. A 79-year-old man with known Paget disease for the past 20 years was diagnosed with prostatic cancer. The anteroposterior radiograph of the lower pelvis and proximal femora shows classic features of Paget disease consisting of thickening of the cortex and coarse trabecular pattern of cancellous bone. Scattered foci of increased bone density represent osseous metastases.

ration pattern of the lesion, which is undifferentiated and cellular in the center, and exhibits an increasingly mature ossification toward the periphery; this is the histologic hallmark of this condition (131,209). On radiography the zoning phenomenon is characterized by a radiolucent center of the lesion and a more dense and sclerotic periphery (Fig. 110) (170). A radiolucent cleft often separates the mass from the adjacent cortex (Fig. 111). The evolution of myositis ossificans can be correlated well with the lapse of time since the trauma (192,209) (see also the discussion on differential diagnosis of juxtacortical periosteal osteosarcoma).

Synovial sarcoma is a lesion with a predilection for younger individuals (13 to 55 years) (165). It is usually located near a joint, especially in the lower extremities and particularly in the area around the knee and foot. The radiologic appearance is that of a lobulated mass, with amorphous calcifications present in 25% of cases. Ossification is extremely rare in the mass of synovial sarcoma (249). In approximately 15% to 20% of patients, a periosteal reaction and/or erosion of adjacent bony structures is noted (see Fig. 9-31). Osteoporosis of the affected limb may be present secondary to disuse.

Chondrosarcoma of soft tissue, a very rare malignant tumor, is much less common than extraskeletal osteosarcoma. It is characterized by a soft tissue mass with ring-like, or

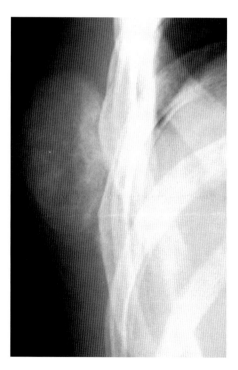

FIG. 110. Juxtacortical myositis ossificans. A coned-down radiograph of the right ribs shows a large focus of juxtacortical myositis ossificans. Note characteristic pattern of zoning phenomenon (i.e., increased density on the periphery of the lesion and more radiolucent center) and the narrow radiolucent cleft separating the ossific mass from the ribs. (Courtesy of Dr. Alex Norman, Valhalla, New York.)

punctate calcifications. It can be radiographically distinguished from osteosarcoma of soft tissues by the lack of bone formation.

Liposarcoma of soft tissues tends to affect older adults, with a higher incidence in men. The lesion may closely mimic osteosarcoma of soft tissues, particularly when ossification is present. The type of ossification, however, is usually more organized, unlike that observed in osteosarcoma of soft tissues, and fatty tissue can usually be identified. The thigh, leg, and gluteal region are commonly affected. Growth of the liposarcoma may be exceedingly slow, over many years, and erosion of adjacent bone is a common feature (165).

Pseudomalignant osseous tumor of soft tissues was first described by Jaffe and later by Fine and Stout (167). These lesions are rare, are more common in females, and are located in the muscles and subcutaneous tissues. They are probably of infective origin, although this has not been unequivocally confirmed. Some lesions may represent unrecognized foci of myositis ossificans (136,177).

Pathology

From the histopathologic standpoint, the differential diagnosis of osteosarcoma should be based on three aspects. First, the differences in histologic and cytologic appearances of malignancy and consecutive grading of the tumor have to be taken into account. Second, the location within a given bone (whether central, intracortical, or surface) is of importance. Finally, different forms of histologic differentiation of osteosarcoma and similarities and differences compared to the other tumors must be considered.

Histology and Cytology

Conventional medullary osteosarcoma (grade 3 or 4) represents the overwhelming majority of all cases, and it is this type that gives rise to the poor prognosis for osteosarcomas in general. Its different histologic types have been discussed above. Because grade 2 tumors still display unequivocal signs of cellular and nuclear malignancy, in most cases the diagnosis is not difficult. Grade 1 tumors, however, exhibit only discrete signs of malignancy; therefore, in the differential diagnosis certain benign tumors and tumor-like lesions must be considered (Fig. 112). One of the tumors that must be distinguished from this malignancy is *osteoblastoma*. Although in most cases the distinction between osteosarcoma and osteoblastoma is straightforward, some osteosarcomas may resemble osteoblastomas (101), and conversely, some osteoblastomas (in particular, the locally aggressive variant also called aggressive osteoblastoma) bear some resemblance to osteosarcoma (see Fig. 51D) (11,123). Probably the best distinction is the lack of cartilage formation by

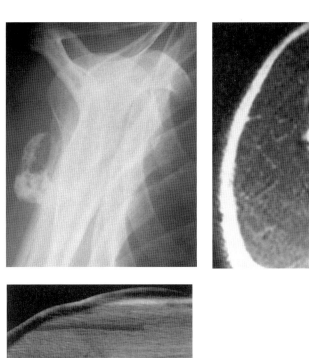

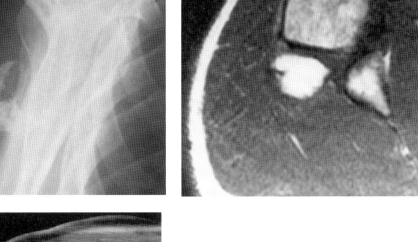

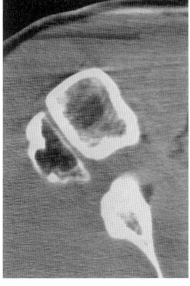

FIG. 111. Juxtacortical myositis ossificans. **A:** An oblique radiograph of the right shoulder shows an ossified lesion abutting lateral cortex of the proximal humeral shaft. **B:** A CT section demonstrates the zoning phenomenon of myositis ossificans. The cleft that separates the lesion from the cortex is shown to the better advantage. **C:** Axial T1-weighted (SE, TR 600, TE 20) MRI shows the center of the lesion to be of high signal intensity, whereas the periphery exhibits low to intermediate signal.

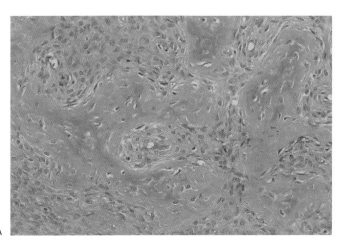

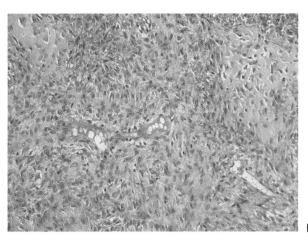

FIG. 112. Histopathology of low-grade central osteosarcoma, resembling fibrous dysplasia. **A:** Irregular woven bone trabeculae in a moderately cellular stroma resemble thos of fibrous dysplasia (hematoxylin and eosin, original magnification ×50) **B:** In another field of view, the high cellularity and pleomorphism of cells allow diagnosis of osteosarcoma (hematoxylin and eosin, original magnification ×50).

osteoblastoma (11,109,205), and the lack of infiltration of the host bone by these tumors (11).

Another good example of this situation is a rare type of central osteosarcoma with a low grade of malignancy, which is well-differentiated, low-grade central osteosarcoma (246). The histologic picture of this tumor resembles *fibrous dysplasia, osteofibrous dysplasia* (Kempson-Campanacci lesion), *adamantinoma, desmoplastic fibroma,* and other lesions (see above). Very discrete focal signs of cellular atypia found in this variant may distinguish this lesion from the above-mentioned benign conditions (Fig. 113). In addition, invasion of bone marrow and permeation of trabeculae of cancellous and cortical bone by the tumor cells are constant features of low-grade osteosarcoma. Desmoplastic fibroma may infiltrate surrounding trabeculae of bone at their periphery, creating a similar picture to that of well-differentiated osteosarcoma (11). However, in the central portions of desmoplastic fibroma there will be no osteoid present and there will be no evidence of tumor bone production. Another low-grade tumor, intracortical osteosarcoma, should also be differentiated from fibrous dysplasia and osteofibrous dysplasia. In this case, the cytologic indicators of malignancy are usually more pronounced.

Location

Within a given bone, osteosarcoma may be located centrally (i.e. in the medullary portion of bone), in the cortical bone, or beneath or outside the periosteum (juxtacortical). Therefore, the radiologic findings are of utmost importance and must always be compared with the histologic sections. An osteosarcoma on the bone surface must be differentiated from several other entities. Periosteal osteosarcoma is usually of a grade 2 malignancy. It differs from p*eriosteal chondrosarcoma* (Fig. 114) by the admixture of tumor bone within the mostly cartilaginous tumor matrix (Fig. 2-114). Fine lace-like osteoid can be demonstrated among the islands of chondroid tissue. In contrast, chondrosarcoma is purely chondroblastic, and may show some reactive bone formation, but there is no tumor bone apposed to malignant cells (**see Fig. 3-92**). *Fracture callus* is occasionally difficult to distinguish from surface osteosarcoma because during the healing stage there is pronounced osteogenesis and new cartilage and bone formation of callus may mimic tumor bone (Fig. 115). In addition, minimal histologic and cytologic signs of malignancy may be present. Therefore, radiography is helpful and the radiographic appearance should take precedence over the histologic findings.

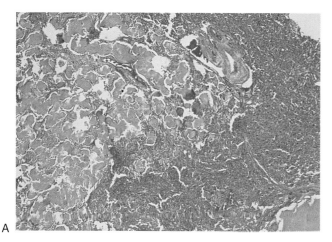

A

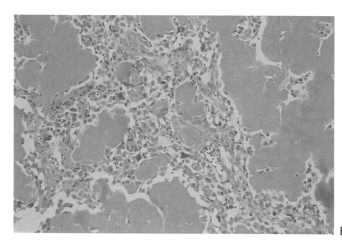

B

C

FIG. 113. Histopathology of low-grade central osteosarcoma resembling fibrous dysplasia. **A:** Densely arranged irregular bone trabeculae (*left*) and almost purely cellular areas (*right*). Bone is denser and cellularity is greater than in fibrous dysplasia (hematoxylin and eosin, original magnification ×12). **B:** At higher magnification, the woven bone trabeculae are clearly broader than in fibrous dysplasia. In contrast to fibrous dysplasia, there are very few osteocytes (hematoxylin and eosin, original magnification ×50). **C:** In more cellular areas, small flecks of tumor osteoid surrounded by densely arranged large, slightly polymorphic cells point to the diagnosis of osteosarcoma (hematoxylin and eosin, original magnification ×50).

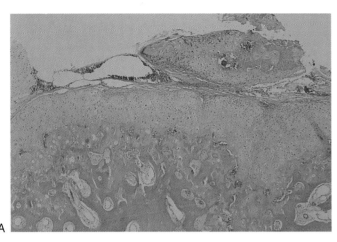
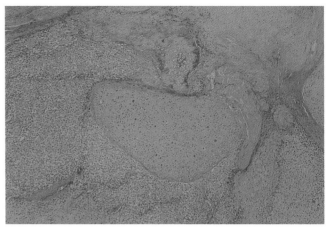

A   B

FIG. 114. Histopathology of periosteal osteosarcoma and periosteal chondrosarcoma. **A:** In periosteal osteosarcoma, the tumor consists of a superficial layer of tumor cartilage and, unlike the case in periosteal chondrosarcoma, a base of partly cancellous tumor bone. The border resembles the zone of endochondral ossification in enchondroma (hematoxylin and eosin, original magnification ×12). **B:** In periosteal chondrosarcoma lobulated chondroblastic tumor tissue partly cellular, partly with matrix resembling hyaline cartilage and with scattered calcifications (*upper center*) is seen. There is no evidence, however, of osteoid formation (hematoxylin and eosin, original magnification ×12).

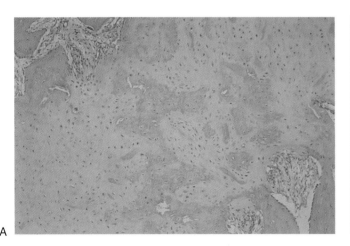
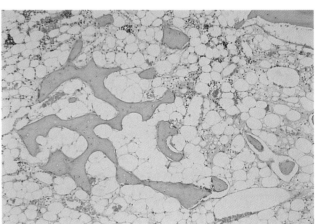

A   B

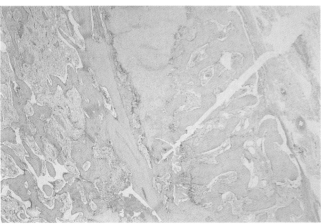

C

FIG. 115. Histopathology of fracture callus. **A:** Callus with irregular arrangement of fibrous cartilage (*clearer areas*) and woven bone (*darker areas*) resembles chondrosteoid of osteosarcoma. Osteoblastic rimming of trabeculae (*upper left and lower right*) and the presence of loose fibrous tissue in the marrow spaces helps in differentiation from low-grade osteosarcoma (hematoxylin and eosin, original magnification ×25). **B:** Marrow at some distance from the fracture line exhibits small foci of necrosis (*right*) and new irregular trabeculae of lamellar bone filling former vascular sinus. These findings constitute an expression of low-grade vascular disturbances after fracture and are not found in osteosarcoma (hematoxylin and eosin, original magnification ×25). **C:** The fracture line is seen crossing the newly formed bone (*upper right to lower middle*). New cancellous bone is present in the marrow space. Here the reparative character of the new bone is obvious (hematoxylin and eosin, original magnification ×25).

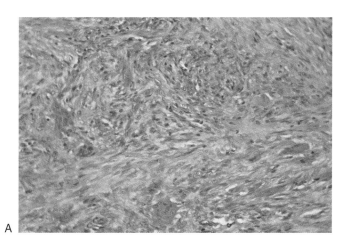

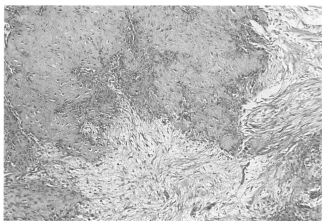

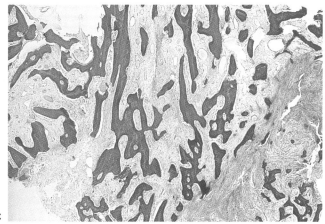

FIG. 116. Histopathology of myositis ossificans. **A:** A central zone of myositis ossificans shows predominantly spindle cell tissue with a disorderly arrangement, producing collagen matrix (hematoxylin and eosin, original magnification ×50). **B:** The intermediate zone reveals immature bone matrix formation. The cellularity of this tissue might cause concern and lead to an erroneous diagnosis of osteosarcoma (hematoxylin and eosin, original magnification ×50). **C:** At the periphery of myositis ossificans, there is mature lamellar bone formation (hematoxylin and eosin, original magnification ×12).

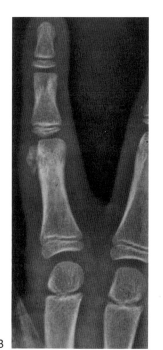

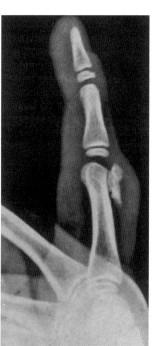

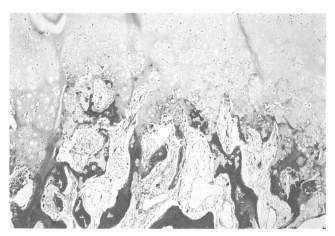

FIG. 117. (**A**) Anteroposterior and (**B**) lateral radiographs of the small finger show an ossific mass adjacent to the posteromedial cortex of the proximal phalanx, representing Nora lesion. (**C**) In Nora lesion, hyaline cartilage (*top*) borders somewhat irregular bone trabeculae formed by endochondral ossification and containing remnants of cartilage matrix, closely resembling osteochondroma. Loose fibrous tissue within the marrow spaces contains wide sinusoid capillaries (hematoxylin and eosin, original magnification ×12).

High-grade surface osteosarcoma is a very rare tumor. It is a grade 3 or 4 malignancy, corresponding to the high-grade osteosarcoma of the central type. Therefore, it is easier to differentiate this variant from other surface lesions, such as periosteal osteosarcoma and fracture callus. Parosteal osteosarcoma, on the other hand, is usually a low-grade tumor. The bone trabeculae usually display a regular alignment and a transformation from woven into lamellar bone. This tumor should be differentiated from myositis ossificans (209), Nora lesion (208), and sessile osteochondroma (208).

Myositis ossificans is fairly easy to distinguish when the lesion has been resected as a whole. The maturation pattern of the bone starting in the periphery (more mature), with fibroblastic tissue in the center producing immature bone by metaplasia, is in sharp contrast to surface osteosarcoma, in which the bone formation starts in the center. In fact, the most prominent feature in the diagnosis of myositis ossificans is the recognition of this zoning pattern, which was first described by Ackerman (131). It consists of a tumor-like structuring in three areas, reflecting different degrees of cellular maturation (**see Fig. 15**). The central zone is composed of an undifferentiated mesenchyme with a high-grade mitotic activity (Fig. 116A); the intermediate zone is composed of a variable amount of unmineralized woven bone intermingled with fibroblasts and osteoblasts (Fig. 116B); and in the peripheral zone the osteoid undergoes calcification and is remodeled into mature lamellar bone (Fig. 116C). The histologic distinction of parosteal osteosarcoma from myositis ossificans is analogous to the radiologic zonal phenomenon. The heterotopic ossification of myositis ossificans matures in a centripetal fashion, the most mature portion of the lesion being the outermost. In parosteal osteosarcoma and higher grade malignant tumors, the outer, advancing portion of the lesion usually is the least mature. As in fracture callus, the problem with the microscopic diagnosis of myositis ossificans involves the interpretation of early stage biopsies when complete maturation has not yet occurred and the tissue resembles that of sarcoma because of slight signs of pleomorphism in the cartilage and the large basophilic osteoblasts. However, in myositis ossificans the cells lack anaplasia, even in the zone where mitotic figures are numerous (7). The other important feature of myositis ossificans is a rather orderly production of bone, especially at the periphery of the lesion (209).

Bizarre parosteal osteochondromatous proliferation (BPOP, Nora lesion) (203,208) is a rare lesion, representing a form of heterotopic ossification, and should not be mistaken for parosteal osteosarcoma. It most commonly affects the bones of the hands and feet, but the long bones are affected in about 25% of reported cases. Radiographs typically show a heavily calcified or ossified mass with a broad base attached to the underlying cortex, which is normal in appearance. The contour of the mass is usually smooth, but it may be slightly lobulated (Fig. 117A, B). In contrast to osteosarcoma, the mass is smaller, shows bizarre cartilage for-

mation and irregular short bone trabeculae, and does not invade the adjacent soft tissues. Histologic examination reveals a large amount of hypercellular cartilage showing transformation to trabecular bone, with frequent spindle cells in the intertrabecular spaces (Fig. 117C). Binucleated cells are common and there may be a considerable osteoblastic activity. This appearance can lead to an incorrect diagnosis of parosteal osteosarcoma.

Occasionally, parosteal osteosarcoma must be differentiated from *osteochondroma*, as this tumor may contain chondroid areas arranged like a cap of an osteochondroma. According to Dahlin and Unni (7), the presence of spindle cells in the former tumor is an important differential point.

Histologic Differentiation

As mentioned above, high-grade central osteosarcoma is by far the most common form of osteosarcoma. It is defined as a tumor with cytologic signs of high-grade malignancy, which forms a tumor bone matrix in very different quantities, from very little, as in telangiectatic osteosarcoma, to abundant, as in the sclerotic osteoblastic form of medullary osteosarcoma.

In osteoblastic osteosarcoma the formation of woven bone occurs in a mostly primitive trabecular or more plate-like manner (**see Fig. 68A**). If bone matrix formation is very conspicuous, resembling that of compact bone (Fig. 118), and with a corresponding radiographic image of very high and homogeneous density, a multicentric osteosarcoma must be suspected and sought by use of various radiologic modalities. It should be kept in mind, however, that in the monostotic osteoblastic form of osteosarcoma the bone matrix is not necessarily mineralized and that this tumor may radio-

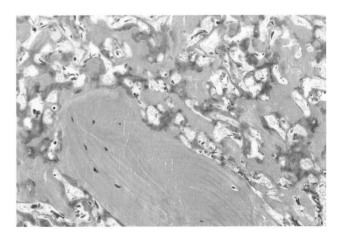

FIG. 118. Histopathology of osteoblastic multicentric osteosarcoma. In the marrow spaces around a trabecula (*lower center*), there are newly formed, irregular, and smaller tumor bone trabeculae, which are fully mineralized and are surrounded by tumor cells (non-decalcified preparation, Goldner trichrome, original magnification ×50).

graphically present as a lytic lesion. *Giant-cell reparative granuloma*, or so-called solid aneurysmal bone cyst, may cause considerable difficulty in differentiation from an osteosarcoma of low or intermediate grade malignancy with moderate bone formation, as the fibroblasts may show some polymorphism and mitoses and the bone formation may appear to be quite irregular. The radiographic features are usually helpful. *Fibrous dysplasia* can be difficult to differentiate from low-grade osteosarcoma with a high grade of differentiation (see above). The lack of osteoblasts rimming trabeculae in fibrous dysplasia is helpful in making this distinction.

In addition to formation of osteoblastic matrix by osteosarcomas, other types of matrix formation may be found. Chondroblastic osteosarcoma usually displays a fairly well-differentiated cartilaginous matrix, often with only moderate cytologic signs of malignancy but without the typical lobular pattern and the hyaline cartilage of *well-differentiated chondrosarcoma*. A characteristic feature is the indistinct transition from the cartilaginous matrix into bony matrix (Fig. 119), the latter pointing to the osteoblastic nature of the tumor. This substance with intermediate characteristics between cartilage and osteoid is called chondrosteoid by most authors (205), and it may be also present in fracture callus. Another tumor that must be differentiated from chondroblastic osteosarcoma is *dedifferentiated chondrosarcoma*, in which features of a high-grade osteosarcoma are found side by side with a well-differentiated chondrosarcoma (Fig. 120). The demarcation is very clearly delineated, unlike chondroblastic osteosarcoma, in which the delineation is not sharp and chondroblastic and osteoblastic matrices may merge into one another (Fig. 119B). In clear cell chondrosarcoma bone formation may be substantial. However, this bone does not represent tumor bone but rather is reactive (Fig. 121). Furthermore, the cartilage cells are larger than those in conventional chondrosarcoma and chondroblastic osteosarcoma, and their cytoplasm ranges from perfectly clear to eosinophilic.

Fibroblastic osteosarcoma consists of a three-dimensional interwoven pattern of collagen fibers formed by malignant fibroblasts of variable pleomorphism and quantity. This tumor must be differentiated from *fibrosarcoma*. In particular, areas of spindle cells and homogeneous eosinophilic material, as encountered in fibroblastic osteosarcoma, may be indistinguishable from fibrosarcoma (142), as the latter occasionally contains areas of homogeneous eosinophilic material that can resemble osteoid. In this situation special stains such as van Gieson or Goldner can be helpful. On the other hand, the formation of tumor osteoid in osteosarcoma may be scant and must be carefully searched for (Fig. 122). Usually, the typical herring-bone pattern of true *fibrosarcoma* is either absent or indistinct, which may be helpful in distinguishing osteosarcoma sparse in osteoid from fibrosarcoma. *Malignant fibrous histiocytoma* (MFH) rarely shows any bone formation and in most cases is characterized by the cartwheel or storiform pattern of fibers and cell arrangement (Fig. 123). In the giant cell–rich variant of MFH, giant cells may be numerous, unlike fibrosarcoma and fibroblastic osteosarcoma, in which they are sparse or absent. In this case, distinction from the giant cell-rich variant of osteosarcoma may create some problems (140). Both giant cell–rich osteosarcoma and MFH may contain giant cells in equal numbers and forms, so that some authors consider MFH to represent only a variant of osteosarcoma. *Desmoplastic fibroma* is easy to differentiate from osteosarcoma because in the former the fibroblasts are monomorphic and very evenly distributed within the tissue, and no tumor bone formation is present (**see Fig. 4-42**).

Telangiectatic osteosarcoma and giant cell–rich osteosarcoma resemble each other in their moderate content of giant

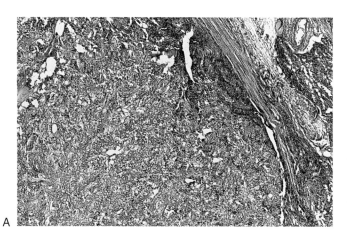
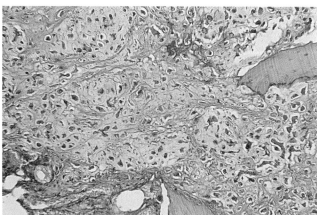

A
B

FIG. 119. Histopathology of chondroblastic osteosarcoma. **A:** Osteoblastic tumor tissue with moderate osteoid formation (*delicate red structures*) extending into the periosteum (*dense, reddish diagonal structure in upper right corner*) (van Gieson, original magnification ×25). **B:** Marrow space with two old trabeculae (*upper right and lower middle*) and tumor chondrosteoid (osteoid and cartilage matrix merging into one another without clear delineation) is typical of many osteosarcomas (hematoxylin and eosin, original magnification ×50).

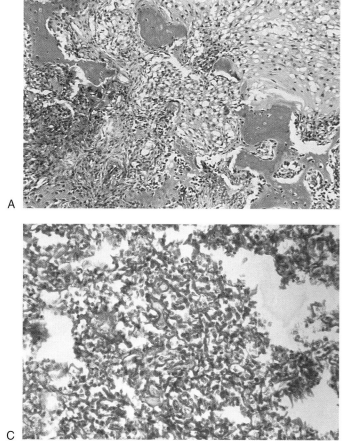

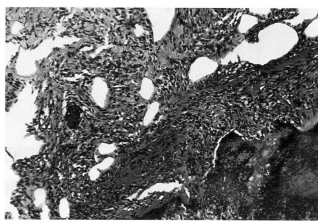

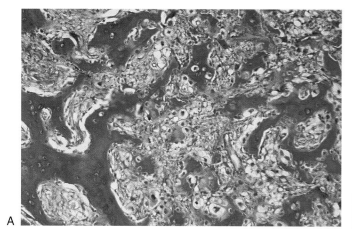

FIG. 120. Histopathology of dedifferentiated chondrosarcoma with an osteosarcoma component. **A:** An area of well-differentiated chondrosarcoma (*upper right*) is sharply demarcated from dedifferentiated tumor showing osteoblastic differentiation within remnants of cancellous bone (*lower left*) (hematoxylin and eosin, original magnification ×25). **B:** Almost entirely cellular, dedifferentiated tumor tissue with scanty tumor bone formation and remnants of cancellous bone (*lower right*) (hematoxylin and eosin, original magnification ×25). **C:** The dedifferentiated portion of tumor exhibits a delicate network of tumor osteoid (*red*) (van Gieson, original magnification ×25).

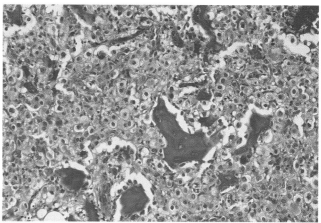

FIG. 121. Histopathology of clear-cell chondrosarcoma resembling osteosarcoma. **A:** A considerable amount of new reactive bone (not produced by tumor cells) makes differentiation from osteosarcoma almost impossible. Meticulous search for areas typical of clear cell chondrosarcoma, such as depicted in **Fig. 3-92**, is essential (hematoxylin and eosin, original magnification ×50). **B:** In other areas there is evidence of small woven bone trabecula formation, mimicking that of osteosarcoma. Identification of cartilage tumor cells is essential for the diagnosis of chondrosarcoma (hematoxylin and eosin, original magnification ×50).

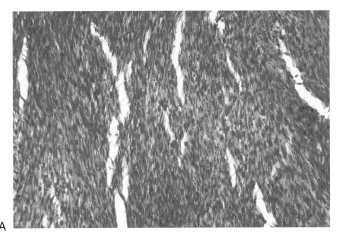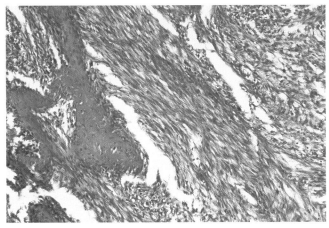

A

B

FIG. 122. Histopathology of fibroblastic osteosarcoma resembling fibrosarcoma. **A:** Areas without bone formation are very much like those of high-grade fibrosarcoma (hematoxylin and eosin, original magnification ×25). **B:** In another section of this tumor, the tumor tissue is composed of spindle cells with distinct pleomorphism (*upper right*). Formation of tumor woven bone trabeculae (*left*) points to the diagnosis of fibroblastic osteosarcoma (hematoxylin and eosin, original magnification ×25).

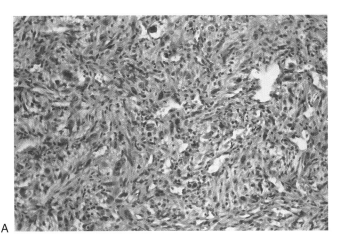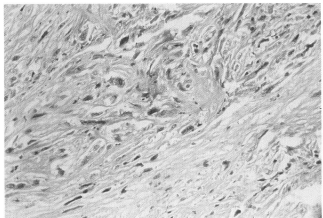

A

B

FIG. 123. Histopathology of malignant fibrous histiocytoma. **A:** Densely arranged spindle cells, showing considerable pleomorphism and hyperchromatism of the nuclei resembling a cartwheel-like pattern (*upper left*), may help to distinguish this tumor from fibroblastic osteosarcoma (hematoxylin and eosin, original magnification ×50). **B:** In another area of this tumor, loose myxoid arrangement of tumor tissue (*middle*) may be helpful in the differential diagnosis (hematoxylin and eosin, original magnification ×50).

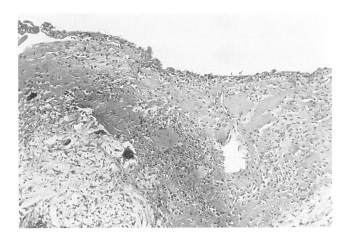

FIG. 124. Histopathology of aneurysmal bone cyst resembling telangiectatic osteosarcoma. A cystic area (*upper*) is bordered by a seam of flat undifferentiated cells intermingled with some small giant cells. Immediately below there is formation of considerable amounts of primitive woven bone rimmed with osteoblasts. Bone formation extends far down into the solid fibrous tissue (*lower left*), which appears myxoid. Here several larger giant cells of the osteoclast type lie near the bone. Bone formation may be erroneously interpreted as osteosarcoma (hematoxylin and eosin, original magnification ×25).

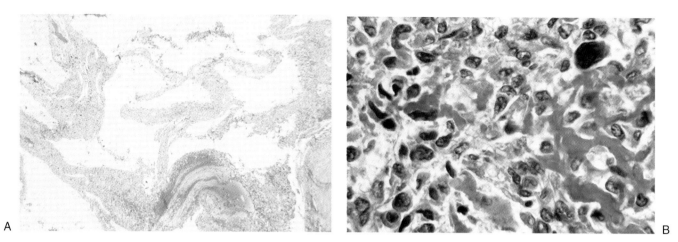

FIG. 125. Histopathology of telangiectatic osteosarcoma resembling aneurysmal bone cyst. **A:** A low-power photomicrograph shows vascular areas very similar to those characteristic of aneurysmal bone cyst (hematoxylin and eosin, original magnification × 15). **B:** At high magnification solid areas of the tumor show significant pleomorphism of malignant cells and hyperchromatism of their nuclei. Also seen is osteoid production by the tumor cells (hematoxylin and eosin, original magnification ×400).

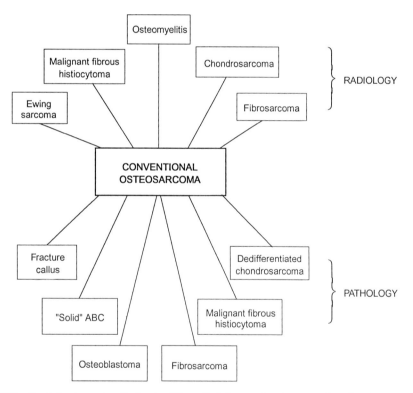

FIG. 126. Radiologic and pathologic differential diagnosis of conventional osteosarcoma.

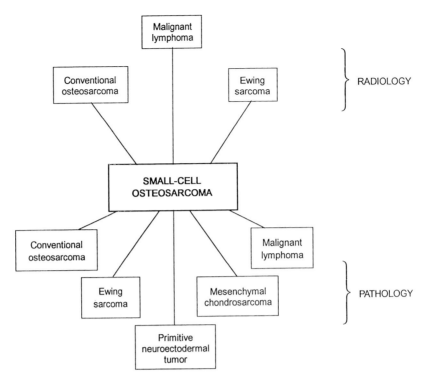

FIG. 127. Radiologic and pathologic differential diagnosis of small cell osteosarcoma.

cells but differ in the number and size of blood-containing spaces resembling blood vessels, which are conspicuous in the former. Both tumors usually contain very little bone. In differentiating giant cell tumor (GCT) from these two malignancies, it is important to note that the number and size of giant cells in grade 1 giant cell tumor are much greater than in the two mentioned variants of osteosarcoma, whereas bone formation in a giant cell tumor is rarely present and is usually scant. In a grade 2 or 3 GCT, however, the number and size of the giant cells may be reduced to the point that makes differentiation extremely difficult. In this situation the radiologic findings are essential. Telangiectatic osteosarcoma contains enlarged capillary vessels surrounded by highly pleomorphic tumor tissue and may also contain elements of a true aneurysmal bone cyst surrounded by normal connective tissue. Differentiation from *aneurysmal bone cyst* may be difficult in such instances. In fact the confusion between telangiectatic osteosarcoma and aneurysmal bone cyst represents one of the most treacherous pitfalls in tumor pathology (11,171,186) (Fig. 124). The hallmark of osteosarcoma is the presence of anaplastic cells, not found to that degree in the aneurysmal bone cyst (Fig. 125). Some authorities suggested that morphometric studies may be of help in differentiating these two entities (223).

Small cell osteosarcoma must be differentiated from Ewing sarcoma, primitive neuroectodermal tumor (PNET), lymphoma, and mesenchymal chondrosarcoma. It is essential to look for a sparse bone formation in osteosarcoma (**see** Figs. 2-71, 5-23). However, in some *Ewing sarcomas*, reactive woven bone formation may be found, and this may be misinterpreted as tumor bone formation, thus causing an erroneous diagnosis of small cell osteosarcoma (38). New immunocytochemical methods may be helpful in distinguishing these tumors from one another.

Mesenchymal chondrosarcoma may contain a population of small cells indistinguishable from that of small cell osteosarcoma. However, according to Fechner and Mills (11), mesenchymal chondrosarcoma has sharply demarcated nests of low-grade cartilage and small cell osteosarcoma contains osteoid. In addition, cartilage markers (S-100) are helpful in this distinction.

Lymphoma can be eliminated by the absence of panleukocytic markers such as leukocyte common antigen, and *primitive neuroectodermal tumor* of bone will demonstrate evidence of neuroendocrine differentiation in the form of positive staining for neuron specific enolase, Leu 7, synaptophysin, chromogranin, or other neural markers, and may demonstrate Homer Wright–type rosettes (11).

Osteosarcomas secondary to Paget disease and those evolving in bone infarcts usually do not cause problems in differential diagnosis, as the primary lesions have characteristic appearances. In some cases, however, these characteristics may be obscured by the tumor tissue and must then be meticulously sought.

The radiologic and pathologic differential diagnosis of various subtypes of osteosarcoma is depicted in Figs. 126 through 133.

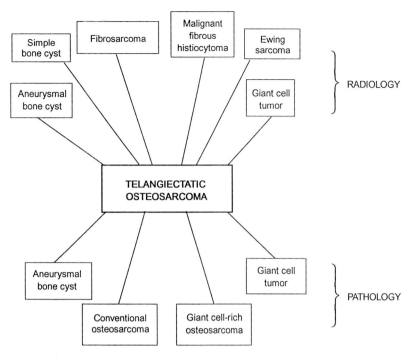

FIG. 128. Radiologic and pathologic differential diagnosis of telangiectatic osteosarcoma.

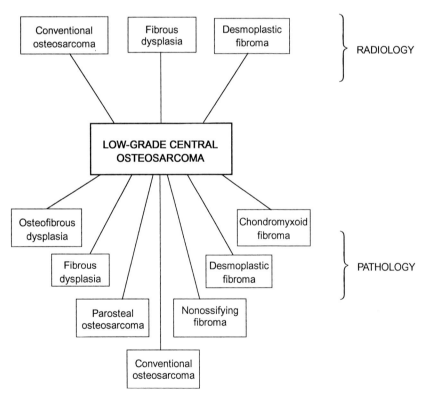

FIG. 129. Radiologic and pathologic differential diagnosis of low-grade central osteosarcoma.

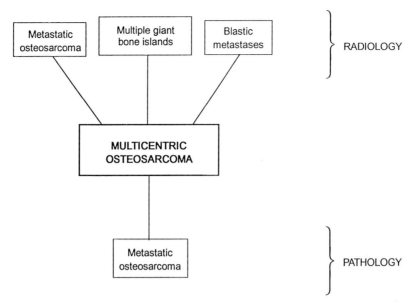

FIG. 130. Radiologic and pathologic differential diagnosis of multicentric osteosarcoma.

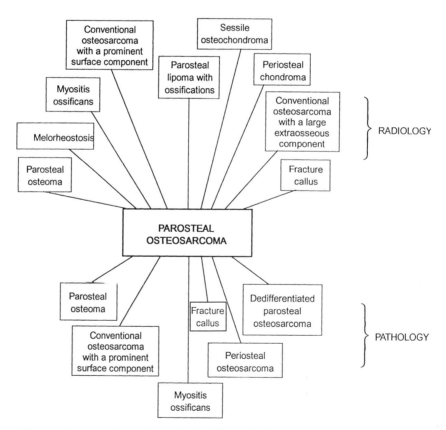

FIG. 131. Radiologic and pathologic differential diagnosis of parosteal osteosarcoma.

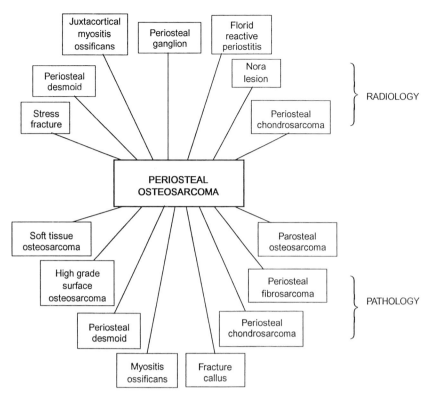

FIG. 132. Radiologic and pathologic differential diagnosis of periosteal osteosarcoma.

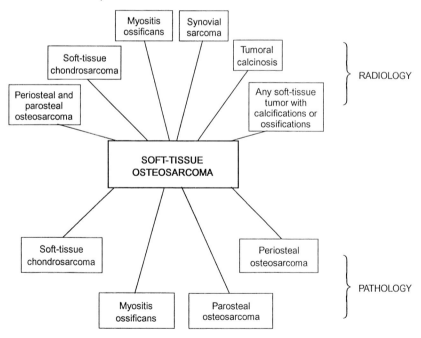

FIG. 133. Radiologic and pathologic differential diagnosis of soft tissue osteosarcoma.

REFERENCES

Osteoma

1. Baum PA, Nelson MC, Lack EE, Bogumill GP. Case report 560. Parosteal osteoma of tibia. *Skeletal Radiol* 1989;18:406–409.
2. Bertoni F, Unni KK, Beabout JW, Sim FH. Parosteal osteoma of bones other than of the skull and face. *Cancer* 1995;75:2466–2473.
3. Bullough PG. *Atlas of orthopedic pathology with clinical and radiologic correlations,* 2nd ed. New York: Gower, 1992.
4. Campbell CJ, Papademetriou T, Bonfiglio M. Melorheostosis. A report of the clinical, roentgenographic, and pathological findings in fourteen cases. *J Bone Joint Surg* 1968;50A:1281–1304.
5. Cervilla V, Haghighi P, Resnick D, Sartoris DJ. Case report 596. Parosteal osteoma of the acetabulum. *Skeletal Radiol* 1990; 19: 135–137.
6. Chang CH, Piatt ED, Thomas KE, Watne AL. Bone abnormalities in Gardner's syndrome. *Am J Roentgenol* 1968;103:645–652.
7. Dahlin DC, Unni KK. Osteoma. In: *Bone tumors. General aspects on 8,542 cases,* 4th ed. Springfield, IL: Charles C Thomas, 1986;84–87, 308–321.
8. Dolan K, Seibert J, Seibert R. Gardner's syndrome. *Am J Roentgenol* 1973;119:359–364.
9. Eckel W, Palm D. Statistische und röntgenologische Untersuchungen zu einigen Fragen des Nebenhöhlenosteoms. *Arch Ohr Nas Kehlkopfheilk* 1959;174:440–457.
10. Enzinger FW, Weiss SW. Osseous tumors and tumor-like lesions of soft tissues. In: *Soft tissue tumors,* 2nd ed. Mosby, St. Louis, 1988, pp. 882–905.
11. Fechner RE, Mills SE. *Tumors of the bones and joints.* Washington, DC: Armed Forces Institute of Pathology, 1993;26–28.
12. Fleming RJ, Alpert M, Garcia A. Parosteal lipoma. *Am J Roentgenol* 1962;87:1075–1084.
13. Gardner EJ, Richards RC. Multiple cutaneous and subcutaneous lesions occurring simultaneously with hereditary polyposis and osteomatosis. *Am J Hum Genet* 1953;5:139–147.
14. Gardner EJ, Plenk HP. Hereditary pattern for multiple osteomas in a family group. *Am J Hum Genet* 1952;4:31–36.
15. Gentry JF, Schechter JJ, Mirra JM. Case report 574. Periosteal osteoblastoma of rib. *Skeletal Radiol* 1989;18:551–555.
16. Geschickter CF, Copeland MM. Parosteal osteoma of bone: a new entity. *Ann Surg* 1951;133:790–807.
17. Greenspan A. Benign bone-forming lesions: osteoma, osteoid osteoma, and osteoblastoma. *Skeletal Radiol* 1993;22:485–500.
18. Greenspan A. Sclerosing bone dysplasias—a target-site approach. *Skeletal Radiol* 1991;20:561–583.
19. Greenspan A. *Orthopedic radiology: a practical approach,* 2nd ed. New York: Lippincott-Raven, 1992;16.1–16.12.
20. Houghton MJ, Heiner JP, DeSmet AA. Osteoma of the innominate bone with intraosseous and parosteal involvement. *Skeletal Radiol* 1995;24:445–457.
21. Huvos AG. *Bone tumors. diagnosis, treatment, and prognosis, 2nd ed.* WB Saunders, Philadelphia, 1991.
22. Jacobs P. Parosteal lipoma with hyperostosis. *Clin Radiol* 1972;23: 196–198.
23. Jacobson HG. Dense bone—too much bone: radiological considerations and differential diagnosis. Part I. *Skeletal Radiol* 1985;13:1–20.
24. Jacobson HG. Dense bone—too much bone: radiological considerations and differential diagnosis. Part II. *Skeletal Radiol* 1985;13: 97–113.
25. Krolls SO, Jacoway JR, Alexander WN. Osseous choristomas (osteomas) of intraoral soft tissues. *Oral Surg* 1971;32:588–595.
26. Lichtenstein L. *Bone tumors* 5th ed. St Louis: CV Mosby, 1977;11.
27. Lichtenstein L, Sawyer WR. Benign osteoblastoma: further observations and report of twenty additional cases. *J Bone Joint Surg* 1964; 46A:755–765.
28. Meltzer CC, Scott WW Jr, McCarthy EF. Case report 698. Osteoma of the clavicle. *Skeletal Radiol* 1991;20:555–557.
29. Mirra JM, Gold RH, Pignatti G, Remotti F. Case report 497. Compact osteoma of iliac bone. *Skeletal Radiol* 1988;17:437–442.
30. Mirra JM, Picci P, Gold RH. Bone tumors: clinical, pathologic, and radiologic correlations. Philadelphia: Lea and Febiger, 1989;226–248.
31. Murphey MD, Johnson DL, Bhatia PS, Neff JR, Rosenthal HG,

Walker CW. Parosteal lipoma: MR imaging characteristics. *Am J Roentgenol* 1994;162:105–110.
32. O'Connell JX, Rosenthal DI, Mankin HJ, Rosenberg AE. Solitary osteoma of a long bone. *J Bone Joint Surg* 1993;75A:1830–1834.
33. Peyser AB, Makley JT, Callewart CC, Brackett B, Carter JR, Abdul-Karim FW. Osteoma of the long bones and the spine: a study of eleven patients and a review of the literature. *J Bone Joint Surg* 1996; 78A:1172–1180.
34. Pool JL, Pontanos JN, Krueger EG. Osteomas and mucoceles of the frontal paranasal sinuses. *J Neurosurg* 1962;19:130–135.
35. Prein J, Remagen W, Spiessl B, Uehlinger E. *Atlas of tumors of the facial skeleton.* Berlin: Springer-Verlag, 1986;99–101.
36. Ramos A, Castello J, Sartoris DJ, Greenway GD, Resnick D, Haghighi P. Osseous lipoma: CT appearance. *Radiology* 1985;157:615–619.
37. Sadry F, Hessler C, Garcia J. The potential aggressiveness of sinus osteomas. A report of two cases. *Skeletal Radiol* 1988;17:427–430.
38. Schajowicz F. *Tumors and tumorlike lesions of bone: pathology, radiology and treatment,* 2nd ed. Berlin: Springer-Verlag, 1994;30–32, 52–56, 406–411.
39. Schajowicz F, Lemos C. Osteoid osteoma and osteoblastoma—closely related entities of osteoblastic derivation. *Acta Orthop Scand* 1970;41:272–291.
40. Schweitzer ME, Greenway G, Resnick D, Haghighi P, Snoots WE. Osteoma of soft parts. *Skeletal Radiol* 1992;21:177–180.
41. Spjut HJ, Dorfman HD, Fechner RE, Ackerman LV. Tumors of bone and cartilage. In: Firminger HI, ed. *Atlas of tumor pathology,* 2nd series, fascicle 5. Washington, DC: Armed Forces Institute of Pathology, 1971;117–119.
42. Spencer MG, Mitchell DB. Growth of a frontal sinus osteoma. *J Laryngol Otol* 1987;101:726–728.
43. Steinberg I. Huge osteoma of the eleventh left rib. *JAMA* 1959;170: 1921–1923.
44. Stern PJ, Lim EVA, Krieg JK. Giant metacarpal osteoma. A case report. *J Bone Joint Surg* 1985;67A:487–489.
45. Sundaram M, Falbo S, McDonald D, Janney C. Surface osteomas of the appendicular skeleton. *Am J Roentgenol* 1996;167:1529–1533.
46. Tamarito LV, Pardo J. Parosteal osteoma: a clinopathological approach. *Pathol Annu* 1977;1:373–387.
47. Unni KK, Dahlin DC, Beabout JW, Ivins JC. Parosteal osteogenic sarcoma. *Cancer* 1976;37:2644–2675.
48. Wilner D. *Radiology of bone tumors and allied disorders.* Philadelphia: WB Saunders, 1982;629–638.

Osteoid Osteoma

49. Adil A, Hoeffel C, Fikry T. Osteoid osteoma after a fracture of the distal radius. *Am J Roentgenol* 1996;167:145–146.
50. Alani WO, Bartal E. Osteoid osteoma of the femoral neck simulating an inflammatory synovitis. *Clin Orthop* 1987;223:308–312.
51. Anderson RB, McAlister JA Jr, Wrenn RN. Case report 585. Intracortical osteosarcoma of tibia. *Skeletal Radiol* 1989;627–630.
52. Assoun J, Richardi G, Railhac J-J, Baunin C, Fajadet P, Giron J, Maquin P, Haddad J, Bonnevialle P. Osteoid osteoma. MR imaging versus CT. *Radiology* 1994;191:217–223.
53. Baron D, Soulier C, Kermabon C, Leroy JP, Le Goff P. Ostéomes ostéoides post-traumatique: à propos de deux cas et revue de la littérature. *Rev Rhum Mal Osteoartic* 1992;59:271–275.
54. Bell RS, O Connor GD, Waddell JP. Importance of magnetic resonance imaging in osteoid osteoma: a case report. *Can J Surg* 1989;32: 276–278.
55. Campanacci M. *Bone and soft tissue tumors.* New York: Springer-Verlag, 1990;355–373.
56. Cohen MD, Harrington TM, Ginsburg WW. Osteoid osteoma: 95 cases and a review of the literature. *Semin Arthritis Rheum* 1983;12: 265–281.
57. Corbett JM, Wilde AH, McCormack LJ, Evarts CM. Intra-articular osteoid osteoma. A diagnostic problem. *Clin Orthop* 1974;98:225–230.
58. Dahlin DC, Unni KK. *Bone tumors: general aspects and data on 8542 cases,* 4th ed. Springfield, IL: Charles C Thomas, 1987;88–101.
59. Dockerty MB, Ghormley RK, Jackson AE. Osteoid osteoma: clinicopathologic study of 20 cases. *Ann Surg* 1951;133:77–89.
60. Edeiken J, DePalma AF, Hodes PJ. Osteoid osteoma. (Roentgenographic emphasis). *Clin Orthop* 1966;49:201–206.

61. Freiberger RH, Loitman BS, Helpern M, Thompson TC. Osteoid osteoma: a report of 80 cases. *Am J Roentgenol* 1959;82:194–205.
62. Gamba JL, Martinez S, Apple J, Harrelson JM, Nunley JA. Computed tomography of axial skeletal osteoid osteomas. *Am J Roentgenol* 1984;142:769–772.
63. Goldberg VM, Jacobs B. Osteoid osteoma of the hip in children. *Clin Orthop* 1975;106:41–47.
64. Glass RB, Poznanski AK, Fisher MR, Shkolnik A, Dias L. MR imaging of osteoid osteoma. *J Comput Tomogr* 1986;10:1065–1067.
65. Goldman AB, Schneider R, Pavlov H. Osteoid osteomas of the femoral neck: report of four cases evaluated with isotopic bone scanning, CT, and MR imaging. *Radiology* 1993;186:227–232.
66. Greenspan A, Steiner G, Knutzon R. Bone island (enostosis): clinical significance and radiologic and pathologic correlations. *Skeletal Radiol* 1991;20:85–90.
67. Greenspan A. Bone island (enostosis): current concept. *Skeletal Radiol* 1995;24:111–115.
68. Greenspan A, Stadalnik RC. Bone island: scintigraphic findings and their clinical application. *Can Assoc Radiol J* 1995;46:368–379.
69. Helms CA. Osteoid osteoma: the double density sign. *Clin Orthop* 1987;222:167–173.
70. Helms CA, Hattner RS, Vogler JB III. Osteoid osteoma: Radionuclide diagnosis. *Radiology* 1984;151:779–784.
71. Herrlin K, Ekelund L, Lövdahl R, Persson B. Computed tomography in suspected osteoid osteomas of tubular bones. *Skeletal Radiol* 1982;9:92–97.
72. Jackson RP, Reckling FW, Mants FA. Osteoid osteoma and osteoblastoma. Similar histologic lesions with different natural histories. *Clin Orthop* 1977;128:303–313.
73. Jaffe HL. Osteoid osteoma of bone. *Radiology* 1945;45:319–334.
74. Keim HA, Reina EG. Osteoid osteoma as a cause of scoliosis. *J Bone Joint Surg* 1975;57-A:159–163.
75. Kendrick JL, Evarts CM. Osteoid osteoma: a critical analysis of 40 tumors. *Clin Orthop* 1967;54:51–59.
76. Klein MH, Shankman S. Osteoid osteoma: radiologic and pathologic correlation. *Skeletal Radiol* 1992;21:23–31.
77. Kransdorf MJ, Stull MA, Gilkey FW, Moser RP Jr. Osteoid osteoma. *RadioGraphics* 1991;11:671–696.
78. Kricun ME. *Imaging of bone tumors.* Philadelphia: WB Saunders, 1993;121–125.
79. Kyriakos M. Intracortical osteosarcoma. *Cancer* 1980;46:2525–2533.
80. Lisbona R, Rosenthall L. Role of radionuclide imaging in osteoid osteoma. *Am J Roentgenol* 1979;132:77–80.
81. Mirra JM, Dodd L, Johnston W, Frost DB. Case report 700. Primary intracortical osteosarcoma of femur, sclerosing variant, grade 1 to 2 anaplasia. *Skeletal Radiol* 1991;20:613–616.
82. Murphey MD, Andrews CL, Flemming DJ, Temple HT, Smith WS, Smirniotopoulos JG. Primary tumors of the spine: radiologic-pathologic correlation. *RadioGraphics* 1996;16:1131–1158.
83. Norman A, Abdelwahab IF, Buyon J, Matzkin E. Osteoid osteoma of the hip stimulating an early onset of osteoarthritis. *Radiology* 1986;158:417–420.
84. Pettine KA, Klassen RA. Osteoid osteoma and osteoblastoma of the spine. *J Bone Joint Surg* 1986;68A:354–361.
85. Picci P, Gherlinzoni F, Guerra A. Intracortical osteosarcoma: rare entity or early manifestation of classical osteosarcoma? *Skeletal Radiol* 1983;9:255–258.
86. Sabanas AO, Bickel WH, Moe JH. Natural history of osteoid osteoma of the spine: review of the literature and report of three cases. *Am J Surg* 1956;91:880–889.
87. Schai P, Friederich NB, Krüger A, Jundt G, Herbe E, Buess P. Discrete synchronous multifocal osteoid osteoma of the humerus. *Skeletal Radiol* 1996;25:667–670.
88. Schlesinger AE, Hernandez RJ. Intracapsular osteoid osteoma of the proximal femur: findings on plain film and CT. *Am J Roentgenol* 1990;154:1241–1244.
89. Sim FH, Dahlin DC, Beabout JW. Osteoid-osteoma: diagnostic problems. *J Bone Joint Surg* 1975;57A:154–159.
90. Smith FW, Gilday DL. Scintigraphic appearances of osteoid osteoma. *Radiology* 1980;137:191–195.
91. Steiner GC. Ultrastructure of osteoid osteoma. *Hum Pathol* 1976;7:309–325.
92. Strach EH. Osteoid osteoma. *Br Med J* 1953;1:1031.
93. Swee RG, McLeod RA, Beabout JW. Osteoid osteoma. Detection, diagnosis, and localization. *Radiology* 1979;130:117–123.
94. Thompson GH, Wong KM, Konsens RM, Vibhakars S. Magnetic resonance imaging of an osteoid osteoma of the proximal femur: a potentially confusing appearance. *J Pediatr Orthop* 1990;10:800–804.
95. Winter PF, Johnson PM, Hilal SK, Feldman F. Scintigraphic detection of osteoid osteoma. *Radiology* 1977;122:177–178.
96. Woods ER, Martel W, Mandell SH, Crabbe JP. Reactive soft-tissue mass associated with osteoid osteoma: correlation of MR imaging features with pathologic findings. *Radiology* 1993;186:221–225.
97. Yamamura S, Sato K, Sugiura H, Asano M, Takahasi M, Iwata H. Magnetic resonance imaging of inflammatory reaction in osteoid osteoma. *Arch Orthop Trauma Surg* 1994;114:8–13.
98. Yeager BA, Schiebler ML, Wertheim SB, Schmidt RG, Torg JS, Perosio PM, Dalinka MK. Case report: MR imaging of osteoid osteoma of the talus. *J Comput Assist Tomogr* 1987;11:916–917.
99. Youssef BA, Haddad MC, Zahrani A, Sharif HS, Morgan JL, Al-Shahed M, Al Sabty A, Choudary R. Osteoid oseoma and osteoblastoma: MRI appearances and the significance of ring enhancement. *Eur Radiol* 1996;6:291–296.

Osteoblastoma

100. Azouz EM, Kozlowski K, Marton D, Sprague P, Zerhouni A, Assalah F. Osteoid osteoma and osteoblastoma of the spine in children. Report of 22 cases with brief literature review. *Pediatr Radiol* 1986;16:25–31.
101. Bertoni F, Unni KK, McLeod RA, Dahlin DC. Osteosarcoma resembling osteoblastoma. *Cancer* 1985;55:416–426.
102. Bettelli G, Tigani D, Picci P. Recurring osteoblastoma initially presenting as a typical osteoid osteoma. Report of two cases. *Skeletal Radiol* 1991;20:1–4.
103. Byers PD. Solitary benign osteoblastic lesions of bone. Osteoid osteoma and benign osteoblastoma. *Cancer* 1968;22:43–57.
104. Crim JR, Mirra JM, Eckardt JJ, Seeger LL. Widespread inflammatory response to osteoblastoma: the flare phenomenon. *Radiology* 1990;177:835–836.
105. Dahlin DC, Johnson EW Jr. Giant osteoid osteoma. *J Bone Joint Surg* 1954;36A:559–572.
106. Della Rocca C, Huvos AG. Osteoblastoma: Varied histological presentations with a benign clinical course. 55 cases. *Am J Surg Pathol* 1996;20:841–850.
107. Denis F, Armstrong GW. Scoliogenic osteoblastoma of the posterior end of the rib: a case report. *Spine* 1984;9:74–76.
108. DeSouza, Diaz L, Frost HM. Osteoid osteoma—osteoblastoma. *Cancer* 1974;33:1075–1081.
109. Dorfman HD, Weiss SW. Borderline osteoblastic tumors: problems in the differential diagnosis of aggressive osteoblastoma and low-grade osteosarcoma. *Semin Diagn Pathol* 1984;1:215–234.
110. Fabris D, Trainiti G, Di Comun M, Agostini S. Scoliosis due to rib osteoblastoma: report of two cases. *J Pediatr Orthop* 1983;3:370–375.
111. Fanning JW, Lucas GL. Osteoblastoma of the scaphoid: A case report. *J Hand Surg* 1993;18A:663–665.
112. Farmlett EJ, Magid D, Fishman EK. Osteoblastoma of the tibia: CT demonstration. *J Comput Assist Tomogr* 1986;10:1068–1070.
113. Gitelis S, Schajowicz F. Osteoid osteoma and osteoblastoma. *Orthop Clin North Am* 1989;20:313–325.
114. Healey HJ: Ghelman B. Osteoid osteoma and osteoblastoma. *Clin Orthop* 1986;204:76–85.
115. Jaffe HL. Benign osteoblastoma. *Bull Hosp Joint Dis* 1956;17:141–151.
116. Jaffe HL, Mayer L. An osteoblastic osteoid tissue-forming tumor of a metacarpal bone. *Arch Surg* 1932;24:550–564.
117. Kenan S, Floman Y, Robin GC, Laufer A. Aggressive osteoblastoma. A case report and review of the literature. *Clin Orthop* 1985;195:294–298.
118. Kroon HM, Schurmans J. Osteoblastoma: clinical and radiologic findings in 98 new cases. *Radiology* 1990;175:783–790.
119. Lichtenstein L. Benign osteoblastoma. A category of osteoid- and bone-forming tumors other than classical osteoid osteoma, which may be mistaken for giant-cell tumor or osteogenic sarcoma. *Cancer* 1956;9:1044–1052.
120. Lucas DR, Unni KK, McLeod RA, O Connor MI, Sim FH. Osteoblastoma: clinicopathologic study of 306 cases. *Hum Pathol* 1994;25:117–134.

121. Marcove RC, Alpert M. A pathologic study of benign osteoblastoma. *Clin Orthop* 1963;30:175–180.
122. Marsh BW, Bonfiglio M, Brady LP, Enneking WF. Benign osteoblastoma: range of manifestations. *J Bone Joint Surg* 1975;57A:1–9.
123. McLeod RA, Dahlin DC, Beabout JW. The spectrum of osteoblastoma. *Am J Roentgenol* 1976;126:321–325.
124. Mirra JM, Dodd L, Johnston W, Frost DB. Case report 700: Primary intracortical osteosarcoma of femur, sclerosing variant, grade 1 to 2 anaplasia. *Skeletal Radiol* 1991;20:613–616.
125. Mitchell ML, Ackerman LV. Metastatic and pseudomalignant osteoblastoma: a report a two unusual cases. *Skeletal Radiol* 1986;15:213–218.
126. Picci P, Campanacci M, Mirra JM. Osteoid osteoma. Differential clinicopathologic diagnosis. In: Mirra JM, ed. *Bone tumors: clinical, radiologic, and pathologic correlations.* Philadelphia: Lea and Febiger, 1989;411–414.
127. Rutter DJ, van Rijssel TG, van der Velde EA. Aneurysmal bone cysts. A clinicopathological study of 105 cases. *Cancer* 1977;39:2231–2239.
128. Schajowicz F, Lemos C. Malignant osteoblastoma. *J Bone Joint Surg* 1976;58B:202–211.
129. Steiner GC. Ultrastructure of osteoblastoma. *Cancer* 1977;39:2127–2136.
130. Tillman BP, Dahlin DC, Lipscomb PR, Stewart JR. Aneurysmal bone cyst: an analysis of ninety-five cases. *Mayo Clin Proc* 1968;43:478–495.

Osteosarcoma

131. Ackerman LV. Extra-osseous localized non-neoplastic bone and cartilage formation (so-called myositis ossificans). *J Bone Joint Surg* 1958;40A:279–298.
132. Allan CJ, Soule EH. Osteogenic sarcoma of the somatic soft tissues. Clinicopathologic study of 26 cases and review of literature. *Cancer* 1971;27:1121–1133.
133. Alpert LI, Abaci IF, Werthamer S. Radiation-induced extraskeletal osteosarcoma. *Cancer* 1973;31:1359–1363.
134. Amendola MA, Glazer GM, Adha FP, Francis IR, Weatherbee L, Martel W. Myositis ossificans circumscripta: computed tomographic diagnosis. *Radiology* 1983;149:775–779.
135. Amstutz HC. Multiple osteogenic sarcomata—metastatic or multicentric? Cancer 1969;24:923–931.
136. Angervall L, Stener B, Stener I, Ahren C. Pseudomalignant osseous tumor of soft tissue. A clinical, radiological and pathological study of five cases. *J Bone Joint Surg* 1969;51Br:654–663.
137. Ayala AG, Ro JY, Raymond AK, Jaffe N, Chawla S, Carrasco H, Link M, Jimenez J, Edeiken J, Wallace S, Murray JA, Benjamin R. Small cell osteosarcoma. A clinicopathologic study of 27 cases. *Cancer* 1989;64:2162–2173.
138. Ballance WA Jr, Mendelsohn G, Carter JR, Abdul-Karim FW, Jacobs G, Makley JT. Osteogenic sarcoma. Malignant fibrous histiocytoma subtype. *Cancer* 1988;62:763–771.
139. Bane BL, Evans HL, Ro JY, Carrasco CH, Grognon DJ, Benjamin RS, Ayala AG. Extra-skeletal osteosarcoma. A clinico-pathologic study of 26 cases. *Cancer* 1990;65:2762–2770.
140. Bathhurst N, Sanerkin N, Watt I. Osteoclast-rich osteosarcoma. *Br J Radiol* 1986;59:667–673.
141. Bertoni F, Present D, Bacchini P, Pignatti G, Picci P, Campanacci M. The Instituto Rizzoli experience with small cell osteosarcoma. *Cancer* 1989;64:2591–2599.
142. Bloem JL, Kroon HM. Osseous lesions. *Radiol Clin North Am* 1993;31:261–278.
143. Bohndorf K, Reiser M, Lochner B, Feaux de Lacroix W, Steinbrich W. Magnetic resonance imaging of primary tumors and tumor-like lesions of bone. *Skeletal Radiol* 1986;15:511–517.
144. Boyko OB, Cory DA, Cohen MD, Provisor A, Mirkin D, DeRosa GP. MR imaging of osteogenic and Ewing's sarcoma. *Am J Roentgenol* 1987;148:317–322.
145. Broders AC. The microscopic grading of cancer. In: Pack CT, Ariel IM, eds. *Treatment of cancer and allied diseases,* 2nd ed., Vol 1. New York: Paul B. Hoeber, 1958;55.
146. Burgener FA, Perry P. Solitary renal cell carcinoma metastasis in Paget s disease simulating sarcomatous degeneration. *Am J Roentgenol* 1977;128:835–855.
147. Campanacci M, Cervellati G. Osteosarcoma: a review of 345 cases. *Ital J Orthop Traumatol* 1975;1:5–22.
148. Campanacci M, Pizzoferrato A. Osteosarcoma emorragico. *Chir Organi Mov* 1971;60:409–421.
149. Chung EB, Enzinger FM. Extraskeletal osteosarcoma. *Cancer* 1987;60:1132–1142.
150. Dardick I, Schatz JE, Colgan TJ. Osteogenic sarcoma with epithelial differentiation. *Ultrastruct Pathol* 1992;16:463–474.
151. Dahlin DC. Malignant osteoblastic tumors. In: Taveras JM, Ferucci JT, eds. *Radiology: Diagnosis, Imaging, Intervention,* vol 5. Philadelphia: JB Lippincott, 1986;1–10.
152. Dahlin DC. Grading of bone tumors. In: Unni KK, ed. *Bone tumors.* New York: Churchill-Livingstone, 1988;35–45.
153. Dahlin DC, Coventry MB. Osteosarcoma: a study of six hundred cases. *J Bone Joint Surg* 1967;49A:101–110.
154. Dahlin DC, Unni KK. Osteosarcoma of bone and its important recognizable varieties. *Am J Surg Pathol* 1977;1:61–72.
155. Dahlin DC, Unni KK, Matsuno T. Malignant (fibrous) histiocytoma of bone—fact or fancy? *Cancer* 1977;39:1508–1516.
156. Dardick I, Schatz JE, Colgan TJ. Osteogenic sarcoma with epithelial differentiation. *Ultrastruct Pathol* 1992;16:463–474.
157. deSantos LA, Edeiken B. Purely lytic osteosarcoma. *Skeletal Radiol* 1982;9:1–7.
158. deSantos LA, Edeiken BS. Subtle early osteosarcoma. *Skeletal Radiol* 1985;13:44–48.
159. deSantos LA, Murray JA, Finkelstein JB, Spjut HJ, Ayala AG. The radiographic spectrum of periosteal osteosarcoma. *Radiology* 1978;127:123–129.
160. DeSmet AA, Norris MA, Fisher DR. Magnetic resonance imaging of myositis ossificans: analysis of seven cases. *Skeletal Radiol* 1992;21:503–507.
161. Dickerson GR, Rosenberg AE. The ultrastructure of small cell osteosarcoma with a review of light microscopy and differential diagnosis. *Hum Pathol* 1991;221:267–275.
162. Doud TM, Moser RP Jr, Giudici MAI, Frauenhoffer EE, Maurer RJ. Case report 704. Extraskeletal osteosarcoma of the thigh with several suspected skeletal metastases and extensive metastases to the chest. *Skeletal Radiol* 1991;20:628–632.
163. Edeiken J, Raymond AK, Ayala AG, Benjamin RS, Murray JA, Carrasco HC. Small-cell osteosarcoma. *Skeletal Radiol* 1987;16:621–628.
164. Ellis JH, Siegel CL, Martel W, Weatherbee L, Dorfman H. Radiologic features of well-differentiated osteosarcoma. *Am J Roentgenol* 1988;151:739–742.
165. Enzinger F, Weiss S. *Soft tissue tumors.* St. Louis: CV Mosby, 1983.
166. Farr GH, Huvos AG, Marcove RC, Higinbotham NL, Foote FW Jr. Telangiectatic osteogenic sarcoma: a review of twenty-eight cases. *Cancer* 1974;34:1150–1158.
167. Fine G, Stout AP. Osteogenic sarcoma of the extraskeletal soft tissues. *Cancer* 1956;9:1027–1043.
168. Gherlinzoni F, Antoci B, Canale V. Multicentric osteosarcomata (osteosarcomatosis). *Skeletal Radiol* 1983;10:281–285.
169. Glicksman AS, Toker C. Osteogenic sarcoma following radiotherapy for bursitis. *Mt Sinai J Med* 1976;43:163–167.
170. Goldman AB. Myositis ossificans circumscripta: a benign lesion with a malignant differential diagnosis. *Am J Roentgenol* 1976;126:32–40.
171. Gomes H, Menanteau B, Gaillard D, Behar C. Telangiectatic osteosarcoma. *Pediatr Radiol* 1986;16:140–143.
172. Greenfield GB, Arrington JA. *Imaging of bone tumors. A multimodality approach.* Philadelphia: JB Lippincott, 1955;48–91.
173. Greenspan A. Osteosarcoma. *Contemp Diagn Radiol* 1993;16:1–6.
174. Greenspan A, Klein MJ. Osteosarcoma: radiologic imaging, differential diagnosis, and pathological considerations. *Semin Orthop* 1991;6:156–166.
175. Greenspan A, Steiner G, Norman A, Lewis MM, Matlen JJ. Case report 436. Osteosarcoma of the soft tissues of the distal end of the thigh. *Skeletal Radiol* 1987;16:489–492.
176. Hall RB, Robinson LH, Malawer MM, Dunham WK. Periosteal osteosarcoma. *Cancer* 1985;55:165–171.
177. Heinrich SD, Zembo MM, MacEwen GD. Pseudomalignant myositis ossificans. *Orthopedics* 1989;12:599–602.
178. Hermann G, Abdelwahab IF, Kenan S, Lewis MM, Klein MJ. Case report 795. High-grade surface osteosarcoma of the radius. *Skeletal Radiol* 1993;22:383–385.
179. Heul RO van der, Ronnen Jr von. Juxtacortical osteosarcoma. Diag-

nosis, differential diagnosis, treatment, and an analysis of eighty cases. *J Bone Joint Surg* 1967;49A:415–439.

180. Hopper KD, Moser RP Jr, Haseman DB, Sweet DE, Madewell JE, Kransdorf MJ. Osteosarcomatosis. *Radiology* 1990;175:233–239.

181. Hudson TM, Springfield DS, Benjamin M, Bertoni F, Present DA. Computed tomography of parosteal osteosarcoma. *Am J Roentgenol* 1985;144:961–965.

182. Huvos AG, Rosen G, Bretsky SS, Butler A. Telangiectatic osteosarcoma: a clinicopathologic study of 124 patients. *Cancer* 1982;49: 1679–1689.

183. Jaffe HL. Intracortical osteogenic sarcoma. *Bull Hosp Joint Dis* 1960; 21:180–197.

184. Jaffe HL. *Tumors and tumorous conditions of the bones and joints.* Philadelphia: Lea and Febiger, 1968.

185. Jelinek JS, Murphey MD, Kransdorf MJ, Shmookler BM, Malawer MM, Hur RC. Parosteal osteosarcoma: value of MR imaging and CT in the prediction of histologic grade. *Radiology* 1996;201: 837–842.

186. Kaufman RA, Towbin RB. Telangiectatic osteosarcoma simulating the appearance of an aneurysmal bone cyst. *Pediatr Radiol* 1981;11: 102–104.

187. Kenan S, Abdelwahab IF, Klein MJ, Hermann G, Lewis MM. Lesions of juxtacortical origin (surface lesions of bone). *Skeletal Radiol* 1993; 22:337–357

188. Kenan S, Abdelwahab IF, Klein MJ, Hermann G, Lewis MM. Case report 835. Parosteal osteosarcoma involving the left radius. *Skeletal Radiol* 1994;22:229–231.

189. Klein MJ, Kenan S, Lewis MM. Osteosarcoma: clinical and pathological considerations. *Orthop Clin North Am* 1989;20:327–345.

190. Kramer K, Hicks D, Palis J, Rosier RN, Oppenheimer J, Fallon MD, Cohen HJ. Epithelioid osteosarcoma of bone. Immunocytochemical evidence suggesting divergent epithelial and mesenchymal differentiation in a primary osseous neoplasm. *Cancer* 1993;71:2977–2982.

191. Kransdorf MJ, Meis JM. Extraskeletal osseous and cartilaginous tumors of the extremities. *RadioGraphics* 1993;13:853–884.

192. Kransdorf MJ, Meis JM, Jelinek JS. Myositis ossificans: MR appearance with radiologic-pathologic correlation. *Am J Roentgenol* 1991; 157:1243–1248.

193. Kumar N, David R, Madewell JE, Lindell MM Jr. Radiographic spectrum of osteogenic sarcoma. *Am J Roentgenol* 1987;148:767–772.

194. Kyriakos M, Gilula LA, Besich MJ, Schoeneker PL. Intracortical small cell osteosarcoma. *Clin Orthop Rel Res* 1992;279:269–280.

195. Lee YY, Van Tassel P, Nauert C, Raymond AK, Edeiken J. Craniofacial osteosarcomas: plain film, CT and MR findings in 46 cases. *Am J Roentgenol* 1988;150:1397–1402.

196. Levine E, De Smet AA, Huntrakoon M. Juxtacortical osteosarcoma: a radiologic and histologic spectrum. *Skeletal Radiol* 1985;14:38–46.

197. Lindell MM Jr, Shirkhoda A, Raymond AK, Murray JA, Harle TS. Parosteal osteosarcoma: radiologic-pathologic correlation with emphasis on CT. *Am J Roentgenol* 1987;148:323–328.

198. Lopez BF, Rodriquez PJL, Gonzalez LJ, Sanchez HS, Sanchez DCM. Intracortical osteosarcoma. A case report. *Clin Orthop Rel Res* 1991; 268:218–222.

199. Malcolm AJ. Osteosarcoma: classification, pathology, and differential diagnosis. *Semin Orthop* 1988;3:1–12.

200. Martinez-Tello FJ, Navas-Palacios JJ. The ultrastructure of conventional, parosteal, and periosteal osteosarcoma. *Cancer* 1982;50: 949–961.

201. Matsuno T, Unni KK, McLeod RA, Dahlin DC. Telangiectatic osteogenic sarcoma. *Cancer* 1976;38:2538–2547.

202. McKenna RJ, Schwinn CP, Soong KY, Higinbotham NL. Osteogenic sarcoma arising in Paget's disease. *Cancer* 1964;17:42–66.

203. Meneses MF, Unni KK, Swee RG. Bizarre parosteal osteochondromatous proliferation of bone (Nora's lesion). *Am J Surg Pathol* 1993; 17:691–697.

204. Mindell ER, Shah NK, Webster JH. Postradiation sarcoma of bone and soft tissues. *Orthop Clin North Am* 1977;8:821–834.

205. Mirra JM, Gold RH, Picci P. Osseous tumors of intramedullary origin. In: Mirra JM, ed. *Bone tumors.* Philadelphia: Lea and Febiger, 1989; 143–438.

206. Moore TE, King AR, Kathol MH, El-Khoury GY, Palmer R, Downey PR. Sarcoma in Paget disease of bone: clinical, radiologic, and pathologic features in 22 cases. *Am J Roentgenol* 1991;156:1199–1203.

207. Mulder JD, Schütte HE, Kroon HM, Taconis WK. *Radiologic atlas of bone tumors.* Amsterdam: Elsevier, 1993;51–76.

208. Nora FE, Dahlin DC, Beabout JW. Bizarre parosteal osteochondromatous proliferations of the hands and feet. *Am J Surg Pathol* 1983; 7:245–250.

209. Norman A, Dorfman H. Juxtacortical circumscribed myositis ossificans: evolution and radiographic features. *Radiology* 1970;96: 301–306.

210. Norton KI, Hermann G, Abdelwahab IF, Klein MJ, Granowetter LF, Rabinowitz JG. Epiphyseal involvement in osteosarcoma. *Radiology* 1991;180:813–816.

211. Nuovo MA, Norman A, Chumas J, Ackerman LV. Myositis ossificans with atypical clinical, radiographic, or pathologic findings: a review of 23 cases. *Skeletal Radiol* 1992;21:87–101.

212. Okada K, Frassica FJ, Sim FH, Beabout JW, Bond JR, Unni KK. Parosteal osteosarcoma. A clinicopathological study. *J Bone Joint Surg* 1994;76A:366–378.

213. Okada K, Kubota H, Ebina T, Kobayashi T, Abe E, Sato K. High-grade surface osteosarcoma of the humerus. *Skeletal Radiol* 1995;24: 531–534.

214. Onikul E, Fletcher BD, Parham DM, Chen G. Accuracy of MR imaging for estimating intraosseous extent of osteosarcoma. *Am J Roentgenol* 1996;167:1211–1215.

215. Partovi S, Logan PM, Janzen DL, O Connell JX, Connell DG. Low-grade parosteal osteosarcoma of the ulna with dedifferentiation into high-grade osteosarcoma. *Skeletal Radiol* 1996;25:497–500.

216. Price CHG, Goldie W. Paget's sarcoma of bone: a study of eighty cases from the Bristol and Leeds bone tumor registries. *J Bone Joint Surg* 1969;51B:205–224.

217. Rao U, Cheng A, Didolkar MS. Extraosseous osteogenic sarcoma: clinicopathological study of eight cases and review of literature. *Cancer* 1978;41:1488–1496.

218. Raymond AK. Surface osteosarcoma. *Clin Orthop Rel Res* 1991;270: 140–148.

219. Ritts GD, Pritchard DJ, Unni KK, Beabout JW, Eckardt JJ. Periosteal osteosarcoma. *Clin Orthop* 1987;219:299–307.

220. Robinson LH, Pitt MJ, Jaffe KA, Siegal GP. Small cell osteosarcoma of the soft tissue. *Skeletal Radiol* 1995;24:462–465.

221. Roessner A, Hobik HP, Grundmann E. Malignant fibrous histiocytoma of bone and osteosarcoma: a comparative light and electron microscopic study. *Pathol Res Pract* 1979;164:385–401.

222. Rosenberg ZS, Leu S, Schmahmann S, Steiner GC, Beltran J, Present D. Osteosarcoma: subtle, rare, and misleading plain film features. *Am J Roentgenol* 1995;165:1209–1214.

223. Ruiter DJ, Cornelisse CJ, van Rijssel TG, van der Velde EA. Aneurysmal bone cyst and telangiectatic osteosarcoma. A histopathological and morphometric study. *Virchows Arch (A)* 1977;373:311–325.

224. Sanerkin NG. Definitions of osteosarcoma, chondrosarcoma and fibrosarcoma of bone. *Cancer* 1980;46:178–185.

225. Sauer DD, Chase DR. Case report 461. Dedifferentiated parosteal osteosarcoma. *Skeletal Radiol* 1988;17:72–76.

226. Schajowicz F, McGuire MH, Araujo ES, Muscolo DL, Gitelis S. Osteosarcomas arising on the surfaces of long bones. *J Bone Joint Surg* 1988;70A:555–564.

227. Schajowicz F, Araujo ES, Berenstein M. Sarcoma complicating Paget s disease of bone: a clinicopathological study of 62 cases. *J Bone Joint Surg* 1983;65B:299–307.

228. Schreiman JS, Crass JR, Wick MR, Maile CW, Thompson RC Jr. Osteosarcoma: role of CT in limb-sparing treatment. *Radiology* 1986; 161:485–488.

229. Seeger LL, Eckardt JJ, Bassett LW. Cross-sectional imaging in the evaluation of osteogenic sarcoma: MRI and CT. *Semin Roentgenol* 1989;24:174–184.

230. Sim FH, Unni KK, Beabout JW, Dahlin DC. Osteosarcoma with small cells simulating Ewing s tumor. *J Bone Joint Surg* 1979; 61A:207–217.

231. Sim FH, Kurt A-M, McLeod RA, Unni KK. Case report 628. Low-grade central osteosarcoma. *Skeletal Radiol* 1990;19:457–460.

232. Simon MA, Bos GD. Epiphyseal extension of metaphyseal osteosarcoma in skeletally immature individuals. *J Bone Joint Surg* 1980; 62A:195–204.

233. Sissons HA, Greenspan A. Paget's disease. In: Taveras JM, Ferrucci JT, eds. *Radiology: diagnosis, imaging, intervention,* vol 5. Philadelphia: JB Lippincott, 1986;1–14.

234. Smith J, Ahuja SC, Huvos AG, Bullough PG. Parosteal (juxtacortical) osteogenic sarcoma: a roentgenological study of 30 patients. *J Can Assoc Radiol* 1978;29:167–174.

235. Smith J, Botet JF, Yeh SDJ. Bone sarcoma in Paget s disease: a study of 85 patients. *Radiology* 1984;152:583–590.
236. Sordillo PP, Hajdu SI, Magill GB, Goldbey RB. Extraosseous osteogenic sarcoma. A review of 48 patients. *Cancer* 1983;51:727–734.
237. Stevens GM, Pugh DG, Dahlin DC. Roentgenographic recognition and differentiation of parosteal osteogenic sarcoma. *Am J Roentgenol* 1957;78:1–12.
238. Sundaram M, McGuire MH, Herbold DR. Magnetic resonance imaging of osteosarcoma. *Skeletal Radiol* 1987;16:23–29.
239. Taconis WK. Osteosarcoma and its variants. *J Med Imag* 1988; 2:276–285.
240. Torres FX, Kyriakos M. Bone infarct-associated osteosarcoma. *Cancer* 1992;70:2418–2430.
241. Tsuneyoshi M, Dorfman HD. Epiphyseal osteosarcoma: distinguishing features from clear cell chondrosarcoma, chondroblastoma and epiphyseal enchondroma. *Hum Pathol* 1987;18:644–651.
242. Unni KK. Osteosarcoma of bone. In: Unni KK, ed. *Bone tumors.* New York: Churchill Livingstone, 1988;107–133.
243. Unni KK, Dahlin DC. Grading of bone tumors. *Semin Diagn Pathol* 1984;1:165–172.
244. Unni KK, Dahlin DC. Premalignant tumors and conditions of bone. *Am J Surg Pathol* 1979;3:47–60.
245. Unni KK, Dahlin DC, Beabout JW. Periosteal osteogenic sarcoma. *Cancer* 1976;37:2476–2485.
246. Unni KK, Dahlin DC, McLeod RA. Intraosseous well-differentiated osteosarcoma. *Cancer* 1977;40:1337–1347.
247. Van Der Heul RO, von Ronnen JR. Juxtacortical osteosarcoma. Diagnosis, differential diagnosis, treatment, and an analysis of eighty cases. *J Bone J Surg* 1967;49A:415–439.
248. Varma DGK, Ayala AG, Guo S-Q, Moulopoulos LA, Kim EE, Charnsangavej C. MRI of extraskeletal osteosarcoma. *J Comput Assist Tomogr* 1993;17:414–417.
249. Verela-Duran J, Enzinger FM. Calcifying synovial sarcoma. *Cancer* 1982;50:345–352.
250. Vigorita VJ, Jones JK, Ghelman B, Marcove RC. Intracortical osteosarcoma. *Am J Surg Pathol* 1984;8:65–71.
251. Waxman M, Vuletin JC, Saxe BI, Monteleone FA. Extraskeletal osteosarcoma. Light and electron microscopic study. *Mt Sinai J Med* 1981;48:322–329.
252. Wold LE. Fibrohistiocytic tumors of bone. In: Unni KK, ed. *Bone tumors.* New York: Churchill Livingstone, 1988;183–197.
253. Wold LE, Unni KK, Beabout JW, Sim FH, Dahlin DC. Dedifferentiated parosteal osteosarcoma. *J Bone Joint Surg* 1984;66A:53–59.
254. Wold LE, Unni KK, Beabout JW, Pritchard DJ. High-grade surface osteosarcomas. *Am J Surg Pathol* 1984;8:181–186.
255. Wong KT, Haygood T, Dalinka MK, Kneeland B. Chondroblastic, grade 3 periosteal osteosarcoma. *Skeletal Radiol* 1995;24:69–71.
256. Wurlitzer F, Ayala A, Romsdahl M. Extraosseous osteogenic sarcoma. *Arch Surg* 1972;105:691–695.
257. Yamaguchi H, Nojima T, Yagi T, Masuda T, Sasaki T. High-grade surface osteosarcoma of the left ilium. A case report and review of the literature. *Acta Pathol Jpn* 1988;38:235–240.
258. Zimmer WD, Berquist TH, McLeod RA, Sim FH, Pritchard DJ, Shives TC, Wold LE, May GR. Magnetic resonance imaging of osteosarcoma. Comparison with computed tomography. *Clin Orthop* 1986;289–299.

CHAPTER 3

Tumors of Cartilaginous Origin

INTRODUCTION

Diagnosis of a bone lesion as originating from cartilage is usually a simple task for the radiologist. The lesion's radiolucent matrix, scalloped margin, and annular, punctate, or comma-shaped calcifications usually suffice to establish its chondrogenic nature (Fig. 1). However, whether a cartilage tumor is benign or malignant is sometimes extremely difficult for the radiologist and the pathologist to determine (30,38,42).

All cartilage tumors, whether benign or malignant, exhibit a positive reaction for S-100 protein (34). This is sometimes diagnostically useful, as most other bone tumors do not display this reaction. Histologically, cartilage tumors are usually recognized by the features of their intercellular matrix, which has a uniformly translucent appearance and contains less collagen compared with the intercellular matrix of osteoblastic tumors, such as osteoblastoma and osteosarcoma. The tumor cells themselves are usually located in rounded spaces (lacunae), as in normal cartilage. In benign cartilage tumors, such as enchondroma, the tissue is sparsely cellular (Fig. 2). The cells, typically with small, dark-staining nuclei, fail to show the cytologic features that are characteristic of chondrosarcoma, such as large nuclei; pleomorphism; large, swollen chondroblastic and double nuclei; and mitoses. The tumor tissue is usually avascular, and areas of degenerate and calcified matrix are common. Calcification is sometimes followed by vascularization and replacement by bone, as in normal endochondral ossification. Because of their slow

growth, enchondromas erode and expand the overlying cortical bone (Fig. 3) but do not invade it, unlike chondrosarcomas. Nevertheless, some slow-growing, low-grade chondrosarcomas can masquerade as enchondromas, and some aggressive-looking benign cartilage lesions may be mistakenly diagnosed as chondrosarcomas. Moreover, it is important to be aware of the capricious biologic behavior displayed by cartilage tumors. Some benign-appearing lesions of cartilage may behave in an aggressive or malignant manner, whereas tumors that present an ominous appearance on radiologic or histologic examination may show limited progression.

Clinically, malignancy is suggested by a variety of signs, including development of pain in a previously asymptomatic lesion (e.g., malignant transformation of enchondroma to chondrosarcoma), development of swelling or a mass at the site of a lesion, or rapid growth of a lesion (e.g., malignant transformation of osteochondroma to chondrosarcoma). Radiologically, the presence of a periosteal reaction, destruction of the cortex, and a soft tissue mass are almost pathognomonic features of malignancy (19). The histopathologic features of a malignant cartilage tumor include the presence of hypercellular and pleomorphic tumor tissue, appreciable numbers of plump cells with large or double nuclei, invasion (permeation) of bony trabeculae, and infiltration of Haversian systems and bone marrow (Fig. 4). However, these obvious features of malignancy may be not so prominent in biopsy specimen, or only a few areas in such a specimen may reveal the diagnostic features of malignancy. As Dahlin

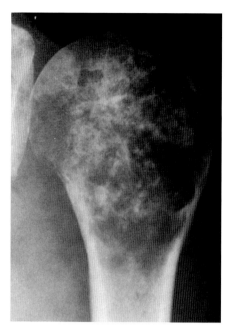

FIG. 1. Cartilage-forming tumor. The radiologic characteristics of a radiolucent matrix, scalloped margin, and annular, and comma-shaped calcifications establish the chondrogenic nature of this lesion (in this example—chondrosarcoma).

pointed out, in the pathologic evaluation it is necessary to examine many fields in these tumors to be certain that there is sufficient evidence for a diagnosis of malignancy because evidence that a tumor is a chondrosarcoma rather than a benign enchondroma is frequently found in isolated areas within the mass (9). Therefore, it is of paramount importance to obtain biopsy specimens from several areas of a tumor. Close cooperation between the clinician, the radiologist, and the pathologist in reviewing the history, the radiologic examination, and the biopsy specimens is crucial to reaching a conclusion on the exact nature of a cartilage lesion.

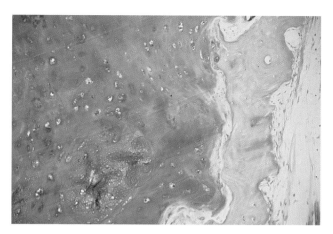

FIG. 3. Histopathology of enchondroma. An enchondroma is eroding the cortex, but there is no evidence of invasion (hematoxylin and eosin, original magnification ×183). (Courtesy Dr. M. J. Klein, New York, NY.)

From the radiologic standpoint, the differential diagnosis of cartilage lesions should focus on the following three points:

1. Distinguishing a benign cartilage tumor from the noncartilaginous lesions (e.g., calcifying enchondroma from bone infarct; enchondroma located near the articular end of bone from giant-cell tumor, osteoarthritic geode, or intraosseous ganglion; or chondromyxoid fibroma from aneurysmal bone cyst).
2. Distinguishing a benign cartilage tumor from a malignant one (e.g., enchondroma from low-grade chondrosarcoma; osteochondroma from exostotic chondrosarcoma; periosteal chondroma from periosteal chondrosarcoma; or synovial chondromatosis from synovial chondrosarcoma).
3. Distinguishing a malignant cartilage tumor from a noncartilaginous lesion (e.g., chondrosarcoma at the articu-

FIG. 2. Histopathology of a benign cartilage tumor. Sparsely cellular tissue and uniform-sized chondrocytes located in rounded lacunae are characteristic features of enchondroma (hematoxylin and eosin, original magnification ×235).

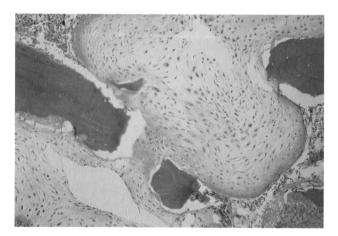

FIG. 4. Histopathology of chondrosarcoma. Invasion of trabeculae by markedly cellular tissue of chondrosarcoma (hematoxylin and eosin, original magnification ×25). (Courtesy Dr. M. J. Klein, New York, NY.)

lar end of bone from giant-cell tumor or from malignant fibrous histiocytoma; or periosteal chondrosarcoma from periosteal osteosarcoma).

From the histopathologic standpoint, because the microscopic features of cartilage lesions are obvious and characteristic, focus should be directed to the following:

1. Recognition of the varieties of benign cartilage tumors (e.g., enchondroma, periosteal chondroma, chondroblastoma, chondromyxoid fibroma) and various subtypes of chondrosarcoma (e.g., clear-cell, mesenchymal, or periosteal).
2. Recognition of benign versus malignant tumor (e.g., enchondroma vs. well-differentiated chondrosarcoma; chondromyxoid fibroma vs. myxoid chondrosarcoma; or chondroblastoma vs. mesenchymal chondrosarcoma).
3. Differentiation of chondrosarcoma from other malignant tumors that contain cartilage (e.g., from chondroblastic osteosarcoma or periosteal osteosarcoma).

BENIGN LESIONS

Enchondroma

Enchondroma is the second most common benign tumor of bone and is characterized by the formation of mature hyaline cartilage. It constitutes about 10% of all benign bone tumors and represents the most common tumor of the phalanges of the hand. Several theories have been postulated regarding its etiology. Among these is that the enchondroma develops from abnormal zones of dysplastic chondrocytes in the growth plate. These abnormal foci fail to undergo normal endochondral ossification; instead, they are deposited within the metaphysis and, as the bone grows, are displaced into the diaphysis (30). Customarily, a lesion located centrally in the bone is called an enchondroma, whereas one located outside the cortex is called a chondroma (periosteal or juxtacortical). Separate groups consist of lesions (a) located in the soft tissues and (b) located in the joint, bursa, or in the tendon sheath. The former are called soft-tissue chondromas and the latter synovial chondromatosis (41).

Clinical Presentation

Although the tumor may occur at any age, most cases arise between the second and fourth decades; there is no sex predilection. The short, tubular bones of the hand and foot (phalanges, metacarpals, and metatarsals) are preferred sites, followed in frequency by the femur, humerus, tibia, and ribs (Fig. 5). The lesion is often asymptomatic and usually is discovered incidentally to a pathologic fracture through the tumor.

The single most important complication of the lesion is malignant transformation to chondrosarcoma. In a solitary enchondroma this occurs predominantly in a long or flat bone, and almost never in a short tubular bone. An important

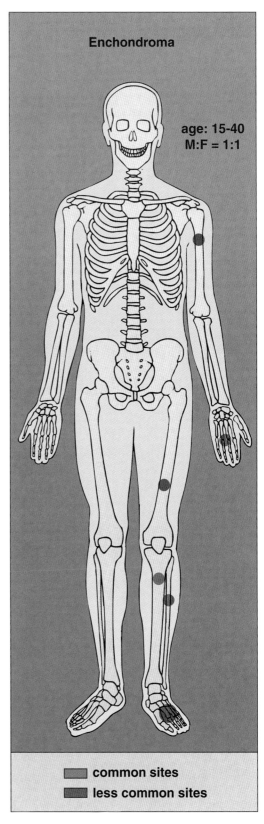

FIG. 5. Enchondroma: skeletal sites of predilection, peak age range, and male-to-female ratio.

clinical sign is development of pain at the site of the lesion in a previously asymptomatic patient and in the absence of a fracture.

Imaging

Plain film radiography and conventional tomography are usually sufficient to demonstrate the lesion and to establish its chondroid character. In short tubular bones the lesion is often entirely radiolucent (Fig. 6), but in long bones it may display visible calcifications (18). This flocculent mineralization usually assumes the form of dots, rings, and arcs, giving a "popcorn" appearance (Fig. 7). If the calcifications are extensive, the lesion is called a calcifying enchondroma (Fig. 8). The cortex is usually thinned and expanded in a symmetric, fusiform fashion. The often cloudy or hazy appearance of a lesion provides a clue to its chondroid composition (15). The lesion can also be recognized by scalloped inner cortical margins, reflecting the lobular growth pattern of cartilage (Fig. 9). Computed tomography (CT) and magnetic resonance imaging (MRI) may further delineate the tumor and more precisely localize it in the bone (Fig. 10). Because in long bones enchondroma may present as a radiolucent lesion with poorly defined margins, particularly in areas where trabeculae are sparse or absent (diaphysis), MRI may be extremely helpful in revealing the exact size

and extent of the tumor (Fig. 11) (45). Like most cartilaginous and fibrous lesions, enchondroma exhibits low to intermediate signal intensity on T1-weighted images and high signal intensity on T2-weighted sequences. On gradient echo sequences the lesion may appear less bright than on conventional T2-weighted images (see Fig. 11E). The calcifications image either as signal void or as low-signal-intensity foci. After administration of gadolinium, enchondroma demonstrates a typical pattern of signal enhancement, which is helpful in distinguishing this lesion from noncartilaginous tumors (33,136).

Histopathology

On histologic examination, enchondroma consists of lobules of hyaline cartilage of variable cellularity and can be recognized by the features of its intercellular matrix, which has a uniformly translucent appearance and contains relatively little collagen (Fig. 12A). The tumor cells are located in lacunae. The tissue is sparsely cellular and the cells contain small, dark-staining nuclei (Fig. 12B). Binucleated cells and small nucleoli are sometimes present (32) (Fig. 12C). Calcifications are common and correspond to matrix calcifications or actual endochondral ossifications at the periphery of cartilage lobules (Fig. 13). Enchondromas located in the

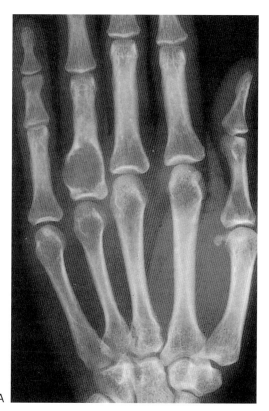
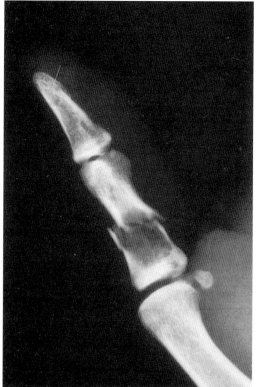

A

B

FIG. 6. Enchondroma in short tubular bones. **A:** A typical, purely radiolucent lesion at the base of the proximal phalanx of the ring finger in a 37-year-old woman. Note the marked attenuation of the ulnar side of the cortex. **B:** A radiolucent lesion at the base of the proximal phalanx of the thumb with a pathologic fracture.

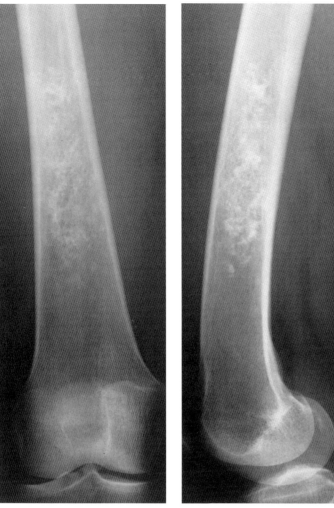

A,B

FIG. 7. Enchondroma in a long bone. (**A**) Anteroposterior and (**B**) lateral radiographs of the femur show a radiolucent lesion with "popcorn" calcifications.

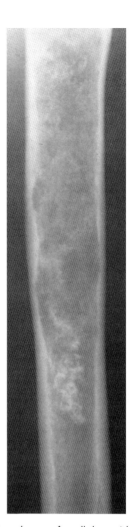

FIG. 9. Enchondroma. A radiolucent lesion exhibits central calcifications and scalloped inner cortical margins, reflecting the lobular growth pattern of cartilage.

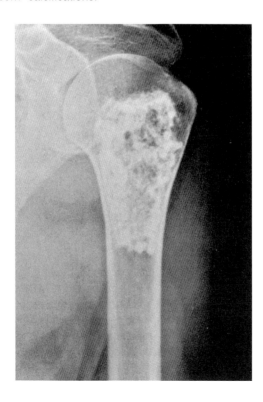

FIG. 8. "Calcifying enchondroma." A heavily calcified lesion in the proximal humerus of a 58-year-old woman.

127

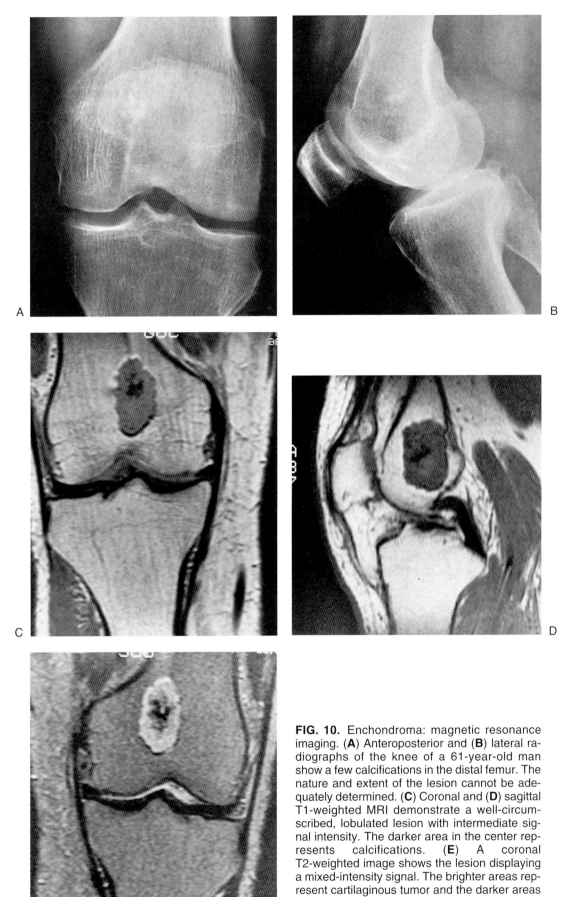

FIG. 10. Enchondroma: magnetic resonance imaging. (**A**) Anteroposterior and (**B**) lateral radiographs of the knee of a 61-year-old man show a few calcifications in the distal femur. The nature and extent of the lesion cannot be adequately determined. (**C**) Coronal and (**D**) sagittal T1-weighted MRI demonstrate a well-circumscribed, lobulated lesion with intermediate signal intensity. The darker area in the center represents calcifications. (**E**) A coronal T2-weighted image shows the lesion displaying a mixed-intensity signal. The brighter areas represent cartilaginous tumor and the darker areas represent calcifications.

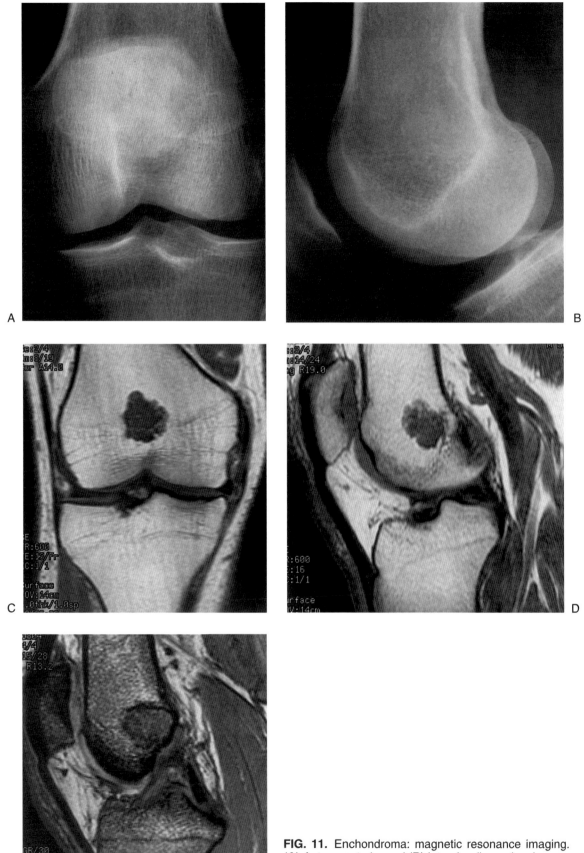

FIG. 11. Enchondroma: magnetic resonance imaging. (**A**) Anteroposterior and (**B**) lateral radiographs show an almost nondiscernible lesion in the distal femur. (**C**) Coronal and (**D**) sagittal T1-weighted sequences reveal the full extent of the lesion. (**E**) On T2* (MPGR) image, enchondroma is not as bright as on conventional T2-weighted images.

129

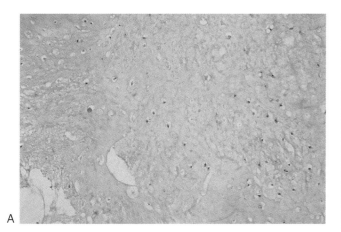

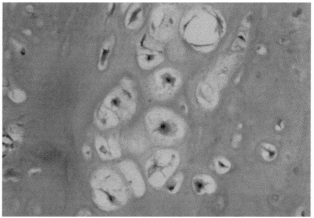

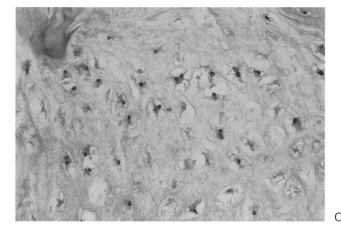

FIG. 12. Histopathology of enchondroma. **A:** At low magnification the lesion exhibits hyaline cartilage of low cellularity (hematoxylin and eosin, original magnification ×40). **B:** At higher magnification the chondrocytes with darkly stained nuclei are seen to be located in the lacunae (hematoxylin and eosin, original magnification ×100). **C:** Occasionally binucleated cells may be present (hematoxylin and eosin, original magnification ×150) (C—courtesy of Dr. K. K. Unni, Rochester, Minnesota.)

short tubular bones of hands and feet may exhibit increased cellularity, plump nuclei, and occasionally even binucleated cells.

Periosteal (Juxtacortical) Chondroma

Periosteal or juxtacortical chondroma, a slow-growing lesion, affects the surface of a bone in or beneath the periosteum. Preferred sites include the proximal humerus, femur, tibia, and the phalanges of the hand (33). This is an uncommon neoplasm, accounting for about only 0.66% of bone tumors in the Mayo Clinic series (35). Periosteal chondroma was first described by Lichtenstein and Hall in 1952 (26). It occurs in children and adults (most commonly in the second and third decades), who usually present with a history of pain and local tenderness, often accompanied by swelling at the involved site.

The radiographic appearance is rather characteristic (5). The lesion is small and is located on the surface of the bone (Fig. 14). As it enlarges, it erodes the underlying cortex in a saucer-like fashion, displaying a sclerotic rim and producing a buttress of periosteal new bone formation (10). The lesion may contain calcifications (Fig. 15). Computed tomography may show the scalloped cortex, matrix calcification (Fig. 16), and cortical shell (21,24). It also may demonstrate the separation of a lesion from the medullary cavity, an impor-

tant feature in differentiation from osteochondroma (20). Magnetic resonance imaging (MRI) findings correspond to radiographic findings, depicting the cartilaginous soft tissue component (47). If periosteal chondroma affects the medullary canal, MRI may be useful in depicting the extent of involvement (Fig. 17). Fat suppression or enhanced gradient echo sequences may improve tumor–marrow contrast

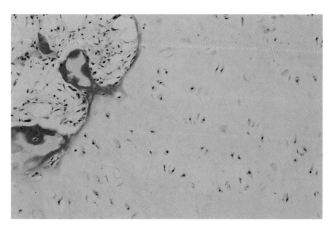

FIG. 13. Histopathology of enchondroma. Cartilage lobules are surrounded by a narrow rim of bone, representing endochondral ossification (hematoxylin and eosin, original magnification ×250).

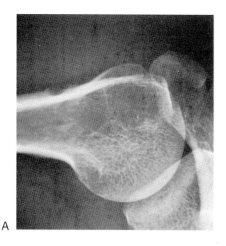

A

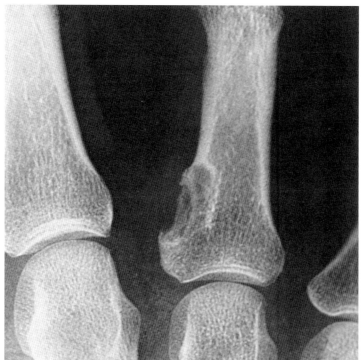

B

FIG. 14. Periosteal chondroma. **A:** A radiolucent lesion erodes the external surface of the cortex of the proximal humerus of a 24-year-old man. **B:** A well-defined, saucer-like erosion of the cortex of the proximal phalanx is characteristic of periosteal chondroma. (Reprinted from Bullough PG. *Atlas of orthopedic pathology,* 2nd ed. New York: Gower, 1992;16.22.) **C:** A metaphyseal periosteal chondroma affecting the fifth metacarpal bone erodes the cortex and evokes the buttress of periosteal reaction.

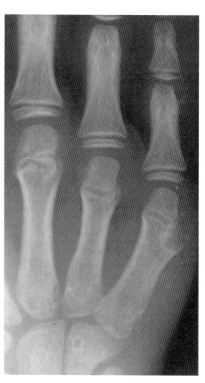

C

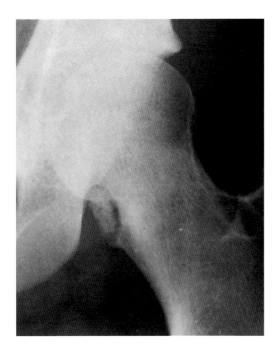

FIG. 15. Periosteal chondroma. A lesion displaying calcifications erodes the medial cortex of the femoral neck. The buttress of a periosteal reaction seen at the inferior border of the lesion is characteristic of periosteal chondroma.

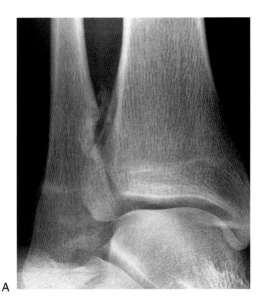

A

FIG. 16. Periosteal chondroma: computed tomography. **(A)** A plain radiograph shows a lesion with calcifications eroding the medial cortex of the distal fibula. **(B)** CT using a bony window and **(C)** a soft tissue window better demonstrates the extent of the lesion and the distribution of the calcifications.

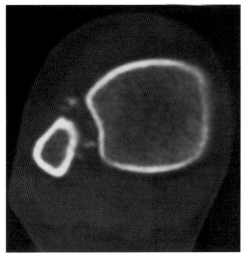

B

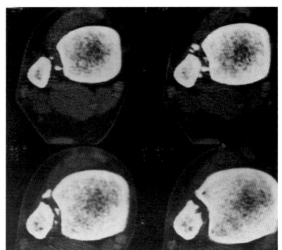

C

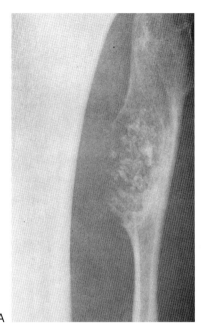

A

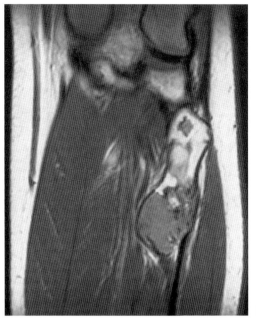

B

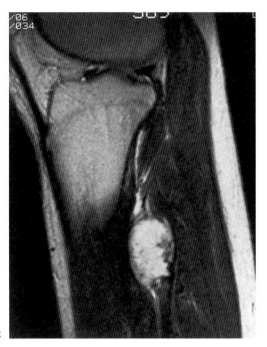

C

FIG. 17. Periosteal chondroma: magnetic resonance imaging. (**A**) A large lesion blends imperceptibly with the medial fibular cortex and extends into the medullary cavity. In such a presentation, differential diagnosis must include enchondroma protuberans and chondrosarcoma. (**B**) Coronal proton-density (SE, TR 2000, TE 19) and (**C**) sagittal T2-weighted (SE, TR 2000, TE 70) MRI show the lesion's extension into the bone marrow.

(4). The potential pitfall of MRI is marrow edema mimicking tumor invasion or vice versa (47). Unlike enchondroma and osteochondroma, periosteal chondroma may continue to grow after skeletal maturation (16). Some lesions may attain a large size (up to 6 cm) and may resemble osteochondromas (20) (Fig. 18 and Fig. 34). Some lesions may mimic an aneurysmal bone cyst (43). Very rarely the lesion may encase itself intracortically, thus mimicking other intracortical lesions (such as intracortical angioma, intracortical fibrous dysplasia, or intracortical bone abscess) (1).

On histologic examination, the findings are identical to those of enchondroma, although the lesion sometimes exhibits a higher level of cellularity, occasionally with atypical and binucleated cells (Fig. 19). Well-formed lamellar bone or fibrous connective tissue separates the cartilaginous nodules, and in some instances deposition of calcium can be observed (13).

Enchondromatosis (Ollier Disease) and Maffucci Syndrome

Enchondromatosis is a condition marked by multiple enchondromas, usually involving the metaphyses and diaphyses. If skeletal involvement is extensive, and particularly if the involvement is unilateral [resembling the original case described by Ollier in 1899 (31)], the term "Ollier disease"

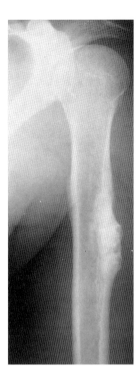

FIG. 18. Periosteal chondroma. A large lesion eroding the cortex of the proximal humerus resembles a sessile osteochondroma. Note the periosteal reaction and separation of the tumor from the medullary cavity by a cortex, features that help in the differentiation from osteochondroma. (Courtesy Dr. K. K. Unni, Rochester, Minnesota.)

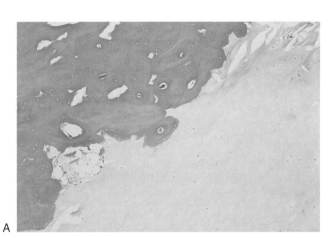

A

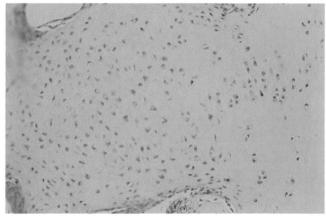

B

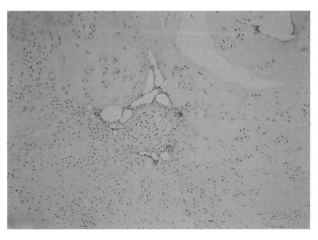

C

FIG. 19. Histopathology of periosteal chondroma. **A:** At the interface with adjacent cortex, the cartilaginous tumor erodes the bone (hematoxylin and eosin, original magnification ×40). **B:** The tumor tissue is more cellular than conventional enchondroma, and some cells appear atypical (hematoxylin and eosin, original magnification ×100). (Reprinted from Bullough PG. *Atlas of orthopedic pathology,* 2nd ed. New York: Gower, 1992;16.22.) **C:** Hyaline cartilage with a rather dense cell population, slight cell pleomorphism, and signs of cell proliferation. These histologic variations are compatible with a benign cartilage lesion in a periosteal location (hematoxylin and eosin, original magnification ×25).

is applied (40). There is no hereditary or familial tendency in this disorder, which some investigators consider to be developmental rather than neoplastic, classifying it as a form of bone dysplasia. The femur, tibia, and ilium are the most commonly affected bones (43), followed by the phalanges, metacarpals, and metatarsals. Much less often the lesions involve the facial bones, skull, spine, carpal, and tarsal bones (14) (Fig. 20).

Maffucci syndrome is a congenital, nonhereditary disorder, characterized by enchondromatosis and soft tissue angiomatosis (hemangiomatosis). The latter may occur anywhere in the skin and subcutaneous tissue. The hemangiomas are usually cavernous and may be unilateral or bilateral, localized or extensive. The skeletal lesions in Maffucci syndrome have the same distribution as those in Ollier disease, with a strong predilection for one side of the body (46).

Clinical Presentation

The condition has a strong preference for involvement of one side of the body. The clinical manifestations, such as knobby swellings of the digits or gross disparities in limb length, are commonly recognized during childhood and adolescence. The affected child often begins to limp during the second year of life as a disparity in leg length becomes apparent (long bones that are affected are always shorter because the growth plate is involved). Pain is uncommon and when present is usually due to a pathologic fracture (33). Ollier disease is often arrested at puberty but may occasionally progress after that time. The most common and severe complication of Ollier disease is malignant transformation of one or more enchondromas to chondrosarcoma (see Figs. 109 and 110) (27). Schajowicz believes that about 30% of the patients with Ollier disease will develop chondrosarcoma (40), but Jaffe (22) and Mirra (30) have estimated that risk to be as high as 50%. However, because patients with enchondromatosis or Ollier disease may develop hundreds of enchondromas, the statistical risk of one given lesion to undergo malignant degeneration is probably not higher than in solitary enchondroma. Unlike solitary enchondromas, in patients with enchondromatosis even lesions in the short tubular bones may undergo sarcomatous changes. This is particularly true in patients with Maffucci syndrome (44).

Imaging

The radiographic appearance of enchondromatosis involving the hands and feet is quite characteristic. Radiolucent masses of cartilage with foci of calcifications closely resembling solitary enchondromas markedly deform the bones (Fig. 21). Enchondromas in this location may be intracortical and periosteal (31). They sometimes protrude from the shaft of the short or long bone, thus resembling osteochondroma (Fig. 22). However, unlike osteochondroma, these

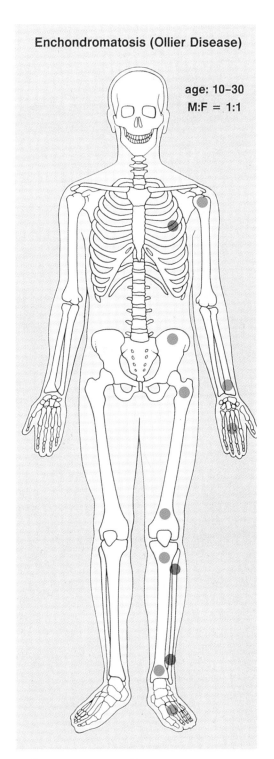

FIG. 20. Enchondromatosis (Ollier disease): skeletal sites of predilection, peak age range, and male-to-female ratio.

protruding enchondromas have neither a cartilaginous cap nor a bony stalk. Also unlike osteochondroma, the protrusions do not point away from the adjacent joint (30). In the long bones, columns of radiolucent streaks extend from the growth plate into the diaphysis. Coalescence of metaphyseal enchondromas often causes asymmetric enlargement of the

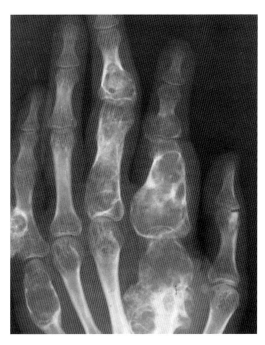

FIG. 21. Enchondromatosis (Ollier disease). Large, lobulated cartilaginous masses markedly deform the bones of the hand.

long bones and flaring of the metaphyses. Interference with the growth plate causes foreshortening and deformity of the bones (Fig. 23). In the pelvis, and particularly in the iliac bones, a fan-like linear pattern is characteristic (Fig. 24). Maffucci syndrome is recognized radiographically by multiple calcified phleboliths in addition to the typical alterations of enchondromatosis (Fig. 25).

Histopathology

Histologically, the lesions in enchondromatosis are essentially indistinguishable from those of solitary enchondromas, although they sometimes tend to be predominantly myxoid, more cellular, and may exhibit more cellular atypia (Fig. 26). Mitoses and prominent nucleoli are uncommon, and anaplasia is not observed (9). However, binucleated cells are often present.

Differential Diagnosis

Radiology

The main differential diagnosis in solitary enchondroma, particularly when it is located in long bones and exhibits substantial calcifications ("calcifying enchondroma") is *medullary bone infarct* (Fig. 27). At times the two lesions are difficult to distinguish from one another because of similar calcifications, particularly when the enchondroma is small.

A number of radiographic features can be helpful in the differential diagnosis. These include lobulation of the margins of an enchondroma, punctate or annular calcifications within the matrix, and absence of the peripheral sclerotic fibro-osseous wall commonly observed in bone infarcts (15). Mineral deposits also tend to exhibit a more central distribution, and the calcifications often have a markedly stippled appearance (Fig. 28). Although the ring-like calcifications typical of enchondroma are occasionally present in medullary bone infarct, they are usually larger and have thicker walls. As a rule, bone infarct, unlike enchondroma, does not expand bone contours (32) except in rare cases of encystification (36) (**see Fig. 7-41**). The distribution of the medullary bone infarcts that commonly affect the proximal and distal femur and the proximal tibia may be helpful in the differential diagnosis.

The most difficult task for the radiologist is to distinguish a large solitary enchondroma from a slowly growing *low-grade chondrosarcoma*. One of the most significant findings pointing to a chondrosarcoma in the early stage of

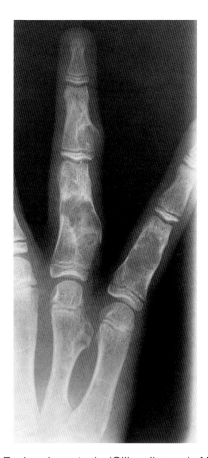

FIG. 22. Enchondromatosis (Ollier disease). Multiple lesions are observed in the phalanges and metacarpals. The intracortical lesion in the metaphysis of the fourth metacarpal protrudes from the bone, thus resembling an osteochondroma.

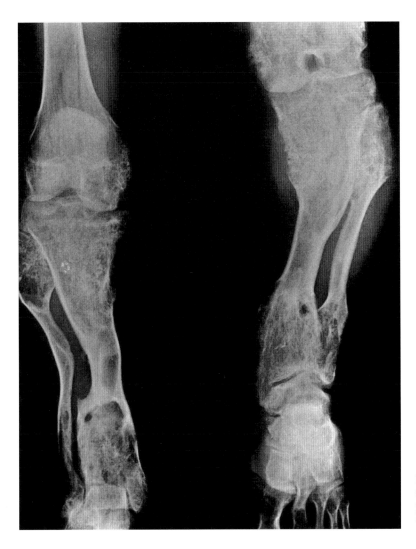

FIG. 23. Enchondromatosis (Ollier disease). An anteroposterior radiograph of both legs of a 17-year-old boy shows growth stunting and marked deformities of the tibiae and fibulae.

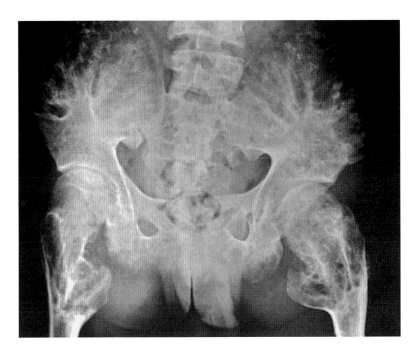

FIG. 24. Enchondromatosis (Ollier disease). An anteroposterior radiograph of the pelvis demonstrates crescent-shaped and ring-like calcifications in tongues of cartilage extending from the iliac crests and the proximal femora, classic features of Ollier disease

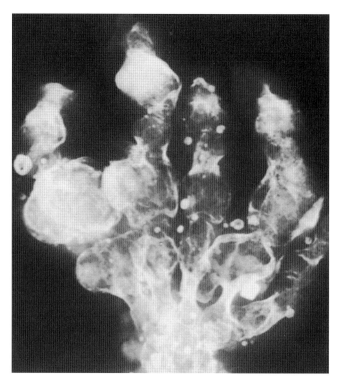

FIG. 25. Maffucci syndrome. A radiograph of the hand of a patient with Maffucci syndrome reveals typical changes of enchondromatosis, accompanied by calcified phleboliths in soft tissue hemangiomas. (Reprinted from Bullough PG. *Atlas of orthopedic pathology,* 2nd ed. New York: Gower, 1992; 14.9).

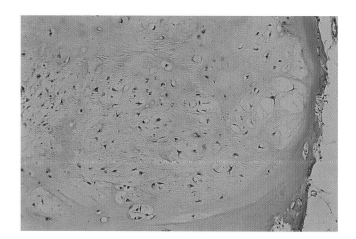

FIG. 26. Histopathology of enchondromatosis. Lobular and cellular appearance of cartilaginous nodules. These lesions usually exhibit more cellularity than is seen in solitary enchondroma (hematoxylin and eosin, original magnification ×50). (Reprinted from Bullough PG. *Atlas of orthopedic pathology,* 2nd ed. New York: Gower, 1992;14.8.)

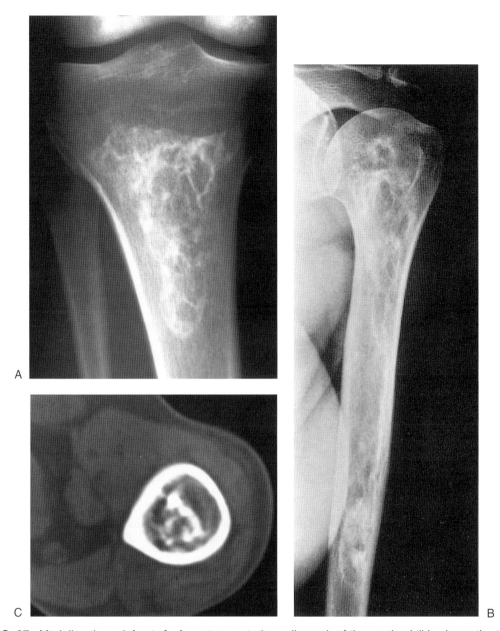

FIG. 27. Medullary bone infarct. **A:** An anteroposterior radiograph of the proximal tibia shows the typical coarse calcifications of bone infarct. Note the sharply defined peripheral margin separating infarcted from viable bone and the lack of characteristic for cartilage tumor annular and comma-shaped calcifications (**compare with Fig. 7**). **B:** In a medullary bone infarct, seen here in the proximal humerus of a 36-year-old man with sickle cell disease, there is no endosteal scalloping of the cortex, and the calcified area is surrounded by a thin, dense sclerotic rim, the hallmark of a bone infarct. **C:** In another patient with a bone infarct in the distal femur, a CT section reveals central calcifications and no endosteal scalloping of the cortex.

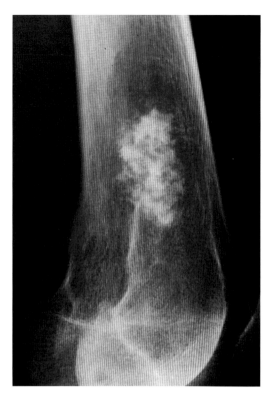

FIG. 28. Enchondroma. Typical appearance of annular and stippled calcifications within a radiolucent lesion.

development is localized thickening of the cortex (Fig. 29). The size of the lesion should also be taken into consideration: lesions longer than 4 cm are suggestive of malignancy (Fig. 30). In more advanced lesions, destruction of the cortex and the presence of a soft tissue mass are the hallmarks of malignancy.

It is equally important to distinguish sarcomatous transformation in patients with multiple enchondromatosis and Ollier disease. Radiography will reveal intralesional radiolucencies and cortical destruction associated with a soft tissue mass (see Fig. 110A).

If enchondroma, particularly in a short tubular bone, extends to the articular end of the bone, *giant-cell tumor* should be included in the differential diagnosis. The latter contains no calcifications, an important differential clue. However, some enchondromas may not display visible calcifications. In addition, giant-cell tumor usually lacks a sclerotic border. In the long tubular bones this distinction is much easier because enchondroma, unlike giant-cell tumor, only rarely extends into the articular end of bone (Fig. 31). Enchondroma may mimic *solitary bone cyst,* although the latter is a rare occurrence in the short tubular bones. If an enchondroma is found in the distal phalanx of the hand and does not contain calcifications, an *epidermoid cyst* is a differential possibility.

An intracortical enchondroma, or an enchondroma that causes nonsymmetric cortical expansion, may be mistaken

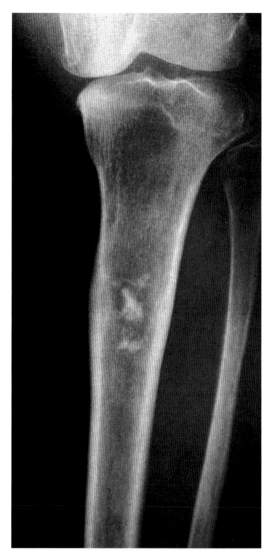

FIG. 29. Low-grade chondrosarcoma. A 48-year-old woman presented with pain in the upper leg. A plain radiograph shows a radiolucent lesion in the proximal tibia with a wide zone of transition and central calcifications. Note the thickening of the cortex, a feature that distinguishes chondrosarcoma from similarly appearing enchondroma.

for *osteochondroma* (**see Fig. 22**). However, the distribution of the mineral matrix visualized within enchondroma usually helps to distinguish the two entities.

Enchondroma protuberans may create a problem in diagnosis (7). Enchondroma protuberans has been defined as an exophytic enchondroma of a long bone, although it may affect a rib as well (23). It arises in the medullary cavity but penetrates the cortex, forming a prominent exophytic mass on the surface of bone, and thus can mimic any surface lesion (e.g., osteoma, osteochondroma, periosteal chondroma, myositis ossificans). It also should be distinguished from chondrosarcoma, either primary or one developing in a preexisting enchondroma. Further distinction must be made

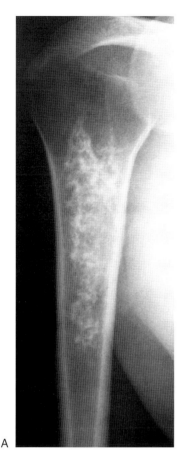

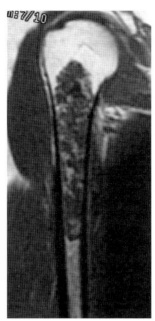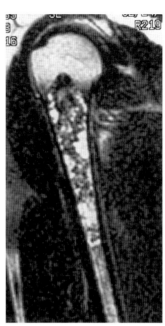

B, C

FIG. 30. Low-grade chondrosarcoma. (**A**) A plain radiograph in a 48-year-old man shows a cartilaginous lesion in the proximal right humerus. Although the cortex is not thickened, the length of the lesion (15 cm) suggests malignancy. (**B**) Coronal T1-weighted. (**C**) T2-weighted MRI show inhomogeneous signal intensity, which may be seen in both enchondroma and chondrosarcoma. On biopsy, the tumor proved to be a low-grade chondrosarcoma.

A

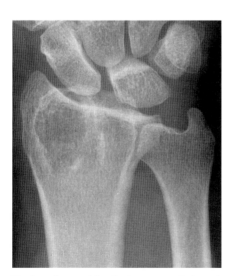

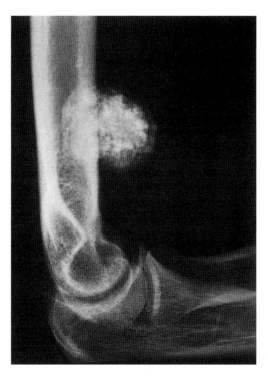

FIG. 31. Enchondroma. The lesion extends into the articular end of the distal radius and therefore may mimic a giant cell tumor. However, unlike the latter, there are a few faintly visualized calcifications and a sclerotic margin.

FIG. 32. Differential diagnosis of periosteal chondroma: tumoral calcinosis. In tumoral calcinosis, although soft tissue calcification may look very similar to that of periosteal chondroma, there is no evidence of periosteal buttress formation.

from the simultaneous occurrence of an osteochondroma and an enchondroma in the same bone (39) (Fig. 32).

Periosteal chondroma should be radiographically differentiated from a variety of other subperiosteal lesions (e.g., *periosteal ganglion, periosteal Ewing sarcoma)*, as well as from *myositis ossificans and tumoral calcinosis.* Features of myositis ossificans have been described in the section on extraskeletal osteosarcoma. The pattern of zoning phenomenon is diagnostic of the former lesion. Features of tumoral calcinosis (Fig. 33) have been described in the section on synovial sarcoma (**see Chapter 9**).

A large periosteal chondroma may closely resemble *sessile osteochondroma* and vice versa. The key to distinguishing between these two lesions is the separation of periosteal chondroma from the medullary portion of the bone by intervening cortex (20) (Fig. 34). Conversely, in a typical osteochondroma the cortex of the host bone merges with the cortex of the lesion, and continuity exists between the medullary cavity of the host bone and the exostosis (see Fig. 38B). Another useful characteristic is the value of attenuation coefficient of the lesion, as determined from CT scans: the base of the osteochondroma, composed mainly of trabecular bone, shows higher numbers for this variable than does the cartilaginous matrix of periosteal chondroma.

Pathology

The main problem is to distinguish benign enchondroma from *low-grade chondrosarcoma.* In the majority of cases, particularly if the histologic picture is typical and the lesion is not cellular, this distinction does not create a problem (Fig. 35). However, if the lesion is cellular, and particularly if it affects the long bones, the pathologist must take care not to confuse an enchondroma with a low-grade chondrosarcoma, and vice versa.

Cell atypias and uneven distribution of cells may be found to a higher degree in enchondromas of the hands and feet without prognostic significance. However, when an enchondroma is located in long tubular bones, particularly in the humerus and femur, or in bones of the trunk, slight histologic atypias have prognostic significance. From observations of large series over long periods of time we know that tumors with these characteristics may recur once or several times and may degenerate to a chondrosarcoma of intermediate or high grade, or even to a dedifferentiated chondrosarcoma.

The microscopic distinction between benign cartilage of enchondromatosis and *low-grade chondrosarcoma* is difficult (13). Necrosis and myxoid stroma strongly favor the diagnosis of chondrosarcoma (17).

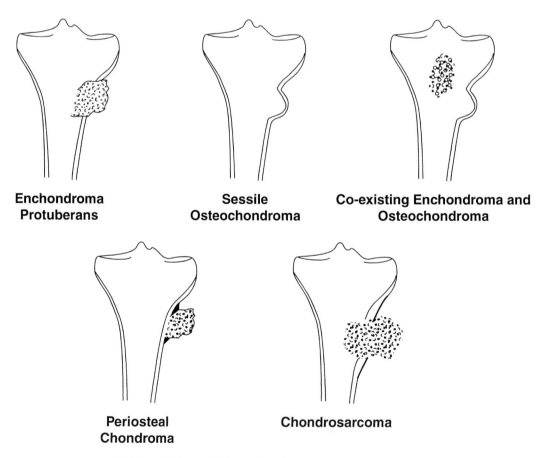

Enchondroma Protuberans **Sessile Osteochondroma** **Co-existing Enchondroma and Osteochondroma** **Periosteal Chondroma** **Chondrosarcoma**

FIG. 33. Differential diagnosis of enchondroma protuberans.

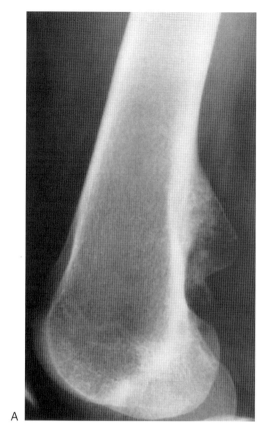

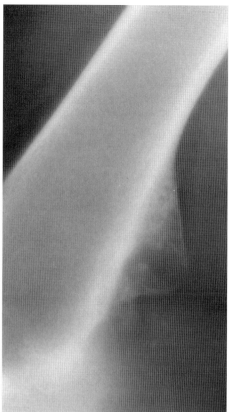

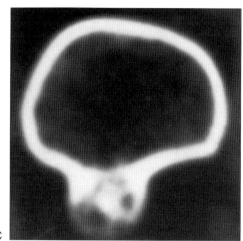

FIG. 34. Periosteal chondroma resembling osteochondroma. **A:** A plain radiograph shows a bony excrescence arising from the posterior cortex of the distal femur that looks like a sessile osteochondroma. **B:** A conventional tomography shows calcifications at the base of the lesion and lack of interruption of the posterior cortex of the femur. **C:** A CT section demonstrates lack of communication between the medullary portion of the femur and the lesion, thus excluding the diagnosis of osteochondroma. *Continued on page 144.* (A and C—reprinted with permission from Greenspan *et al. Can Assoc Radiol J,* 1993; 44:205–208.)

Histologically, *periosteal chondroma* must be differentiated from *periosteal chondrosarcoma* and *periosteal osteosarcoma* (**see Figs. 2-94, 2-95**). The latter lesion, however, is usually grade 2 or 3, exhibits a diaphyseal location, and contains osteoid or less commonly, mature bone.

Radiologic and pathologic differential diagnosis of enchondroma and periosteal chondroma is depicted in Fig. 36.

Soft-Tissue Chondroma

These rare lesions occur preferentially in the soft tissues of hands and feet. A soft-tissue chondroma located close to a joint is known as a para-articular chondroma (29). Because these lesions exhibit a wide range of cytologic variations, as in the case of cartilage tumors of bone, they are commonly misdiagnosed as chondrosarcomas (15). They have no

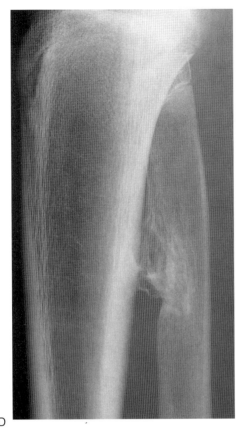

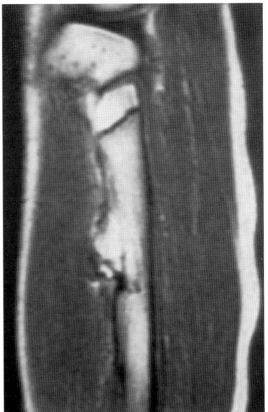

D

E

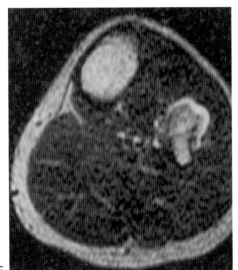

F

FIG. 34. *Continued.* **D:** In another patient the lateral radiograph of the proximal leg demonstrates a lesion that may represent either a sessile osteochondroma or a periosteal chondroma. **E:** A sagittal T1-weighted (SE, TR 600, TE 20) MRI reveals that the lesion is brighter than the fibula's bone marrow and the anterior fibular cortex does not interrupt medullary continuity, suggesting a diagnosis of osteochondroma. **F:** This diagnosis is further confirmed with an axial T2-weighted (SE, TR 2000, TE 80) MRI that shows unequivocally not only the merging of the medullary portions of the lesion and the host bone, but a cartilaginous cap (*bright signal*), characteristic of osteochondroma.

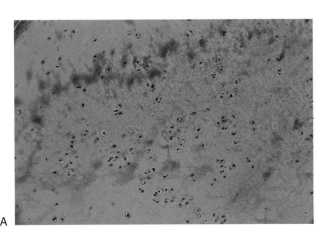

A

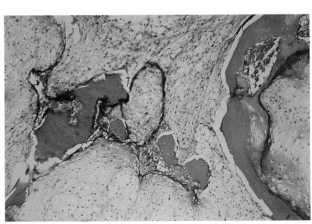

B

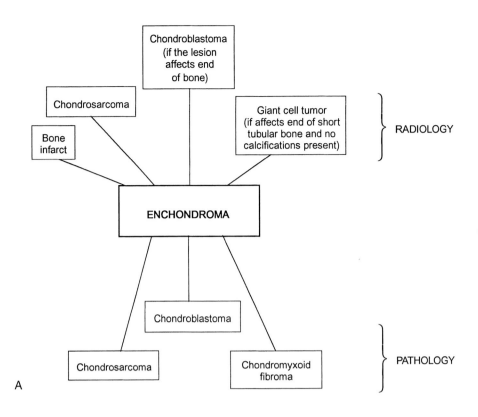

A

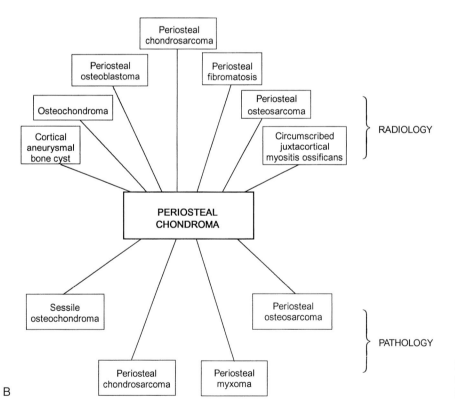

B

FIG. 36. Radiologic and pathologic differential diagnosis of (**A**) enchondroma and (**B**) periosteal chondroma.

FIG. 35. Low-grade chondrosarcoma. **A:** Chondrocytes with a moderate degree of pleomorphism and irregularly distributed within a chondroid matrix point to a low-grade malignancy (van Gieson's original magnification ×25). **B:** Resorption of the bone trabeculae surrounded by chondroblastic tumor tissue that infiltrates the marrow spaces, and a dense arrangement of chondrocytes correspond to grade 2 tumor (hematoxylin and eosin, original magnification ×25).

predilection for either gender and most patients are 20 years or older, with a mean occurrence during the fourth and fifth decades (6). These lesions are usually small, ranging from 2 cm to 4 cm. On radiographic studies they present as well-defined soft tissue masses, often (33% to 77%) with calcifications similar to those seen in enchondroma (48). They are not attached to the periosteum or cortex of a bone and are not found within the confines of a joint capsule or tendon sheath (2,8,11). On histopathologic examination they consist of masses of hyaline cartilage, which are commonly lobulated and sometimes partially myxoid (15). They may contain focal areas of fibrosis, hemorrhage, necrosis, calcification, ossification, or granuloma formation (2,11).

Differential Diagnosis

Radiology

The main differential possibility is *periosteal chondroma*. This lesion is, however, attached to the periosteum or cortex and usually produces a cortical erosion and buttress of periosteal reaction. *Myositis ossificans* can result in a mineralized mass; however, it exhibits a classic zoning phenomenon while calcifications in the soft-tissue chondroma are distributed in a haphazard pattern. *Synovial chondromatosis* is a condition affecting joints and tendon sheaths, and CT or MRI is usually able to identify intraarticular or within the tendon sheath location. *Benign mesenchymoma* of soft tissue may contain calcifications. These lesions are composed primarily of mature hyaline cartilage. The difference between soft-tissue chondroma and mesenchymoma is that the latter may also contain adipose and vascular elements (28). Lesions reported in the literature as soft tissue osteochondromas may appear similar to soft-tissue chondromas although in addition to calcifications they also may contain bony elements (25).

Tumoral calcinosis usually presents on radiography as a well-defined lobulated calcific mass, exhibiting a layering effect when imaged with a horizontal beam (3,37).

Soft-tissue chondrosarcomas are rare lesions (11). Unlike soft tissue chondromas they almost never occur in the hands and feet, their preferred sites being in the proximal parts of extremities and buttocks. *Synovial sarcoma* exhibits a soft tissue mass and, in approximately 25% to 30% of reported cases, calcifications. It is usually accompanied by destruction of adjacent bones.

The radiologic and pathologic differential diagnosis of soft-tissue chondroma is depicted in Fig. 37.

Osteochondroma (Osteocartilaginous Exostosis)

Clinical Presentation

Osteochondroma, the most common benign bone lesion (representing 45% of all benign bone tumors and 12% of all bone tumors) (9), is a cartilage-capped bony projection on the external surface of a bone. Usually diagnosed before the third decade, it most commonly involves the metaphyses of long bones, particularly around the knee and the proximal humerus. In general, the lower extremities are more often af-

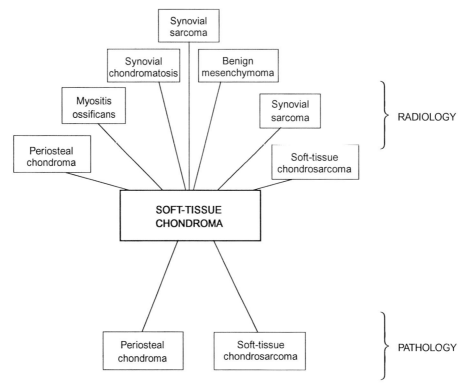

FIG. 37. Radiologic and pathologic differential diagnosis of soft-tissue chondroma.

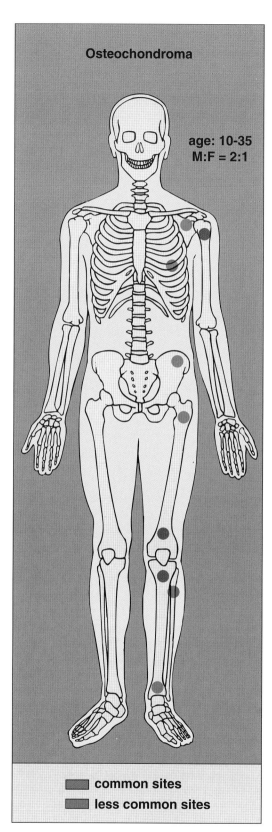

FIG. 38. Osteochondroma: skeletal sites of predilection, peak age range, and male-to-female ratio.

fected than the upper extremities. The flat bones, including the scapula, ilium, and clavicle, are much less commonly affected (Fig. 38). The lesion, which possesses its own growth plate, usually stops growing at skeletal maturity. Osteochondroma is usually asymptomatic unless it causes pressure on adjacent muscles, nerves, or blood vessels (61), as well as on adjacent bone, occasionally with consequent fracture (70). Other complications have been reported, such as fracture of the lesion itself (51) and inflammatory changes of the bursa exostotica covering the cartilaginous cap (49,52,56) (**see Figs. 51 and 52**). Malignant transformation to chondrosarcoma is very rare, occurring in <1% of solitary lesions (**see Fig. 49**). Pain (in the absence of a fracture, bursitis, or pressure on nerves) and a growth spurt or continued growth of the lesion beyond skeletal maturity are highly suspicious for this complication (68) (Table 1).

Imaging

Radiographic presentation of osteochondroma depends on the type of lesion. The pedunculated osteochondroma manifests with a slender pedicle, which is usually directed away from the neighboring growth plate or joint (Fig. 39A). The sessile osteochondroma exhibits a broad base attached to the cortex (Fig. 39B). In either type, the most important identifying features are that the cortex of the host bone merges without interruption with the cortex of the osteochondroma and that the cancellous portion of the lesion is continuous with the medullary cavity of the adjacent diaphysis. Calcifications in the chondro-osseous portion of the stalk of the lesion are also typical features. CT scanning can establish unequivocally the continuity of cancellous portions of the lesion and the host bone (Fig. 40). These characteristics distinguish this lesion from the occasionally similar-appearing bone masses of osteoma, juxtacortical osteosarcoma, soft tissue osteosarcoma, and juxtacortical myositis ossificans (**see Fig. 2-6**). CT or MRI examination will demonstrate the cartilaginous cap (32) (Fig. 41). On MRI the cartilaginous cap shows a high signal intensity on T2-weighted and gradient echo sequences. A narrow band of low signal intensity surrounding the cap represents the perichondrium (56,65) (Fig. 42). Small areas of various degrees of signal void and low signal intensity represent cartilage calcifications. Gadolinium-enhanced MRI may be helpful in demonstrating peripheral enhancement in osteochondroma, corresponding to fibrovascular tissue covering the nonenhancing cartilage cap (55).

Scintigraphy will show variably increased uptake by the lesion (12). The intensity of activity is directly correlated with the degree of chondral ossification (64). However, the main use of scintigraphy is to search for multiple lesions, when only a single osteochondroma has been discovered by radiography.

Histopathology

Histologically, the cap of the osteochondroma is composed of hyaline cartilage arranged similarly to a growth plate. A zone of provisional calcification is present, corresponding to the areas of calcifications in the chondro-

TABLE 1. *Clinical and radiologic features suggesting malignant transformation of osteochondroma*

Clinical features	Radiologic findings	Imaging modality
Pain (in the absence of feature, bursitis, or pressure on nearby nerves)	Enlargement of the lesion	Plain films (comparison with earlier radiographs)
Growth spurt (after skeletal maturity)	Development of a bulky cartilaginous cap, usually 2–3 cm thick	CT, MRI
	Dispersed calcifications in the cartilaginous cap	Plain films Conventional tomography
	Development of a soft tissue mass with or without calcifications	Plain films, CT, MRI
	Increased uptake of isotope after closure of growth plate (not always reliable)	Scintigraphy (planar and SPECT)

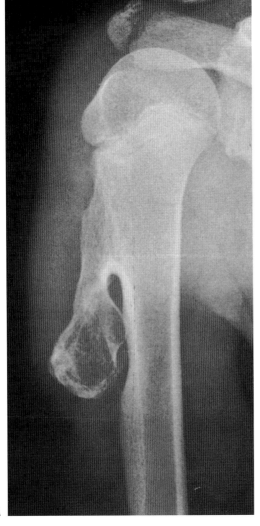

A

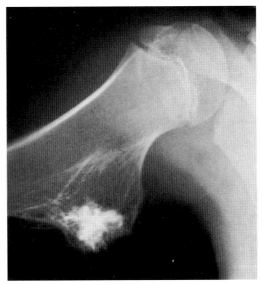

B

FIG. 39. Osteochondroma. **A:** Pedunculated osteochondroma. The typical pedunculated type of osteochondroma is seen arising near the proximal growth plate of the right humerus in a 13-year-old boy. **B:** Sessile osteochondroma. Broad-based variant of osteochondroma is seen here arising from the medial cortex of the proximal diaphysis of the right humerus in a 14-year-old boy. Note that in both lesions the cortex of the host bone merges, without interruption, with the cortex of the lesion, and the medullary portion of both lesions and the medullary cavities of the adjacent bones communicate

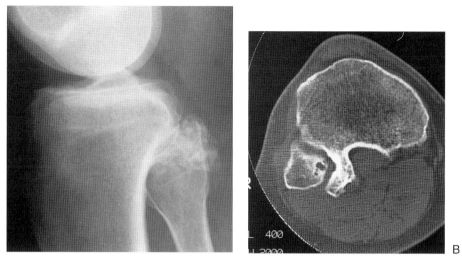

FIG. 40. Osteochondroma: computed tomography. **A:** A lateral radiograph of the knee shows a calcified lesion at the posterior aspect of the proximal tibia. The exact nature of this lesion can not be ascertained. **B:** CT clearly establishes the continuity of the cortex, which extends without interruption from the osteochondroma into the tibia. Note also that the medullary portion of the lesion and the tibia communicate.

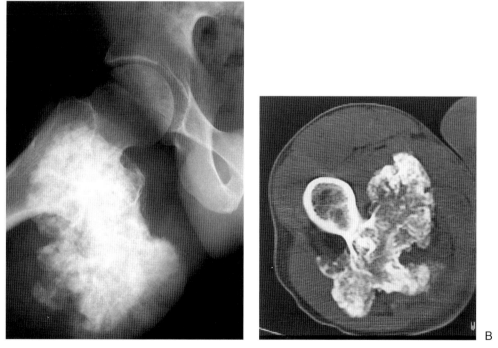

FIG. 41. Osteochondroma: computed tomography. **A:** A plain radiograph shows a large osteochondroma arising at the intertrochanteric area of the right femur. **B:** CT section shows the heavily calcified, cauliflower-like mass and a thin, cartilaginous cap.

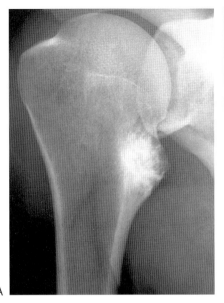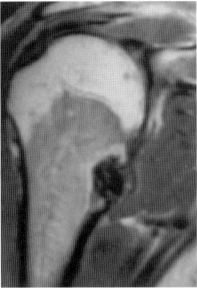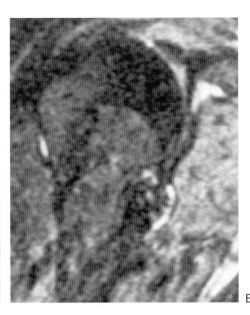

A   B, C

FIG. 42. Osteochondroma: magnetic resonance imaging. **A:** A plain radiograph shows a sessile lesion at the medial aspect of the proximal humeral diaphysis. **B:** T1-weighted coronal MRI reveals that the lesion exhibits a low signal intensity because of significant mineralization. **C:** T2-weighted image shows the thin, cartilaginous cap as an area of high signal intensity, covered by a linear area of low signal intensity representing perichondrium.

osseous portion of the stalk (Fig. 43). The thickness of the cartilaginous cap ranges from 1 mm to 3 mm and rarely up to 1 cm. Greater thickness may imply the possibility of transformation to chondrosarcoma (15). A delicate, fibrous membrane known as the perichondrium, representing a continuation of the periosteum of the adjacent bony cortex, overlies the cartilaginous cap **(see Fig. 43D)**. With age the cap atrophies and in some instances disappears completely (32).

Multiple Hereditary Osteochondromata

Classified by some authorities among the bone dysplasias, multiple osteochondromata, also known as multiple osteocartilaginous exostoses, familial osteochondromatosis, or diaphyseal aclasis, represent an autosomal dominant, hereditary disorder (60). There is a decided 2:1 male predilection (Fig. 44). The lesions are usually discovered at about 2 years of age. The knees, hips, ankles, and shoulders are the most commonly affected sites and growth disturbances are often present, primarily in the forearms and legs (Fig. 45) (69). There is evidence of defective metaphyseal remodeling with deformation of affective bones, and asymmetric retardation of longitudinal bone growth (13). The radiologic features are similar to those of a solitary osteochondroma; the sessile form of the lesion is more common (Figs. 46 to 48).

The pathologic features of multiple osteochondromata are the same as those of solitary lesions. Malignant transformation to chondrosarcoma in osteochondromatosis is more common (5% to 15%) than in solitary lesions, not only because of the greater number of lesions present but because of the higher risk for malignant transformation of each lesion.

Lesions at the shoulder girdle and around the pelvis are usually at greater risk for this complication.

Differential Diagnosis

Radiology

The most important differential diagnosis is the distinction between benign osteochondroma and *exostotic chondrosarcoma* arising in previous exostosis. It is important to recognize early the features that suggest malignant transformation of osteochondroma to chondrosarcoma. Radiographic evaluation may reveal a constellation of features suggesting this complication: development of a thick, bulky cartilaginous cap (usually more than 2 to 3 cm in thickness) (59,66); development of a soft tissue mass with or without calcifications; and dispersed calcifications within the cartilaginous cap, separate from those contained in the stalk (Fig. 49), a sign described by Norman and Sissons (68). The most reliable imaging modalities for evaluating possible malignant transformation are plain radiography, conventional tomography, CT, and MRI (50,94). Plain films usually demonstrate containment of the calcifications of osteochondroma within the stalk of the lesion, but occasionally conventional tomography can also be helpful (Fig. 50). Dispersement of the calcifications in the cartilaginous cap and increased thickness of the cap, the cardinal signs of malignant degeneration, can be demonstrated by any of the above-mentioned modalities. Radionuclide bone scan can also be performed and may reveal increased uptake of radiopharmaceutical agent at the site of a lesion. Exostotic chondrosar-

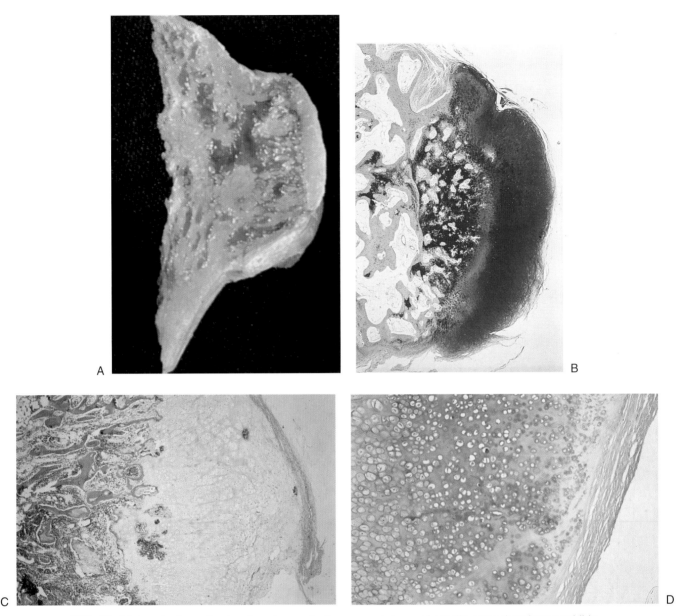

FIG. 43. Histopathology of osteochondroma. **A:** A gross specimen of sessile osteochondroma exhibits characteristic features of the lesion: continuity of the cortex and medullary cavity and a thin, cartilaginous cap. (Reprinted with permission from Bullough PG. *Atlas of orthopedic pathology,* 2nd ed. New York: Gower, 1992;14.10.) **B:** The tumor consists of the hyaline cartilage cap with strong metachromasia of the matrix. A broad zone of endochondral ossification borders the cancellous bone containing the remnants of cartilaginous matrix (*center*) (Giemsa, original magnification ×6). **C:** At higher magnification areas of calcification are seen in the chondro-osseous portion of the lesion. These areas correspond to a zone of provisional calcification in the growth plate (hematoxylin and eosin, original magnification ×30). **D:** A hyaline cartilage cap is seen at the periphery of the lesion, and beneath it transformation of cartilage into bone by endochondral ossification. A thin fibrous membrane (perichondrium) loosely overlies the cartilage (hematoxylin and eosin, original magnification ×60).

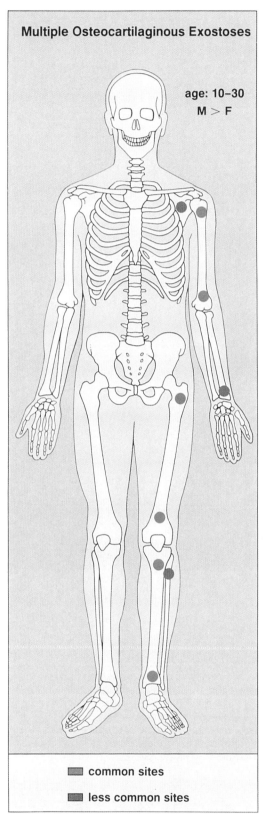

Multiple Osteocartilaginous Exostoses

age: 10–30
M > F

■ common sites

▦ less common sites

FIG. 44. Multiple osteocartilaginous exostoses: skeletal sites of predilection, peak age range, and male-to-female ratio.

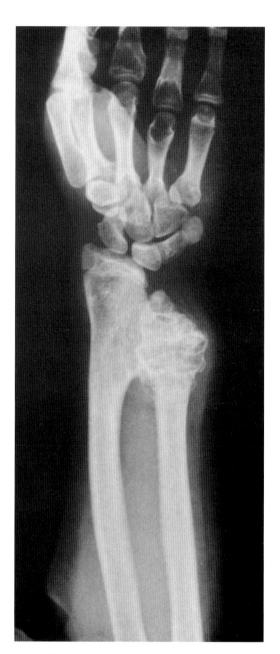

FIG. 45. Multiple osteocartilaginous exostoses. A radiograph of the distal forearm of an 8-year-old boy with multiple osteochondromas shows growth disturbance in the distal radius and ulna.

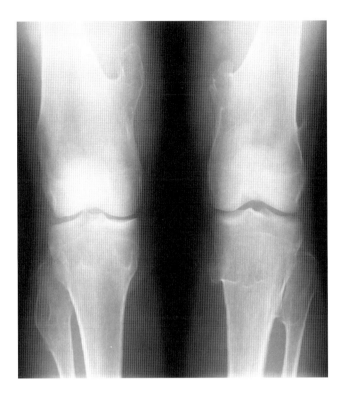

FIG. 46. Multiple osteocartilaginous exostoses. An anteroposterior radiograph of both knees of a 17-year-old boy shows numerous sessile and pedunculated lesions.

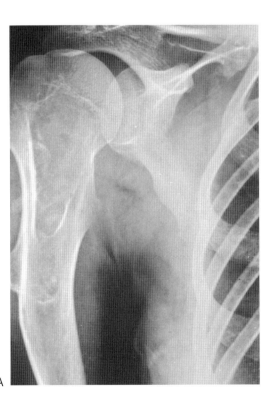

A

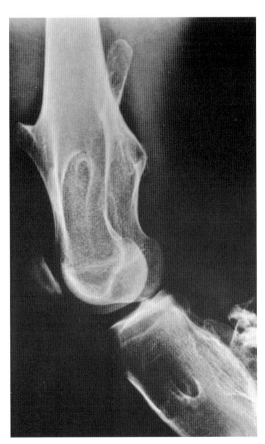

B

FIG. 47. Multiple osteocartilaginous exostoses. **A:** An anteroposterior radiograph of the shoulder of a 22-year-old man with familial multiple osteochondromas demonstrates multiple sessile lesions involving the proximal humerus and scapula. **B:** Involvement of the distal femur and proximal tibia in the same patient is characteristic of this disorder.

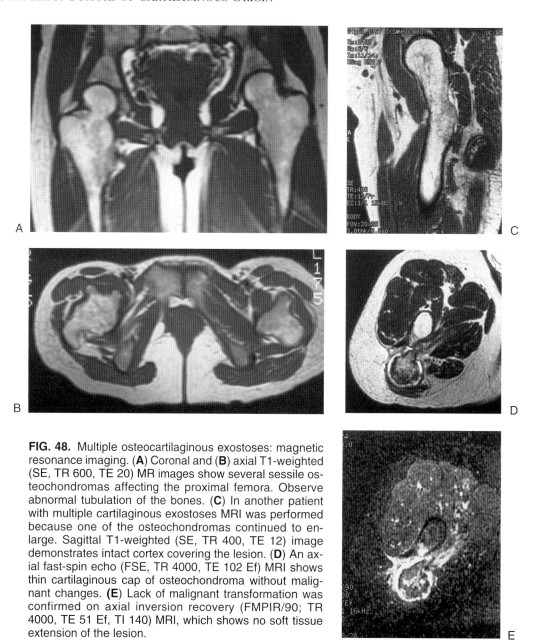

FIG. 48. Multiple osteocartilaginous exostoses: magnetic resonance imaging. (**A**) Coronal and (**B**) axial T1-weighted (SE, TR 600, TE 20) MR images show several sessile osteochondromas affecting the proximal femora. Observe abnormal tubulation of the bones. (**C**) In another patient with multiple cartilaginous exostoses MRI was performed because one of the osteochondromas continued to enlarge. Sagittal T1-weighted (SE, TR 400, TE 12) image demonstrates intact cortex covering the lesion. (**D**) An axial fast-spin echo (FSE, TR 4000, TE 102 Ef) MRI shows thin cartilaginous cap of osteochondroma without malignant changes. (**E**) Lack of malignant transformation was confirmed on axial inversion recovery (FMPIR/90; TR 4000, TE 51 Ef, TI 140) MRI, which shows no soft tissue extension of the lesion.

coma often exhibits greater intensity of uptake than a benign exostosis. However, a number of investigators believe that this is not always a reliable distinguishing feature of malignant transformation (58). The increased activity of a benign exostosis on bone scan is related to endochondral ossification within the cartilaginous cap, whereas that of exostotic chondrosarcoma represents active ossification, osteoblastic activity, and hyperemia within the cartilage and bony stalk of the tumor (58). Occasionally the clinical and radiologic features of inflammatory changes occurring in bursa exostotica that covers the cartilaginous cap of osteochondroma can mimic malignant transformation to chondrosarcoma (Figs. 51 and 52).

On radiographic examination, the signs pointing to malignant transformation of multiple cartilaginous exostoses to

chondrosarcoma are identical with those present in malignant transformation of solitary osteochondroma (54). After skeletal maturation has occurred, alteration in lesion's size must be considered a potential indicator of malignant transformation. Particularly suggestive are alterations in the size and irregularity of contour of the cartilage cap, or the presence of mineral deposition beyond the previous contour as documented by radiography (15). When such signs are associated with signs of bone destruction at the base or neck, or when a soft tissue mass is present, the diagnosis of malignancy is certain (Fig. 53).

An interesting lesion that can be confused with osteochondroma is the so-called epiphyseal or intraarticular osteochondroma, better known as *Trevor-Fairbank disease or dysplasia epiphysealis hemimelica* (53,62). This is a devel-

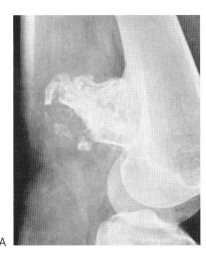
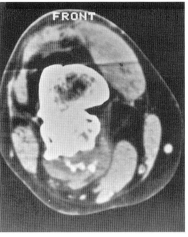

A   B

FIG. 49. Exostotic chondrosarcoma. A 28-year-old man developed pain in the popliteal region and also noted an increase in a mass of which he had been aware for 15 years. **A:** A lateral radiograph of the knee shows a sessile-type osteochondroma arising from the posterior cortex of the distal femur. Calcifications are present not only in the stalk of the lesion but are also dispersed in the cartilaginous cap. **B:** CT section confirms the increased thickness of the cartilaginous cap (2.5 cm) and dispersed calcifications within the cap. These features are consistent with a diagnosis of malignant transformation to chondrosarcoma, which was confirmed by histopathologic examination.

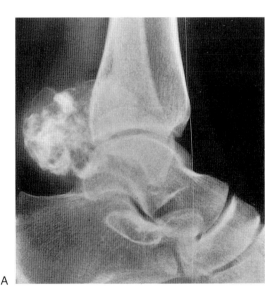
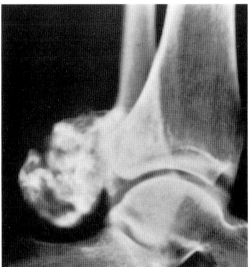

A   B

FIG. 50. Osteochondroma. **A:** A lateral radiograph of the ankle of a 26-year-old woman with a painful osteochondroma shows a sessile lesion arising from the posterior aspect of the distal tibia. In the interpretation of this radiograph, uncertainties were raised that some of the calcifications might not be contained within the stalk, and tomographic examination was suggested. **B:** Tomographic section demonstrates lack of separation of calcifications from the main mass, suggesting a benign lesion. The osteochondroma was resected and histopathologic examination confirmed the lack of malignant transformation.

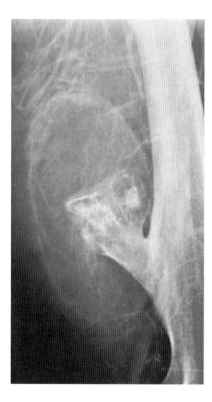

FIG. 51. Bursa exostotica. A 25-year-old man with a known solitary osteochondroma of the distal right femur presented with gradually increasing pain. Malignancy was suspected and arteriography was performed. The capillary phase of the arteriogram reveals a huge bursa exostotica. Inflammation of the bursa, with accumulation of a large amount of fluid (bursitis), was the cause of the patient's symptoms.

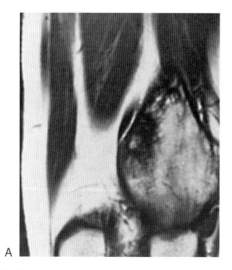

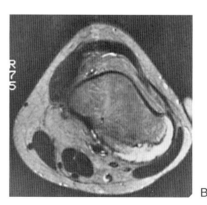

A   B

FIG. 52. Bursa exostotica. A 12-year-old girl presented with pain in the popliteal fossa. **A:** Coronal T1-weighted (SE, TR 650, TE 25) MRI demonstrates a large osteochondroma arising from the posterolateral aspect of the distal femur. **B:** Axial T2-weighted (SE, TR 2200, TE 70) MRI shows a bursa exostotica distended with fluid.

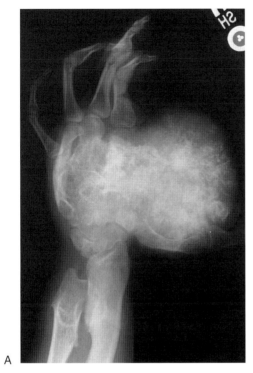
A

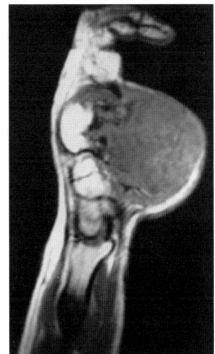
B

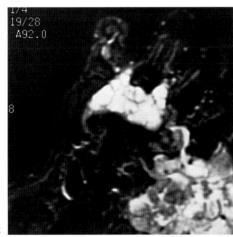
C

FIG. 53. Multiple cartilaginous exostoses: malignant transformation to chondrosarcoma. **A:** An oblique radiograph of the hand of a 22-year-old man shows multiple osteochondromas. A large soft tissue mass with chondroid calcifications indicates malignant transformation. **B:** Sagittal T1-weighted (SE, TR 600, TE 16) MRI reveals volar extension of a large soft tissue mass. **C:** Coronal inversion recovery (FMPIR/90, TR 4000, TE 64/Ef) MRI demonstrates malignant lobules of the cartilage invading the bones and soft tissues of the hand.

opmental disorder characterized by asymmetric cartilaginous overgrowth of one or more epiphyses in the lower and occasionally the upper extremities. The talus, distal femur, and distal tibia are the most common sites of involvement (62). The lesion typically arises on one side of the affected limb and deforms the bone. The basic pathologic process is abnormal cartilage proliferation in an epiphysis, and on histologic examination the lesion is almost identical with osteochondroma. Dysplasia epiphysealis hemimelica has been noted in association with conventional osteochondroma and chondroma (57). The clinical features are pain, deformity, and restricted motion in the affected joints. Radiography reveals an irregular, bulbous overgrowth of the epiphysis to one side of the ossification center (Fig. 54). As the lesion enlarges the joint deformity increases (63).

An osteochondroma in which intracartilaginous ossifica-

tion has completely consumed the cartilage may be mistaken for an *osteoma* if the base of the stem is not available for histologic examination.

Finally, *sessile osteochondroma* should be differentiated from *periosteal chondroma* (20). The latter is separated from the host bone by intervening cortex (see also section on differential diagnosis of periosteal chondroma).

Pathology

Malignant transformation of *osteochondroma* to *chondrosarcoma* is the most important histopathologic differential diagnosis. On histologic examination, malignant transformation is recognized by greater cellularity of the cartilage tissue, uneven distribution of cells, pleomorphism, and cellular and nuclear atypia (Fig. 55).

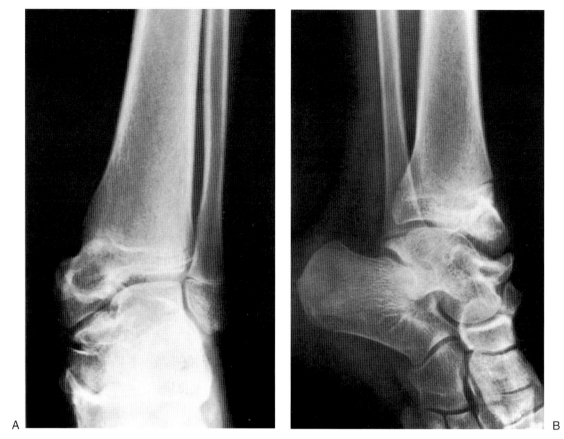

FIG. 54. Dysplasia epiphysealis hemimelica. A 12-year-old girl presented with pain and limitation of motion in the ankle joint. (**A**) Anteroposterior and (**B**) lateral radiographs of the ankle demonstrate deformity and enlargement of the medial malleolus, talus, and navicular bone, features typical of Trevor-Fairbanks disease.

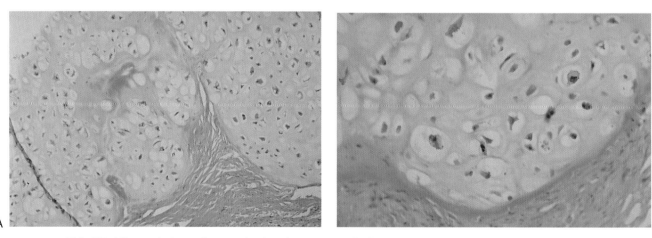

FIG. 55. Histopathology of exostotic chondrosarcoma. **A:** A photomicrograph (same patient as in Fig. 53) shows cellular chondroid tissue exhibiting slight increase in size and variation in shape of the nuclei, consistent with grade-1 chondrosarcoma (hematoxylin and eosin, original magnification ×100). **B:** At higher magnification the malignant cells are clearly depicted (hematoxylin and eosin, original magnification ×300).

The other differential possibility of osteochondroma is so-called *reactive cartilaginous exostosis,* which differs from the former by its smaller size and the metaplastic formation of cartilage from the fibrous tissue covering a bone (67) (Fig. 56). The resulting fibrocartilage undergoes endochondral ossification, as in osteochondroma. Continuing formation is the result of ongoing metaplasia from the surrounding fibrous tissue on its surface, whereas in osteochondroma growth is generated by mitotic division of the chondrocytes.

Chondroblastoma (Codman Tumor)

Clinical Presentation

Representing <1% of all primary bone tumors and 9% of benign bone tumors, this rare lesion typically presents in the epiphysis of long bones, such as the humerus, tibia, and femur (73,113,114). The proximal humerus, distal femur, and proximal tibia are the preferred sites of involvement (95) (Fig. 57). Occasionally the patella, which is considered equivalent to an epiphysis, is involved (103). Ten percent of chondroblastomas involve the small bones of the hands and feet, the talus and calcaneus representing the most common sites (76,96). The lesion is usually seen before skeletal maturity, but some cases have been reported after obliteration of

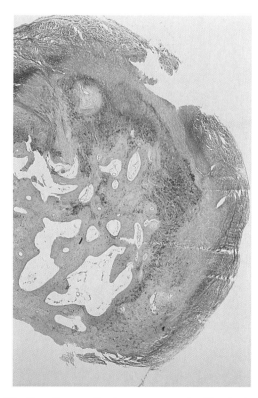

FIG. 56. Reactive cartilaginous exostosis. The lesion consists of a cap of fibrocartilage exhibiting weak metachromatism of the matrix. It is formed and grows by metaplasia from the overlying fibrous connective tissue, with a zone of endochondral ossification against the base of cancellous bone that contains some remnants of cartilage matrix (*center*) (compare this lesion with osteochondroma, **Fig. 43B**) (Giemsa, original magnification ×6).

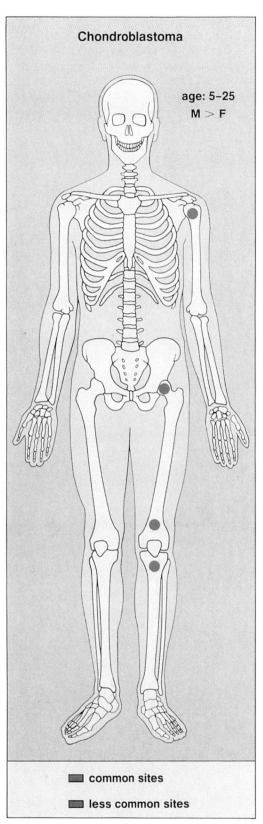

FIG. 57. Chondroblastoma: skeletal sites of predilection, peak age range, and male-to-female ratio.

the growth plate (80). Males are almost twice as frequently affected as females (33), although in the series from AFIP the ratio was 3:1 (103). In general, the clinical symptoms are nonspecific: pain, often related to the nearest joint, and swelling, usually lasting for several months, are the most common complaints (75). Approximately one third of patients exhibit joint effusion (110). Pathologic fractures occur only rarely.

Imaging

Radiographically, the lesion is usually located eccentrically (105). It is radiolucent and well defined, with a thin sclerotic border, and it exhibits a geographic pattern of bone destruction (Fig. 58) (88). The margins are smooth in 63% of cases, scalloped in 27%, and lobulated in 10% (100). Internal trabeculation can sometimes be observed (98). In 25% to 50% of cases, stippled calcifications are present (Fig. 59). If calcifications are not apparent on standard radiographs, con-

ventional tomography or CT can be helpful (85) (Fig. 60; see also Fig. 58C). The latter modality may also assess the extent of the lesion (107). The presence of a solid or layered periosteal reaction, usually located in some distance from the tumor, was reported on plain radiographs in more than 50% of 214 cases in the series by Brower *et al.* (77) (Fig. 60A; **see also Fig. 61A**). These authors suggest an inflammatory response to the tumor as the cause of this phenomenon. MRI usually reveals a larger area of involvement than can be seen on plain radiography, including prominent soft tissue and regional bone marrow edema (79,86,116) (Fig. 61). This strikingly, aggressive appearance can lead to an incorrect diagnosis of a malignant tumor (97,115). The combination of highly cellular chondroid matrix and calcification in chondroblastoma presumably accounts for the observed decrease in relaxation time on T2-weighted imaging (79). Low to intermediate heterogeneous signal intensity, lobular internal architecture, and fine lobular margins were detected with high-resolution, T2-weighted MRI (115). Focal lobules of

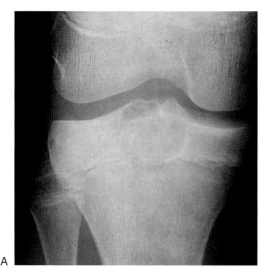

A

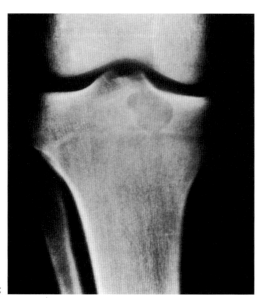

C

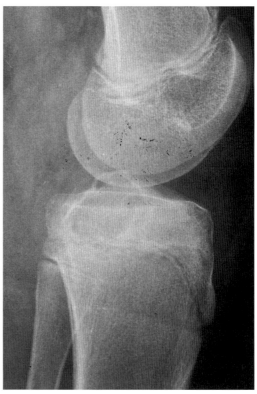

B

FIG. 58. Chondroblastoma. (**A**) Anteroposterior and (**B**) lateral radiographs of the right knee of a 14-year-old boy show the typical appearance of this tumor in the proximal epiphysis of the tibia. Note the radiolucent, eccentrically located lesion with a thin, sclerotic margin. (**C**) A frontal tomogram in another patient with chondroblastoma reveals faint calcifications.)

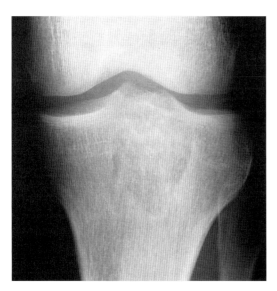

FIG. 59. Chondroblastoma. An anteroposterior radiograph of the left knee of a 17-year-old boy show a large lesion crossing the scarred growth plate of the proximal tibia. The lesion is sharply demarcated and exhibits calcifications of the matrix.

low, intermediate, and high signal intensity are superimposed and most likely correspond to calcification, chondroid matrix, and fluid in the lesion. In addition, MRI may demonstrate a rare extension of tumor to the soft tissues and may also reveal a joint effusion (Fig. 62).

Histopathology

Before the recognition of chondroblastoma by Jaffe and Lichtenstein (1942), this tumor was usually referred to as epiphyseal chondromatous giant-cell tumor (78). The tumor does contain giant cells and in fact is still occasionally misdiagnosed as giant-cell tumor. However, Jaffe and Lichtenstein felt that these giant cells were not part of the primary tumor pattern and instead pointed out its relationship to cartilage (91).

Histologically, chondroblastoma is composed of nodules of fairly mature cartilage matrix surrounded by a highly cellular, relatively undifferentiated tissue comprising round and polygonal chondroblast-like cells, sometimes having indistinct outlines. At the borders of the differentiated areas, giant cells of the osteoclast or chondroclast type are usually found (110). The nuclei of the cells are of uniform shape and moderate size (76) (Fig. 63). They may be round but usually are indented. Mitotic figures are occasionally observed (101). Foci of intercellular calcifications are typically present. Particularly characteristic are fine, lattice-like matrix calcifications surrounding apposing chondroblasts and having a spatial arrangement that resembles the hexagonal configuration of chicken wire (76,85), a diagnostically useful feature but not mandatory for diagnosis (Fig. 63C). Although chondroid matrix is relatively scant in chondroblastoma, the cells exhibit immunocytologic staining reaction for S-100 protein identical to that of other cartilage tumors. Larger tumors may break into the metaphysis or through the cortex without signs of malignancy.

Pulmonary metastases have been reported in a minority of cases of chondroblastoma (30,80,84), but no histologic evidence of malignancy has been reported in either the primary bone tumor or the pulmonary metastases (89,90). However, single cases with a spontaneous malignant transformation of chondroblastoma have been reported (106,214).

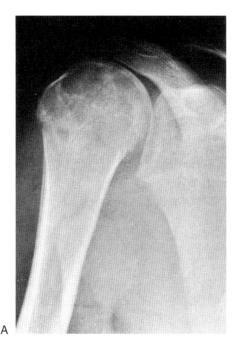

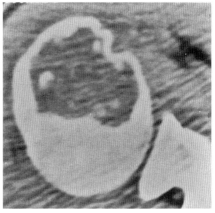

FIG. 60. Chondroblastoma. **A:** An anteroposterior radiograph of the right shoulder of a 16-year-old boy shows a lesion in the proximal humeral epiphysis, but calcifications are not well demonstrated. Note the well-organized layer of periosteal reaction at the lateral cortex. **B:** CT section shows the calcifications clearly.

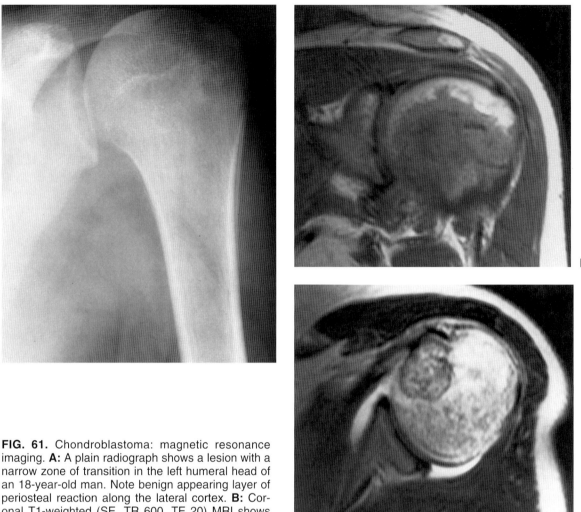

FIG. 61. Chondroblastoma: magnetic resonance imaging. **A:** A plain radiograph shows a lesion with a narrow zone of transition in the left humeral head of an 18-year-old man. Note benign appearing layer of periosteal reaction along the lateral cortex. **B:** Coronal T1-weighted (SE, TR 600, TE 20) MRI shows significant amount of perilesional edema. **C:** Axial T2-weighted (SE, TR 2000, TE 80) MRI shows the lesion exhibiting an inhomogeneous signal.

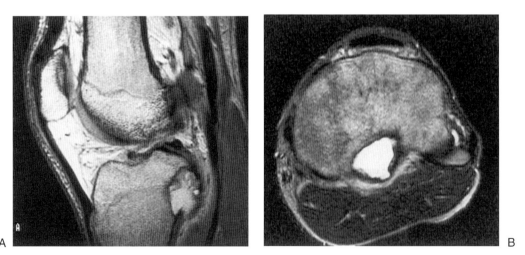

FIG. 62. Chondroblastoma: magnetic resonance imaging. (**A**) Sagittal proton-density (SE, TR 2000, TE 28) and (**B**) axial T2-weighted (SE, TR 2000, TE 80) MRI of the lesion depicted in Fig. 59 show extension of the tumor posteriorly into the soft tissues.

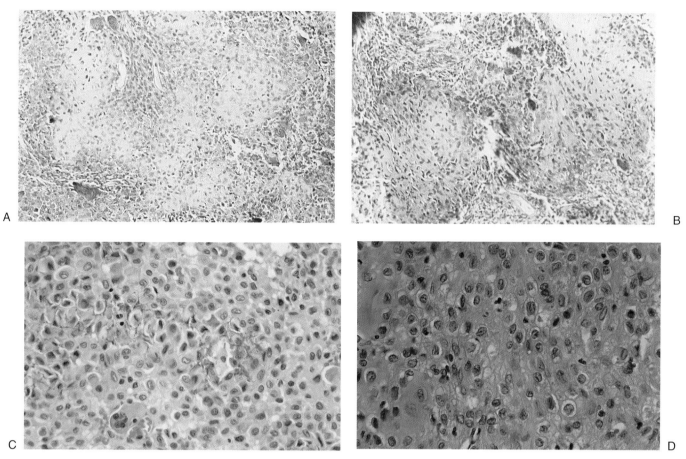

FIG. 63. Histopathology of chondroblastoma. **A:** Primitive chondroblastic tissue is seen in islands surrounded by densely arranged roundish cells. Note also many giant cells of osteo- and chondroclastic type (Giemsa, original magnification ×25). **B:** At higher magnification, there is pleomorphism of chondrocytes within the cartilaginous matrix, with signs of resorption by giant cells (Giemsa, original magnification ×50). **C:** The chondrocytes, some with ovoid and some with elongated nuclei are embedded in a chondroid matrix. Surrounding the cells are fine, intercellular calcifications forming a chicken-wire image (hematoxylin and eosin, original magnification ×235). **D:** At high magnification the chondroblasts, some well-demarcated, and some with ill-defined borders, display nuclei of various sizes, mostly roundish in shape. (Hematoxylin and eosin, original magnification ×400.)

Differential Diagnosis

Radiology

If the lesion is in the classic epiphyseal location, only a few possibilities may be included in the radiographic differential diagnosis. The radiographic findings in chondroblastoma may be nonspecific when calcifications are not visible or when atypical features, such as extension into the metaphysis after closure of the growth plate, are encountered (82). *Clear-cell chondrosarcoma* may be indistinguishable from chondroblastoma because it may exhibit the same benign pattern and, moreover, like chondroblastoma the former tumor may be seen in the immature skeleton (72).

Bone abscess is rare in an epiphyseal location (79,81) (**see Fig. 2-33**). It may demonstrate extension into the growth plate through a serpentine, radiolucent tract. The surrounding zone of sclerosis is usually thicker than that observed in chondroblastoma. In addition, no calcifications are present in this lesion and periosteal reaction is noted only in exceptional cases.

Osteonecrosis of either the humeral or the femoral head, although occasionally resembling chondroblastoma, usually exhibits classic radiographic findings, such as a crescent sign and a rather homogeneous density adjacent to it (83). MRI findings are also typical, although they vary depending on the stage of osteonecrosis.

Intraosseous ganglion is a rare lesion near the articular surface, invariably eccentric in location, with knee, ankle, and shoulder joints being preferred sites (Figs. 64 and 65). It is almost never seen before skeletal maturation.

Giant-cell tumor, with very few exceptions, is a lesion of the mature skeleton, and if seen before skeletal maturity it is metaphyseal in location (74,104,111). In addition, it shows no calcifications (92).

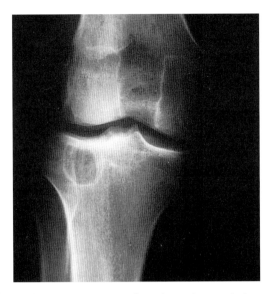

FIG. 64. Intraosseous ganglion. An anteroposterior radiograph of the right knee shows a radiolucent lesion with a sclerotic border eccentrically located in the articular end of the proximal tibia, resembling a chondroblastoma.

Osteoblastoma of the epiphysis is extraordinarily rare (99,108), its usual location being the metaphysis or diaphysis. *Enchondroma* is rare in the epiphysis but at times may appear similar to chondroblastoma. *Langerhans cell granuloma,* like osteoblastoma and enchondroma, is extremely rare in the epiphysis and, unlike chondroblastoma, never presents with central calcifications.

Occasionally, a normal radiolucency in the proximal humerus (representing an increased amount of cancellous bone in the region of greater tuberosity seen on end) may be mistakenly diagnosed as chondroblastoma (87,93,109) (Fig. 66). Knowledge of the existence of this normal variant may prevent radiologist from making this erroneous diagnosis.

Pathology

Histologically, chondroblastoma must be differentiated from *chondrosarcoma* and *giant-cell tumor*. Because large nuclei of variable size and shape are occasionally present in chondroblastoma, this and the presence of mitotic figures may suggest malignancy. Overall low-power histopathologic appearance and correlation with radiography should help in arriving at the correct diagnosis (76).

Because osteoclast-like giant cells usually form a part of the histologic pattern of chondroblastoma, being present particularly at the border of the chondroid areas of this tumor, it may be mistaken for giant-cell tumor. The giant cells of chondroblastoma, however, can be distinguished from the same cells in giant-cell tumor by the rounded appearance of the intervening cells, in contrast to the spindle-shaped stromal cells of giant-cell tumor. The presence of the chondroid areas indicates the true nature of the tumor (Fig. 67). When further doubt exists, the matrix stain aldehyde-fuchsin at pH 1.0 is useful, especially when combined with immunostaining for S-100 protein (102). The chondroid matrix of chondroblastoma is stained by aldehyde-fuchsin purple, as are the "chicken wire" calcifications often present around the tumor cells. Staining for S-100 protein is present in the cytoplasm of chondroblastoma but is absent in giant cell tumor mononuclear cells (76).

The radiologic and pathologic differential diagnosis of chondroblastoma is depicted in Fig. 68.

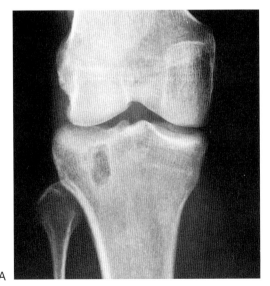
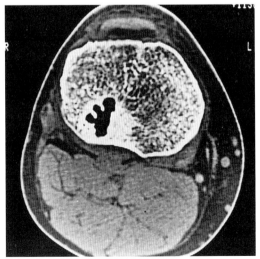

A   B

FIG. 65. Intraosseous ganglion. **A:** An anteroposterior radiograph of the right knee of a 24-year-old man with an 8-week history of pain shows an oval, radiolucent eccentric lesion in the proximal tibia, resembling a chondroblastoma. **B:** CT section shows a low-attenuation area with ramifications, surrounded by a zone of reactive sclerosis.

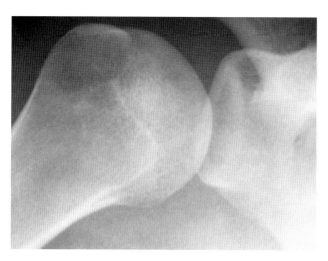

FIG. 66. Pseudotumor of the greater tuberosity of the humerus. A radiolucent area in the region of the greater tuberosity is a normal variant that resembles a chondroblastoma.

Chondromyxoid Fibroma

Clinical Presentation

This rare cartilage tumor, consisting of a mixture of fibromyxoid tissue and cartilage tissue in variable proportions and accounting for 0.5% of all primary bone tumors and 2% of benign bone tumors, occurs predominantly in adolescents and young adults (most patients are <30 year of age) and more commonly in males than in females (2:1) (9). This tumor has a predilection for the bones of the lower extremities, usually the proximal tibia (Fig. 69), and the clinical symptoms include the presence of a peripherally located mass, together with local pain and swelling (117,119,129).

Imaging

On radiographic imaging, the lesion may range from 1 to 10 cm in size, with an average of 3 to 4 cm (9,119). It is a round or ovoid, lucent, and eccentrically located lesion ex-

hibiting a geographic pattern of bone destruction and a scalloped, sclerotic margin (Fig. 70) (122,130). Occasionally, ridges or septa are present within the lesion (33) (Fig. 71). It often erodes or balloons out from the cortex (119), and often a buttress of periosteal new bone can be observed (85) (Fig. 72). Calcifications are not apparent on radiography. MRI reveals characteristics of most cartilaginous tumors: intermediate to low signal intensity on T1-weighted and high signal intensity on T2-weighted sequences (Fig. 73). This technique can also effectively demonstrate soft tissue extension of chondromyxoid fibroma (123). Recently, a few cases of chondromyxoid fibroma have been reported that exhibited predominantly cortical involvement (125).

Histopathology

Chondromyxoid fibroma is characterized by large lobulated areas of spindle-shaped or stellate cells distributed within abundant myxoid or chondroid intercellular material. They are separated by septum-like zones of more cellular tissue that may contain variable numbers of giant cells (Fig. 74) (131). A characteristic finding is the increased cellularity of the tissue near the septa (9) (Fig. 75). As the term "chondromyxoid fibroma" implies, the variety of tissues are characteristic of this lesion. Two types of matrix can be identified: dense chondroid matrix, which stains basophilic, and loose myxoid matrix, which stains eosinophilic, the latter being predominant in most chondromyxoid fibromas. Genuine hyaline cartilage is not seen in these tumors. Mild nuclear atypia may be observed. Large pleomorphic and hyperchromatic cells are sometimes observed and can lead to confusion in diagnosis with chondrosarcoma (127). Before the description of this entity by Jaffe and Lichtenstein in 1948 (120), many examples had probably been regarded as chondrosarcomas. Some cases reported as myxomas or myxofibromas of long bones are probably chondromyxoid fibromas (119). Histochemical studies demonstrate glycogen granules in many chondroblastic elements and in the stellate cells of the

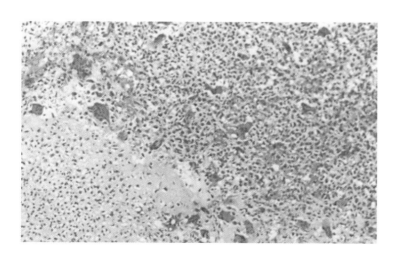

FIG. 67. Chondroblastoma. A highly cellular area of the tumor contains several giant cells (*upper right*). However, the juxtaposition of an area of chondroid matrix (*lower left*) indicates the true nature of this tumor (hematoxylin and eosin, original magnification ×100). (Reprinted with permission from Bullough PG. *Atlas of orthopedic pathology,* 2nd ed. New York: Gower, 1992;16.24.)

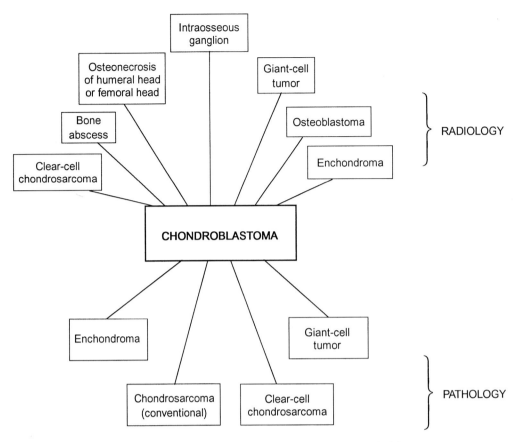

FIG. 68. Radiologic and pathologic differential diagnosis of chondroblastoma.

myxoid areas. The cytoplasm of giant cells of the osteoclast type exhibits a discrete amount of periodic acid-Schiff–positive material that is resistant to ptyalin digestion, and is strongly positive for acid phosphatase, as has been observed in other giant cell lesions (126). Ultrastructural studies of the stellate cells in this lesion reveal irregular cell processes, scalloping of the cell membrane, and frequently the presence of abundant cytoplasmic fibrils (128).

Differential Diagnosis

Radiology

The classic radiographic findings, including round or oval shape, eccentric metaphyseal location, lobulation, septation, and peripheral sclerosis, are usually diagnostic of chondromyxoid fibroma. Occasionally, however, the lesion may be radiographically indistinguishable from an *aneurysmal bone cyst* (see **Fig. 72**). Other differential possibilities include nonossifying fibroma and fibrous dysplasia.

Nonossifying fibroma, unlike chondromyxoid fibroma, rarely displays cortical ballooning or cortical destruction, and a periosteal reaction is present only in lesions that have sustained a pathologic fracture. *Fibrous dysplasia,* in contrast to chondromyxoid fibroma, is centrally located rather than eccentric, rarely shows internal septations, and does not elicit a periosteal reaction.

In the tibia, adamantinoma and osteofibrous dysplasia (Kempson-Campanacci lesion) are the main differential possibilities, and when the lesion extends to the articular end of bone, giant-cell tumor should be considered.

Adamantinoma is usually a much more destructive lesion, composed of multiple, sharply defined, radiolucent foci interspersed with sclerotic changes. It frequently involves the anterior cortex. Almost all cases of adamantinoma of long bones have been reported in the tibia and fibula. Periosteal reaction is usually much more aggressive than that observed in chondromyxoid fibroma. In addition, the peak age incidence of adamantinoma is between 30 and 50 years, in contrast to chondromyxoid fibroma, which occurs mostly in children and adolescents.

Osteofibrous dysplasia is usually limited in extent to the anterior cortex of the tibia (rarely in the fibula), is much more sclerotic than chondromyxoid fibroma, and does not elicit a periosteal reaction. The tibia is usually anteriorly bowed. The peak incidence of osteofibrous dysplasia is in the first decade, whereas that of chondromyxoid fibroma is in the second decade.

In the mature skeleton, particularly if the lesion extends to the articular end of the bone, *giant-cell tumor* should be a

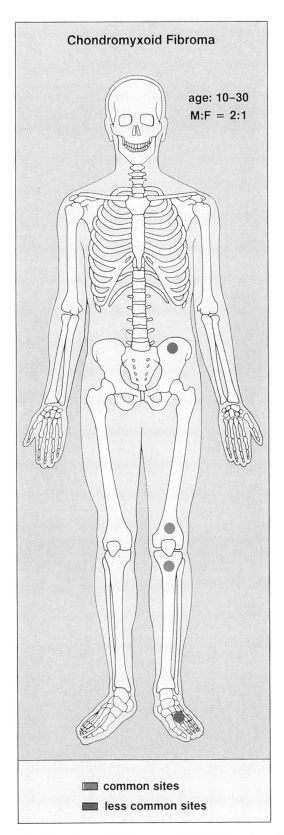

FIG. 69. Chondromyxoid fibroma: skeletal sites of predilection, peak age range, and male-to-female ratio.

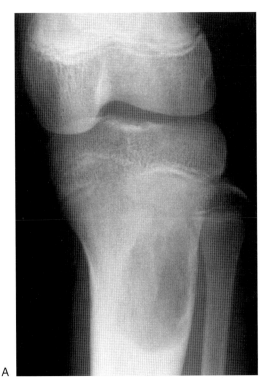

A

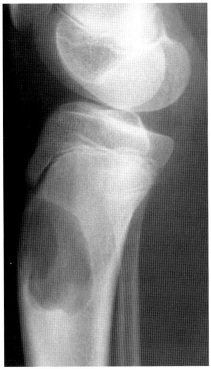

B

FIG. 70. Chondromyxoid fibroma. (A) Anteroposterior and (B) lateral radiographs of the knee of a 12-year-old girl show a radiolucent, slightly lobulated lesion with a thin sclerotic margin in the proximal tibial diaphysis. Note the lack of visible calcifications.

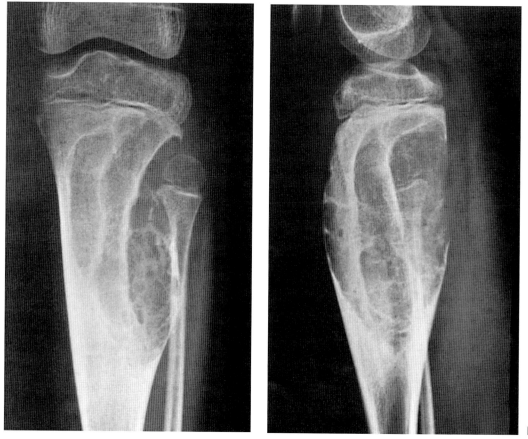

FIG. 71. Chondromyxoid fibroma. **(A)** Anteroposterior and **(B)** lateral radiographs of the proximal left leg of an 8-year-old girl demonstrate a radiolucent lesion extending from the metaphysis into the diaphysis of the tibia, exhibiting a geographic type of bone destruction, a sclerotic scalloped border, and internal septa.

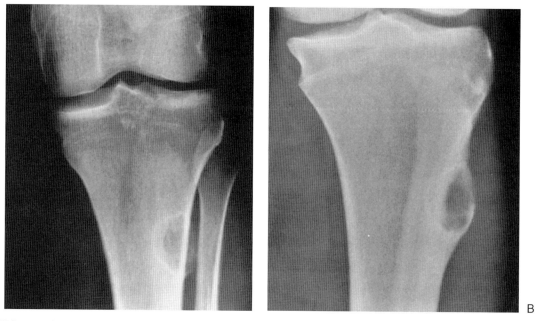

FIG. 72. Chondromyxoid fibroma. **(A)** An anteroposterior radiograph of the knee of an 18-year-old woman shows a lesion located in the lateral aspect of the proximal tibia. **(B)** The lesion balloons out from the cortex and is supported by a solid periosteal buttress, better appreciated on a tomographic cut.

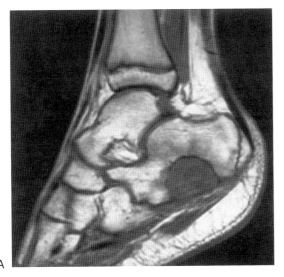

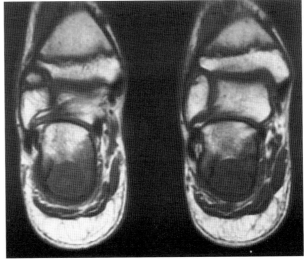

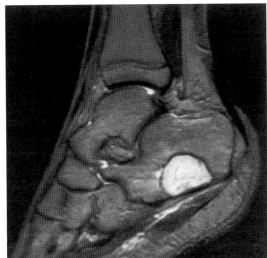

FIG. 73. Chondromyxoid fibroma: magnetic resonance imaging. **A:** Sagittal T1-weighted (SE, TR 600, TE 19) MRI in a 10-year-old girl shows a well-demarcated lesion in the plantar aspect of the calcaneus, displaying low signal intensity. **B:** Two axial T1-weighted (SE, TR 600, TE 17) images show significant amount of peritumoral edema. **C:** Sagittal T2-weighted (SE, TR 2000, TE 80) MRI shows the lesion displaying high signal intensity. A sclerotic border is imaged as a rim of low signal intensity.

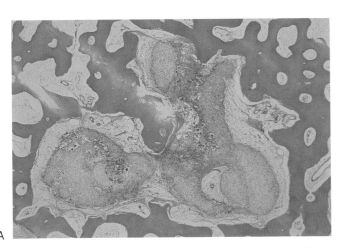

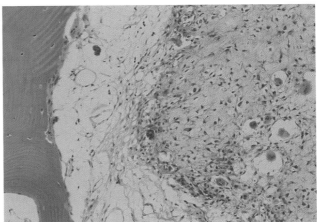

FIG. 74. Histopathology of chondromyxoid fibroma. **A:** Cancellous bone with dilated marrow space (center) contains tumor tissue separated from bone by a layer of connective tissue (hematoxylin and eosin, original magnification ×6). **B:** At higher magnification, the edge of the tumor (*right*) exhibits a denser arrangement of cells than the central portion. Several giant cells are scattered within a loose fibrous stroma. Resorption of the trabecula is seen at left (hematoxylin and eosin, original magnification ×50) *Continued on page 170.*

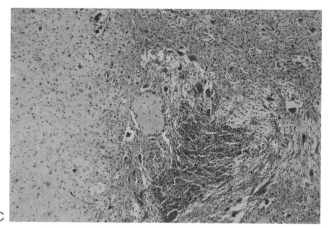

C

FIG. 74. (*Continued.*) **C:** In another area, less cellular stroma (*left*) merges with more cellular tissue containing several giant cells and extravasated red blood cells (hematoxylin and eosin, original magnification ×50).

consideration in the differential diagnosis. The latter lesion, however, normally presents with no sclerotic margin (unlike chondromyxoid fibroma, which is demarcated from normal bone by a distinct sclerotic border).

Smaller lesions, particularly those located in the metaphysis, should be differentiated from *bone abscess* (Brodie abscess).

Pathology

On histologic examination, chondromyxoid fibroma may resemble myxoid chondrosarcoma, chondroblastoma, and enchondroma (118,120). However, in chondromyxoid fibroma the stellate cells on the myxoid background lack mitotic activity, and the cells at the periphery of the lobules are

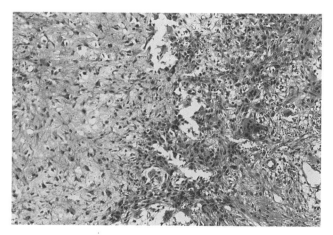

FIG. 75. Histopathology of chondromyxoid fibroma. A photomicrograph reveals the typical lobulated appearance of this tumor. Lobules of chondromyxoid tissue (*left and right*) are separated by a septum (*center*) of cellular fibrous tissue, with occasional giant cells (hematoxylin and eosin, original magnification ×50).

usually similar in shape to chondroblastoma cells. Conversely, in *myxoid chondrosarcoma* the mitotic activity is found at the peripheries of the lobules. In addition, myxoid chondrosarcoma exhibits intranuclear details such as a fine chromatin pattern and nucleoli (124). When large areas of chondroid matrix are present, chondrosarcoma is suggested, but the absence of such matrix has no significance (13). Small areas that resemble *chondroblastoma* are sometimes observed in chondromyxoid fibroma. However, the diagnosis can be confirmed by the lack of calcifications and the presence of a myxoid component in the latter tumor.

Radiologic and pathologic differential diagnoses of chondromyxoid fibroma is depicted in Fig. 76.

Synovial (Osteo)Chondromatosis

Synovial chondromatosis (also known as synovial osteochondromatosis or synovial chondrometaplasia) is an uncommon benign disorder marked by metaplastic proliferation of multiple cartilaginous nodules in the synovial membrane of the joint, bursa, or tendon sheath. It is almost invariably monoarticular; rarely, multiple joints may be affected. This condition is discussed in **Chapter 9**.

MALIGNANT LESIONS

Chondrosarcoma

Chondrosarcoma, a malignant tumor of the connective tissue, is characterized by formation of cartilage matrix by the tumor cells (166). Chondrosarcomas comprise the third most common primary malignant tumors of bone, after multiple myeloma and osteosarcoma. Accounting for approximately 10% of all primary bone sarcomas, chondrosarcoma is twice as common in men as in women (9). The peak age of incidence is late adulthood, and very few cases of chondrosarcoma have been reported in children and adolescents (137,165,230). These tumors, when they occur in young people, often appear in unusual sites and may have a more ominous prognosis (137,170,230).

Chondrosarcoma preferentially affects the flat bones, limb girdles, and proximal portions of long tubular bones. Anatomic location can be classified as either intramedullary (central) or surface (peripheral). It is rare for central chondrosarcomas to develop in preexisting benign lesions; they are therefore referred to as primary chondrosarcomas. Peripheral chondrosarcomas, conversely, often arise from underlying benign lesions, such as osteochondroma, and are termed secondary chondrosarcomas (Fig. 77) (177).

Clinical Presentation

In primary chondrosarcomas, pain usually develops insidiously but no mass is apparent. Conversely, secondary chondrosarcomas arising at peripheral sites may be asymptomatic despite the presence of a large mass. Peripheral chondrosar-

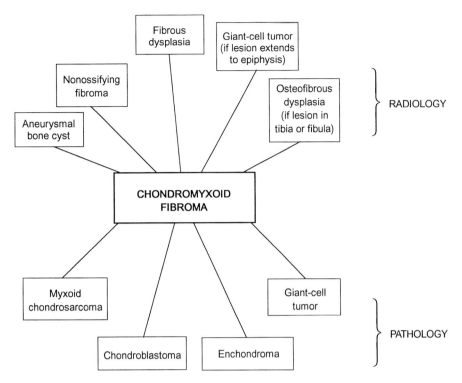

FIG. 76. Radiologic and pathologic differential diagnosis of chondromyxoid fibroma.

comas that occur at sites with large potential spaces (e.g., the pelvis) may not be clinically detected until they reach an immense size.

Chondrosarcomas exhibit a wide range of behaviors (206). Some are slow growing and relatively benign, whereas others are highly malignant neoplasms with associated metastases. Most of these tumors, however, are indolent and of low grade. They tend to recur locally, and metastases are uncommon or occur late in the course of disease. Nevertheless, because they are often located close to the trunk, abdomen, or pelvis, a fatal outcome resulting from repeated local recurrence associated with compromise of vital functions is not unusual. In contrast to low-grade tumors, metastasis is common with high-grade chondrosarcomas (158).

Imaging

Radiologic evaluation of a chondrosarcoma may require a range of imaging modalities (82), including conventional radiography and tomography, arteriography, radionuclide imaging (scintigraphy, bone scan), CT, and MRI (133, 174,220). The single most important modality for establishing the diagnosis is plain radiography, which provides the most useful diagnostic information about radiologic morphology of the tumor, including the specific type of bone destruction, endosteal scalloping, calcifications, and periosteal reaction. Conventional tomography may help to better delineate the matrix calcifications, evaluate the cortex and periosteal reaction, and detect occult pathologic fracture. Arteriography is an essential technique for mapping the tumor and its vascular supply, and for choosing the area most suitable for open biopsy.

In the evaluation of intra- and extraosseous extension of a tumor, CT and MRI are crucial (144,146,156,188,203). Both modalities are highly accurate in determining the presence or absence of soft tissue invasion by tumor (50,198). MRI may be superior to CT, particularly in the coronal plane, for delineating the intramedullary extent of tumor and its relationship to surrounding structures (133). Because it reveals a sharper demarcation between normal and abnormal bone tissue than CT, MRI, particularly in evaluation of the extremities, can reliably identify the spatial boundaries of tumor masses, encasement and displacement of major neurovascular bundles, and the extent of joint involvement (169). Axial and coronal images in combination have been employed to determine the extent of soft tissue invasion in relation to important vascular structures (133,220). Compared with CT, however, MR images do not clearly depict or allow characterization of calcification in the tumor matrix; in fact, large amounts of calcification or ossification may be almost undetectable (197,198). Moreover, MRI is less satisfactory than CT, or even plain films and tomography, for demonstration

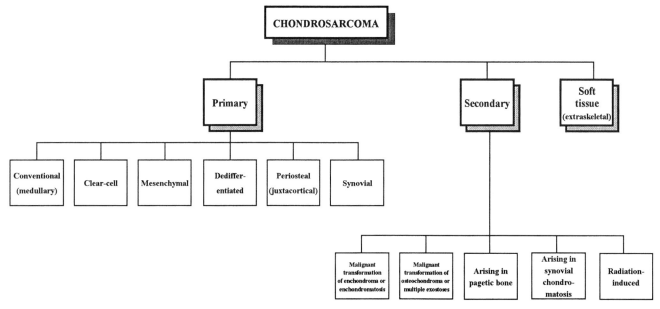

FIG. 77. Classification of the types of chondrosarcoma.

of cortical destruction (146,155). The use of the inversion recovery mode to obtain strongly T1-weighted images and the development of the spin-echo mode with variation of the pulse sequences have improved the evaluation of chondrosarcoma by MRI (55,156,172).

Histopathology

The histologic hallmark of chondrosarcoma is production of malignant cartilage by the tumor cells. Assessment of the degree of malignancy of cartilage tumors is difficult. This reflects the lack of precisely defined criteria for grading the malignancy, as many tumors exhibit overlapping of the features used for gradation. Therefore each histologic appearance of a cartilage lesion should be correlated with the radiographic appearance. The degree of malignancy of chondrosarcoma is determined by several histologic criteria. These include structural characteristics (numbers of cells and appearance of matrix), cytologic findings (size of cells, pleomorphism, nuclear detail, and presence or absence of bizarre cell forms), and replicate activity (bizarre forms, mitotic figures, and binucleated or multinucleated cells).

There is a decided correlation between the histologic structure and the clinical behavior of these tumors (207). It is therefore important to differentiate among borderline, low-grade, intermediate, and high-grade chondrosarcomas (grades 0.5, 1, 2, and 3, respectively). Such differentiation is based on several histologic characteristics, including the cellularity of the tumor tissue (e.g., hypocellular, hypercellular), the degree of pleomorphism observed in cells and nuclei

(e.g., the presence of double- and multinucleated cells, bizarre-shaped nuclei, large nuclei), and the degree of hyperchromasia of the nuclei (e.g., hyperchromatism) (Table 2 and Fig. 78). Certain other histologic signs are also indicative of malignancy, such as invasion of trabeculae by tumor tissue, infiltration of bone marrow and Haversian systems, and permeation through the cortex. These features, however, are not an integral part of an accepted grading system.

Some investigators distinguish only two grades of chondrosarcoma, low grade and high grade (184,204). Low-grade tumors have lower cell density, abundant matrix, limited pleomorphism, minimal mitotic activity, and few bizarre cells. High-grade tumors are characterized by hypercellularity (often in myxoid, fibrous, or mixed stroma), moderate to marked pleomorphism, double nuclei, bizarre forms, and high mitotic activity.

On histologic examination, so-called pushing margins distinguish low-grade chondrosarcoma from high-grade chondrosarcoma that exhibits infiltrative margins (15,184).

Several types of chondrosarcoma are recognized, each having particular clinical, radiologic, and pathologic features (210).

Primary Chondrosarcomas

Conventional Medullary Chondrosarcoma

This is the most common type of chondrosarcoma, accounting for about 80% of all cases. It usually occurs in men over the age of 30 (217). The sites most commonly affected

TABLE 2. *Histologic grading of chondrosarcoma*

Grade	Histologic features
0.5 (borderline)	Histologic features similar to enchondroma, but radiographic features more aggressive.
1 (low-grade)	Cellularity: slightly increased. Cytologic atypia: slight increase in size and variation in shape of the nuclei; slightly increased hyperchromasia of the nuclei. Binucleation: few binucleate cells are present. Stromal myxoid change: may or may not present.
2 (intermediate)	Cellularity: moderately increased. Cytologic atypia: moderate increase in size and variation in shape of the nuclei; moderately increased hyperchromasia of the nuclei. Binucleation: large number of double- and trinucleated cells. Stromal myxoid change: focally present.
3 (high-grade)	Cellularity: markedly increased. Cytologic atypia: marked enlargement and irregularity of the nuclei; markedly increased hyperchromasia of the nuclei. Binucleation: large number of double- and multinucleated cells. Stromal myxoid change: commonly present. Other: small foci of spindling at the periphery of the lobules of chondrocytes.

Modified from Dahlin and Unni, 1988.

are the pelvis and the long bones, particularly the femur and the humerus, but the tumor may develop in any part of the skeleton (Fig. 79) (167,192).

Imaging

Plain radiography is usually sufficient to establish the diagnosis. The typical chondrosarcoma exhibits a characteristic expansion of the medullary portion of the bone (Fig. 80) (228). Thickening of the cortex and endosteal scalloping are frequently observed, often associated with popcorn-like, comma-shaped, arc-like, or annular calcifications (Fig. 81) (186). The periosteal reaction may be absent, may have a noninterrupted benign appearance, or may display very aggressive features, including Codman triangle and sunburst characteristics (200). Endosteal scalloping is a frequent finding. In some instances a soft tissue mass is present (Figs. 82 and 83). In exceptional cases, particularly in the early stage, the tumor may be indistinguishable from an enchondroma. Therefore, all central cartilage tumors that affect the long bones, particularly those in adults, should be considered malignant until they have been proven benign (200).

Computed tomography and magnetic resonance imaging are invaluable techniques for evaluation and staging of primary chondrosarcomas, particularly in determining tumor extension in the bone marrow and the extent of soft tissue involvement (Figs. 84 and 85) (188). On CT examination, chondrosarcoma usually appears as a lobulated, intramedullary mass with scattered low-attenuation calcifications (Fig. 86). The Hounsfield values of the bone marrow affected by the tumor are in the positive range (high attenuation) in contrast to the negative values of normal fatty bone marrow (low attenuation) (see Fig. 84B).

The MRI appearance of chondrosarcoma is not specific (169). In general, the tumor appears to be lobulated, with intermediate to low signal intensity on T1-weighted images (167,226) and high signal intensity on T2-weighted images.

Calcifications display low signal or signal void (Fig. 87). The hyperintense, usually homogeneous signal corresponds to areas of hyaline cartilage matrix with uniform composition and high water content (114). Visual analysis of signal characteristics on routine MR images usually does not enable the histologic type or grade of chondrosarcoma to be distinguished. MRI in the coronal plane provides a more graphic and precise definition of the intramedullary extent of the tumor, with a sharper demarcation between normal and abnormal bone tissue, than does CT (see Fig. 87C). For determination of the extent of tumor in the soft tissue and its relationship to important vascular structures, axial images are more effective (see Fig. 84). Intravenous administration of Gd-DTPA before T1-weighted spin-echo images are obtained can demonstrate enhancement of scalloped margins (reflecting hyaline cartilage lobules surrounded by fibrovascular bundles) and enhanced curvilinear septa with a distinct ring and arc pattern (reflecting the typical lobulated growth pattern of chondrosarcoma), yielding an appearance similar to that of enchondroma (136). The nonenhancing areas consist of paucicellular hyaline cartilage, cystic mucoid tissue, and necrosis (55). Some authorities point to the fact that septal enhancement of chondrosarcoma is more common in low-grade tumors (55); however, the validity of this has been challenged (152).

Scintigraphy of chondrosarcoma invariably shows increased uptake of radiotracer (Fig. 88) (168). This technique may demonstrate the extent of intramedullary involvement of the cartilage tumor better than plain film radiography or conventional tomography. However, it is not as accurate as MRI because the exact level of intramedullary spread of the tumor cannot be adequately evaluated. A radionuclide bone scan usually shows the extent of the bone lesion to be larger than it actually is because the areas of hyperemia and edema adjacent to the tumor also demonstrate increased activity.

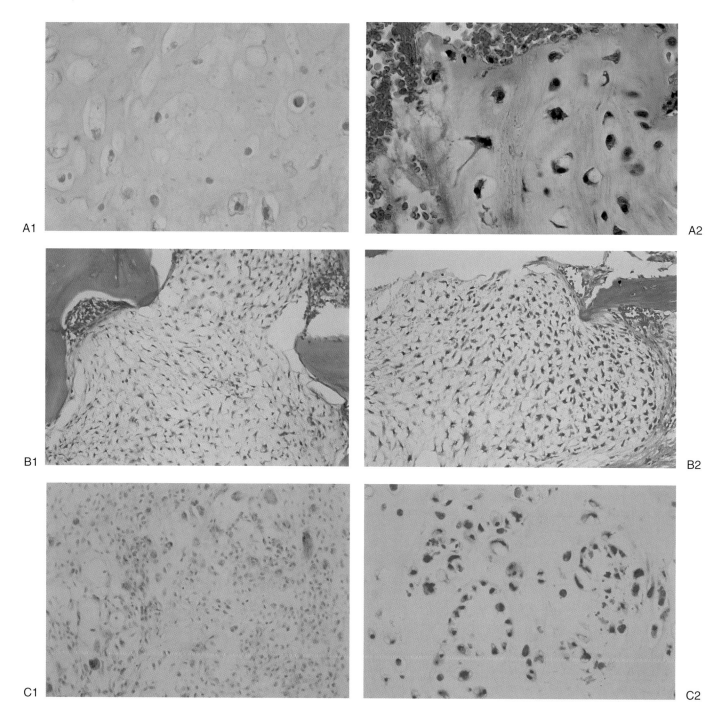

FIG. 78. Histologic grades of chondrosarcoma. (**A1**) Grade 1. Low-cellular tumor shows slightly abnormal nuclei (hematoxylin and eosin, original magnification ×156). (**A2**) Grade 1. At high magnification the variation in shape of the nuclei and hyperchromasia are evident (hematoxylin and eosin, original magnification ×400). (**B1**) Grade 2. The tumor exhibits moderately increased cellularity and several double-nucleated cells are present (hematoxylin and eosin, original magnification ×25). (**B2**) Grade 2. At high magnification focal myxoid changes of the stroma are evident (hematoxylin and eosin, original magnification ×50). (**C1**) Grade 3. The tumor is markedly cellular showing pleomorphism and hyperchromatism of the nuclei. In addition to crowding of the cells, they are lying in a myxoid matrix (hematoxylin and eosin, original magnification ×50). (**C2**) Grade 3. Irregularly distributed cells with marked pleomorphism of nuclei. Numerous bi-and trinucleated cells are present (hematoxylin and eosin, original magnification ×50).

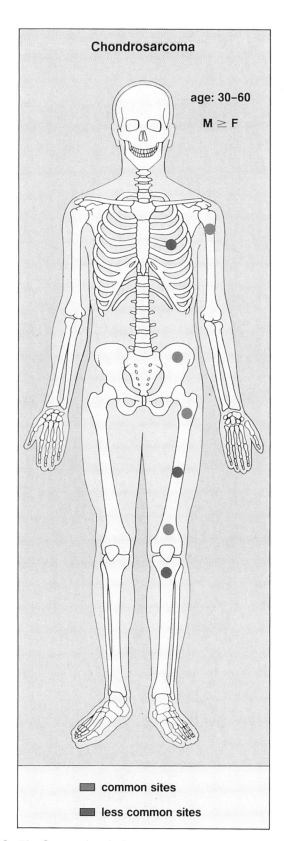

FIG. 79. Conventional chondrosarcoma: skeletal sites of predilection, peak age range, and male-to-female ratio.

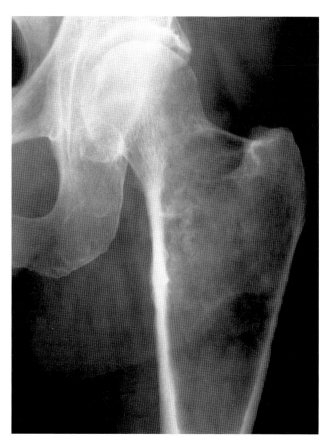

FIG. 80. Chondrosarcoma. An anteroposterior radiograph of the proximal left femur in a 52-year-old woman shows, typical for this tumor, expansion of the medullary portion of the bone due to destruction of the endocortex and periosteal new bone apposition.

Clear-Cell Chondrosarcoma

This rare variant of chondrosarcoma was first described in 1976. It is considered a low-grade malignant tumor that exhibits clinical behavior less aggressive than that of conventional chondrosarcoma (138). Accounting for only 2% of all chondrosarcomas (180), it is more common in males than in females (2:1) and usually affects patients in the third to fifth decades (72). Clear-cell chondrosarcoma preferentially affects the articular ends (epiphysis) of long tubular bones (the femur and the humerus are most commonly involved), with resultant joint pain, effusions, and a limited range of motion. On radiography the lesion is predominantly lytic, and sometimes expansive. There is often a sharp interface between tumor and surrounding normal bone, with a sclerotic border and occasionally with central calcifications and ossifications (Figs. 89 and 90). Endosteal scalloping is occasionally seen. Periosteal reaction is rare, as is soft tissue extension of the tumor (72,225). Because of its location and the narrow zone of transition with normal bone, the tumor resembles chondroblastoma. However, MRI appearance of clear-cell chon-

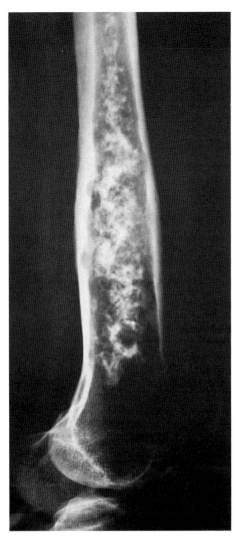

FIG. 81. Conventional chondrosarcoma. An oblique radiograph in a 46-year-old man shows the characteristic features of this tumor, located in the right femur. Within the destructive lesion in the medullary portion of the bone noted are annular and comma-shaped calcifications. The thickened cortex, which is due to periosteal new bone formation in response to invasion of the cortex by the chondroblastic tumor, shows the typical endosteal scalloping.

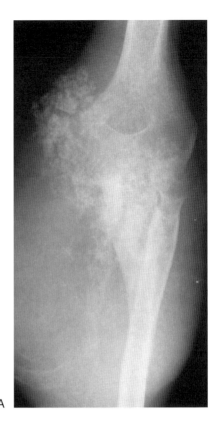

A

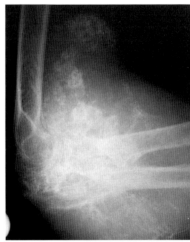

B

FIG. 83. Conventional chondrosarcoma. **(A)** Anteroposterior and **(B)** lateral radiographs of the right elbow in a 55-year-old man show a tumor arising from the proximal ulna that is accompanied by a huge soft tissue mass.

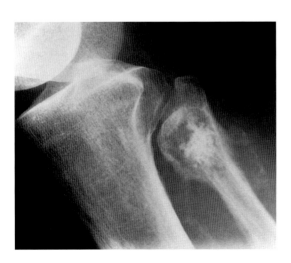

FIG. 82. Conventional chondrosarcoma. Oblique radiograph of the knee in a 58-year-old woman shows a tumor in the proximal fibula and a soft tissue mass containing chondroid calcifications.

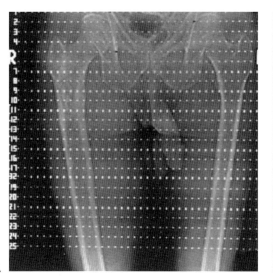

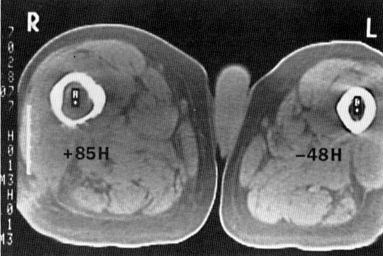

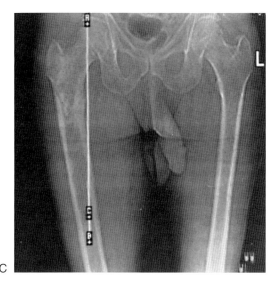

FIG. 84. Chondrosarcoma: computed tomography. CT evaluation of intraosseous extension of chondrosarcoma includes the following: **A:** Several contiguous axial sections, preferably 1 cm in thickness, of both affected and unaffected limbs are obtained. **B:** Hounsfield values of bone marrow are measured to determine the distal extent of tumor in the medullary cavity. A value of +85 in this example indicates the presence of tumor; a value of −48 is normal for fatty marrow. **C:** The linear measurement is obtained from proximal articular end of the bone (A) to the point located 5 cm distally to the tumor margin (B). Point C corresponds to the most distal axial section that still shows tumor in the marrow.

drosarcoma differs from that of chondroblastoma, which usually shows low signal intensity on T1- and T2-weighted sequences. Clear-cell chondrosarcoma, on the other hand, exhibits intermediate signal intensity on T1 weighting, which becomes bright on T2-weighted images (159). Histologic study reveals regions of obvious cartilaginous matrix and clusters of large chondrocytes with distinct cell boundaries. These chondrocytes possess rather small nuclei and abundant clear or eosinophilic cytoplasm (Fig. 91) (150). Osteoclast-like giant cells and foci of reactive bone formation are also observed. Since osteoid trabeculae are occasionally present in clear cell chondrosarcoma (Fig. 92), this tumor should not be diagnosed as atypical osteoblastoma (9). A review by Weiss and Dorfman states that metastases develop in only 10% of patients with clear cell chondrosarcomas (227). However, in an earlier published series, late local recurrence and pulmonary and bone metastases were not uncommon.

Mesenchymal Chondrosarcoma

Mesenchymal chondrosarcoma is a rare lesion, representing <1% of all chondrosarcomas, with a peak incidence in the second and third decades (140). Long-standing pain, swelling, and a soft tissue mass are typical clinical findings. This tumor exhibits no characteristic radiologic pattern. In some instances it may resemble conventional chondrosarcoma or another type of more highly malignant tumor, characterized by aggressive, lytic bone destruction or a permeative pattern of bony infiltration (Figs. 93 and 94). It appears to have a predilection for the mandible, femur, fibula, and ribs (194). On histologic examination, mesenchymal chondrosarcoma consists of two components: (a) small, round, uniform-sized cells of mesenchymal tissue with round or ovoid nuclei that resemble those seen in Ewing sarcoma, occasionally intermingled with spindle-shaped cells, alternating with (b) areas of well-differentiated cartilage containing foci of calcification and occasionally meta-

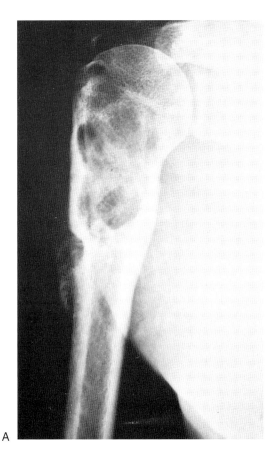

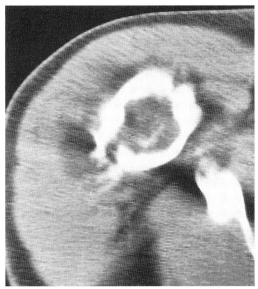

A

B

FIG. 85. Chondrosarcoma: computed tomography. **A:** A plain radiograph of the right shoulder of a 62-year-old man is not adequate for demonstrating the soft tissue extension of the chondrosarcoma in the proximal humerus. **B:** CT section through the lesion demonstrates cortical destruction and an extensive soft tissue mass.

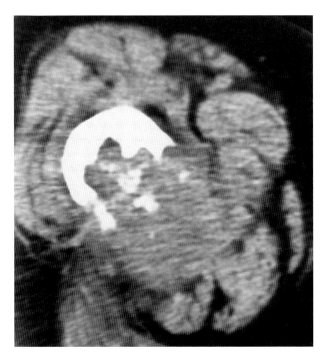

FIG. 86. Chondrosarcoma: computed tomography. CT section through the lesion in the proximal femur of a 69-year-old man with chondrosarcoma shows thickening of the cortex, endosteal scalloping, and a large soft tissue mass. The calcifications of the tumor image as low-attenuation foci.

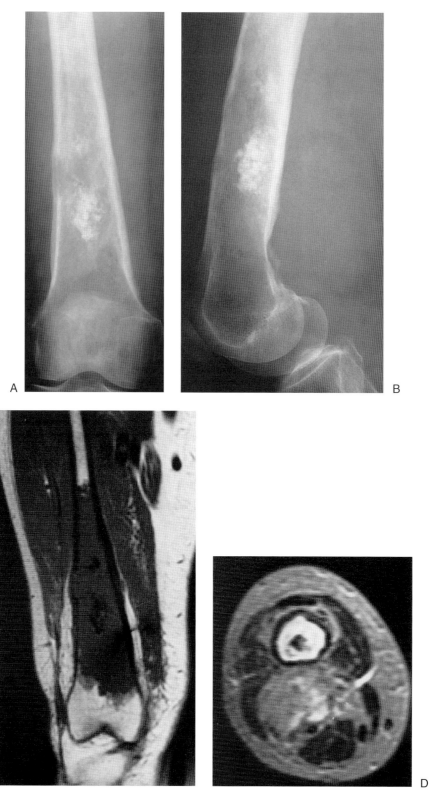

FIG. 87. Chondrosarcoma: magnetic resonance imaging. (**A**) Anteroposterior and (**B**) lateral radiographs of the distal femur show typical appearance of central medullary chondrosarcoma. The cortex is destroyed, and there is a large soft tissue mass projecting posteriorly. (**C**) Coronal T1-weighted (SE, TR 700, TE 20) MRI shows the tumor to be of low signal intensity. The calcifications display signal void. (**D**) Axial T2-weighted (SE, TR 2000, TE 80) image shows intramedullary tumor displaying a high signal intensity, whereas calcifications are of low signal. The soft tissue mass shows heterogeneous signal.

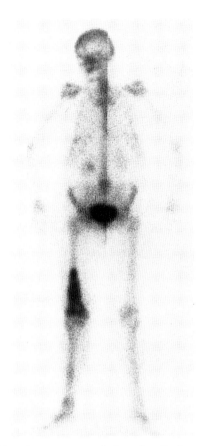

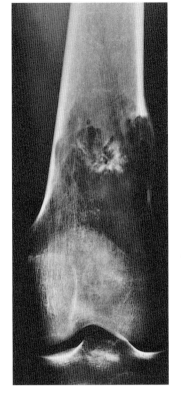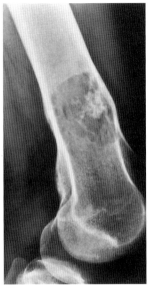

A,

FIG. 88. Chondrosarcoma: scintigraphy. Radionuclide bone scan obtained after intravenous injection of 15 mCi (555 MBq) of ^{99m}Tc-MDP (technetium-labeled methylene diphosphonate) shows increased uptake of tracer localized to the site of the tumor (same patient as in Fig. 3-87).

FIG. 90. Clear cell chondrosarcoma. (**A**) Anteroposterior and (**B**) lateral radiograph of the distal femur show unusual diaphyseal location of the tumor in a 32-year-old man. Note sharp demarcation of the lesion from the normal bone (narrow zone of transition) and its lytic character with central calcifications. (Courtesy of Dr. G. Jundt, Basel, Switzerland.)

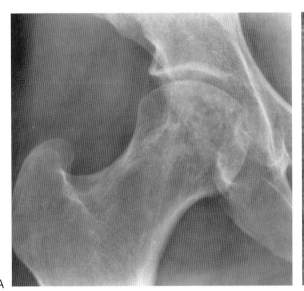

A

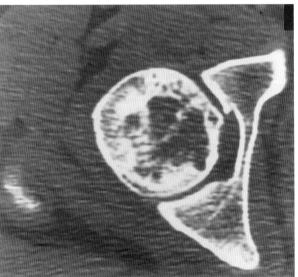

B

FIG. 89. Clear cell chondrosarcoma. **A:** An anteroposterior radiograph of the right hip shows a radiolucent lesion with calcifications in the femoral head. **B:** CT section shows a lytic character of the tumor and central chondroid calcifications.

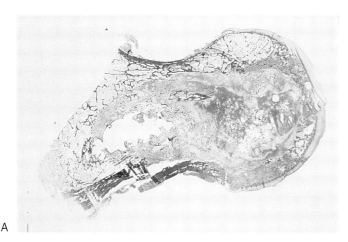

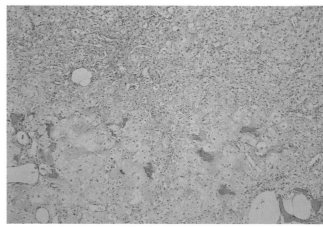

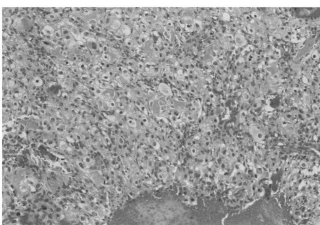

FIG. 91. Histopathology of clear-cell chondrosarcoma. **A:** Coronal section of resected femoral head and neck (same patient as in Fig. 89) shows extension of the tumor from articular cartilage to the base of the neck. In the proximal part of the femoral head some uninvolved cancellous bone is seen (hematoxylin and eosin, original magnification × 0.2). **B:** Large cells with clear or slightly eosinophilic cytoplasm and small nuclei are typical for this variant of chondrosarcoma (hematoxylin and eosin, original magnification ×25). **C:** Homogeneous area of large polygonal cells is in solid arrangement displaying a clear or slightly eosinophilic cytoplasm and small, dark, roundish nuclei. Some giant cells *(left and right middle)* are also present. Note small areas of necrosis *(center and bottom.)* (Hematoxylin and eosin, original magnification ×50).

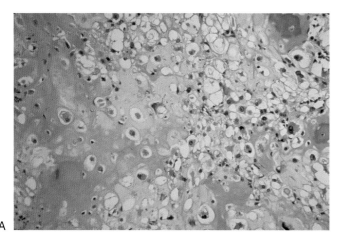

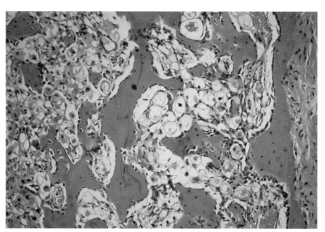

FIG. 92. Histopathology of clear cell chondrosarcoma. **A:** Large and vacuolated cells interspersed in the intercellular cartilaginous matrix. Note small osteoid trabeculae (hematoxylin and eosin, original magnification ×150). **B:** In another area, vacuolated cells are seen in close proximity of reactive bone trabeculae (hematoxylin and eosin, original magnification ×75).

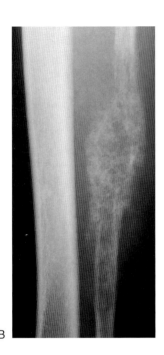
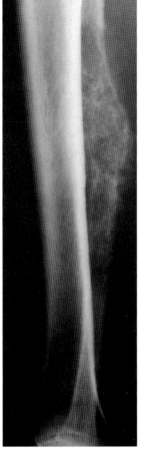

A, B

FIG. 93. Mesenchymal chondrosarcoma. (**A**) Anteroposterior and (**B**) lateral coned-down radiographs of the right leg of a 43-year-old woman with a 6-month history of intermittent pain in the right calf show a destructive lesion at the midportion of the fibula. The central portion of the lesion exhibits annular and comma-shaped calcifications typical of a cartilage tumor, but its periphery shows a permeative type of bone destruction characteristic of round cell tumors.

plastic bone encasement (205), representing endochondral ossification. The microscopic appearances of these components are strikingly different (Fig. 95). An electron microscopic study by Steiner (218) confirmed the bistructural characteristics of this tumor. In some portions the cells may be clustered, often arranged in an alveolar pattern resembling that observed in malignant lymphoma or in embryonal rhabdomyosarcoma and other small cell tumors (15), or may have the antler-like arrangement of capillary vessels seen in hemangiopericytoma. However, the chondroid component is the differentiating feature.

Biologically, the behavior of mesenchymal chondrosarcoma is unpredictable. Although it tends to be aggressive and to exhibit a high rate of metastasis, some patients may not develop metastatic spread for 15 to 20 years after removal of the tumor, whereas other patients develop distant metastases soon after diagnosis. At present, no clinicopathologic features have been described that can distinguish this different biologic behavior for these histologically identical tumor types.

Dedifferentiated Chondrosarcoma

This tumor represents approximately 10% of all chondrosarcomas and overall has the worst prognosis (154). Histologically it is characterized by a relatively low-grade chondrosarcoma with juxtaposed dedifferentiated, i.e., less differentiated, noncartilaginous sarcomatous component including osteosarcoma, fibrosarcoma, MFH, rhabdomyosarcoma, angiosarcoma, and undifferentiated sarcoma (141,149,171,173,191,222). The age group affected and the anatomic predilection are the same as that of conventional chondrosarcoma (189). Patients with this tumor often present with rapid onset of swelling and local tenderness, superimposed on a long history of less severe pain (160). The chronic pain may be associated with a low-grade malignant lesion, and the sudden change in the pattern of symptoms probably reflects the emergence of a more malignant tumor (201). Pathologic fractures are not uncommon, and metastasis to distant organs is common. Radiography often reveals remodeling expansion of the involved segment with variable

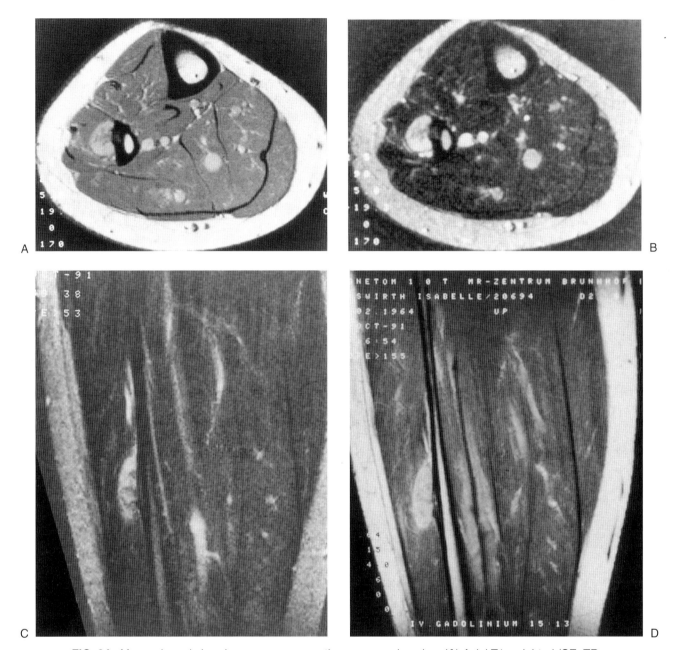

FIG. 94. Mesenchymal chondrosarcoma: magnetic resonance imaging. (**A**) Axial T1-weighted (SE, TR 600, TE 20) MRI shows a focus of intermediate signal within low signal of the lateral cortex of the fibula. A soft tissue mass displays a signal slightly higher than muscles but lower than subcutaneous fat. (**B**) Axial and (**C**) coronal T2-weighted (SE, TR 2000, TE 80) images better demonstrate a destruction of the fibular cortex. On these sequences the soft tissue mass becomes bright. (**D**) On T1-weighted image after intravenous administration of gadolinium there is enhancement of the tumor.

degrees of mineralization; evidence of a long-standing, low-grade cartilage tumor; and a superimposed, more destructive moth-eaten or permeative pattern (Fig. 96). Often, there is an accompanying soft tissue mass (196,215). Histologic studies demonstrate that the tumor usually arises from the site of a Grade 1 chondrosarcoma, either spontaneously or after surgical treatment and recurrence of the latter. It is composed of low-grade cartilage tissue surrounded by a high-grade sarcomatous component, with a clear delineation between the two components (Fig. 97). The high-grade tumor tissue is usually a fibrosarcoma, malignant fibrous histiocytoma, or osteosarcoma (Figs. 98 and 99) (181). The problem is further complicated by the fact that in a considerable number of cases (up to 33% in larger series) the chondrosarcoma arises on the

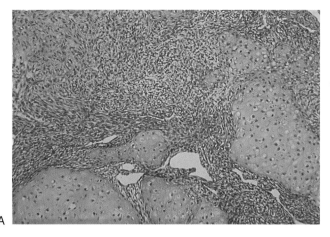

A

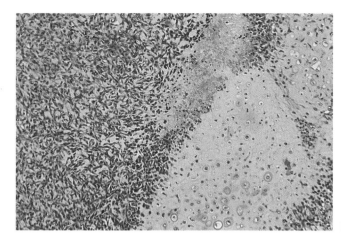

B

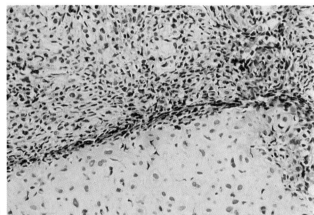

C

FIG. 95. Histopathology of mesenchymal chondrosarcoma. **A:** Islands of fairly well differentiated chondroblastic tissue are surrounded by densely arranged small spindle cells (hematoxylin and eosin, original magnification ×25). **B:** At higher magnification the clear-cut distinction between two components, spindle cell (*left*) and chondroblastic (*right*) is obvious. A narrow band of necrotic tissue lies side-by-side with the chondroblastic area (*middle top*) (hematoxylin and eosin, original magnification ×50). **C:** A high magnification photomicrograph shows the interface between cartilaginous and mesenchymal components of the tumor (hematoxylin and eosin, original magnification ×50).

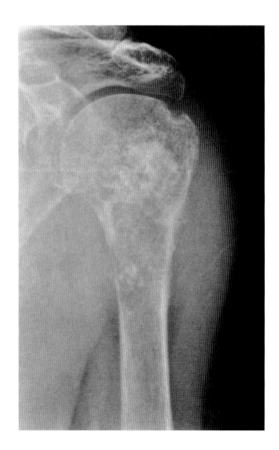

FIG. 96. Dedifferentiated chondrosarcoma. An anteroposterior radiograph of the left shoulder in a 70-year-old woman shows a lytic lesion with chondroid calcifications in the humeral neck extending into the proximal shaft. The proximal part of the lesion is consistent with a slow-growing tumor, whereas the distal part exhibits more aggressive appearance including cortical destruction and a soft tissue mass.

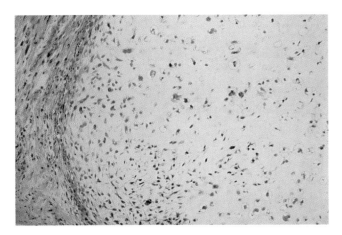

FIG. 97. Histopathology of dedifferentiated chondrosarcoma. A photomicrograph shows low-grade chondrosarcoma (*right*) that is clearly separated from the pleomorphic spindle-cell tissue (*left*) (hematoxylin and eosin, original magnification ×50) (Courtesy of Prof. Hubert A. Sissons, London.)

site of a usually calcified enchondroma, so that the manifestations of all three tumors, one benign and two malignant (enchondroma, chondrosarcoma, and dedifferentiated chondrosarcoma) may be present side by side (Fig. 100). Although the term "dedifferentiation" implies that the high-grade tumor elements arise from genetic alterations in the chondrocytes of the low-grade cartilage that cause them to grow more rapidly, most investigators now believe that these tumors may in fact derive from synchronous neoplastic cell clones, one of which does not have the capacity to differentiate (185). The former theory that an already well-differentiated cell may dedifferentiate is no more accepted. Instead, the general opinion holds that phenotypically distinct primitive cell clones are present within a chondrosarcoma and that these are capable of differentiating into separate cell lines in which different histologic characteristics exist (e.g., fibrosarcoma, osteosarcoma, malignant fibrous histiocytoma,

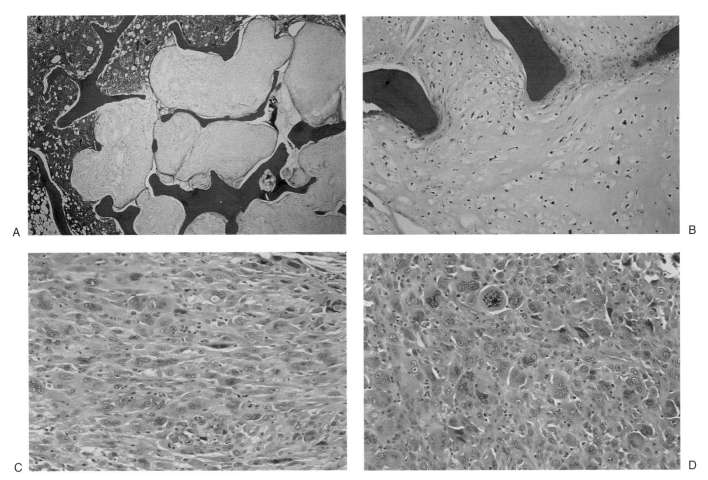

FIG. 98. Histopathology of dedifferentiated chondrosarcoma. **A:** Grade 1 chondrosarcoma invades marrow spaces of cancellous bone (right 75%). Purely cellular dedifferentiated tumor tissue is present on the left (van Gieson, original magnification ×12). **B:** Low-grade chondrosarcoma tissue flowing within the marrow spaces of cancellous bone (van Gieson, original magnification ×50). **C:** In another field spindle-cell part of dedifferentiated tumor exhibits conspicuous cell and nuclear pleomorphism (hematoxylin and eosin, original magnification ×50). **D:** Yet in another field the dedifferentiated tissue represents a giant cell-rich variant of malignant fibrous histiocytoma (hematoxylin and eosin, original magnification ×50).

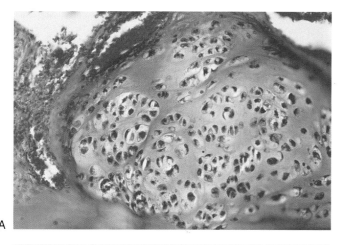

A

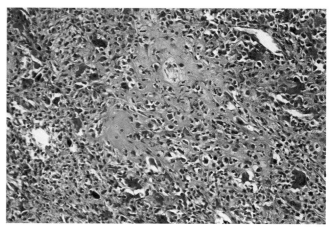

B

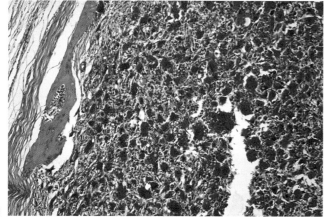

C

FIG. 99. Histopathology of dedifferentiated chondrosarcoma. **A:** In one part of the tumor there is a grade 2 chondrosarcoma with irregular distribution of chondrocytes (hematoxylin and eosin, original magnification ×50). **B:** The other areas show dedifferentiated part of tumor with spindle-cell tissue and tumor-bone formation (*center*) typical for osteosarcoma. Some giant cells are also present (hematoxylin and eosin, original magnification ×50). **C:** Another field of view shows differentiation of giant cell-containing spindle cell tissue, consistent with malignant giant-cell tumor (hematoxylin and eosin, original magnification ×50).

and rhabdomyosarcoma) (40). Support for this hypothesis has come from an immunohistochemical and biochemical study of cultured human chondrosarcoma, in which the existence of four different clonal cell lines within a parent tumor was demonstrated (161). Patients with dedifferentiated chondrosarcoma usually do not survive for more than 2 years after diagnosis.

Periosteal (Juxtacortical) Chondrosarcoma

Although most primary chondrosarcomas arise centrally in bone, in rare instances a tumor originates in a periosteal (juxtacortical) location (139). A periosteal chondrosarcoma arises from the surface of a bone to which it is firmly attached, but with no associated exostosis (Figs. 101 and 102). Only exceptionally it invades the medullary cavity (164). These tumors present as an asymptomatic or a slightly painful, slowly growing mass. On radiologic and pathologic studies, they exhibit the same general features as a central chondrosarcoma (208)

(Fig. 103). Most of them represent well-differentiated grade 1 or 2 cartilage malignancy (Fig. 104), and the prognosis after surgical excision is therefore good. Metastases develop only rarely. On radiography they are occasionally mistaken for periosteal osteosarcomas, which also occur on the external surface of long bones and consist largely of cartilage.

Synovial Chondrosarcoma

This exceptionally rare tumor, which arises from the synovial membrane, may be primary or secondary. Primary lesions arise *de novo* in the joint synovium without evidence of previous synovial chondromatosis (143). In radiographic studies, synovial chondrosarcoma may mimic synovial chondromatosis or periosteal chondrosarcoma. Secondary tumors are believed to arise from malignant transformation of synovial chondromatosis (163) **(see Chapter 9)**.

Because very few cases of synovial chondrosarcoma have been documented, it is difficult to compare the behavior of

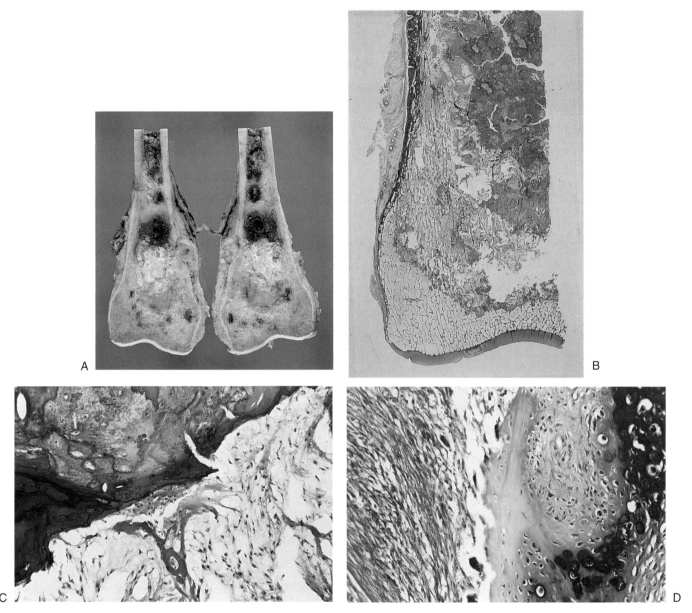

FIG. 100. Histopathology of dedifferentiated chondrosarcoma. **A:** Coronal section of the specimen of the distal femur shows calcified enchondroma (*round whitish area in center*), well-differentiated chondrosarcoma (*darker area medially*), and dedifferentiated tumor (*rose area distally*). Site of the biopsy is marked by hemorrhagic area proximally. **B:** Histologic overview of the medial half of the distal femur shows three different tumors: calcified enchondroma (*proximal middle*), well-differentiated chondrosarcoma (*section close to the medial cortex on the left*), and dedifferentiated tumor with osteoblastic differentiation (*distal middle*) (hematoxylin and eosin, original magnification ×0.2). The details of osteoblastic differentiations are depicted in FIG 2.120. **C:** Calcified enchondroma (*upper half*) is bordered by well-differentiated chondrosarcoma with myxoid component (*lower half*) (hematoxylin and eosin, original magnification ×25). **D:** Two different tissues are clearly separated: on the left dedifferentiated part of tumor formed of spindle cells and some giant cells, abutting the well-differentiated chondrosarcoma on the right (Giemsa, original magnification ×50).

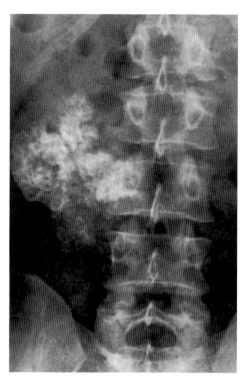

FIG. 101. Periosteal chondrosarcoma. Anteroposterior radiograph of the lumbar spine shows a large calcified mass attached to the lateral aspect of the third lumbar vertebra. (Reprinted with permission from Bullough PG. *Atlas of orthopedic pathology,* 2nd ed. New York: Gower, 1992;16.31.)

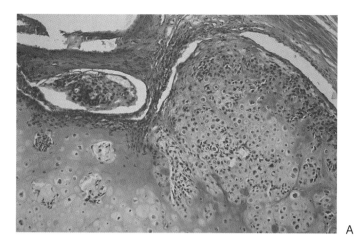

A

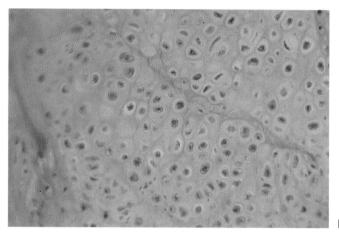

B

FIG. 103. Histopathology of periosteal chondrosarcoma. A: Lobulated chondroblastic tumor is clearly separated from adjacent connective tissue (*top*) (hematoxylin and eosin, original magnification ×12). **B:** At higher magnification there is obvious pleomorphism of the cells and hyperchromatism of the nuclei, proving malignancy (hematoxylin and eosin, original magnification ×50).

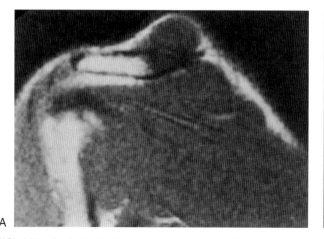

A

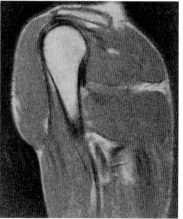

B

FIG. 102. Periosteal chondrosarcoma: magnetic resonance imaging. **A:** A sagittal T1-weighted MRI shows an intermediate signal intensity lesion arising from the cortex of the clavicle and extending into the soft tissues. **B:** A proton-density MRI demonstrates that the lesion now exhibits a bright signal.

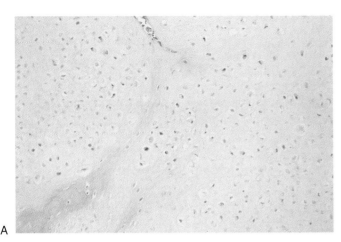
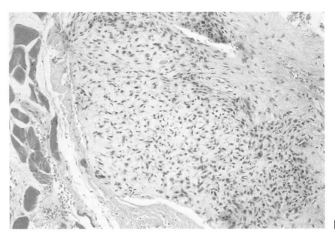

A

B

FIG. 104. Histopathology of periosteal chondrosarcoma. **A:** Hyaline cartilage with irregular cell arrangement and pleomorphic ("chondroblastic") cell nuclei betray malignant character of the tumor (hematoxylin and eosin, original magnification ×25). **B:** At higher magnification in another area high cellularity, conspicuous pleomorphism of the cells and nuclei, some mitoses, and partly myxoid matrix are consistent with grade 1 to 2 chondrosarcoma (hematoxylin and eosin, original magnification ×50).

these tumors to that of chondrosarcoma of bone. However, the former appears to be characterized by a spectrum ranging from low-grade neoplasms to high-grade tumors (162,176,182,183).

Soft-Tissue (Extraskeletal) Chondrosarcoma

This tumor, first described by Stout and Verner in 1953 (219), is derived from multipotential mesenchymal progenitor cells. It develops in the soft tissues and is independent of bone, periosteum, or cartilage. It represents about 2% of all soft tissue sarcomas (179). More than 80% of soft tissue chondrosarcomas affect the lower extremities, particularly in the regions of the thigh and knee (135,229). These tumors have a predilection for middle-aged men. It is usually not possible to determine the exact site at which they arise. However, it appears that they originate in muscle, fascia, bursa, and other connective tissue structures. Patients typically present with a slowly enlarging soft tissue mass, and approximately one third of cases are characterized by pain or tenderness (134, 157). On radiography, this type of chondrosarcoma appears as a soft tissue mass with mineralization similar to that observed in conventional intramedullary chondrosarcomas. However, calcifications occur only in 30% of cases. Adjacent bone destruction may or may not be present (Fig. 105). On MRI examination, the mass is usually isointense to the surrounding tissues on T1-weighted sequences, and of a high signal intensity on T2 weighting (153). After administration of Gd-DTPA, inhomogeneous enhancement of the tumor is observed on T1-weighted images (178). Aohi et al. proposed a term of rings and arcs enhancement to describe the phenomenon that reflects the lobulated growth pattern of this tumor (136). Scintigraphy demonstrates increased uptake of ^{99m}Tc-MDP

that is related to hyperemia, calcifications, endochondral ossification, and reactive new bone formation in these tumors (132,181).

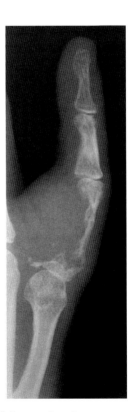

FIG. 105. Soft-tissue chondrosarcoma. A dorsovolar radiograph of a fifth finger of the left hand of a 47-year-old woman shows a soft-tissue mass invading and destroying the proximal phalanx. There are no visible calcifications. The biopsy revealed myxoid chondrosarcoma.

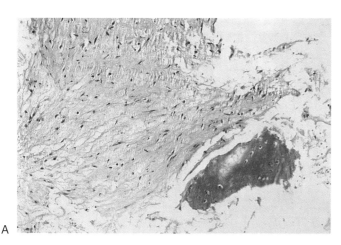
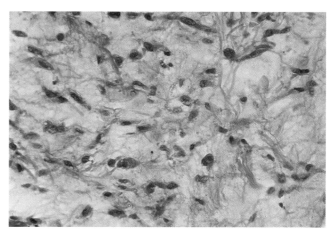

A   B

FIG. 106. Histopathology of soft tissue myxoid chondrosarcoma. **A:** Cartilaginous tissue with malignant cells is seen invading a bone trabecula (hematoxylin and eosin, original magnification ×25). **B:** At higher magnification the myxoid character of the tumor is conspicuous (hematoxylin and eosin, original magnification ×50).

On histologic examination, the lesion is characterized by undifferentiated mesenchymal cells with islands of well-differentiated cartilage (221). This tumor is typically surrounded by a pseudocapsule, which is formed by compression of normal connective tissue. In some instances lobulation is observed. The nodules sometimes consist of well-formed hyaline cartilage in which connective tissue septa are present. The septa may exhibit invasion by malignant cells with bizarre hyperchromatic and multiple nuclei of irregular size and shape (15). The tumor may consist of well- or poorly differentiated hyaline cartilage (conventional soft tissue chondrosarcoma) may be partially or entirely myxoid in appearance (myxoid chondrosarcoma) (Fig. 106), or may contain mesenchymal tissue (mesenchymal chondrosarcoma) (11,213).

Secondary Chondrosarcomas

The term secondary chondrosarcoma is applied to any tumor that arises as a result of malignant transformation of a benign cartilaginous lesion, such as osteochondroma or enchondroma. It also applies to the rare cases of Paget disease (216) or irradiated bone that lead to development of a cartilaginous malignancy. These tumors, which constitute about 20% of all chondrosarcomas, may be either central or peripheral. The most common are peripheral lesions, which develop as malignant transformation of either hereditary multiple exostoses **(see Fig. 53)** (10% to 15% of patients with this condition develop chondrosarcoma) or solitary osteochondroma (Fig. 107) (<1% of patients are at risk). Central secondary chondrosarcomas develop as malignant transformation of enchondroma (rarely in patients with a solitary lesion and much more commonly in patients with multiple enchondromatosis, e.g., Ollier disease and Maffucci syn-

drome). Exceptionally, secondary chondrosarcoma develops in the joint as a malignant transformation of synovial chondromatosis (193).

In malignant transformation of osteochondroma to chondrosarcoma, the most reliable clinical and radiologic features include pain (in the absence of fracture, bursitis, or pressure on nearby nerves), the growth spurt of osteochondroma (after skeletal maturity), development of a bulky cartilaginous cap (thicker than 2 cm), dispersed calcifications in the cartilaginous cap (which in benign exostosis are confined to the osteochondral junction), and development of a soft tissue mass (68) (Fig. 107; **see also Figs. 49, 53, and Table 2**). Scintigraphy is not a reliable modality for differentiation of benign exostoses from exostotic chondrosarcoma.

Some chondrosarcomas are believed to originate from benign enchondromas (15,201,202). However, it is almost impossible to establish the evolution of a preexisting enchondroma to a chondrosarcoma by histologic means alone, particularly when the former is a solitary lesion. Some investigators believe that in these rare cases the preexisting enchondroma may in fact represent a low-grade chondrosarcoma that masquerades as a benign lesion. Nevertheless, malignant transformation of a calcified enchondroma has been well documented in patients with dedifferentiated chondrosarcoma, with Ollier disease, and with Maffucci syndrome (148) (Figs. 108 and 109).

The radiographic signs of malignant transformation of enchondroma to chondrosarcoma include thickening or destruction of the adjacent cortex, appearance of a periosteal reaction without evidence of a pathologic fracture, and development of a soft tissue mass. Pain at the site of the lesion in the absence of fracture is an important clinical sign of evolving malignancy.

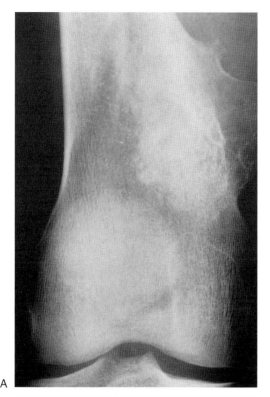
A

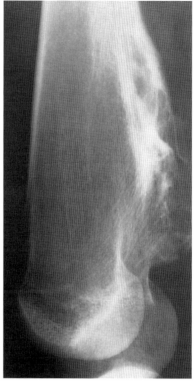
B

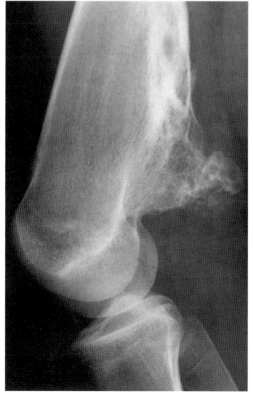
C

FIG. 107. Malignant transformation of osteochondroma. A 28-year-old man had been diagnosed of having osteochondroma since age 14. Recently he developed pain in the popliteal fossa and noticed a growing mass. (A) Anteroposterior and (B) lateral radiographs obtained in the past show a sessile osteochondroma arising from the posteromedial cortex of the distal femur. (C) Current lateral radiograph of the distal femur shows that the osteochondroma has enlarged. Also seen are dispersed calcifications in the cartilaginous cap pointing to the malignant transformation to chondrosarcoma.

Differential Diagnosis

Radiology

Radiologic differential diagnosis of conventional chondrosarcoma includes mainly an *enchondroma*. Among other clinical signs, the malignancy of a lesion is suggested by the development of pain in a previously asymptomatic lesion (e.g., malignant transformation of enchondroma to chondrosarcoma) or by development of swelling at the site of a lesion. The most obvious signs of malignancy are thickening of the cortex, cortical destruction, periosteal reaction, and a soft tissue mass **(see Figs. 80 to 83)**. If any of these features are present the diagnosis can be made unequivocally. A more difficult task is to differentiate low-grade chondrosarcoma from enchondroma. In some cases this is almost impossible, although the focally thickened cortex may point to the former tumor (Fig. 110; **see also Fig. 29**). It must be stressed that neither CT nor MRI is usually suitable for establishing the precise nature of a cartilage lesion. In particular, too

much faith has been placed in MRI as a method helpful in distinguishing benign cartilage lesions from malignant ones. Despite the use of various criteria, the application of MRI to tissue diagnosis has rarely achieved satisfactory results (231) because benign and malignant chondrogenic lesions have the same MR characteristics. Both exhibit a low to intermediate signal intensity compared with normal bone marrow on T1-weighted images and a high signal intensity on T2-weighted images (79,145). Quantitative determination of relaxation times is of little clinical value in identifying cartilage tumor types (156), although it is an important technique in the staging of chondrosarcoma (142).

Occasionally, central chondrosarcoma located in the proximal femur or humerus may mimic *osteonecrosis*. Careful examination of the plain radiograph for the presence of cartilage calcification and MRI findings typical of an osteonecrotic pattern (i.e., a clear demarcation at the reactive interface between live and dead bone), as well as MRI characteristics for each class of osteonecrosis (151), should help

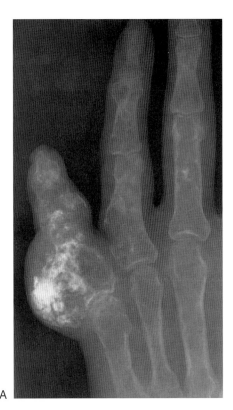

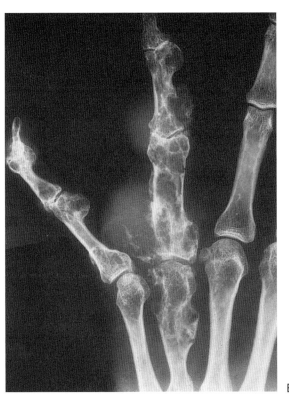

A

B

FIG. 108. Malignant transformation of Ollier disease. **A:** A 38-year-old woman with known long-standing Ollier disease since childhood presented with pain and a slowly enlarging mass at the dorsomedial aspect of the fifth finger of the right hand. The radiograph shows typical changes of enchondromatosis in the hand. Also noted is destruction of the cortex of the proximal phalanx of the small finger and a soft tissue mass containing chondroid calcifications, indicating malignant transformation to chondrosarcoma. **B:** A 30-year-old man with enchondromatosis presented with pain and an enlarging mass at the base of the ring finger of the right hand. A plain radiograph shows typical changes of enchondromatosis. Also noted is destruction of the cortex of the proximal and distal phalanges of the ring finger associated with adjacent soft tissue masses. The open biopsy revealed malignant transformation of enchondroma into chondrosarcoma.

in making this distinction. Clear cell chondrosarcoma may be difficult to differentiate from *chondroblastoma* and from giant cell tumor (Fig. 111), as both of the latter lesions also preferentially affect the articular end of a bone. Furthermore, because clear-cell chondrosarcoma can arise before skeletal maturity, it may be indistinguishable from chondroblastoma. *Giant-cell tumor* may be distinguished by the lack of matrix calcifications (although clear cell chondrosarcoma sometimes presents also as a purely lytic lesion). Mesenchymal chondrosarcoma, because of a permeative or moth-eaten type of bone destruction, may be mistaken for a round cell tumor. Periosteal chondrosarcoma may be indistinguishable from *periosteal osteosarcoma* (see text on osteosarcoma).

Soft-tissue chondrosarcoma may mimic soft-tissue osteosarcoma, *myositis ossificans,* and *tumoral calcinosis,* and vice versa. Although *synovial chondrosarcoma* may be difficult to distinguish from synovial chondromatosis, MRI is occasionally helpful in this respect (195) (see Fig. 9-38).

Pathology

Histopathologic differential diagnosis of chondroblastic tumors is sometimes difficult because some tumors may exhibit indistinct histologic and cellular characteristics (190). The diagnosis is, however, dependent on the location of a given tumor within the skeleton.

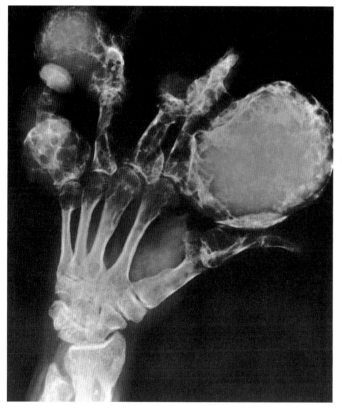

A

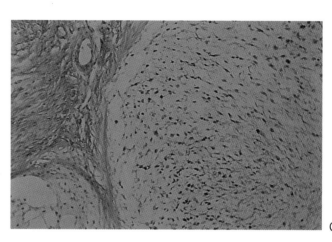

C

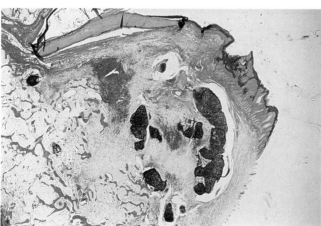

B

FIG. 109. Malignant transformation of Ollier disease. **A:** A 48-year-old watchmaker with a long history of Ollier disease developed pain in the ring finger. An oblique radiograph of the right hand demonstrates characteristic changes of this disorder consisting of multiple enchondromas and large lobulated cartilaginous masses in all fingers. The lesion of the middle phalanx of the ring finger shows destruction of the cortex and the extension of the tumor into the soft tissues. Biopsy revealed chondrosarcoma. **B:** Longitudinal section of the distal phalanx of the left thumb with nail (*clear blue lamella*) of another patient shows cancellous bone with large islands of chondrosarcoma (*purple*) proliferating into the surrounding soft tissue (*center*) (Giemsa, original magnification ×1). **C:** At a higher magnification, the malignant cartilage exhibiting spindle cells in dense arrangement, with clearly polymorphous, hyperchromatic nuclei and a myxoid matrix, borders the fibrous connective tissue of the distal phalanx (*upper left*) Giemsa, original magnification ×20).

The pathologic features of a malignant cartilage tumor which include the presence of hypercellular areas and pleomorphic cells are not unequivocal. The diagnosis is then dependent on the anatomic location of a given tumor. Appreciable numbers of plump cells with large vesicular ("chondroblastic"), or double nuclei, and invasion (permeation) of bone marrow and trabeculae, as well as infiltration of compact bone are clear signs of malignancy.

A cartilage tumor with histologic signs that clearly indicate malignancy, such as marked atypia of chondrocytes, cells arranged densely in clusters, and hyperchromasia of nuclei (grades 2 and 3), is easy to diagnose, as there are no reasonable differential problems. An important differentiation point is the relation between cartilage tissue and trabecular bone. In *enchondroma* the lobuli are usually surrounded by a narrow rim of bone (Fig. 112A) or dense fibrous tissue, whereas the cartilage of a chondrosarcoma "flows" into the marrow spaces of the trabecular bone, with secondary induction of bone resorption (Fig. 112B). Differentiation of chondrosarcoma from *chondroblastic osteosarcoma* may be difficult if the latter shows only scant bone formation. In such instances the presence of hyaline matrix in chondrosarcoma (at least in the grade 1 and 2 tumors) may be helpful, in contrast to the fibrocartilage of osteosarcoma. Myxoid transformation of the matrix is in itself not a sign of malignancy. However, differentiation from *chondromyxoid fibroma* may cause a problem if the cell atypias of the malignant tumor are not clear-cut.

A special histopathologic problem in differential diagnosis is posed by dedifferentiated chondrosarcoma. This tumor may be confused with high-grade chondrosarcoma contain-

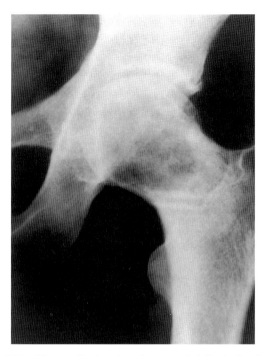

FIG. 111. Clear-cell chondrosarcoma. A lytic lesion in the femoral head in a 39-year-old woman was thought to represent a giant-cell tumor. Biopsy revealed clear-cell chondrosarcoma.

ing areas of spindle cells, mesenchymal chondrosarcoma, chondroblastic osteosarcoma, malignant fibrous histiocytoma, and fibrosarcoma (13). The two latter diagnoses can be eliminated by the presence of cartilage in dedifferentiated chondrosarcoma. The areas of spindle cells seen in high-grade chondrosarcomas exhibit multiple zones of transition and intermingling of the spindle cell foci with the hyaline cartilage. Conversely, in dedifferentiated chondrosarcoma the foci of spindle cells and the hyaline cartilage are juxtaposed at the interface between the two tumor components, with no intermingling of components throughout the lesion. In a similar manner, the cartilaginous component of mesenchymal chondrosarcoma appears as specks throughout the tumor and is mingled with the major component of spindle cells or small round cells (13). In *chondroblastic osteosarcoma,* tumor bone or tumor osteoid is usually irregularly mixed with cartilage and the two malignant elements are not as distinctly separated as in dedifferentiated chondrosarcoma, but may merge onto one another in the form of chondrosteoid. Differentiation of these tumors is further complicated by the fact that in a number of cases dedifferentiated chondrosarcoma arises at the site of a usually calcified enchondroma or a low-grade chondrosarcoma, so that all three tumor manifestations, one benign and two malignant, may be found side by side. It therefore follows that the term "dedifferentiated chondrosarcoma" is not accurate, although well established.

Clear-cell chondrosarcoma consists of rather large cells with a water-clear or more eosinophilic cytoplasm and fairly small nuclei. They are arranged in clusters, with intermin-

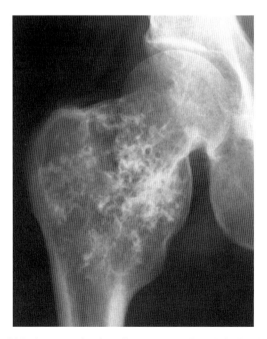

FIG. 110. Low-grade chondrosarcoma. Focal thickening of the cortex at the greater trochanter and expanded character of the lesion point to malignancy.

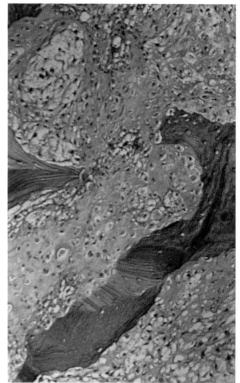

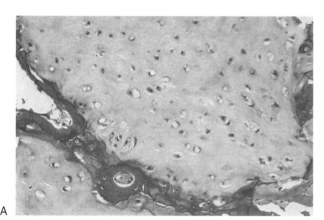

A   B

FIG. 112. Histopathology of enchondroma: distinction from chondrosarcoma. **A:** In enchondroma, the cartilage lobules are commonly surrounded by a narrow rim of bone (hematoxylin and eosin, original magnification ×250). (Reprinted with permission from Bullough PG. *Atlas of orthopedic pathology,* 2nd ed. New York: Gower, 1992;16.21.) **B:** In chondrosarcoma the tumor is more cellular and invades the bone trabeculae (hematoxylin and eosin, original magnification ×100). (Reprinted with permission from Bullough PG. *Atlas of orthopedic pathology,* 2nd ed. New York: Gower, 1992;16.32.)

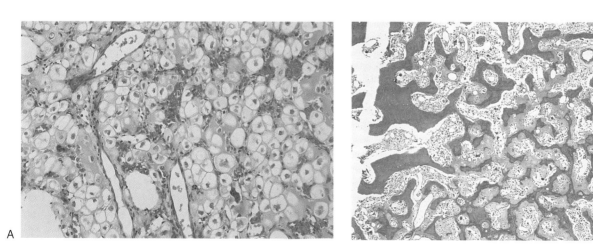

A   B

FIG. 113. Histopathology of clear-cell chondrosarcoma resembling osteosarcoma. **A:** Clear-cell chondrosarcoma exhibiting bundles and cords of fairly large, slightly polymorphic cells with water-clear cytoplasm and small hardly polymorphic nuclei. Minimal reactive bone is present (*right upper corner*) (hematoxylin and eosin, original magnification ×50). **B:** Tumor with extremely marked bone formation mimics osteosarcoma. Clear cells in small clusters within the marrow spaces identify this lesion as clear-cell chondrosarcoma (hematoxylin and eosin, original magnification ×25).

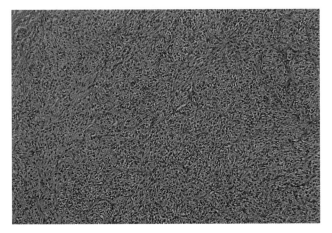

FIG. 114. Histopathology of mesenchymal chondrosarcoma resembling fibrosarcoma. In areas without chondroblastic differentiation and capillaries, distinction from low-grade fibrosarcoma may be difficult (hematoxylin and eosin, original magnification ×25).

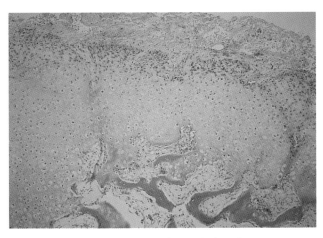

FIG. 115. Histopathology periosteal chondrosarcoma resembling periosteal osteosarcoma. Fairly regularly appearing chondroblastic tissue borders loose connective tissue (*top*) and is supported by trabecular bone (*below*) with features of endochondral ossification, which is not part of the tumor. That reactive bone formation mimics tumor bone of osteosarcoma (hematoxylin and eosin, original magnification ×6).

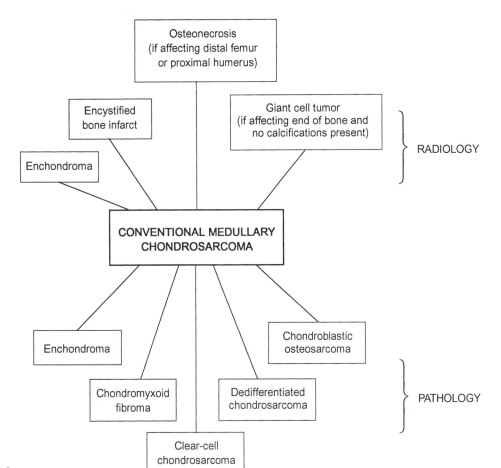

A

FIG. 116. A: The radiologic and pathologic differential diagnosis of conventional medullary chondrosarcoma.

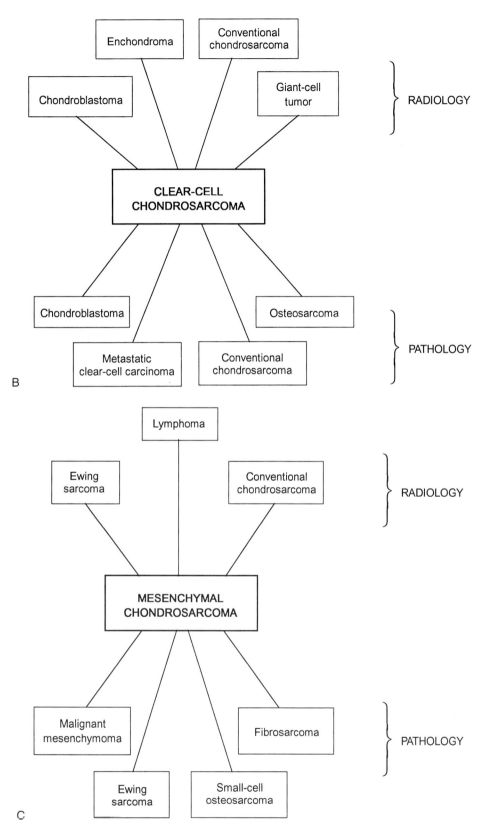

FIG. 116. *Continued.* **B:** The radiologic and pathologic differential diagnoses of clear-cell chondrosarcoma. **C:** The radiologic and pathologic differential diagnoses of mesenchymal chondrosarcoma. (*Figure continues on page 198.*)

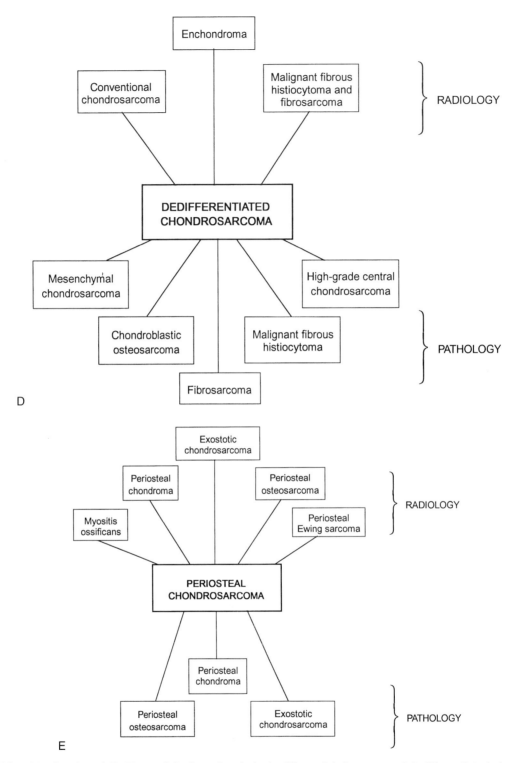

FIG. 116. *Continued.* **D:** The radiologic and pathologic differential diagnoses of dedifferentiated chondrosarcoma. **E:** The radiologic and pathologic differential diagnoses of periosteal chondrosarcoma.

gled small trabeculae or newly built reactive bone (Fig. 113A). Bone formation may be so extensive as to mimic an osteosarcoma (Fig. 113B) (147). In such instances, the location in the epiphysis and the size and characteristics of the cartilage cells are helpful. However, sporadic cases located in the diaphysis have recently been observed (Jundt, unpublished observations, 1995). Histologic differential diagnosis should also include *chondroblastoma.* This tumor may have cells with clear cytoplasm, although they are not a predominant feature. In addition, in the latter tumor the cell nuclei are indented or cleaved, whereas in clear-cell chondrosarcoma they are round (199). Furthermore, in most cases of clear-cell chondrosarcomas areas typical of conventional chondrosarcoma are present.

Metastatic clear-cell carcinoma (such as from the kidneys) may be difficult to distinguish from clear cell chondrosarcoma solely on the basis of its histologic appearance. The glandular architecture or lumen formation are characteristic features of the former and are not seen in clear cell chondrosarcoma. The clinical setting and the presence of chondroid differentiation are essential in confirming the latter diagnosis (199).

Mesenchymal chondrosarcoma may be difficult to distinguish from *malignant mesenchymoma of bone* because both tumors demonstrate the same biphasic pattern (209,211). In malignant mesenchymoma, however, a third component (osteosarcoma) is always present, whereas in mesenchymal chondrosarcoma the matrix-producing component is always chondrosarcoma. The nonmatrix cellular component of malignant mesenchymoma consists of either liposarcoma, rhabdomyosarcoma, or both (175). The nonmatrix component of mesenchymal chondrosarcoma consists of undifferentiated round or spindle cells, frequently arranged in a hemangiopericytomatous pattern.

Areas containing broad sheaths of small cells may mimic *Ewing sarcoma* (13). Moreover, both tumors contain cytoplasmic glycogen. In Ewing sarcoma, however, spindle cells and cartilage formation are absent. Areas containing primarily spindle cell tissue may resemble low-grade fibrosarcoma (Fig. 114).

Small-cell osteosarcoma may occasionally mimic mesenchymal chondrosarcoma because the background population of small cells in both tumors may be indistinguishable. However, the presence of osteoid in osteosarcoma is diagnostic.

Periosteal chondrosarcoma is occasionally difficult to distinguish from the malignant transformation of solitary osteochondroma to chondrosarcoma. In such cases the continuity of the cancellous bone of osteochondroma with that of the adjacent host bone may indicate malignant transformation rather than a periosteal tumor.

To make a distinction between periosteal chondrosarcoma and periosteal osteosarcoma is extremely difficult. In fact, some investigators (40) have previously considered these lesions to be identical. Although periosteal osteosarcoma is predominantly a chondroblastic tumor, unlike the large low-grade cartilage present in periosteal chondrosarcoma, the chondroid element in periosteal osteosarcoma is usually high grade (13). Moreover, tumor osteoid is formed by the malignant neoplastic cells of periosteal osteosarcoma, a feature that is absent in *periosteal chondrosarcoma* (Fig. 115) (224).

Periosteal chondroma may mimic periosteal chondrosarcoma and vice versa. There is overlap in the histologic appearance of both lesions. Mirra contended that periosteal chondrosarcomas are usually wider than they are long, in contrast to periosteal chondromas (30).

The radiologic and pathologic differential diagnosis of conventional chondrosarcoma, clear cell chondrosarcoma, mesenchymal chondrosarcoma, dedifferentiated chondrosarcoma, and periosteal chondrosarcoma are depicted in Fig. 116, respectively.

REFERENCES

Enchondroma, Periosteal Chondroma, Enchondromatosis, Soft-Tissue Chondroma

1. Abdelwahab IF, Hermann G, Lewis MM, Klein MJ. Case report 588. Intracortical chondroma of the left femur. *Skeletal Radiol* 1990;19:59–61.
2. Bansal M, Goldman AB, DiCarlo EF, McCormack R. Soft tissue chondromas: diagnosis and differential diagnosis. *Skeletal Radiol* 1993;22:309–315.
3. Barton DL, Reeves RJ. Tumoral calcinosis. Report of three cases and review of the literature. *Am J Roentgenol* 1961;86:351–358.
4. Beltran J, Chandnani V, McGhee RA Jr, Kursunoglu-Brahme S. Gadopentetate dimeglumine-enhanced MR imaging of the musculoskeletal system. *Am J Roentgenol* 1991;156:457–466.
5. Boriani S, Bacchini P, Bertoni F, Campanacci M. Periosteal chondroma. A review of twenty cases. *J Bone Joint Surg* 1983;65A:205–212.
6. Chung EB, Enzinger FM. Chondromas of soft parts. *Cancer* 1978;41:1414–1424.
7. Crim JR, Mirra JM. Enchondroma protuberans. Report of a case and its distinction from chondrosarcoma and osteochondroma adjacent to an enchondroma. *Skeletal Radiol* 1990;19:431–434.
8. Dahlin DC, Salvador AH. Cartilaginous tumors of the soft tissues of the hands and feet. *Mayo Clin Proc* 1974;49:721–726.
9. Dahlin DC, Unni KK. *Bone tumors. General aspects and data on 8542 cases,* 4th ed. Springfield, IL: Charles C Thomas, 1986;18, 33–51, 227–259.
10. deSantos LA, Spjut HJ. Periosteal chondroma: a radiographic spectrum. *Skeletal Radiol* 1981;6:15–20.
11. Enzinger FM, Weiss SW. Cartilaginous tumors and tumor-like lesions of soft tissue. In: *Soft tissue tumors,* 2nd ed. St. Louis: CV Mosby, 1988;861.
12. Epstein DA, Levin EJ. Bone scintigraphy in hereditary multiple exostoses. *Am J Roentgenol* 1978;130:331–333.
13. Fechner RE, Mills SE. *Tumors of the bones and joints.* Washington, DC: Armed Forces Institute of Pathology, 1993.
14. Feldman F. Cartilaginous lesions of bones and soft tissues. *CRC Crit Rev Clin Radiol Nucl Med* 1974;4:477–554.
15. Feldman F. Cartilaginous tumors and cartilage-forming tumor-like conditions of the bones and soft tissues. In: Ranniger K, ed. *Bone tumors.* Berlin: Springer-Verlag, 1977;83–242.
16. Freiberg TA, Hembree JL, Laine W. Periosteal chondroma: a review of the literature and case report. *J Foot Surg* 1986;25:54–57.
17. Goodman SB, Bell RS, Fornasier VS, De Demeter D, Bateman JE. Ollier's disease with multiple sarcomatous transformation. *Hum Pathol* 1984;15:91–93.

18. Greenfield GB, Arrington JA. *Imaging of bone tumors. A multimodality approach.* Philadelphia: JB Lippincott, 1995.
19. Greenspan A. Tumors of cartilage origin. *Orthop Clin North Am* 1989; 20:347–366.
20. Greenspan A, Unni KK, Matthews J II. Periosteal chondroma masquerading as osteochondroma. *Can Assoc Radiol J* 1993;44:205–210.
21. Holder SF, Grana WA. Periosteal chondroma. *Orthopaedics* 1987;10: 1997–1998.
22. Jaffe HL. *Tumors and tumorous conditions of the bones and joints.* Philadelphia: Lea and Febiger, 1968.
23. Keating RB, Wright PW, Staple TW. Enchondroma protuberans of the rib. *Skeletal Radiol* 1985;13:55–58.
24. Lewis MM, Kenan S, Yabut SM, Norman A, Steiner G. Periosteal chondroma. A report of ten cases and review of the literature. *Clin Orthop* 1990;256:185–192.
25. Li C, Arger PH, Dalinka MK. Soft tissue osteochondroma. A report of three cases. *Skeletal Radiol* 1989;18:435–437.
26. Lichtenstein L, Hall JE. Periosteal chondroma: a distinctive benign cartilage tumor. *J Bone Joint Surg* 1952;34A:691–697.
27. Liu J, Hudkins PG, Swee RG, Unni KK. Bone sarcomas associated with Ollier's disease. *Cancer* 1987;59:1376–1385.
28. Milchgrub S, McMurry NK, Vuitch F, Dorfman HD. Chondrolipoangioma. A cartilage-containing benign mesenchymoma of soft tissue. *Cancer* 1990;66:2636–2641.
29. Milgram JW, Dunn EJ. Para-articular chondromas and osteochondromas. A report of three cases. *Clin Orthop* 1980;148:147–151.
30. Mirra JM, Picci P, Gold RH. *Bone tumors: clinical, radiologic and pathologic correlations.* Philadelphia: Lea and Febiger, 1989.
31. Mitchell ML, Ackerman LV. Case report 405. Ollier disease (enchondromatosis). *Skeletal Radiol* 1987;16:61–66.
32. Moser RP, Gilkey FW, Madewell JE. Enchondroma. In: Moser RP,, ed. *Cartilaginous tumors of the skeleton. AFIP Atlas of Radiologic-Pathologic Correlation*, vol 2. Philadelphia: Hanley and Belfus, 1990; 8–34.
33. Mulder JD, Schütte HE, Kroon HM, Taconis WK. *Radiologic atlas of bone tumors.* Amsterdam: Elsevier, 1993.
34. Nakamura Y, Becker LE, Marks A. S-100 protein in tumors of cartilage and bone: an immunohistochemical study. *Cancer* 1983;52: 1820–1824.
35. Nojima T, Unni KK, McLeod RA, Pritchard DJ. Periosteal chondroma and periosteal chondrosarcoma. *Am J Surg Pathol* 1985;9:666–677.
36. Norman A, Steiner GC. Radiographic and morphological features of cyst formation in idiopathic bone infarction. *Radiology* 1983;146: 335–338.
37. Palmer PES. Tumoral calcinosis. *Br J Radiol* 1966;39:518–525.
38. Ragsdale BD, Sweet DE, Vinh TN. Radiology as gross pathology in evaluating chondroid tumors. *Hum Pathol* 1989;20:930–951.
39. Resniek CS, Levine AM, Aisner SC, Young JW, Dorfman HD. Case report 522. Concurrent adjacent osteochondroma and enchondroma. *Skeletal Radiol* 1989;18:66–69.
40. Schajowicz F. Cartilage-forming tumors. In: Schajowicz F,, ed. *Tumors and tumorlike conditions of bone.* New York: Springer-Verlag, 1994;141–256.
41. Schajowicz F, Ackerman LV, Sissons HA. *Histological typing of bone tumours.* International Histological Classification of Tumors, No. 6. Geneva: World Health Organization, 1972.
42. Schajowicz F, McGuire M. Diagnostic difficulties in skeletal pathology. *Clin Orthop* 1989;240:281–308.
43. Shapiro F. Ollier's disease. An assessment of angular deformity, shortening, and pathological fracture in twenty-one patients. *J Bone Joint Surg* 1982;64A:95–103.
44. Sun TC, Swee RG, Shives TC, Unni KK. Chondrosarcoma in Maffucci's syndrome. *J Bone J Surg* 1985;67A:1214–1219.
45. Sundaram M, McLeod RA. MR imaging of tumor and tumor-like lesions of bone and soft tissue. *Am J Roentgenol* 1990;155:817–824.
46. Unger EC, Kessler HB, Kowalyshyn MJ, Lackman RD, Morea GT. MR imaging of Maffucci syndrome. *Am J Roentgenol* 1988;150: 351–353.
47. Varma DGK, Kumar R, Carrasco CH, Guo S-Q, Richli WR. MR imaging of periosteal chondroma. *J Comput Assist Tomogr* 1991;15: 1008–1010.
48. Zlatkin MB, Lander PH, Begin LR, Hadjipavlou A. Soft-tissue chondromas. *Am J Roentgenol* 1985;144:1263–1267.

Osteochondroma, Multiple Hereditary Osteochrondromatosis

49. Borges AM, Huvos AG, Smith J. Bursa formation and synovial chondrometaplasia associated with osteochondromas. *Am J Clin Pathol* 1981;75:648–653.
50. Cohen EK, Kressel HY, Frank TS, Fallon M, Burk DL Jr, Dalinka MK, Schiebler ML. Hyaline cartilage-origin bone and soft-tissue neoplasms: MR appearance and histologic correlation. *Radiology* 1988; 167:477–481.
51. Davids JR, Glancy GL, Eilert RE. Fracture through the stalk of pedunculated osteochondromas. A report of three cases. *Clin Orthop Rel Res* 1991;271:258–264.
52. El-Khoury GY, Bassett GS. Symptomatic bursa formation with osteochondromas. *Am J Roentgenol* 1979;133:895–898.
53. Fairbank TJ. Dysplasia epiphysealis hemimelica (tarso-epiphyseal aclasis). *J Bone Joint Surg* 1956;38 Br:237–257.
54. Garrison RC, Unni KK, McLeod RA, Pritchard DJ, Dahlin DC. Chondrosarcoma arising in osteochondroma. *Cancer* 1982;49:1890–1897.
55. Geirnaerdt MJA, Bloem JL, Eulderink F, Hogendoorn PCW, Taminiau AH. Cartilaginous tumors: correlation of gadolinium-enhanced MR imaging and histopathologic findings. *Radiology* 1993; 186:813–817.
56. Griffiths HJ, Thompson RC Jr, Galloway HR, Everson LI, Suh J-S. Bursitis in association with solitary osteochondromas presenting as mass lesions. *Skeletal Radiol* 1991;20:513–516.
57. Hensinger RN, Cowell HR, Ramsey PL, Leopold RG. Familial dysplasia epiphysealis hemimelica associated with chondromas and osteochondromas. Report of a kindred with variable presentations. *J Bone Joint Surg* 1974;56A:1513–1516.
58. Hudson TM, Chew FS, Manaster BJ. Scintigraphy of benign exostoses and exostotic chondrosarcomas. *Am J Roentgenol* 1983;140: 581–586.
59. Hudson TM, Spriengfield DS, Spanier SS, Enneking WF, Hamlin DJ. Benign exostoses and exostotic chondrosarcomas: evaluation of cartilage thickness by CT. *Radiology* 1984;152:595–599.
60. Jaffe HL. *Tumors and tumorous conditions of the bones and joints.* Philadelphia: Lea and Febiger, 1968.
61. Karasick D, Schweitzer ME, Eschelman DJ. Symptomatic osteochondromas: imaging features. *Am J Roentgenol* 1997; 68:1507–1512.
62. Kettelkamp DB, Campbell CJ, Bonfiglio M. Dysplasia epiphysealis hemimelica. A report of fifteen cases and a review of the literature. *J Bone Joint Surg* 1966;48A:746–766.
63. Lang IM, Azuuz EM. MRI appearance of dysplasia epiphyealis heminelisa of Nu Knee. *Skeletal Radiol* 1997;26:226–229.
64. Lange RH, Lange TA, Rao BK. Correlative radiographic, scintigraphic, and histological evaluation of exostoses. *J Bone Joint Surg* 1984;66A:1454–1459.
65. Lee JK, Yao L, Wirth CR. MR imaging of solitary osteochondromas: report of eight cases. *Am J Roentgenol* 1987;149:557–560.
66. Malghem J, Vande Berg B, Noël H, Maldague B. Benign osteochondromas and exostotic chondrosarcomas: evaluation of cartilage cap thickness by ultrasound. *Skeletal Radiol* 1992;21:33–37.
67. Nidecker A, Remagen W, Elke M. Korrelation radiologischer und pathologischer Befunde bei Tumoren und tumorähnlichen Läsionen der Hand. *Radiologe* 1982;22:222–229.
68. Norman A, Sissons HA. Radiographic hallmarks of peripheral chondrosarcoma. *Radiology* 1984;151:589–596.
69. Peterson HA. Multiple hereditary osteochondromata. *Clin Orthop* 1989;239:222–230.
70. Uri DS, Dalinka MK, Kneeland JB. Muscle impingement: MR imaging of a painful complication of osteochondromas. *Skeletal Radiol* 1996;25:689–692.

Chondroblastoma

71. Azouz EM, Greenspan A, Marton D. CT evaluation of primary epiphyseal bone abscesses. *Skeletal Radiol* 1993;22:17–23.
72. Björnsson J, Unni KK, Dahlin DC, Beabout JW, Sim FH. Clear-cell chondrosarcoma of bone: observation in 47 cases. *Am J Surg Pathol* 1984;8:223–230.

73. Bloem JL, Mulder JD. Chondroblastoma: a clinical and radiological study of 104 cases. *Skeletal Radiol* 1985;14:1–9.

74. Bogumill GP, Schultz MA, Johnson LC. Giant-cell tumor - a metaphyseal lesion. (Scientific exhibit). *J Bone Joint Surg* 1972;54A:1558.

75. Braunstein E, Martel W, Weatherbee L. Periosteal bone apposition in chondroblastoma. *Skeletal Radiol* 1979;4:34–36.

76. Brower AC, Moser RP, Gilkey FW, Kransdorf MJ. Chondroblastoma. In: Moser RP, ed. *Cartilaginous tumors of the skeleton. AFIP Atlas of Radiologic-Pathologic Correlation*, vol 2. Philadelphia: Hanley and Belfus, 1990;74–113.

77. Brower AC, Moser RP, Kransdorf MJ. The frequency and diagnostic significance of periostitis in chondroblastoma. *Am J Roentgenol* 1990; 154:309–314.

78. Codman EA. Epiphyseal chondromatous giant cell tumors of the upper end of the humerus. *Surg Gynecol Obstet* 1931;52:543– 548.

79. Cohen EK, Kressel HY, Frank TS, Fallon M, Burk DL Jr, Dalinka MK, Schiebler ML. Hyaline cartilage-origin bone and soft-tissue neoplasms: MR appearance and histologic correlation. *Radiology* 1988; 167:477–481.

80. Dahlin DC, Ivins JC. Benign chondroblastoma: a study of 125 cases. *Cancer* 1972;30:401–413.

81. Gardner DJ, Azouz EM. Solitary lucent epiphyseal lesions in children. *Skeletal Radiol* 1988;17:497–504.

82. Giudici MA, Moser RP Jr, Kransdorf MJ. Cartilaginous bone tumors. *Radiol Clin North Am* 1993;31:237–259.

83. Gohel VK, Dalinka MK, Edeiken J. Ischemic necrosis of the femoral head simulating chondroblastoma. *Radiology* 1973;107:545–546.

84. Green P, Wittaker RP. Benign chondroblastoma. Case report with pulmonary metastasis. *J Bone Joint Surg* 1975;57A:418–420.

85. Greenspan A, Klein MJ. Radiology and pathology of bone tumors. In: Lewis MM, ed. *Musculoskeletal oncology. A multidisciplinary approach*. Philadelphia: WB Saunders, 1992;13–72.

86. Hayes CW, Conway WF, Sundaram M. Misleading aggressive MR imaging: appearance of some benign musculoskeletal lesions. *Radio-Graphics* 1992;12:1119–1134.

87. Helms C. Pseudocyst of the humerus. *Am J Roentgenol* 1979;131:287–292.

88. Hudson TM, Hawkins IF Jr. Radiological evaluation of chondroblastoma. *Radiology* 1981;139:1–10.

89. Huvos AG. Chondroblastoma and clear cell chondrosarcoma. In: Huvos AG, ed. *Bone tumors. Diagnosis, treatment and prognosis*, 2nd ed. Philadelphia, WB Saunders, 1991;295–318.

90. Huvos AG, Higinbotham NL, Marcove RC, O Leary P. Aggressive chondroblastoma: Review of the literature on aggressive behavior and metastases with a report of one new case. *Clin Orthop* 1977;126:266–272.

91. Jaffe HL, Lichtenstein L. Benign chondroblastoma of bone: Reinterpretation of so-called calcifying or chondromatous giant cell tumor. *Am J Pathol* 1942;18:969–991.

92. Kaufman RA, Wakely PE, Greenfield DJ. Case report 224. Giant cell tumor of ossification center of the distal end of the fibula, growing into the metaphysis. *Skeletal Radiol* 1983;9:218–222.

93. Keats TE. *Normal Roentgen variants that may simulate disease*. Chicago: Year Book Medical, 1980.

94. Kenney PJ, Gilula LA, Murphy WA. The use of computed tomography to distinguish osteochondroma and chondrosarcoma. *Radiology* 1981;139:129–137.

95. Kricun ME. *Imaging of bone tumors*. Philadelphia: WB Saunders, 1993.

96. Kricun ME, Kricun R, Haskin ME. Chondroblastoma of the calcaneus: radiographic features with emphasis on location. *Am J Roentgenol* 1977;128:613–616.

97. Kroon HM, Bloem JL, Holscher HC, van der Woude HJ, Reijnierse M, Taminiau AHM. MR imaging of edema accompanying benign and malignant bone tumors. *Skeletal Radiol* 1994;23:261–269.

98. Kurt AM, Unni KK, Sim FH, McLeod RA. Chondroblastoma of bone. *Hum Pathol* 1989;20:965–976.

99. Marsh BW, Bonfiglio M, Brady LP, Enneking WF. Benign osteoblastoma: range of manifestations. *J Bone Joint Surg* 1975;57A:1–9.

100. McLeod RA, Beabout JW. The roentgenographic features of chondroblastoma. *Am J Roentgenol* 1973;118:464–471.

101. Mirra JM, Ulich TR, Eckardt JJ, Bhuta S. "Aggressive" chondroblastoma. Light and ultramicroscopic findings after en bloc resection. *Clin Orthop* 1983;178:276–284.

102. Monda L, Wick MR. S-100 protein immunostaining in the differential diagnosis of chondroblastoma. *Hum Pathol* 1985;16:287–293.

103. Moser RP, Brockmole DM, Vinh TN, Kransdorf MJ, Aoki J. Chondroblastoma of the patella. *Skeletal Radiol* 1988;17:413–419.

104. Picci P, Manfrini M, Zucchi V, Gherlinzoni F, Rock M, Bertoni F, Neff JR. Giant-cell tumor of bone in skeletally immature patients. *J Bone Joint Surg* 1983;65A:486–490.

105. Plum GE, Pugh DG. Roentgenologic aspects of benign chondroblastoma of bone. *Am J Roentgenol* 1958;79:584–591.

106. Pösl M, Werner M, Amling M, Ritzel H, Delling G. Malignant transformation of chondroblastoma. *Histopathology* 1996;29:477–480.

107. Quint LE, Gross BH, Glazer GM, Braunstein EM, White SJ. CT evaluation of chondroblastoma. *J Comput Assist Tomogr* 1984;8:907–910.

108. Raymond AK, Raymond PG, Edeiken J. Case report 531. Epiphyseal osteoblastoma distal end of femur. *Skel Radiol* 1989;18:143–146.

109. Resnick D, Cone RO III. The nature of humeral pseudocyst. *Radiology* 1984;150:27–28.

110. Schajowicz F, Gallardo H. Epiphyseal chondroblastoma of bone: a clinicopathological study of sixty-nine cases. *J Bone Joint Surg* 1970; 52B:205–226.

111. Schütte HE, Taconis WK. Giant cell tumor in children and adolescents. *Skeletal Radiol* 1993;22:173–176.

112. Sissons HA, Murray RO, Kemp HBS. *Orthopaedic diagnosis*. Berlin: Springer-Verlag, 1984.

113. Springfield DS, Capanna R, Gherlinzoni F, Picci P, Campanacci M. Chondroblastoma: a review of seventy cases. *J Bone Joint Surg* 1985; 67A:748–755.

114. Steiner GC. Benign cartilage tumors. In: Taveras JM, Ferrucci JT, eds. *Radiology: diagnosis, imaging, intervention*, vol 5. Philadelphia: JB Lippincott, 1986; chap 78.

115. Weatherall PT, Maale GE, Mendelsohn DB, Sherry CS, Erdman WE, Pascoe HR. Chondroblastoma: classic and confusing appearance at MR imaging. *Radiology* 1994;190:467–474.

116. Yamamura S, Sato K, Sugiura H, Iwata H. Inflammatory reaction in chondroblastoma. *Skeletal Radiol* 1996;25:371–376.

Chondromyxoid Fibroma

117. Beggs IG, Stoker DJ. Chondromyxoid fibroma of bone. *Clin Radiol* 1982;33:671–679.

118. Dahlin DC. Chondromyxoid fibroma of bone, with emphasis on its morphological relationship to benign chondroblastoma. *Cancer* 1956; 9:195–203.

119. Feldman F, Hecht HL, Johnston AD. Chondromyxoid fibroma of bone. *Radiology* 1970;94:249–260.

120. Jaffe HL, Lichtenstein L. Chondromyxoid fibroma of bone: a distinctive benign tumor likely to be mistaken especially for chondrosarcoma. *Arch Pathol* 1948;45:541–551.

121. Mitchell ML, Sartoris DJ, Resnick D. Case report 713. Chondromyxoid fibroma of the third metatarsal. *Skeletal Radiol* 1992;21:252–255.

122. Murphy NB, Price CHG. The radiological aspects of chondromyxoid fibroma of bone. *Clin Radiol* 1971;22:261–269.

123. O'Connor PJ, Gibbon WW, Hardy G, Butt WP. Chondromyxoid fibroma of the foot. *Skeletal Radiol* 1996;25:143–148.

124. Ribalta T, Ro JY, Carrasco CH, Heffelman C, Ayala AG. Case report 638. Chondromyxoid fibroma of a sesamoid bone. *Skeletal Radiol* 1990;19:549–551.

125. Schajowicz F. Chondromyxoid fibroma: report of three cases with predominant cortical involvement. *Radiology* 1987;164:783–786.

126. Schajowicz F, Cabrini RL. Histochemical studies on glycogen in normal ossification and calcification. *J Bone Joint Surg* 1958; 40A:1081–1092.

127. Schajowicz F, Gallardo H. Chondromyxoid fibroma (fibromyxoid chondroma) of bone. *J Bone Joint Surg* 1971;53B:198–216.

128. Ushigome S, Takakuwa T, Shinagawa T, Kishida H, Yamazaki M. Chondromyxoid fibroma of bone. An eletron microscopic obversations. *Acta Pathol Jpn* 1982;32:113–122.

129. White PG, Saunders L, Orr W, Friedman L. Chondromyxoid fibroma. *Skeletal Radiol* 1996;25:79–81.

130. Wilson AJ, Kyriakos M, Ackerman LV. Chondromyxoid fibroma: Radiographic appearance in 38 cases and in a review of the literature. *Radiology* 1991;179:513–518. Also Erratum. *Radiology* 1991;180:586.

131. Zillmer DA, Dorfman HD. Chondromyxoid fibroma of bone: thirty-six cases with clinicopathologic correlation. *Hum Pathol* 1989;20: 952–964.

Chondrosarcoma

132. Abello R, Lomena F, Garcia A, Herranz R, Fernandez SJ, Plaza V, Sole M, Setoain J. Unusual metastatic chondrosarcoma detected with bone scintigraphy. *Eur J Nucl Med* 1986;12:306–308.
133. Aisen AM, Martel W, Braunstein EM, McMillin KI, Phillips WA, Kling TF. MRI and CT evaluation of primary bone and soft-tissue tumors. *Am J Roentgenol* 1986;146:749–756.
134. Amir D, Amir G, Mogle P, Pogrund H. Extraskeletal soft tissue chondrosarcoma. Case report and review of the literature. *Clin Orthop* 1985;198:219–223.
135. Angervall L, Enerback L, Knutson H. Chondrosarcoma of soft tissue origin. *Cancer* 1973;32:507–513.
136. Aoki JA, Sone S, Fujioka F, Terajama K, Ishii K, Karakida O, Imai S, Sakai F, Imai Y. MR of enchondroma and chondrosarcoma: rings and arcs of Gd-DTPA enhancement. *J Comput Assist Tomogr* 1991;15: 1011–1016.
137. Aprin H, Riseborough EJ, Hall JE. Chondrosarcoma in children and adolescents. *Clin Orthop Rel Res* 1982;166:226–232.
138. Bagley L, Kneeland JB, Dalinka MK, Bullough P, Brooks J. Unusual behavior of clear cell chondrosarcoma. *Skeletal Radiol* 1993;22: 279–282.
139. Bertoni F, Boriani S, Laus M, Campanacci M. Periosteal chondrosarcoma and periosteal osteosarcoma. Two distinct entities. *J Bone Joint Surg* 1982;64B:370–376.
140. Bertoni F, Picci P, Bacchini P, Capanna R, Innao V, Bacci G, Campanacci M. Mesenchymal chondrosarcoma of bone and soft tissues. *Cancer* 1983;52:533–541.
141. Bertoni F, Present D, Bacchini P, Picci P, Pignatti G, Gherlinzoni F, Campanacci M. Dedifferentiated peripheral chondrosarcomas. A report of seven cases. *Cancer* 1989;63:2054–2059.
142. Bertoni F, Present DA, Enneking WF. Staging of bone tumors. In: Unni KK, ed. *Bone tumors*. New York: Churchill Livingstone, 1988; 47–83.
143. Bertoni F, Unni KK, Beabout JW, Sim FH. Chondrosarcomas of the synovium. *Cancer* 1991;67:155–162.
144. Berquist TH. Magnetic resonance imaging of primary skeletal neoplasms. *Radiol Clin North Am* 1993;31:411–424.
145. Bloem JL, Bluemm RG, Taminiau AH, van Oesterom AT, Stolk J, Doornbos J. Magnetic resonance imaging of primary malignant bone tumors. *RadioGraphics* 1987;7:425–445.
146. Bohndorf K, Reiser M, Lochner B, Feaux de Lacroix W, Steinbrich W. Magnetic resonance imaging of primary tumors and tumor-like lesions of bone. *Skeletal Radiol* 1986;15:511–517.
147. Brien EW, Mirra JM, Ippolito V, Vaughn L. Clear-cell chondrosarcoma with elevated alkaline phosphatase, mistaken for osteosarcoma on biopsy *Skeletal Radiol* 1996;25:770–774.
148. Brien EW, Mirra JM, Herr R. Benign and malignant cartilage tumors of bone and joints: Their anatomic and theoretical basis with an emphasis on radiology, pathology, and clinical biology. Skel Radiol 1997;26:325–353.
149. Capanna R, Bertoni F, Bettelli G, Picci P, Bacchini P, Present D, Giunti A, Campanacci M. Dedifferentiatated chondrosarcoma. *J Bone Joint Surg* 1988;70A:60–69.
150. Chan YF, Yeung SH, Chow TC, Ma L. Clear cell chondrosarcoma: case report and ultrastructural study. *Pathology* 1989;21:134–137.
151. Chang CC, Greenspan A, Gershwin ME. Osteonecrosis: current perspectives on pathogenesis and treatment. *Semin Arthritis Rheum* 1993; 23:47–69.
152. Crim JR, Seeger LL. Diagnosis of low-grade chondrosarcoma. *Radiology* 1993;189:503–504.
153. Crim JR, Seeger LL, Yao L, Chandnani V, Eckardt JJ. Diagnosis of soft-tissue masses with MR imaging: can benign masses be differentiated from malignant ones? *Radiology* 1992;185:581–586.
154. Dahlin DC, Beabout JW. Dedifferentiation of low-grade chondrosarcomas. *Cancer* 1971;28:461–466.
155. De Beuckeleer LHL, De Schepper AMA, Ramon F. Magnetic resonance imaging of cartilaginous tumors: is it useful or necessary? *Skeletal Radiol* 1996;25:137–141.

156. Ehman RL, Berquist TH, McLeod RA. MR imaging of the musculoskeletal system: a 5-year appraisal. *Radiology* 1988;166:313–320.
157. Enzinger FM, Shiraki M. Extraskeletal myxoid chondrosarcoma: an analysis of 34 cases. *Hum Pathol* 1972;3:421–435.
158. Evans HL, Ayala AG, Romsdahl MM. Prognostic factors in chondrosarcoma of bone. *Cancer* 1977;40:818–883.
159. Fobben ES, Dalinka MK, Schiebler ML, Burk DL, Fallon MD, Schmidt RG, Kressel HY. The MRI appearance at 1.5 tesla of cartilaginous tumors involving the epiphysis. *Skeletal Radiol* 1987;16: 647–651.
160. Frassica FJ, Unni KK, Beabout JW, Sim FH. Dedifferentiated chondrosarcoma. A report of the clinicopathological features and treatment of seventy-eight cases. *J Bone Joint Surg* 1986;68A:1197–1205.
161. Gitelis S, Block JA, Inerot SE. Clonal analysis of human chondrosarcoma. The 35th Annual Meeting, Orthop Research Society. *Orthop Trans* 1989;13:443.
162. Goldman RL, Lichtenstein L. Synovial chondrosarcoma. *Cancer* 1964;17:1233–1240.
163. Hamilton A, Davis RI, Hayes D, Mollan RA. Chondrosarcoma developing in synovial chondromatosis. *J Bone Joint Surg* 1987; 69Br:137–140.
164. Hatano H, Ogose A, Hotta T, Otsuka H, Takahashi HE. Periosteal chondrosarcoma invading the mediallary cavity. *Skel Radiol* 1997;26: 375–378.
165. Haygood TM, Teot L, Ward WG, Allen A, Monu JUV. Low-grade chondrosarcoma in a 12-year-old boy. *Skeletal Radiol* 1995;24: 466–468.
166. Henderson ED, Dahlin DC. Chondrosarcoma of bone: a study of 280 cases. *J Bone Joint Surg* 1963;45A:1450–1458.
167. Hudson TM. Medullary (central) chondrosarcoma. In: Hudson TM, ed. *Radiologic pathologic correlations of musculoskeletal lesions*. Baltimore: Williams and Wilkins, 1987;153–175.
168. Hudson TM, Chew FS, Manaster BJ. Radionuclide scanning of medullary chondrosarcoma. *Am J Roentgenol* 1982;139:1071–1076.
169. Hudson TM, Hamlin DJ, Enneking WF, Petterson H. Magnetic resonance imaging of bone and soft-tissue tumors: early experience in 31 patients compared with computed tomography. *Skeletal Radiol* 1985; 13:134–146.
170. Huvos AG, Marcove RC. Chondrosarcoma in the young: a clinicopathologic analysis of 79 patients younger than 21 years of age. *Am J Surg Pathol* 1987;11:930–942.
171. Ishida T, Dorfman HD, Habermann ET. Dedifferentiated chondrosarcoma of humerus with giant cell tumor-like features. *Skeletal Radiol* 1995;24:76–80.
172. Janzen L, Logan PM, O'Connel JX, Conne DG, Mark PL. Intramedullary chondroid tumors of loose: correlation of abnormal peritoneal narrow and soft tissue MRI signal with tumor type. *Skel Radiol* 1997; 26: 100–106.
173. Johnson S, Tetu B, Ayala AG, Chawla SP. Chondrosarcoma with additional mesenchymal component (dedifferentiated chondrosarcoma). A clinical study of 26 cases. *Cancer* 1986;58:278–286.
174. Kaufman JH, Cedermark BJ, Parthasarathy KL, Didolkar MS, Bakshi SP The value of 67Ga scintigraphy in soft-tissue sarcoma and chondrosarcoma. *Radiology* 1977;123:131–134.
175. Kessler S, Mirra JM, Ishii T, Thompson JC, Brien EW. Primary malignant mesenchymoma of bone: case report, literature review, and distinction of this entity from mesenchymal and dedifferentiated chondrosarcoma. *Skeletal Radiol* 1995;24:291–295.
176. King JW, Spjut HJ, Fechner RE, Vanderpool DW. Synovial chondrosarcoma of the knee joint. *J Bone Joint Surg* 1967; 49A:1389–1396.
177. Klein MJ. Chondrosarcoma. *Semin Orthop* 1991;6:167–176.
178. Kransdorf MJ, Jelinek JS, Moser RP Jr, Utz JA, Brower AC, Hudson TM, Berrey BH Jr. Soft-tissue masses: diagnosis using MR imaging. *Am J Roentgenol* 1989;153:541–547.
179. Kransdorf MJ, Meis JM. Extraskeletal osseous and cartilaginous tumors of the extremities. *RadioGraphics* 1993;13:853–884.
180. Kumar R, David R, Cierney G III. Clear cell chondrosarcoma. *Radiology* 1985;154:45–48.
181. Lin W-Y, Wang S-J, Yeh S-H. Radionuclide imaging in extraskeletal myxoid chondrosarcoma. *Clin Nucl Med* 1995;20:524–527.
182. Mahajam H, Lorigan JG, Shirkhoda A. Synovial sarcoma: MR imaging. *Magn Reson Imag* 1989;7:211–216.
183. Manivel JC, Dehner LP, Thompson R. Case report 460. Synovial chondrosarcoma of left knee. *Skeletal Radiol* 1988;17:66–71.
184. Mankin JH, Cantley KP, Lippiello L, Schiller AL, Campbell CJ. The

biology of human chondrosarcoma. I. Description of the cases, grading, and biochemical analyses. *J Bone Joint Surg* 1980;62A:160–176.

185. McCarthy EF, Dorfman HD. Chondrosarcoma of bone with dedifferentiation: a study of eighteen cases. *Hum Pathol* 1982;13:36–40.

186. McFarland GB, McKinley LM, Reed RJ. Dedifferentiation of low-grade chondrosarcomas. *Clin Orthop* 1977;122:157–164.

187. McLeod RA. Chondrosarcoma. In: Taveras JM, Ferrucci JT, eds. *Radiology: diagnosis, imaging, intervention,* vol 5. Philadelphia: JB Lippincott, 1993;1–12.

188. McLeod RA, Berquist TH. Bone tumor imaging: contribution of CT and MRI. In: Unni KK, ed. *Bone tumors.* New York: Churchill Livingstone, 1988;1–34.

189. Mercuri M, Picci P, Campanacci M, Rulli E. Dedifferentiated chondrosarcoma. *Skeletal Radiol* 1995;24:409–416.

190. Mirra JM, Gold R, Downs J, Eckardt JJ. A new histologic approach to the differentiation of enchondroma and chondrosarcoma of the bones. *Clin Orthop Rel Res* 1:214–237.

191. Mirra JM, Marcove RC. Fibrosarcomatous dedifferentiation of primary and secondary chondrosarcomas. *J Bone Joint Surg* 1974; 56A:285–296.

192. Moser RP. Cartilaginous tumors of the skeleton. *AFIP Atlas of Radiologic-Pathologic Correlation,* vol 2. Philadelphia: Hanley and Belfus.

193. Mullins, F, Berard CW, Eisenberg SH. Chondrosarcoma following synovial chondromatosis. A case study. *Cancer* 1965;18:1180–1188.

194. Nakashima Y, Unni KK, Shives TC, Swee RG, Dahlin DC. Mesenchymal chondrosarcoma of bone and soft tissue. A review of 111 cases. *Cancer* 1986;57:2444–2453.

195. Ontell F, Greenspan A. Chondrosarcoma complicating synovial chondromatosis: findings with magnetic resonance imaging. *Can Assoc Radiol J* 1994;45:318–323.

196. Park Y-K, Yang MH, Ryu KN, Chung DW. Dedifferentiated chondrosarcoma arising in an osteochondroma. *Skeletal Radiol* 1995;24: 617–619.

197. Pettersson H, Gillespy T III, Hamlin DJ, Enneking WF, Springfield DS, Andrew ER, Spanier S, Slone R. Primary musculoskeletal tumors: examination with MR imaging compared with conventional modalities. *Radiology* 1987;164:237–241.

198. Pettersson H, Slone RM, Spanier S, Gillespy T III, Fitzsimmons JR, Scott KN. Musculoskeletal tumors: T1 and T2 relaxation times. *Radiology* 1988;167:783–785.

199. Present DA, Bacchini P, Pignatti G, Picci P, Bertoni F, Campanacci M. Clear cell chondrosarcoma of bone. A report of eight cases. *Skeletal Radiol* 1991;20:187–191.

200. Reiter FB, Ackerman LV, Staple TW. Central chondrosarcoma of the appendicular skeleton. *Radiology* 1972;105:525–530.

201. Remagen W, Nidecker A, Dolanc B. Case report 368. Enchondroma of the tibia with extensive myxoid degeneration.Recurrence with secondary highly differentiated chondrosarcoma. *Skeletal Radiol* 1986; 15:330–333.

202. Resnick D, Kyriakos M, Greenway GD. Tumors and tumor-like lesions of bone: imaging and pathology of specific lesions. In: Resnick D, Niwayama G, eds. *Diagnosis of bone and joint disorders,* 3rd ed. Philadelphia: WB Saunders, 1988.

203. Richardson ML, Kilcoyne RF, Gillespy T III, Helms CA, Genant HK. Magnetic resonance imaging of musculoskeletal neoplasms. *Radiol Clin North Am* 1986;24:259–267.

204. Rosenthal DJ, Schiller AL, Mankin HJ. Chondrosarcoma: correlation of radiological and histological grade. *Radiology* 1984;150:21–26.

205. Salvador AH, Beabout JW, Dahlin DC. Mesenchymal chondrosarcoma—observations on 30 new cases. *Cancer* 1971;28:605–615.

206. Sanerkin NG, Gallagher P. A review of the behaviour of chondrosarcoma of bone. *J Bone Joint Surg* 1979;61B:395–400.

207. Sanerkin NG. The diagnosis and grading of chondrosarcoma of bone. *Cancer* 1980;45:582–594.

208. Schajowicz F. Juxtacortical chondrosarcoma. *J Bone Joint Surg* 1978; 59B:473–480.

209. Schajowicz F, Cuevillos AR, Silberman FS. Primary malignant mesenchymoma of bone. *Cancer* 1966;19:1423–1428.

210. Schajowicz F, Sissons HA, Sobin LH. The World Health Organization's histologic classification of bone tumors. A commentary on the second edition. *Cancer* 1995;75:1208–1214.

211. Scheele PM, von Kuster LC, Krivchenia G. Primary malignant mesenchymoma of bone. *Arch Pathol Lab Med* 1990;114:614–617.

212. Schiller AL. Diagnosis of borderline cartilage lesions of bone. *Semin Diagn Pathol* 1985;1:42–62.

213. Shapeero LG, Vanel D, Couanet D, Contesso G, Ackerman LV. Extraskeletal mesenchymal chondrosarcoma. *Radiology* 1993;186: 819–826.

214. Sirsat MV, Doctor VM. Benign chondroblastoma of bone. Report of a case of malignant transformation. *J Bone Joint Surg* 1970; 52B:741–745.

215. Sissons HA, Matlen JA, Lewis MM. Dedifferentiated chondrosarcoma. Report of an unusual case. *J Bone Joint Surg* 1991; 73A:294–300.

216. Smith J, Botet JR, Yeh SDJ. Bone sarcomas in Paget's disease. A study of 85 patients. *Radiology* 1984;152:583–590.

217. Spjut HJ, Dorfman HD, Fechner RE, Ackerman LV. Tumors of bone and cartilage. In: *Atlas of tumor pathology,* 2nd series, fascicle 5. Washington, DC: Armed Forces Institute of Pathology, 1971.

218. Steiner GC, Mirra JM, Bullough PG. Mesenchymal chondrosarcoma. A study of the ultrastructure. *Cancer* 1973;32:926–939.

219. Stout AP, Verner EW. Chondrosarcoma of the extraskeletal soft tissues. *Cancer* 1953;6:581–590.

220. Sundaram M, McGuire MH, Herbold DR, Wolverson MK, Heiberg E. Magnetic resonance imaging in planning limb-salvage surgery for primary malignant tumors of bone. *J Bone Joint Surg* 1986; 68A:809–819.

221. Sundaram M, Percelay S, McDonald DJ, Janney C. Case report 799. Extraskeletal chondrosarcoma. *Skeletal Radiol* 1993;22:449–451.

222. Tetu B, Ordonez NG, Ayala AG, Mackay B. Chondrosarcoma with additional mesenchymal component (dedifferentiated chondrosarcoma). *Cancer* 1986;58:287–298.

223. Unni KK. *Dahlin's Bone Tumors. General Aspects and Data on 11,087 Cases.* 5th ed. Philadelphia, Lippincott-Raven, 1996.

224. Unni KK, Dahlin DC, Beabout JW. Periosteal osteosarcoma. *Cancer* 1976;37:2476–2485.

225. Unni KK, Dahlin DC, Beabout JW, Sim FH. Chondrosarcoma: Clear-cell variant: a report of 16 cases. *J Bone Joint Surg* 1976; 58A:676–683.

226. Varma DGK, Ayala AG, Carrasco CH, Guo S-Q, Kumar R, Edeiken J. Chondrosarcoma: MR imaging with pathologic correlation. *Radio-Graphics* 1992;12:687–704.

227. Weiss AC, Dorfman HD. Clear cell chondrosarcoma: a report of 10 cases and review of the literature. *Surg Pathol* 1988;1:123–129.

228. West OC, Reinus WR, Wilson AJ. Quantitative analysis of the plain radiographic appearance of central chondrosarcoma of bone. *Invest Radiol* 1995;30:440–447.

229. Wu KK, Collon DJ, Guise ER. Extra-osseous chondrosarcoma. Report of five cases and review of the literature. *J Bone Joint Surg* 1980; 62A:189–194.

230. Young CL, Sim FH, Unni KK, McLeod RA. Chondrosarcoma of bone in children. *Cancer* 1990;66:1641–1648.

231. Zimmer WD, Berquist TH, McLeod RA, Sim FH, Pritchard DJ, Shives TC, Wold LE, May GR. Bone tumors: magnetic resonance imaging versus computed tomography. *Radiology* 1985;155:709–718.

CHAPTER 4

Fibrous and Fibrohistiocytic Lesions

INTRODUCTION

Fibrous and fibrohistiocytic lesions of bone represent a clinical spectrum, ranging from very innocent lesions requiring no treatment at all to highly malignant neoplasms (27) (Table 1). All of these lesions have a common dominant constituent cell, the fibroblast (7,15). In general, fibrous lesions are composed of spindle cells and produce a collagenous matrix, whereas fibrohistiocytic lesions may or may not produce a collagenous matrix (26).

BENIGN LESIONS

Fibrous Cortical Defect and Nonossifying Fibroma

Fibrous cortical defect (also called metaphyseal defect) and nonossifying fibroma (formerly called nonosteogenic fibroma) are the most common fibrous lesions of bone and have histologically identical characteristics. Some authors prefer the term fibroxanthoma for both lesions (15), whereas Schajowicz prefers the term histiocytic xanthogranuloma (22). These lesions are not true neoplasms but are considered developmental defects (12), arising in the region of the primary trabeculae of a tubular bone and wandering toward the diaphysis as the bone grows in length (19).

Clinical Presentation

Seen predominantly in childhood and adolescence and more commonly (2:1) in boys (5), both lesions have a predilection for the long bones, particularly the femur and the tibia (Fig. 1) (7). Fibrous cortical defect is a small, asymptomatic lesion (24) that occurs in 30% of the normal population during the first and second decades of life (6,8,16). The term nonossifying fibroma is applied to this lesion if it enlarges and encroaches on the medullary portion of the bone (21). Depending on age, the distance of these lesions from the growth plate varies (19). When the longitudinal axis of a fibrous metaphyseal defect projects in the direction of the epiphysis it encounters a tendon or ligamentous structure that inserts at the epiphyseal line (20). On the basis of this finding, some investigators believe that such an insertion, along with additional pathogenetic factors, may be related in some degree to the development of this lesion (20). Recent investigations have demonstrated characteristic radiomorphologic stages of progression and regression of fibrous cortical defects (19). At stage A they are located near the growth plate (24), have a round to oval shape, and exhibit a fine sclerotic margin. In stage B the lesion has wandered into the metaphysis and represents a polycyclic form, also delineated by a distinct sclerotic margin, giving the lesion a grape-like appearance. Stage C represents the beginning of the healing process and shows increased mineralization, which characteristically begins at the diaphyseal end of the lesion and progresses toward the growth plate (14,19). Stage D represents complete healing, and the lesion becomes sclerotic.

Most nonossifying fibromas are asymptomatic, but larger ones may undergo a pathologic fracture (1). Although multifocal presentation is rare (3,9), Moser et al. found that about 8% of patients exhibit a multicentric localization (18). The multiple lesions occur in four patterns: (a) clustered together, usually around the knee; (b) nonclustered, at opposite ends

TABLE 4-1. *Spectrum of fibrous and fibrohistiocytic lesions of bone*

Condition	Histopathology
Fibrous cortical defect (metaphyseal defect)	Benign
Nonossifying fibroma	Benign
Benign fibrohistiocytoma (fibroxanthoma)	Benign
Congenital fibromatosis	Benign
Periosteal desmoid	Benign
Fibrous dysplasia	Benign
Monostotic	
Polyostotic	
Osteofibrous dysplasia (Kempson-Campanacci lesion)	Benign
Desmoplastic fibroma	Intermediate
Fibrosarcoma	Malignant
Malignant fibrous histiocytoma	Malignant

of long bones; (c) several small lesions gradually coalescing into one large lesion; and (d) a metachronous appearance, with new lesions eventually appearing near the original lesion (18). Occasionally such multiple nonossifying fibromas are associated with neurofibromatosis (Jaffe-Campanacci syndrome) (17,23).

Imaging

Plain film radiography is usually diagnostic (10). Nonossifying fibromas present as elliptic, radiolucent defects confined to the cortex of a long bone near the growth plate, frequently resembling a bunch of grapes and demarcated by a thin sclerotic margin (Fig. 2). They range in size from 0.5 to 7 cm, with their long axes aligned with the long axis of the affected bone (12). The larger defects are usually scalloped and have a wider zone of sclerosis. Most foci undergo spontaneous involution (healing) by the remodeling process of the tubular bone with diaphyseal diminution of the diameter finally resulting in osteosclerosis. A few lesions may continue to grow and as they encroach on the medullary cavity they characteristically display a scalloped, sclerotic border and are located eccentrically within the bone (Fig. 3). Some of the larger lesions may be complicated by a fracture (Fig. 4).

Skeletal scintigraphy shows a minimal to mild increase in activity (4). During the healing phase, mild hyperemia may be seen on the blood pool image, and the positive delayed scan reflects the osteoblastic activity (11). Computed tomography (CT) may demonstrate to better advantage the cortical thinning and medullary involvement, and may more precisely delineate early pathologic fracture. Hounsfield attenuation values for nonossifying fibroma are higher than for normal bone marrow. Magnetic resonance imaging (MRI), usually performed for another reason, shows a low signal intensity on both T1- and T2-weighted sequences (12). After gadolinium-DTPA injection, fibrous cortical defects invari-

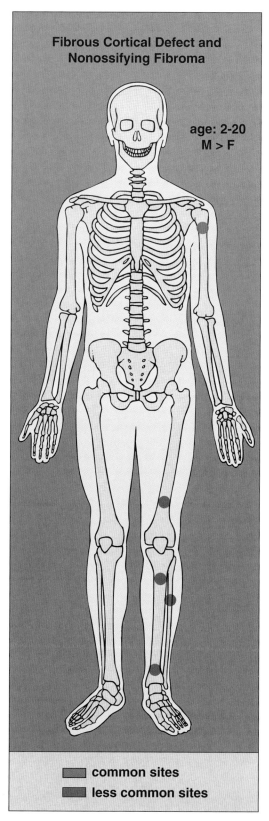

Fibrous Cortical Defect and Nonossifying Fibroma

age: 2-20
M > F

common sites
less common sites

FIG. 1. Fibrous cortical defect and nonossifying fibroma: skeletal sites of predilection, peak age range, and male-to-female ratio.

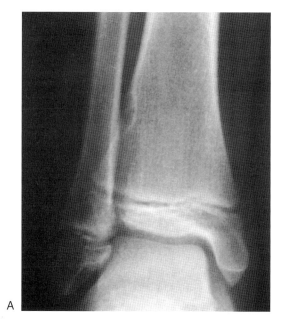
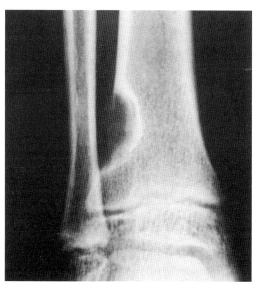

A

B

FIG. 2. Fibrous cortical defect and nonossifying fibroma. **A:** Fibrous cortical defect, seen here in the lateral cortex of the distal tibia in a 13-year-old boy, typically presents as a radiolucent lesion demarcated by a thin zone of sclerosis. **B:** When a fibrous cortical defect encroaches on the medullary cavity, it is called a nonossifying fibroma. Note the similarity of the lesion to that in A. The only difference is the size.

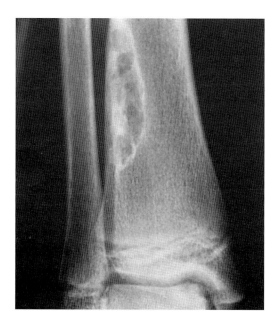

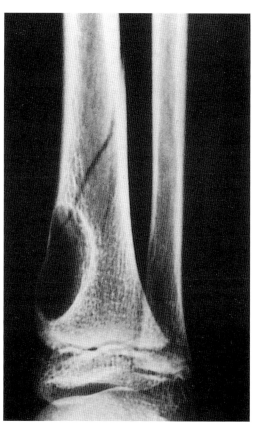

FIG. 3. Nonossifying fibroma. The lesion, seen here in the distal tibia in an asymptomatic 15-year-old boy, appears eccentrically located in the bone and has a scalloped sclerotic border.

FIG. 4. Nonossifying fibroma: a pathologic fracture. A large radiolucent lesion in the distal tibia of a 10-year-old boy is complicated by a pathologic fracture.

ably exhibit a hyperintense border and signal enhancement (20). Mineralization of the lesion during healing (stages C and D) appears predominantly as low signal intensity on MR images.

Histopathology

Histologically identical regardless of size, fibrous cortical defect and nonossifying fibroma are composed of rather bland monomorphous spindle cells admixed with histiocytic cells that often possess a clear or foamy cytoplasm (25). The cells are frequently arranged in a swirling storiform pattern (derived from Greek and implying resemblance to a woven mat), typical of fibrohistiocytic lesions, but a fascicular arrangement may also be seen (Fig. 5). A variable number of lipid-bearing xanthomatous cells and of hemosiderin pigment-laden histiocytes may be present **(see Fig. 5C)** (22). In some cases, unusually heavily lipidized fibroxanthomatous areas are predominant. Such lesions have been referred to as xanthoma or fibroxanthoma by some investigators (2). Usually, osteoclast-like giant cells are present (Fig. 6) and, when numerous, may lead to confusion of the lesion with giant-cell tumor of bone (13). Typically, variable numbers of inflammatory cells, especially lymphocytes, and a few plasma cells

are scattered in the background. The amount of collagen production may vary, but no bone or cartilage formation should be present unless a fracture or previous surgical disruption of the lesion has occurred.

Differential Diagnosis

Radiology

Both fibrous cortical defect and nonossifying fibroma have rather characteristic radiographic features (see above) that make plain film radiography diagnostic. Rarely, a fibrous cortical defect affecting the posterior aspect of the distal femur may be mistaken for *periosteal desmoid*, and a nonossifying fibroma in long or flat bones may be mistaken for a focus of *fibrous dysplasia or desmoplastic fibroma*. An atypical sclerotic presentation of nonossifying fibroma or healing stage of this lesion may occasionally be confused with a *medullary bone infarct, sclerotic metastasis*, or a *giant bone island* (Fig. 7). If a lesion is located in thin bones (e.g., fibula, ulna) and occupies the entire diameter of the bone, its characteristic eccentric location is lost and it may therefore mimic a *simple bone cyst*, an *aneurysmal bone cyst* (Fig. 8), or a *Langerhans cell granuloma*.

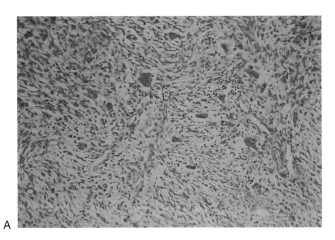

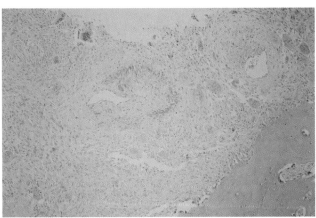

A

B

C

FIG. 5. Histopathology of nonossifying fibroma. **A:** Fibrous stroma displays a storiform arrangement. Several giant cells are present (hematoxylin and eosin, original magnification ×100). **B:** At the lesion–bone interface the fibrous stroma exhibits a mostly fascicular arrangement. Bone resorption is minimal. Small aggregates of giant cells are also present (hematoxylin and eosin, original magnification ×25). **C:** At high magnification several foam cells are conspicuous (hematoxylin and eosin, original magnification ×400).

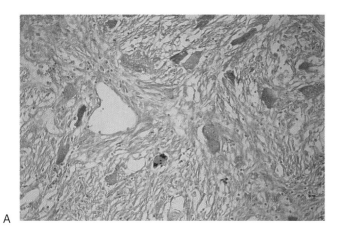

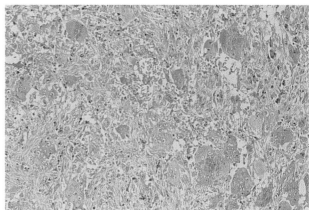

A

B

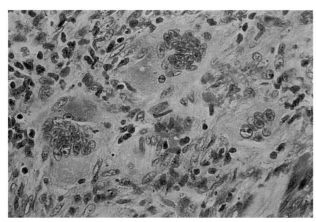

C

FIG. 6. Histopathology of nonossifying fibroma. **A:** Many giant cells are scattered within a fairly dense spindle cell tissue. (Giemsa, original magnification ×50). **B:** In another area the number and the size of the giant cells containing up to 50 nuclei resemble that of a true giant-cell tumor of bone (hematoxylin and eosin, original magnification ×50). **C:** At high magnification the resemblance of giant cells to those of a giant cell tumor is striking (hematoxylin and eosin, original magnification ×400).

Pathology

Nonossifying fibroma can be confused with *benign fibrous histiocytoma* because both lesions have almost identical histopathologic features, differing mainly in their clinical and radiologic presentation. A storiform architecture in a hypercellular nonossifying fibroma can lead to confusion with *malignant fibrous histiocytoma* if the pathologist is unfamiliar with the clinicopathologic spectrum of fibrous cortical defect and nonossifying fibroma. Less likely differential possibilities are *giant-cell tumor, fibrous dysplasia, osteofibrous dysplasia*, or *low-grade intraosseous osteosarcoma*. Although giant cells are almost always present in nonossifying fibroma, they are not uniformly distributed throughout the lesion as in giant cell tumor **(see Figs. 6 and 7–11A)**. Because bone formation is not a feature of nonossifying fibroma, all three lesions—fibrous dysplasia, osteofibrous dysplasia, and low-grade osteosarcoma—can easily be distinguished.

The radiologic and pathologic differential diagnosis of nonossifying fibroma are depicted in Fig. 9.

Benign Fibrous Histiocytoma

The term *benign fibrous histiocytoma* (sometimes called xanthofibroma or fibrous xanthoma) may be controversial

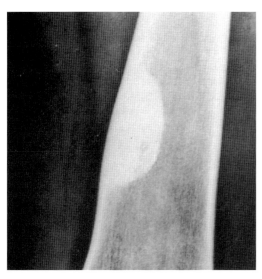

FIG. 7. Nonossifying fibroma: differential diagnosis. A lesion that healed spontaneously may persist as a sclerotic patch. In this sclerosing phase, nonossifying fibroma should not be mistaken for osteoblastic tumor or bone island.

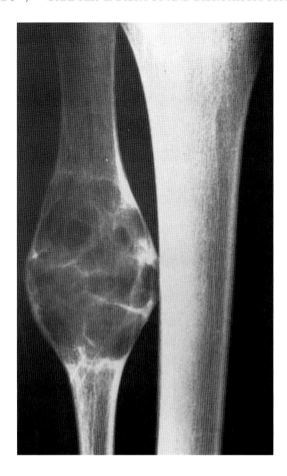

FIG. 8. Nonossifying fibroma: differential diagnosis. A large lesion in the fibula exhibits an expansive character and thus resembles an aneurysmal bone cyst. Note, however, the absence of a periosteal reaction that is invariably present in the latter lesion.

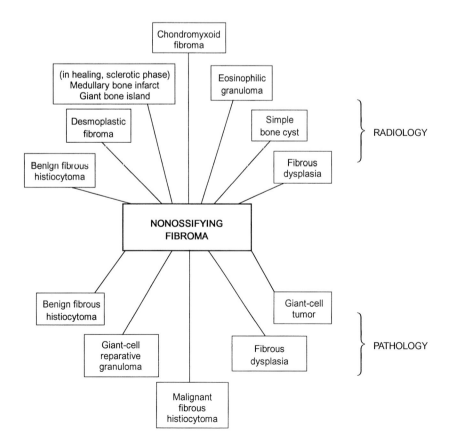

FIG. 9. Radiologic and pathologic differential diagnosis of nonossifying fibroma.

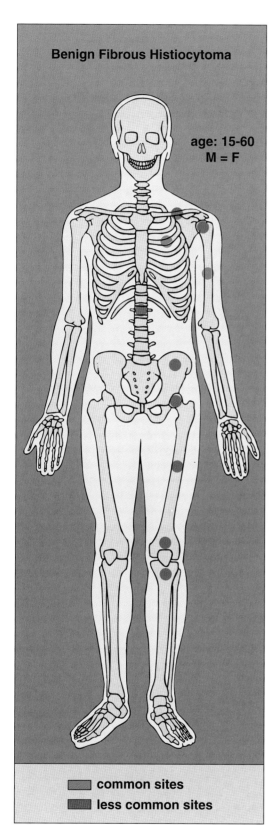

Benign Fibrous Histiocytoma

age: 15-60
M = F

☐ common sites
☐ less common sites

FIG. 10. Benign fibrous histiocytoma: skeletal sites of predilection, peak age range, and male-to-female ratio.

(27), but it is useful in an organizational sense for subclassification of lesions with histologic features similar to those of nonossifying fibroma but having an atypical location and an atypical clinical or radiographic pattern (36, 37). This is a rare lesion characterized by a spindle cell fibrous tissue arranged in a storiform pattern. The tissue contains variable numbers of giant cells, hemosiderin, and lipid-laden histiocytes (36).

Clinical Presentation

The lesion, which is often symptomatic (painful), is usually diagnosed in older patients in the age range from 15 to 60 years. The usual location is the shaft or (in contrast to nonossifying fibroma) the articular end of a long bone, the pelvis, and the ribs. Rarely the clavicle, spine, or skull is affected (22) (Fig. 10). Clinically, the lesion can exhibit a locally aggressive behavior, with recurrences after curettage or excision.

Imaging

Radiographically, benign fibrous histiocytoma may also appear to be more aggressive than nonossifying fibroma, although some features are similar. Plain radiographs show a well-defined, radiolucent lesion with sclerotic borders, occasionally exhibiting some degree of expansion (Fig. 11). Internal trabeculations may also be present (29). The lesion may be situated either centrally in the bone or eccentrically, the latter presentation being more common at the articular end of bone (34). In this location it may mimic a giant-cell tumor. On skeletal scintigraphy, benign fibrous histiocytoma exhibits a moderately increased uptake (32). Magnetic resonance imaging shows the lesion to be of intermediate signal intensity (isointense with the muscles) on SE T1-weighted sequences and of a high signal intensity on T2- and TI-IR images (28,32).

Histopathology

Benign fibrous histiocytoma usually has histologic features quite similar to those of nonossifying fibroma, although the storiform spindle cell stroma is more distinctive (22,35) (Fig. 12). The background may contain larger numbers of histiocytic cells and Touton-type giant cells seen in xanthomatous tissue reactions (30) or in malignant fibrous histiocytoma. Although the cell of origin of fibrous histiocytoma has not been ascertained, at least three cell types have been proposed (39). These include the histiocytic type, which is capable of acting as a facultative fibroblast; the fibroblastic type capable of acting as a facultative histiocyte (38); and an undifferentiated stem cell type (29). Although frankly malignant histologic criteria are absent and no cytologic atypia is seen, mitotic activity may be present (31). Reactive bone formation may be seen at the periphery of the lesion or in association with a pathologic fracture through the lesion (27).

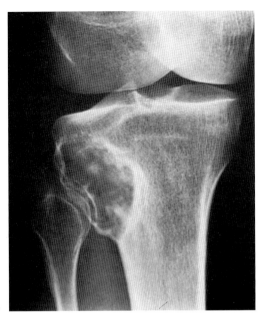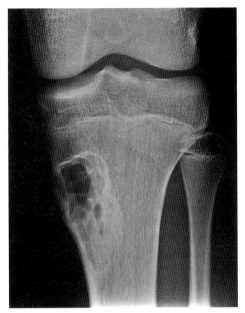

A

B

FIG. 11. Benign fibrous histiocytoma. **A:** A 37-year-old man presented with occasional pain in the right knee. An oblique radiograph of the knee shows a lobulated radiolucent lesion with a well-defined sclerotic border, located eccentrically in the proximal tibia. **B:** A 16-year-old boy presented with a painful tibial lesion that on radiography looked like a nonossifying fibroma. Because of persistent symptoms the lesion was biopsied and proved to be consistent with a benign fibrous histiocytoma.

Differential Diagnosis

Radiology

From the radiologic standpoint, the main differential possibilities include *nonossifying fibroma* and giant-cell tumor. The radiographic features of nonossifying fibroma may be indistinguishable from those of benign fibrous histiocytoma, although the more aggressive appearance of the latter (such as an expanding border) and the location, which is atypical for nonossifying fibroma, are the clues to the diagnosis. *Giant-cell tumor* only rarely exhibits a rim of reactive sclerosis, whereas this is a common feature of benign fibrous histiocytoma. Although *intraosseous ganglion* is usually much smaller than the average size of benign fibrous histiocytoma, the former should be considered in differential diagnosis if the lesion occurs at the articular end of a bone. *Osteoblastoma*, unlike benign fibrous histiocytoma, usually evokes a periosteal reaction and exhibits central opacities of bone formation.

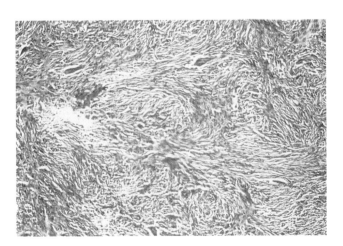

FIG. 12. Histopathology of benign fibrous histiocytoma. Benign-appearing fibrous tissue displays a storiform arrangement (hematoxylin and eosin, original magnification ×100).

Pathology

The differentiation of *nonossifying fibroma* and *fibrous cortical defect* from benign fibrous histiocytoma must be made on a clinical and radiographic basis rather than on histologic grounds (27) because the microscopic appearance of all three lesions is almost identical (Fig. 13).

Giant-cell tumor always must be considered in the differential diagnosis. It is particularly difficult to distinguish a giant cell tumor that undergoes regressive changes and, conversely, some giant-cell tumors with regressive features may erroneously be diagnosed as benign fibrous histiocytoma (29). Furthermore, the healing reaction associated with a pathologic fracture in a giant-cell tumor can lead to proliferation of spindle cells with associated lipid- and hemosiderin-laden macrophages, giving the appearance of benign fibrous histiocytoma (27). Finally, some investigators consider benign fibrous histiocytoma a regressive stage of a burned-out giant-cell tumor (34).

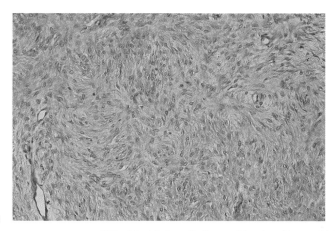 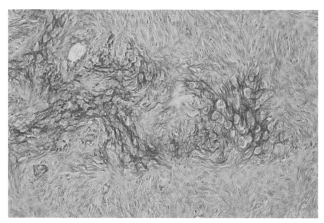

A   B

FIG. 13. Histopathology of benign fibrous histiocytoma. **A:** Densely arranged spindle cells exhibit cartwheel-like arrangement (*center*). In contrast to nonossifying fibroma, giant cells are rarely encountered (hematoxylin and eosin, original magnification ×50). **B:** Spotty increase of collagen fiber formation (red) resembles primitive osteoid (van Gieson, original magnification ×20).

The radiologic and pathologic differential diagnosis of benign fibrous histiocytoma are depicted in Fig. 14.

Periosteal Desmoid

Periosteal desmoid (also known as avulsive cortical irregularity, distal metaphyseal femoral defect, cortical desmoid, or medial supracondylar defect of the femur) (42,44) is a tumor-like fibrous proliferation of the periosteum, which has a striking predilection for the posteromedial cortex of the medial femoral condyle (12,40). Although the term *periosteal desmoid* is widely accepted, it has an unfortunate similarity to the term *desmoid tumor* of soft tissue and therefore is suggestive of an aggressive lesion (26). Periosteal desmoid usually occurs between the ages of 12 and 20 years, mainly in boys, and most lesions disappear spontaneously by the end of the second decade. It is considered to represent an asymptomatic normal variant that does not require biopsy or treatment. Although many patients have a history of injury, trauma does not necessarily predispose to the development of this lesion (46). The radiologic features of periosteal desmoid are similar to those of fibrous cortical defect, except for the specificity of its location. Its radiographic hallmarks are a saucer-like radiolucent defect with sclerosis at its base. The lesion may erode the cortex (45) and appear as a cortical

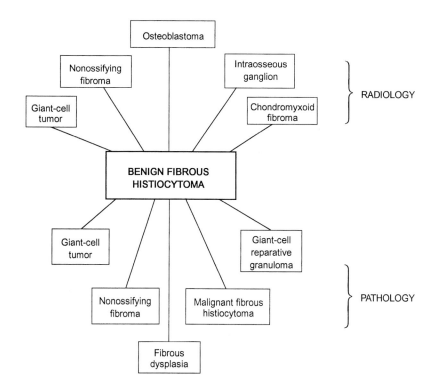

FIG. 14. Radiologic and pathologic differential diagnosis of benign fibrous histiocytoma.

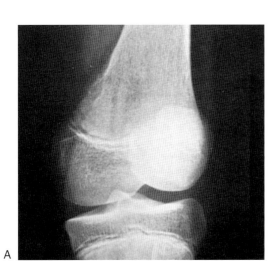
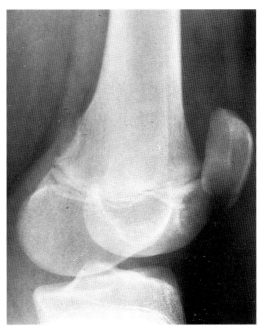

A   B

FIG. 15. Periosteal desmoid. **A:** An oblique radiograph of the left knee of a 12-year-old boy shows the classic appearance of periosteal desmoid. Note the elliptical radiolucency eroding the medial border of the distal femoral metaphysis at the linea aspera and producing cortical irregularity. **B:** In another patient, an 11-year-old boy, a saucer-like defect is present in the medial cortex of the distal femoral metaphysis.

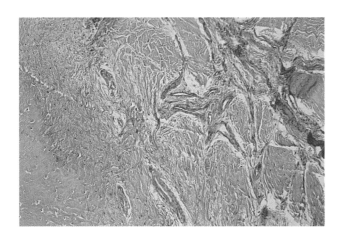

FIG. 16. Histopathology of periosteal desmoid. The cortical bone (*lower left*) is made up of coarse plates of cell-rich woven bone merging with benign-appearing fibrous tissue (hematoxylin and eosin, original magnification ×12).

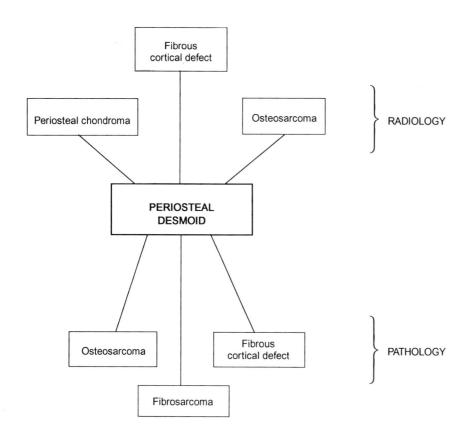

FIG. 17. Radiologic and pathologic differential diagnosis of periosteal desmoid.

irregularity (Fig. 15). Occasionally, because of its poorly defined and irregular bony margin and the presence of small bony spiculae at the cortical surface, it may simulate an aggressive or even a malignant tumor. The bone scan usually is normal (12,43,47). On MRI the lesion appears hypointense on T1- and hyperintense on T2-weighted images, with a dark rim on both sequences at or near the sites of the bony attachment of the medial head of the gastrocnemius muscle (48). Histopathologic examination of the lesion demonstrates fibroblastic spindle cells that produce large amounts of collagen (41) (Fig. 16). Large areas of hyalinization and fibrocartilage and small fragments of bone may be scattered within the fibrous tissue. Unlike nonossifying fibroma or fibrous cortical defect, giant cells or xanthomatous cells are not present. The most important point in the differential diagnosis is not to mistake this lesion for a malignancy. Its characteristic radiographic appearance and location should serve as clues to the correct diagnosis.

The radiologic and pathologic differential diagnosis of periosteal desmoid is depicted in Fig. 17.

Fibrous Dysplasia

Fibrous dysplasia is a fibro-osseous lesion that may affect one bone (monostotic form) or several bones (polyostotic form) (66). Classified as a developmental abnormality by some authorities, it is characterized by the replacement of normal lamellar cancellous bone by an abnormal fibrous tissue that contains small, abnormally arranged trabeculae of immature woven bone (12), formed by metaplasia of the fibrous stroma.

Monostotic Fibrous Dysplasia

Clinical Presentation

Most commonly affecting the femur (with a predilection for the femoral neck), the tibia, the ribs (representing the most common benign lesion of the rib), and the base of the skull, the lesion of monostotic fibrous dysplasia arises centrally in the bone (Fig. 18); it usually spares the epiphysis in children and the articular end of the bone in adults (59). Because these lesions are usually asymptomatic, most of them are discovered incidentally on radiographs obtained for other reasons. Rarely, pain accompanied by local swelling and deformity is present. The most common complication is a pathologic fracture through the structurally weakened bone. This may be the initial presentation particularly for lesions located in the lower extremity (22).

Imaging

The radiographic appearance of the lesion depends on the proportion of osseous to fibrous tissue. Lesions with higher degrees of ossification appear more dense and sclerotic. More fibrous lesions exhibit a greater radiolucency, with a

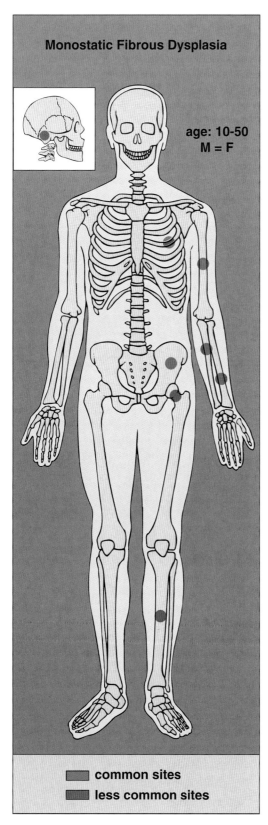

Monostatic Fibrous Dysplasia

age: 10-50
M = F

■ common sites
▪ less common sites

FIG. 18. Monostotic fibrous dysplasia: skeletal sites of predilection, peak age range, and male-to-female ratio.

characteristic "ground-glass" or even cystic appearance (Fig. 19). Some lesions may contain scattered calcifications similar to those of chondroid lesions. A solitary focus of fibrous dysplasia may be surrounded by a characteristic thick band of reactive bone, creating a rind sign (Fig. 20). This appearance of fibrous dysplasia must be differentiated from the very similar presentation of a bone infarct (see Fig. 32). When the lesion enlarges, it expands the medullary cavity. Although the cortex may be attenuated and even remodeled around the lesion, it is rarely directly involved by the lesion. In extremely rare instances, lesions of fibrous dysplasia may protrude from the bone (the so-called exophytic variant of fibrous dysplasia) (55).

Scintigraphy is helpful in determining the activity (Fig. 21) and the potential multicentricity of the lesion (61). Machida et al. reported that although a high incidence of increased uptake of radiopharmaceutical was seen in 59 patients with fibrous dysplasia, 10% of the lesions with a ground-glass appearance failed to show similarly increased uptake (67).

The lesion of fibrous dysplasia shows a variety of appearances on magnetic resonance imaging (65). Some lesions show a decreased signal on both T1 and T2 sequences, and some low signal on T1 but either mixed or high signal on T2 images (64). The sclerotic rim ("rind sign") is invariably imaged as a band of low signal intensity on both T1 and T2 sequences (77).

Histopathology

Histologically, fibrous dysplasia consists of an aggregate of moderately dense fibrous connective tissue composed of spindle cells arrayed in intersecting, whorled bundles containing haphazardly distributed bone trabeculae. Rather than being stress oriented, as in normal cancellous bone, these trabeculae tend to be irregularly curved and branching with sparse interconnections (49,68). The collagen fibers of the stroma are characteristically continuous with those of the bone trabeculae. The low-power photomicrographic picture has been likened to Chinese characters or even alphabet soup (Fig. 22). Although bony trabeculae contain osteocytes, they exhibit no evidence of osteoblastic activity. In some areas, cement-like rounded trabeculae may be present (Fig. 23) and scattered osteoclasts may be found. Areas of hyaline cartilage may also be present. Under polarized light, the bone trabeculae are seen to be composed of woven immature bone (Fig. 24). The cells of the stroma and of the trabeculae show a strong alkaline phosphatase activity, indicating that they are all potential osteoblasts. It appears that an enzymatic or some other organizational defect prevents them from differentiating into fully mature, polarized osteoblasts capable of forming normal lamellar bone. The lack of seams of polarized osteoblasts at any stage in their maturation ("naked trabeculae") and the direct passage of the collagen fibers from the stroma into the bone trabeculae are the most important

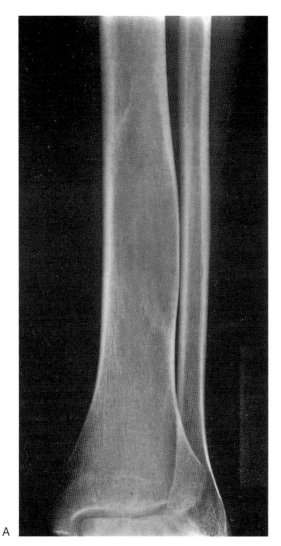

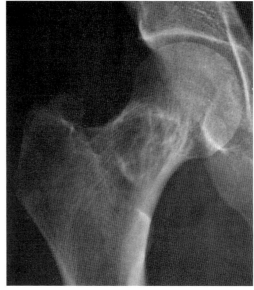

FIG. 19. Monostotic fibrous dysplasia. **A:** An anteroposterior radiograph of the distal leg of a 17-year-old girl shows a monostotic focus of fibrous dysplasia in the diaphysis of the tibia. Observe the slight expansion and thinning of the cortex and the partial loss of trabecular pattern in the cancellous bone, which gives the lesion a "ground-glass" or "smoky" appearance. **B:** An anteroposterior radiograph of the right hip in a 25-year-old man shows the focus of fibrous dysplasia in the femoral neck that exhibits a more sclerotic appearance than that seen in **A**.

characteristics in differential diagnosis **(see Fig. 23)**. Therefore, the bone formed is considered metaplastic **(see Fig. 24)**. Furthermore, typical findings on electron microscopy are fairly extended areas with collagen fibrils in the precollagen stage and in continuation with normal-appearing mature collagen fibrils and calcification (Remagen, unpublished observations) (Fig. 25).

Polyostotic Fibrous Dysplasia

Clinical Presentation

Although radiographically similar to the monostotic form, polyostotic fibrous dysplasia often exhibits a somewhat more aggressive appearance. Moreover, the lesions are distributed differently in the skeleton, showing a striking predilection (more than 90% of cases) for one side of the body. They often involve the pelvis, followed in frequency by the long bones, skull, and ribs; the proximal end of the femur is a common site of occurrence (Fig. 26). In general, the lesions of polyostotic fibrous dysplasia progress in number and size until skeletal maturity is reached, after which they become quiescent. Only 5% of lesions continue to enlarge. Unlike the monostotic form, this variant of fibrous dysplasia is usually symptomatic. In most patients the presenting symptoms, such as a limp, leg pain, or a pathologic fracture, result from skeletal involvement. However, at a very early age associated endocrine abnormalities (such as vaginal bleeding) usually appear first (75).

Polyostotic fibrous dysplasia that is associated with endocrine disturbances (i.e., premature sexual development, acromegaly, hyperthyroidism, hyperparathyroidism, and Cushing syndrome) and skin pigmentation (café-au-lait spots) constitute the disorder called Albright-McCune syndrome. This condition almost exclusively affects girls, who exhibit true sexual precocity resulting from an accelerated gonadotropin release by the anterior lobe of the pituitary. Typically, the café-au-lait spots of Albright-McCune syndrome show irregular, ragged ("coast of Maine") borders, in contrast to the smoothly marginated ("coast of California")

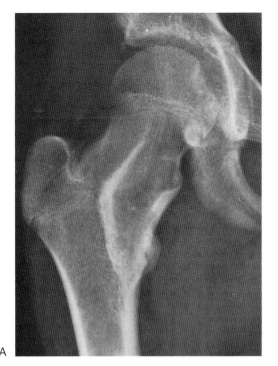

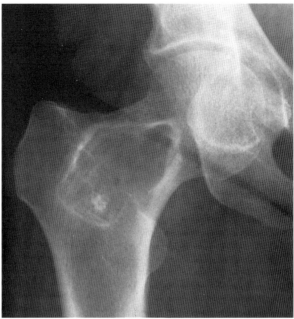

A

B

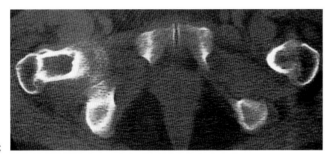

C

FIG. 20. Monostotic fibrous dysplasia. **A:** In this presentation of fibrous dysplasia the thick peripheral rim and a radiolucent center creates the image of a "rind" sign. **B:** In another patient a similar rind sign marks a focus of fibrous dysplasia. **C:** CT section through the lesion shows a thick rim of peripheral sclerosis.

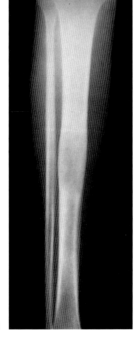

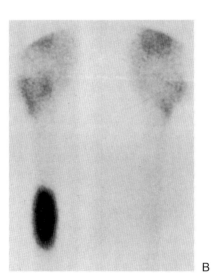

A

B

FIG. 21. Monostotic fibrous dysplasia: scintigraphy. **A:** A 24-year-old woman presented with mild discomfort in the right leg. An anteroposterior radiograph shows a radiolucent lesion with "smoky" appearance in the midshaft of the tibia, associated with thinning of the cortex and slight expansion. **B:** Radionuclide bone scan shows markedly increased uptake of the radiopharmaceutical agent indicating activity of fibrous dysplasia.

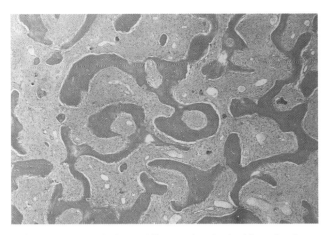

FIG. 22. Histopathology of fibrous dysplasia. Metaplastic trabeculae are haphazardly arranged in loose, fibrous stroma. Note lack of osteoblastic activity (hematoxylin and eosin, original magnification ×20).

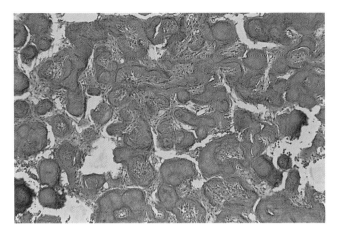

FIG. 23. Histopathology of fibrous dysplasia. Variant of classic histologic appearance with small, discrete, almost osteocyte-free foci of calcified matrix resemble the cementicles usually seen in cementifying fibromas of the jaw. The scanty spindle cell stroma shows the typical passing of the collagen fibers into the bone (hematoxylin and eosin, original magnification ×25).

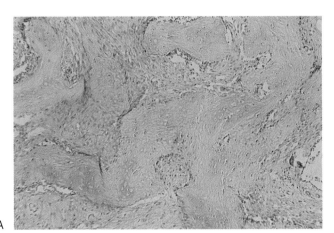

A

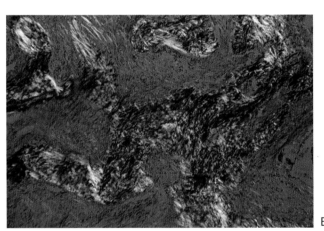

B

FIG. 24. Histopathology of fibrous dysplasia. **A:** In a background of collagenized fibrous tissue, irregularly shaped spicules of immature woven bone have been formed by metaplasia. No polarized differentiated osteoblasts are seen (hematoxylin and eosin, original magnification ×25). **B:** Under polarized light the woven structure of the collagen fibers within the bone matrix is conspicuous (hematoxylin and eosin, polarized light, original magnification ×25).

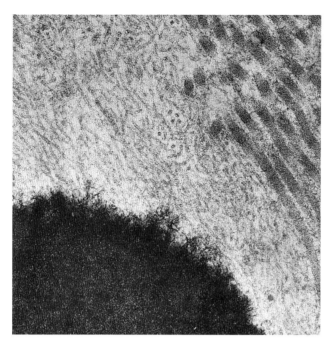

FIG. 25. Electron microscopy of fibrous dysplasia. Mature cross-striated collagen fibrils are seen (*upper right corner*) and extended area with immature collagen fibrils. Mineralization of the matrix progresses (*lower left*) regardless of the structure and maturation of the collagen.

café-au-lait markings seen in neurofibromatosis. Mazabraud syndrome is a condition in which multiple fibrous and fibromyxomatous soft tissue tumors occur in association with polyostotic fibrous dysplasia (58,76).

The most common complication of polyostotic fibrous dysplasia is a pathologic fracture that, when it occurs in the femoral neck, frequently leads to a "shepherd's crook" deformity (Fig. 27). Occasionally, accelerated growth of a bone or hypertrophy of a digit may be observed. The development of a sarcoma in fibrous dysplasia is extremely rare, but it may occur either spontaneously (72,74,78) or, more commonly, after radiation therapy (73,78).

Imaging

The characteristic radiographic changes of polyostotic fibrous dysplasia may occur in any portion of the long bones, and involvement of the bone by the lesion may be limited or extensive. The lower extremities are most commonly affected, with a preferentially unilateral distribution. As in the monostotic form, the articular ends of bones are usually unaffected. This latter phenomenon has given rise to speculations that a defect of the primary ossification center may lead to impairment of the production and maintenance of mature cancellous bone. The cortex, as in the solitary form, is usually intact but is often thinned because of the expansive nature of the lesion. The borders of the lesion are well defined and the inner cortical margins may exhibit scalloping. The

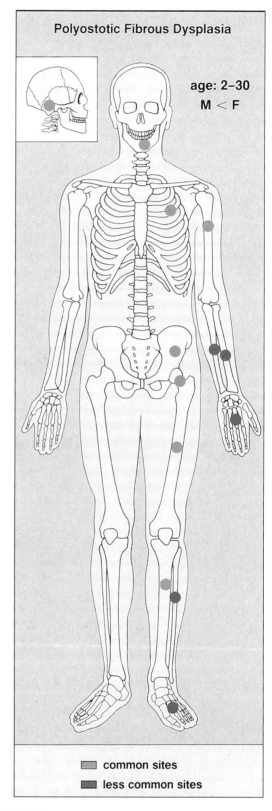

FIG. 26. Polyostotic fibrous dysplasia: skeletal sites of predilection, peak age range, and male-to-female ratio.

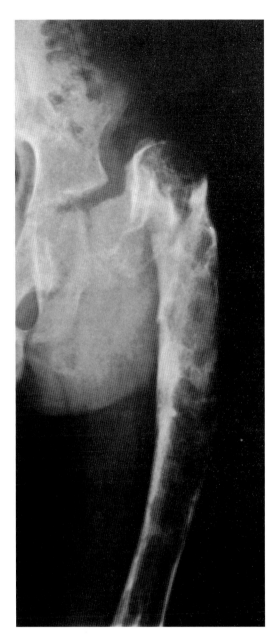

FIG. 27. Polyostotic fibrous dysplasia. A "shepherd's-crook" deformity, seen here in the proximal femur in a 12-year-old boy, is often the result of multiple, pathologic fractures.

and sclerosis of the sphenoid wings, sella, and the vertical portion of the frontal bone (12,50). Less commonly, the vault of the skull is affected (71).

Because of increased uptake on skeletal scintigraphy, radionuclide bone scanning is the most rapid way to determine the distribution of skeletal lesions (51). This examination may also disclose unsuspected sites of involvement (Fig. 30). Computed tomography can accurately delineate the extent of bone involvement (52). Tissue attenuation values, as measured by Hounsfield units, are usually within the 70- to 400-HU range (12), apparently reflecting the presence of calcium and microscopic ossification throughout the abnormal tissue. On MRI, fibrous dysplasia exhibits homogeneous, moderately low signal intensity on T1-weighted images, whereas on T2 weighting the signal is bright (77,74) or mixed (57,62,64). After gadolinium infusion, the majority of lesions show central contrast enhancement and some peripheral rim enhancement (64). In general, signal intensity on T1- and T2-weighted images and the degree of contrast enhancement on T1 sequences depends on the amount and degree of bone trabeculae, collagen, and cystic and hemorrhagic changes (64).

Histopathology

The histologic appearance of polyostotic fibrous dysplasia is identical to that of the monostotic form. The presence of small trabeculae of woven bone of various sizes and shapes, scattered within a fibrous tissue without evidence of osteoblastic activity, is diagnostic for this disorder (12,33,38).

Differential Diagnosis

Radiology

If the lesion of fibrous dysplasia contains cartilage (fibrocartilaginous dysplasia) and displays visible calcifications, the differential diagnosis includes *enchondroma* (if the lesion is solitary) or *enchondromatosis* (if the lesion is polyostotic). In exceptional circumstances, a monostotic presentation of fibrous dysplasia may mimic *desmoplastic fibroma* (Fig. 31). If a solitary focus is present in the tibia, *osteofibrous dysplasia* and *adamantinoma* are the diagnostic possibilities. In the early phase of development, particularly if the lesion is entirely radiolucent and is situated in the proximal humerus or proximal femur, *a simple bone cyst* should be considered. When the lesion markedly expands the cortex, an *aneurysmal bone cyst* is a possibility. On those rare occasions when the lesion exhibits an eccentric location,   must be excluded. Monostotic presentation with a thick sclerotic rim at the periphery (rind sign), particularly in the proximal femur, must not be mistaken for *medullary bone infarct* (Fig. 32) (70).

Polyostotic fibrous dysplasia should be mainly differentiated from enchondromatosis and neurofibromatosis. In *en-*

variable amount of bone in the fibrous tissue that replaces the cancellous bone imparts a radiographic picture that ranges from lucency to increased density (Fig. 28A). More fibrous lesions exhibit greater lucency, occasionally with a loss of the trabecular pattern and a ground-glass, milky, or smoky appearance (Fig. 28B). Massive formation of cartilage may be observed in the lesion, accompanied by secondary calcification and ossification patterns (so-called fibrocartilaginous dysplasia) (56,60,63) that can easily be confused radiographically with a cartilaginous neoplasm (Fig. 29) (53,54). Skull lesions affect primarily the base, causing thickening

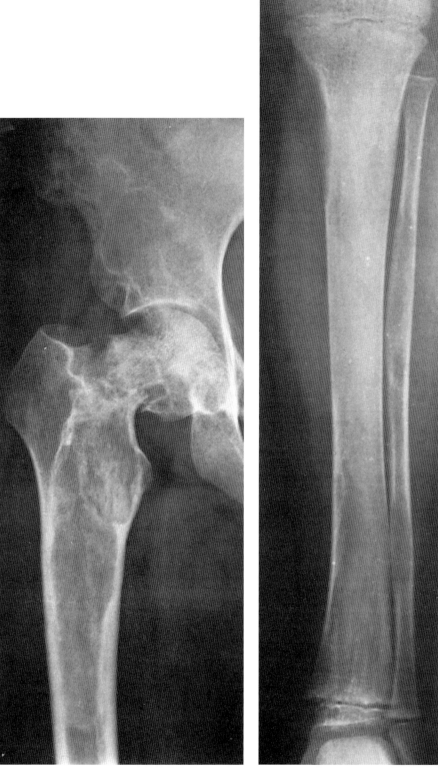

FIG. 28. Polyostotic fibrous dysplasia. **A:** Anteroposterior radiograph of the right hip of an 18-year-old woman shows unilateral involvement of the ilium and femur. Some lesions are more radiolucent, some more sclerotic. **B:** In this anteroposterior radiograph of the left leg of a 5-year-old girl with precocious puberty whose left upper and lower extremities were affected (Albright-McCune syndrome), note slight expansion of the tibia and fibula associated with thinning of the cortex and "ground-glass" appearance of the medullary portion of these bones.

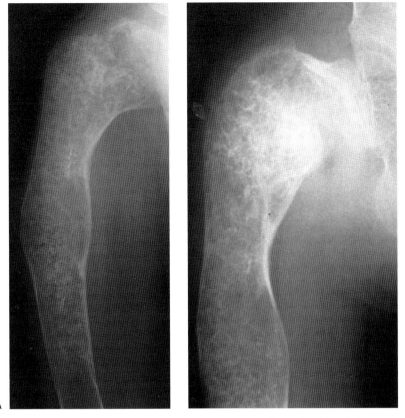

FIG. 29. Fibrocartilaginous dysplasia. **A:** An anteroposterior radiograph of the right femur in a 10-year-old boy with polyostotic fibrous dysplasia exhibits typical appearance of a massive formation of cartilage. **B:** A coned-down view of the proximal femur displays annular calcifications typical for a cartilaginous matrix.

chondromatosis, unlike in polyostotic fibrous dysplasia, the lesions may extend into the articular ends of the bone, and columns of radiolucent streaks extending from the growth plate into the metaphyses are characteristic of the former disorder. *Neurofibromatosis* affecting the skeleton usually exhibits long bone deformities without intramedullary changes typical of fibrous dysplasia. A problem in differential diagnosis may arise if neurofibromatosis is associated with multiple nonossifying fibromas (Jaffe-Campanacci syndrome), which can mimic the lesion of fibrous dysplasia (23).

Pathology

Although in most cases fibrous dysplasia exhibits a very characteristic histologic picture, occasionally it can mimic *fibroblastic osteosarcoma* and *fibrosarcoma.* In osteosarcoma the cells and nuclei are usually distinctly pleomorphic and mitoses are frequent. In addition, tumor bone formation is more amorphous, without a distinctive trabecular structure. However, low-grade central osteosarcoma may present a real challenge to the pathologist (see section "Osteosar-

coma"). *Adamantinoma* may resemble fibrous dysplasia when it is accompanied by abundant fibroblastic tissue. However, the distinct epithelial cells of the former (which in more obscure cases can be identified using immunohistochemistry with epithelial markers) are characteristic and diagnostic.

When the formation of bone is limited, as in some cases of fibrous dysplasia, there may be a problem with the differential diagnosis of *nonossifying fibroma* (69). In such instances, the absence of groups of osteoclast-like giant cells and of hemosiderin may be helpful.

The radiologic and pathologic differential diagnosis of monostotic and polyostotic fibrous dysplasia is depicted in Fig. 33A and B, respectively.

Osteofibrous Dysplasia (Kempson-Campanacci Lesion)

Osteofibrous dysplasia or Kempson-Campanacci lesion (formerly called ossifying fibroma) is a rare disorder with a decided preference for the tibia (81,87). It is characterized by the presence of fibrous connective tissue and trabeculae of immature nonlamellar bone rimmed by osteoblasts.

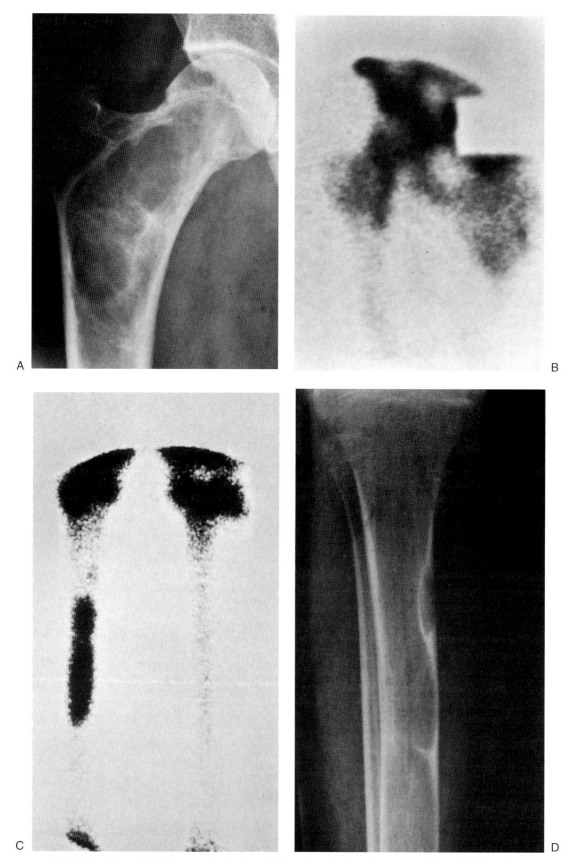

FIG. 30. Polyostotic fibrous dysplasia: scintigraphy. **A:** A radiograph of the right hip, obtained to exclude a fracture, demonstrates an asymptomatic focus of fibrous dysplasia in the femoral neck. **B, C:**. To determine other sites of involvement, a radionuclide bone scan was obtained. In addition to the focus in the femoral neck, increased uptake of the tracer was demonstrated at various other sites, but predominantly in the right leg. **D:** Subsequent plain radiograph of the right lower leg confirmed the presence of multiple foci of polyostotic fibrous dysplasia.

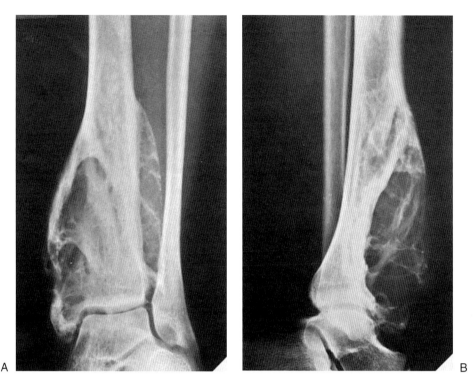

A   B

FIG. 31. Fibrous dysplasia: differential diagnosis. (**A**) Oblique and (**B**) lateral radiographs of the left lower leg of a 32-year-old woman demonstrate a large, trabeculated radiolucent lesion in the distal tibia. Because of its aggressive features, it was thought to be a desmoplastic fibroma. However, biopsy proved it to be a fibrous dysplasia, a rare lesion at this location in adults.

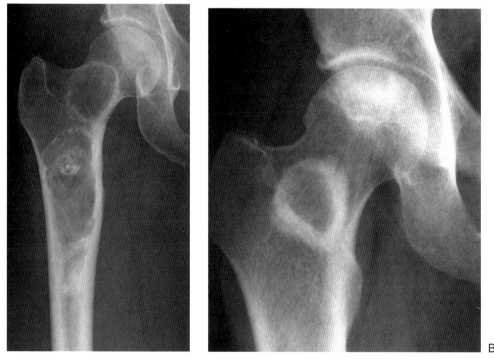

A   B

FIG. 32. Fibrous dysplasia: differential diagnosis. **A:** Two separate foci of fibrous dysplasia affecting the right femur display a rind sign (proximal lesion) and central calcifications (distal lesion). This presentation resembles a bone infarct. **B:** Bone infarct located in the neck of the right femur exhibits a rind sign. Observe also osteonecrosis of the femoral head.

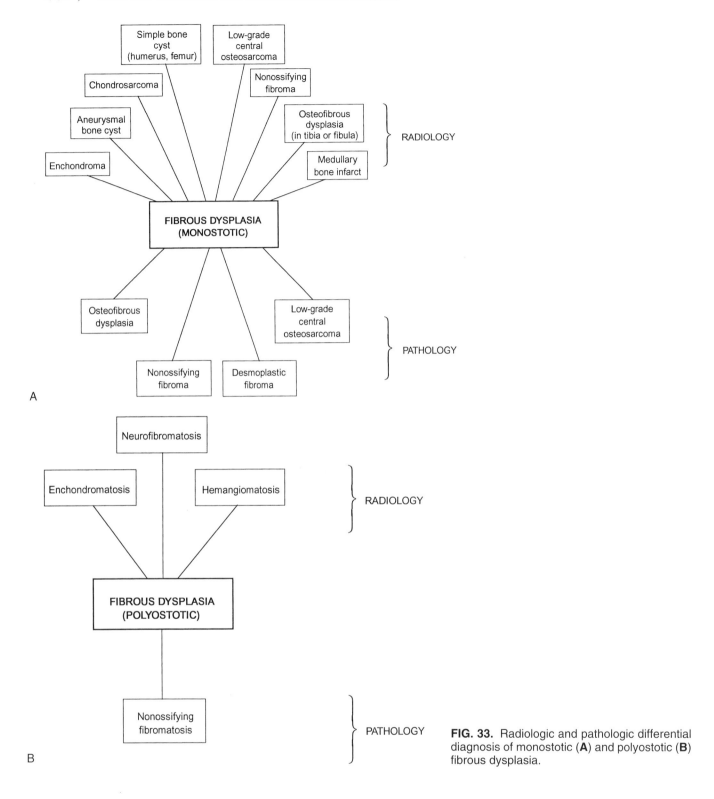

FIG. 33. Radiologic and pathologic differential diagnosis of monostotic (**A**) and polyostotic (**B**) fibrous dysplasia.

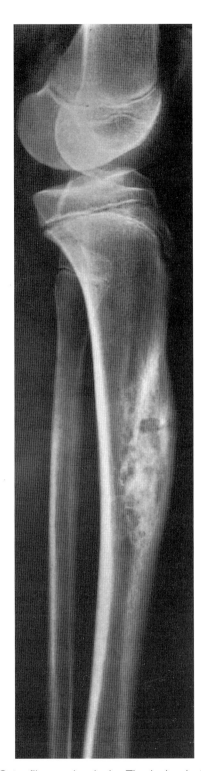

FIG. 34. Osteofibrous dysplasia. The lesion in the anterior aspect of the right tibia of a 14-year-old girl was originally diagnosed as nonossifying fibroma. Although it is similar to a nonossifying fibroma and fibrous dysplasia, its site is typical of osteofibrous dysplasia, which was confirmed by biopsy.

Clinical Presentation

With rare exceptions, the lesion is situated in the proximal or middle third of the tibia and is often localized to the anterior cortex (80,81). In >80% of patients, some degree of anterior bowing is observed. When the fibula is affected, the distal third of the diaphysis is usually involved (83). This lesion occurs predominantly in childhood (>60% of the patients affected are <5 years of age), but occasionally it is first discovered in adolescence. Boys are slightly more commonly affected (81).

Osteofibrous dysplasia is usually asymptomatic but occasionally may be revealed clinically by the enlargement and bowing of the tibia (95). The disorder may sometimes be locally aggressive. It frequently recurs after local excision and, according to some authors, may coexist with the malignant lesion adamantinoma (79,91). Other investigators have suggested that osteofibrous dysplasia may be a precursor to adamantinoma (84,93,94). Weiss and Dorfman, and later Czerniak et al., suggested that adamantinoma and osteofibrous dysplasia are on a continuum, with osteofibrous dysplasia on one end and adamantinoma on the other (85,96).

Imaging

Radiographically, the Kempson-Campanacci lesion bears a striking similarity to nonossifying fibroma and fibrous dysplasia. It is radiolucent and possesses lobulated sclerotic margins, usually confined to the cortex (Fig. 34). Larger lesions may destroy the cortical bone and invade the medullary cavity (Fig. 35) (97). In the tibia the lesion rarely involves the entire circumference of the shaft, but in the fibula this may occur (79). Rarely, there are multiple osteolytic lesions over a large part of the diaphysis, simulating adamantinoma.

Histopathology

Osteofibrous dysplasia and fibrous dysplasia, as the similarity in their names suggests, have a remarkable histopathologic resemblance. Like fibrous dysplasia, osteofibrous dysplasia is characterized by a fibrous background containing a rather haphazard arrangement of incomplete trabeculae (89). In osteofibrous dysplasia, however, these bony trabeculae often show appositional activity by polarized osteoblasts ("dressed trabeculae") (Fig. 36A). Such activity, which can sometimes be seen at the earliest stages of bone development, more often occurs surrounding larger trabeculae (88). Viewed under polarized light, these trabeculae consist of an inner portion of woven bone surrounded by an outer zone of lamellar transformation (Fig. 36B), a pattern sometimes referred to as zonal architecture (80,81). Because osteofibrous dysplasia and fibrous dysplasia exhibit almost identical radiographic and very similar histologic features, with the exception of the former lesion's predilection for the cortex of the tibia, the differences in the light and electron microscopy findings must be meticulously sought. Nevertheless, some

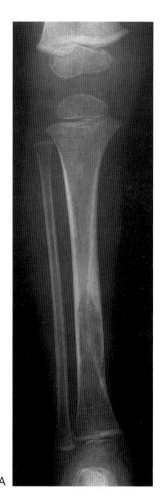
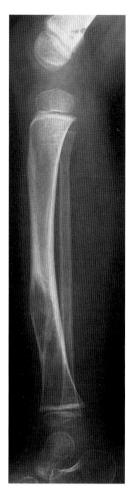

FIG. 35. Osteofibrous dysplasia. **A, B:** A cortical lesion in the distal tibia invades the medullary portion of the bone in a 2-year-old boy.

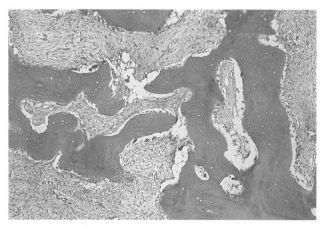
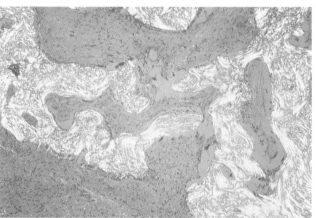

FIG. 36. Histopathology of osteofibrous dysplasia. **A:** Plump, irregular bone trabeculae scattered in a moderate density spindle cell stroma are made up in part of a cell-rich woven bone, but at the periphery display lamellar bone rimmed by the osteoblasts (hematoxylin and eosin, original magnification ×25). **B:** Viewed under polarized light, lamellar (*light green*) and woven (*darker areas*) bone is better discernible (polarized light, original magnification ×25).

TABLE 2. *Differential features of various fibro-osseous lesions with similar radiographic appearance*

Sex	Age	Location	Radiographic appearance	Histopathology
		Fibrous Dysplasia		
M/F	Any age (monostotic) First to third decades (polyostotic)	Femoral neck (frequent) Long bones Pelvis Ends of bones usually spared Polyostotic: unilateral in skeleton (frequent)	Radiolucent, ground glass, or smoky lesion Thinning of cortex with endosteal scalloping "Shepherd's crook" deformity Accelerated growth	Woven (nonlamellar) type of bone in loose to dense fibrous stroma; bony trabeculae lacking osteoblastic activity ("naked trabeculae")
		Nonossifying Fibroma		
M/F	First to third decades	Long bones (frequently posterior femur)	Radiolucent, eccentric lesion Scalloped, sclerotic border	Whorled pattern of fibrous tissue containing giant cells, hemosiderin, and lipid-filled histiocytes
		Osteofibrous Dysplasia (Kempson-Campanacci Lesion)		
M/F	First to second decades	Tibia (frequently anterior aspect) Fibula Intracortical (frequent)	Osteolytic, eccentric lesion Scalloped, sclerotic border Anterior bowing of long bone	Woven and mature (lamellar) type of bone surrounded by cellular fibrous spindle cell growth in whorled or matted pattern; bony trabeculae rimmed by differentiated osteoblasts ("dressed trabeculae")
		Ossifying Fibroma of Jaw		
F	Third to fourth decades	Mandible (90%) Maxilla	Expansive radiolucent lesion Sclerotic, well-defined borders	Uniformly cellular fibrous spindle cell growth with varying amounts of woven bone formation and small, round cementum-like bodies
		Ossifying Fibroma (Sissons Lesion)		
M/F	Second decade	Tibia Humerus	Radiolucent lesion Sclerotic border Similar to osteofibrous dysplasia	Fibrous tissue containing rounded and spindle-shaped cells with scant intercellular collagen and small, partially calcified spherules resembling cementum-like bodies of ossifying fibroma of jaw

investigators have speculated that osteofibrous dysplasia represents a regional or localized presentation of fibrous dysplasia (82). This, however, is unlikely in view of the histomorphologic findings.

Sissons and colleagues reported two cases of fibro-osseous lesions containing smaller aggregates of osseous material resembling cementum. They proposed the term "ossifying fibroma" for this lesion (90). The term "osteofibrous dysplasia," they suggested, should be reserved for fibrous cortical lesions of the tibia and fibula. To avoid confusion in terminology, the differential features of the various lesions are summarized in Table 2.

Differential Diagnosis

Radiology

The main differential possibilities include *fibrous dysplasia* and *nonossifying fibroma*. If the lesion is confined to the cortex and there is associated anterior bowing of the tibia, osteofibrous dysplasia is more likely. Conversely, particularly in older children and adolescents, if the lesion extends into the medullary portion of the bone and is bordered with a sclerotic rim, nonossifying fibroma is a more probable diagnosis. Centrally located lesions that exhibit thinning of the cortex rather than an intracortical multiloculated bubbly appearance more likely represent fibrous dysplasia. Finally, osteofibrous dysplasia should be differentiated from *adamantinoma*. The latter lesion is usually more extensive, with a more aggressive appearance. A helpful hint is that patients with adamantinoma are much older than those with osteofibrous dysplasia.

Pathology

The main differential diagnoses include fibrous dysplasia and adamantinoma. *Fibrous dysplasia* shows the characteristic absence of osteoblasts at the surface of trabeculae,

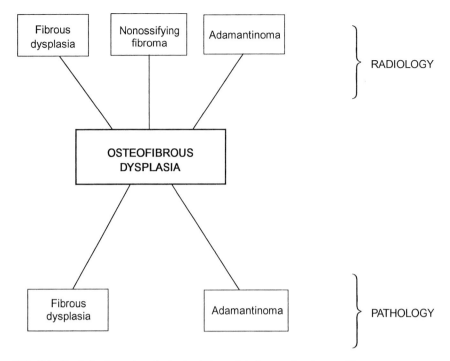

FIG. 37. Radiologic and pathologic differential diagnosis of osteofibrous dysplasia.

whereas osteofibrous dysplasia exhibits dressed trabeculae. Adamantinoma is distinguished from osteofibrous dysplasia by the presence of single or small nests of epithelial cells within the fibro-osseous stroma (86). More problems are encountered in distinguishing osteofibrous dysplasia from so-called osteofibrous dysplasia-like adamantinoma (91). From a practical standpoint, a diagnosis of osteofibrous dysplasia made on the basis of tissue removed by a small incisional biopsy cannot be certain because the biopsy material may not be representative, and one cannot rule out an osteofibrous dysplasia-like adamantinoma (91). In such cases, immunohistochemical staining for markers of epithelial tissues can be helpful.

Radiologic and pathologic differential diagnosis of osteofibrous dysplasia is depicted in Fig. 37.

Desmoplastic Fibroma

Desmoplastic fibroma is a rare, locally aggressive tumor, closely related to the desmoid tumor of abdominal wall, characterized by the formation of abundant collagen fibers by the tumor cells (36). Although generally classified as a benign bone tumor, some investigators classify this lesion in a so-called intermediate category between benign and malignant lesions (22).

Clinical Presentation

Desmoplastic fibroma accounted for only about 0.06% of all bone tumors and 0.3% of benign bone tumors in the Mayo

Clinic series (7). It usually arises in individuals younger than 40 years; half of the cases occur during the second decade (7). There is no sex predominance (Fig. 38). The clinical signs and symptoms are nonspecific (98). Because the onset is often insidious, the lesion tends to be relatively large before the patient begins to experience symptoms (69). In symptomatic patients, pain or swelling, sometimes of long duration, is the most common complaint (101). Rarely (in about 10% of cases), a pathologic fracture through the lesion is the first presenting symptom (106). The long bones (humerus, femur, tibia), mandible, and pelvis are the most common sites of involvement (105). In the long bones the lesion is diaphyseal, sparing the epiphysis, but it often extends into the metaphysis and may even extend into the articular end of the bone after closure of the growth plate (107).

Imaging

There are no characteristic radiographic features of this tumor. In general, it is an expansive, radiolucent lesion, usually with nonsclerotic but sharply defined borders (Fig. 39A). Occasionally a wide zone of transition is present (104). The cortex is either thinned or thickened, but there is no significant periosteal response (100). Internal septation or trabeculation is observed in approximately 75% of cases, yielding a honeycomb pattern of bone destruction (102) (Fig. 39B). Locally aggressive variants, which may simulate malignant bone tumors, are marked by bone destruction and invasion of the soft tissues.

In addition to plain films, radiologic evaluation of desmoplastic fibroma should include bone scintigraphy, CT, and

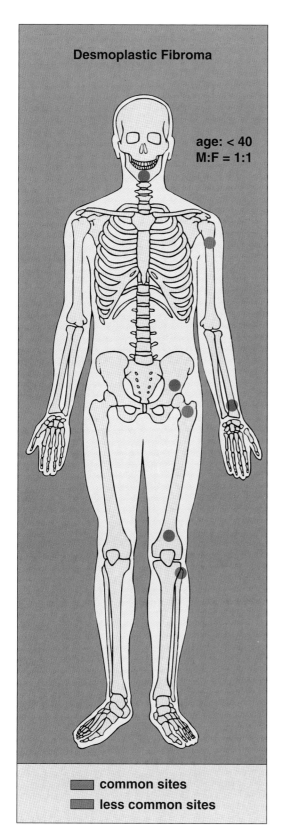

Desmoplastic Fibroma

age: < 40
M:F = 1:1

common sites
less common sites

FIG. 38. Desmoplastic fibroma: skeletal sites of predilection, peak age range, and male-to-female ratio.

MRI. Radionuclide bone scan shows an increase in the uptake of the radiopharmaceutical agent at the site of the lesion (109). CT is useful for evaluating cortical breakthrough and tumor extension into the soft tissues (108, 110). MRI, also helpful in assessing intra- and extraosseous extension, can further characterize the tumor (Figs. 40 and 41). The lesion appears well defined on MR images, exhibiting an intermediate signal intensity on T1 weighting and a heterogeneous pattern on T2 weighting, marked by an area of increased signal intensity mixed with foci of intermediate and low signal intensity (100,102). The hypointensity of the signal reflects the dense connective tissue matrix and relative acellularity of the tumor (109).

Histopathology

Histologically, the lesion is composed of very regular bundles of normal-looking, spindle-shaped, and occasionally stellate fibroblasts with elongated or ovoid nuclei interspersed within a densely collagenized matrix (Fig. 42). There is no evidence of mitotic activity (103). Although cellularity is variable, the collagenous matrix almost always constitutes the greater portion of the tumor. For this reason, the biopsy specimen, resembling scar tissue, is identical in appearance to a desmoid tumor of soft tissue. Large, thin-walled vessels similar to those observed in soft tissue desmoid tumors are usually apparent (26). On purely histologic grounds, the lesion most closely resembles periosteal desmoid, but correlation with the radiographs clarifies its true nature. As with desmoids of soft tissue, in desmoplastic fibroma of bone it is difficult to distinguish the tumor tissue from the surrounding normal connective tissue.

Differential Diagnosis

Radiology

Desmoplastic fibroma is frequently difficult to distinguish radiographically from similar-appearing lesions. These include s*imple bone cyst, aneurysmal bone cyst, fibrous dysplasia, chondromyxoid fibroma, giant-cell tumor, fibrosarcoma, malignant fibrous histiocytoma,* and *chondrosarcoma.* Giant cell tumor, fibrosarcoma, and malignant fibrous histiocytoma can be excluded if the lesion possesses sclerotic margins. A purely lytic appearance of desmoplastic fibroma excludes simple and aneurysmal bone cyst and chondromyxoid fibroma, as these entities possess sclerotic borders.

Pathology

Histopathologic differential diagnosis must include *nonossifying fibroma* and *fibrous dysplasia* (99). However, unlike the former, abundant intercellular substance is ob-

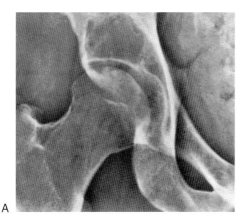

A

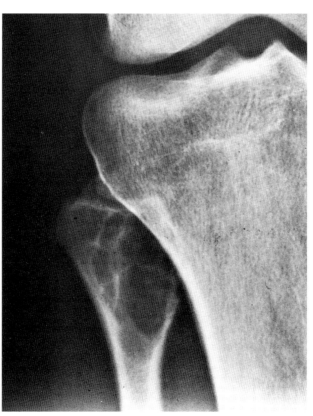

B

FIG. 39. Desmoplastic fibroma. A: A radiolucent lesion with nonsclerotic, sharply defined borders is seen in a supra-acetabular region of the right ilium. (Reprinted from Bullough PG, *Atlas of orthopedic pathology,* 2nd ed. New York: Gower, 1992;17.2.) B: A radiolucent, trabeculated lesion occupies the proximal end of the right fibula in a 17-year-old girl. Note lack of periosteal reaction.

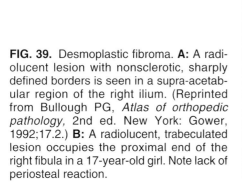

A

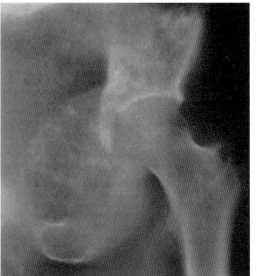

B

FIG. 40. Desmoplastic fibroma. A: An anteroposterior radiograph of the pelvis in a 67-year-old man demonstrates an expansive, lytic lesion that involves left ischium and pubis and extends into the supraacetabular portion of the ilium. B: Conventional tomography shows the lytic nature of the tumor and its expansive character. The involvement of the ilium is better demonstrated.

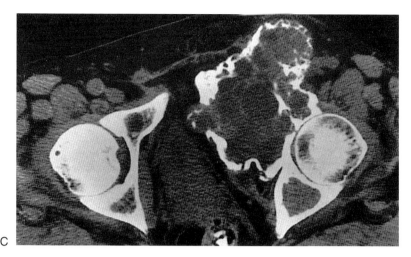

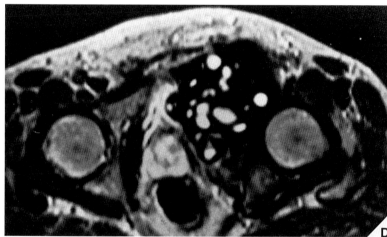

FIG. 40. *Continued.* **C:** CT section through the hip joint shows a lobulated appearance of the tumor and a thick, sclerotic margin. **D:** Axial T2-weighted (SE, TR 2000, TE 80) MRI demonstrates nonhomogeneity of the signal from tumor. The bulk of the lesion displays low-to-intermediate signal intensity with central areas of high signal.

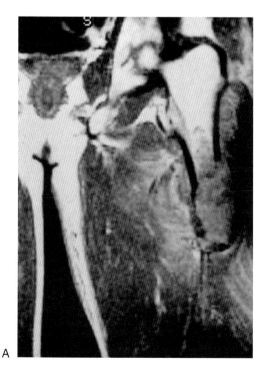

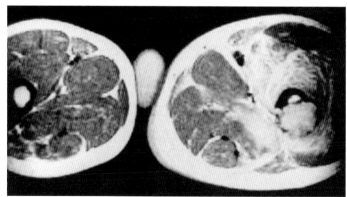

FIG. 41. Desmoplastic fibroma: magnetic resonance imaging. **A:** Coronal T1-weighted MRI shows the lesion in the left femoral shaft breaking through the cortex and extending into the soft tissues. **B:** Axial proton density image demonstrates replacement of the bone marrow by the tumor, extension into the soft tissues, and peritumoral edema.

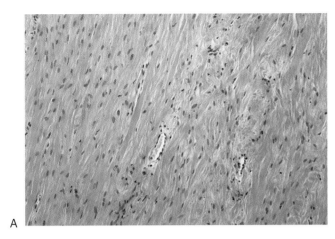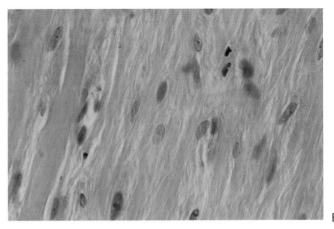

A   B

FIG. 42. Histopathology of desmoplastic fibroma. **A:** Densely collagenized hypocellular stroma contains spindle-shaped fibroblasts with uniformly appearing nuclei (hematoxylin and eosin, original magnification ×40). **B:** At higher magnification the cells producing the abundant collagen show no evidence of atypia (hematoxylin and eosin, original magnification ×150).

served, and giant cells and lipid-bearing histiocytes are absent (22); lack of metaplastic bone formation distinguishes desmoplastic fibroma from the latter. In addition, the structure of the fibrous tissue in nonossifying fibroma, with its typical cartwheel or storiform pattern, as well as its content of giant cells and foam cells, makes the distinction easy. A very cellular lesion may be confused with *low-grade fibrosarcoma* or *malignant fibrous histiocytoma,* although the absence of mitotic activity and the lack of nuclear hyperchromatism and atypia in desmoplastic fibroma may help in this differentiation. In fibrosarcoma, the cells are usually

more densely arranged, and slight pleomorphism and hyperchromatism of the nuclei should point to the correct diagnosis, although in a low-grade tumor the distinction may be very difficult. If the radiographs are confusing, the distinction usually can be made histologically on the basis of the quantity of collagen, the lack of nuclear atypia and hyperchromatism, and the paucity of mitotic activity in desmoplastic fibroma.

Fibroblastic osteosarcoma can be distinguished from desmoplastic fibroma by the tumor bone production in the former tumor.

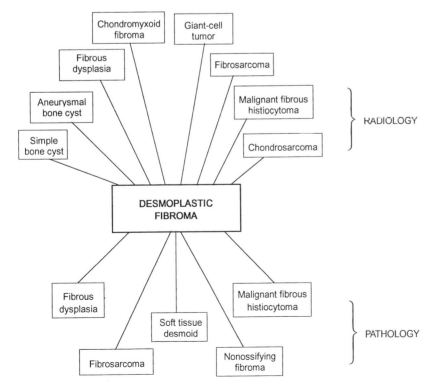

FIG. 43. Radiologic and pathologic differential diagnosis of desmoplastic fibroma.

The distinction between *desmoid of soft tissues* and desmoplastic fibroma of bone must be made on the basis of the clinical and radiologic features (104).

The radiologic and pathologic differential diagnosis of desmoplastic fibroma is depicted in Fig. 43.

MALIGNANT LESIONS

Fibrosarcoma and Malignant Fibrous Histiocytoma

Fibrosarcoma and malignant fibrous histiocytoma (MFH) are malignant fibrous tumors with similar radiographic presentations and similar histologic features. Fibrosarcoma is a malignant tumor characterized by the formation of interlacing bundles of collagen fibers by the spindle-shaped tumor cells and by the absence of bone or cartilage formation. Malignant fibrous histiocytoma is a malignant tumor with a pleomorphic spindle-cell structure producing varying amounts of collagen fibers but devoid of any specific pattern of histologic differentiation (21,22,37,145). Because there is no essential difference in the radiologic features, clinical behavior, and survival data for these tumors, it is justified to regard them as a single group (140,151).

Both fibrosarcoma and MFH can be either primary tumors or secondary to a preexisting benign condition, such as Paget disease, fibrous dysplasia, bone infarct, or chronic draining sinuses of osteomyelitis (119,124,125,137,138). These lesions may also arise in bones that were previously irradiated (135,139,146). Such lesions are termed secondary fibrosarcomas (or secondary MFH).

Rarely fibrosarcoma can arise in a periosteal location (periosteal fibrosarcoma). Some investigators postulate, however, that these lesions in fact represent primary soft tissue tumors abutting the bone and invading the underlying periosteum (112).

Clinical Presentation

Both fibrosarcoma and MFH usually occur in the third to sixth decades and represent about 11% of all cases of malignant bone tumors (69). Their sites of predilection are the femur, humerus, tibia, and pelvic bones (121,129,156) (Fig. 44). Clinically, the most common symptoms are pain and localized swelling, ranging in duration from a few weeks to several months (123). In about 23% of reported cases a pathologic fracture led to detection of the tumor (69,147).

Imaging

Radiographically, both lesions are marked either by an osteolytic area of destruction surrounded by a wide zone of transition or by a moth-eaten or permeative type of bone destruction (125). There is little or no reactive sclerosis, and usually no periosteal reaction (Figs. 45 and 46) (115). The

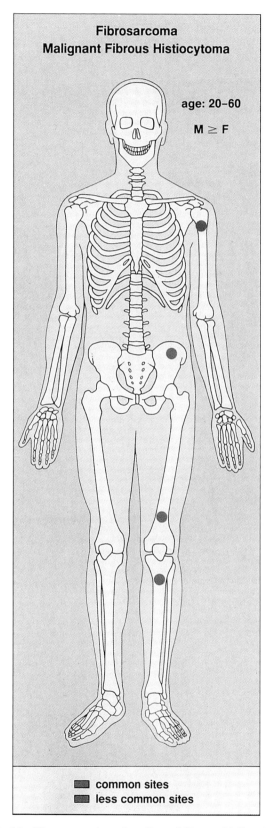

FIG. 44. Fibrosarcoma and malignant fibrous histiocytoma: skeletal sites of predilection, peak age range, and male-to-female ratio.

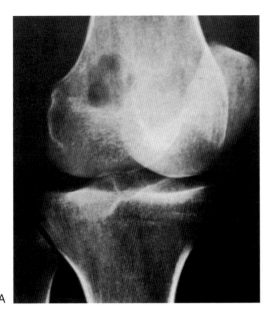
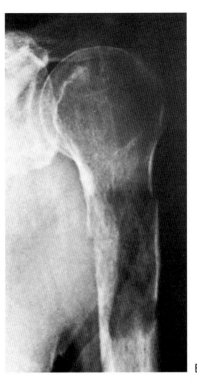

A   B

FIG. 45. Fibrosarcoma. **A:** An oblique radiograph of the right knee of a 28-year-old woman shows a purely destructive osteolytic lesion in the intercondylar fossa of the distal femur. Note the absence of reactive sclerosis and lack of periosteal reaction. **B:** An anteroposterior radiograph of the left proximal humerus in a 62-year-old man shows an osteolytic lesion in the shaft of the bone with a pathologic fracture. A metastatic lesion was suspected but biopsy revealed a fibrosarcoma.

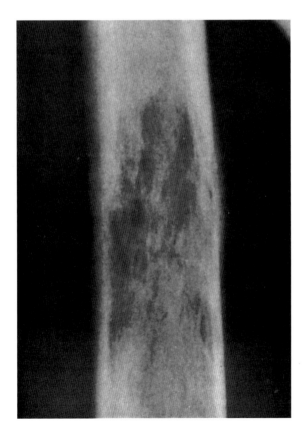

FIG. 46. Malignant fibrous histiocytoma. A destructive osteolytic lesion in the distal femoral shaft shows poorly defined margins. (Reprinted from Greenfield GB, *Imaging of bone tumors,* p. 113).

lesions are often eccentrically located, close to or within the articular end of the bone. Pathologic fractures are not uncommon. A soft tissue mass is frequently present (122). These lesions may resemble giant-cell tumor of bone or telangiectatic osteosarcoma, and they may be mistaken for metastatic carcinoma because of the age group in which they usually occur. Some authorities believe that an almost pathognomonic sign of fibrosarcoma is its tendency to allow the preservation of small sequestrum-like fragments of cor-

tical bone and spongy trabeculae, which can be demonstrated on conventional radiographs or CT examination. On scintigraphy, both lesions typically exhibit an area of increased uptake (113,135), often around the periphery of the tumor (12).

On CT examination, both fibrosarcoma and MFH show a predominant density similar to that of normal muscle (144) and exhibit the nonspecific tissue attenuation values of Hounsfield units encountered in most nonmineralized tis-

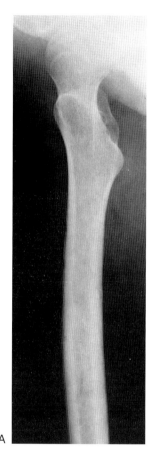
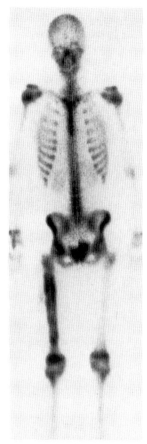

A

B

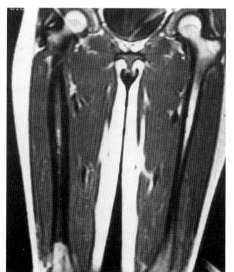
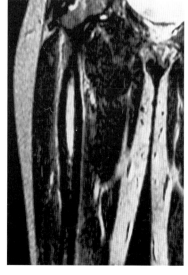

C

D

FIG. 47. Malignant fibrous histiocytoma: magnetic resonance imaging. A: An oblique radiograph of the right femur of a 16-year-old girl shows fusiform thickening of the cortex and permeative type of medullary bone destruction. B: A radionuclide bone scan (^{99}Tc-MDP) shows increased uptake of the tracer in the right femur. C: A coronal T1-weighted (SE, TR 500, TE 20) MRI demonstrates the extent of the tumor that involves about 75% of the length of the femur. D: A coronal T2-weighted (SE, TR 2000, TE 80) MRI shows that the tumor exhibits high signal intensity. The soft tissue extension medially is also accurately depicted.

sues. Hypodense areas reflect areas of necrosis within tumor. MRI is useful to outline the intraosseous and extraosseous extension of these tumors, but there are no characteristic MRI findings for either one (111,113,126,141) (Fig. 47). Some investigators found the signal characteristics comparable to those of other lytic bone tumors (142,150). Signal intensity is intermediate to low on T1-weighted images and high on T2 weighting, frequently inhomogeneous and varying with the degree of necrosis and hemorrhage within the tumor (12).

Histopathology

The histologic criteria for the diagnosis of MFH for soft tissue lesions were outlined by Stout and Lattes in 1967 and by Kempson and Kyriakos in 1972, and have been applied to tumors arising in bone (120,133,148). These include (a) bundles of fibers and of spindle-shaped, fibroblast-like cells arranged in a cartwheel or storiform pattern, exhibiting mitotic

activity and features of atypia; (b) rounded cells with histiocytic features, exhibiting ovoid, and often grooved or indented nuclei and well-defined cytoplasmic borders. These cells often display phagocytic activity with cytoplasmic inclusions of red blood cells, hemosiderin, and/or lipids. They may become transformed into foam cells that contain bizarre and pleomorphic frequently multiple nuclei; (c) typical and atypical giant cells of the osteoclastic type; and (d) a relatively conspicuous infiltration of inflammatory cells, predominantly lymphocytes (22).

Fibrosarcomas are graded from 1 to 4, depending on their cellularity and their nuclear atypia. The higher grade lesions are very cellular and show a greater mitotic activity, nuclear hyperchromatism, and variation in nuclear size and shape (116). The low-grade lesions are less cellular, show only slight anaplasia of the collagen-producing spindle cells, and demonstrate considerable fibrogenesis (143). Other investigators divide these tumors into three grades: well differentiated, moderately differentiated, and poorly differentiated (22,152). In well differentiated tumors, the cells are elon-

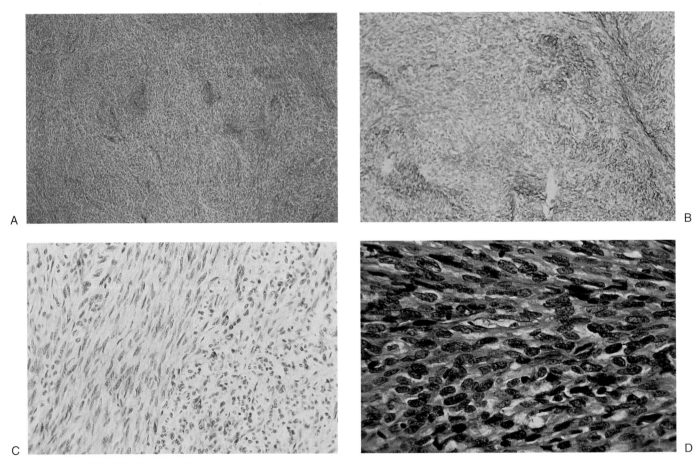

FIG. 48. Histopathology of fibrosarcoma. **A:** Interwoven bundles of spindle cells with a moderate degree of pleomorphism characterize this grade 2 fibrosarcoma (hematoxylin and eosin, original magnification ×25). **B:** With a reticulin fiber stain the uneven distribution of the fibers is obvious (Novotny reticulin stain, original magnification ×50). **C:** The cells and fiber bundles are cut longitudinally (*center*) and across the axis (*left and right*), producing a herring-bone pattern (Giemsa, original magnification ×50). **D:** At high magnification the herringbone pattern is conspicuous (hematoxylin and eosin, original magnification ×400).

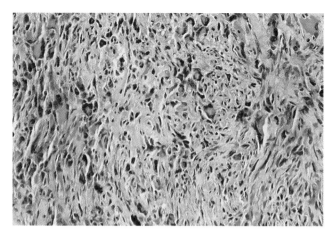

FIG. 49. Histopathology of malignant fibrous histiocytoma. Marked nuclear pleomorphism of malignant fibroblasts and scattered giant cells form the typical storiform or "starry-night" pattern (hematoxylin and eosin, original magnification ×50).

of tumor cells running transversely and others running longitudinally (Fig. 48A, B). In some areas of sectioning all bundles may lie longitudinally, forming a "herringbone tweed" pattern in their spatial relationship (117) (Fig. 48C, D). The spindle cells have hyperchromatic nuclei with an increased ratio of nucleus to cytoplasm. Mitotic activity, including bizarre mitoses, may be present. Collagen production is usually evident in parts of the neoplasm, but it tends to be sparse compared with that of the benign fibroblastic tumors. It is important that there is no evidence of osteoid or bone formation, a feature that distinguishes fibrosarcoma from fibroblastic variants of osteosarcoma (153).

In contrast to the long fascicles of tumor cells in fibrosarcoma, the spindle cells of MFH tend to be arranged in sweeping, curved fascicles and expanding nodules (136). Their histologic appearance has been compared to pinwheels, spiral nebulae, or cut, matted straw (storiform pattern) (118) (Fig. 49). Believed to represent histiocytes acting as "facultative" fibroblasts, the cells of this tumor therefore tend to be more pleomorphic than the simple fibroblasts of fibrosarcoma (Fig. 50). Support for a histiocytic origin of this tumor also lies in the phagocytic activity of occasional tumor cells and the usual presence of giant cells, sometimes in large numbers. Although predominantly spindle-shaped, the tumor cells may also be round or polyhedral. In addition to the usual hyperchromatic nuclei, vesicular nuclei (as found in histiocytes) may be identified. Areas of necrosis are a common finding, and it is not unusual to observe a background with scattered chronic inflammatory cells. Occasionally, collagen production by the fibroblastic type of tumor cells of MFH may be seen in broader hyaline-appearing bands resembling osteoid, which may lead to diagnostic confusion with osteosarcoma. In such cases, experience is necessary to make the differentiation from true osteosarcoma (27,153). Immunohistochemical studies have been helpful in the diagnosis of MFH by demonstrating the presence of certain non-

gated and spindle-shaped, with ovoid or elongated nuclei (114). Sometimes nuclei are hyperchromatic and plump, but no mitotic activity is present. The tumor cells are sparse compared with the relatively abundant intercellular collagen fibers, which are sometimes dense and hyalinized. The poorly differentiated type of tumor is highly cellular, with a marked cellular atypia and a high mitotic activity. The cells possess one or more bizarre, hyperchromatic nuclei. The intercellular matrix is also sparse and occasionally consists only of reticulin fibers (22).

Although both fibrosarcoma and MFH are composed of sarcomatous spindle cells that form variable amounts of collagen, each tumor has certain distinguishing features. The spindle-shaped cells of fibrosarcoma are largely arranged in long fascicles. These fascicles usually run at right angles to one another, so that any plane of section shows some bundles

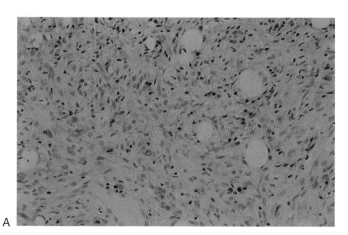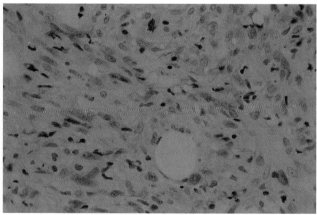

A B

FIG. 50. Histopathology of malignant fibrous histiocytoma. **A:** Moderately cellular tumor, predominantly composed of spindle cells exhibits an allusively storiform pattern. Some preserved fat cells are seen within the tumor tissue (*upper right*) (Giemsa, original magnification ×50). **B:** At higher magnification the pleomorphism of the spindle cells is obvious. In the center seen is one preserved fat cell (Giemsa, original magnification ×100).

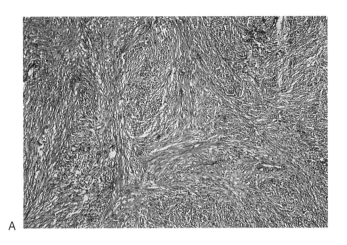

A

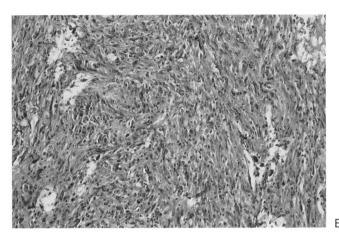

B

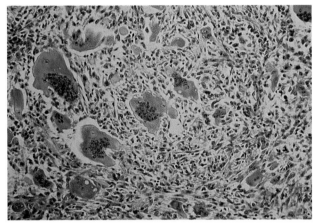

C

FIG. 51. Histopathology of malignant fibrous histiocytoma. **A:** Fibroblastic pattern with typical storiform arrangement (van Gieson, original magnification ×25). **B:** Histiocytic pattern with giant cells (hematoxylin and eosin, original magnification ×25). **C:** Giant cell-rich pattern (hematoxylin and eosin, original magnification ×250).

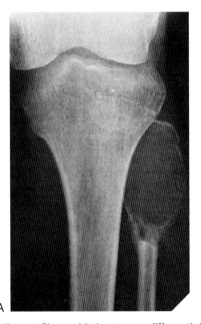

A

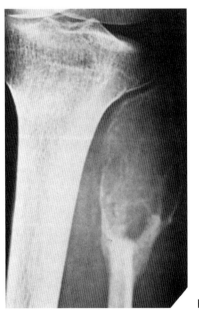

B

FIG. 52. Malignant fibrous histiocytoma: differential diagnosis. **(A)** An anteroposterior radiograph of the left knee and **(B)** a magnification study in the oblique projection show an expanding, lytic lesion in the proximal end of the fibula in a 13-year-old girl. There is a buttress of periosteal new bone formation at the distal extent of the tumor. A giant-cell tumor or an aneurysmal bone cyst have been suspected, but a biopsy revealed a malignant fibrous histiocytoma.

specific markers for histiocytic enzymes (e.g., lysozyme, α_1-antitrypsin) in the tumor. On the other hand, studies of direct immunologic markers for the monocyte-macrophage lineage have yielded somewhat mixed results (149,154,155). The problem with many immunologic studies is that they have

been performed on MFH of soft tissue, and these tumors have not been subjected to the cellular alterations inherent in decalcification.

Huvos et al subdivide the histologic pattern seen in MFH into several variants, according to the predominant patho-

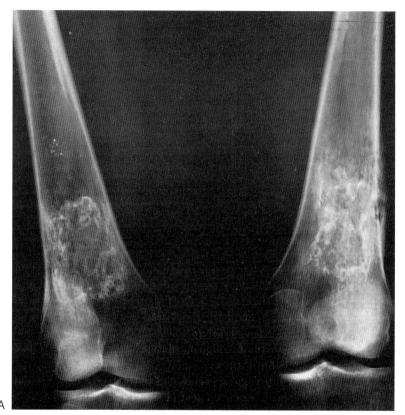

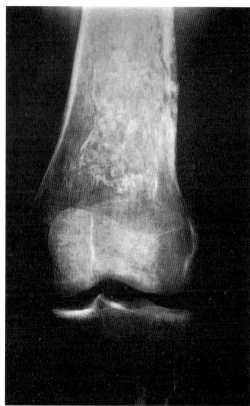

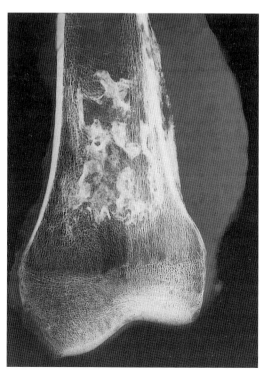

FIG. 53. Malignant fibrous histiocytoma: differential diagnosis. **A:** An anteroposterior radiograph of both knees in a 39-year-old woman with known multiple idiopathic bone infarcts shows the typical appearance of this condition in the distal femora. In the left femur there is, however, evidence of a lamellated periosteal reaction along the lateral cortex. **B:** Magnification study shows cortical destruction. On biopsy the suspicious lesion proved to be a malignant fibrous histiocytoma complicating a bone infarct. **C:** A radiograph of the resected specimen shows the aggressive periosteal reaction and a soft tissue mass more clearly. Note typical serpentine coarse calcifications of the medullary bone infarct.

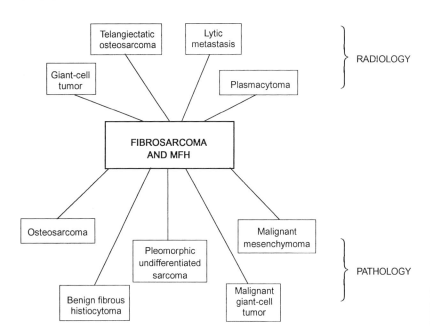

FIG. 54. Radiologic and pathologic differential diagnosis of fibrosarcoma and malignant fibrous histiocytoma.

logic appearance, although in clinical practice these patterns frequently overlap: (a) a predominantly fibroblastic pattern (Fig. 51A), in which the fibroblast-like spindle cells are arranged in whorls of cartwheel or storiform pattern with only occasional giant cells of the osteoclastic type; (b) a predominantly histiocytic or xanthomatous morphologic variant, in which giant cells of the osteoclastic type, frequently with foamy cytoplasm, predominate (Fig. 51B); and (c) the malignant giant-cell tumor type, in which there is an intimate admixture of fibroblasts, mononuclear histiocytes, and giant cells of the osteoclastic type (127,128) (Fig. 51C).

Differential Diagnosis

Radiology

Because fibrosarcoma and MFH have an almost identical radiologic appearance, both lesions will be considered as one in the differential diagnosis. All purely lytic lesions without marginal sclerosis should be considered in the differential diagnosis, including *giant-cell tumor, lymphoma, solitary myeloma, metastasis,* and *brown tumor of hyperparathyroidism.* Giant-cell tumor must be particularly considered in lesions affecting the articular end of a bone (Fig. 52). Occasionally, *chondrosarcoma* with minimal or no central calcification and lack of peripheral sclerosis may look like fibrosarcoma or MFH. In lesions located in the tibia, *adamantinoma* should be excluded. In the younger age group, osteolytic (either fibroblastic or telangiectatic) *osteosarcoma* may be a differential consideration and for the patients in the first two decades, *Ewing sarcoma.*

The presence of calcifications at the periphery or within the tumor is strongly suggestive of secondary fibrosarcoma or secondary MFH resulting from malignant complications of a bone infarct (Fig. 53).

Pathology

Because fibrosarcoma and malignant fibrous histiocytoma represent closely related entities, their differential diagnosis may be extremely difficult (134). Their histopathologic differences, in particular the characteristic herringbone tweed pattern of a well-differentiated fibrosarcoma and the storiform pattern of malignant fibrous histiocytoma (132), have been outlined above.

The histologic appearance of fibrosarcoma may resemble *fibroblastic osteosarcoma* (153). However, the distinctive difference is the absence of bone or osteoid formation in the former tumor. *Desmoplastic fibroma* may be a differential possibility when a well-differentiated type of fibrosarcoma is being examined, although this lesion is less cellular than fibrosarcoma and its mitotic activity is very low.

The radiologic and pathologic differential diagnosis of fibrosarcoma and malignant fibrous histiocytoma is depicted in Fig. 54.

REFERENCES

Fibrous Cortical Defect and Nonossifying Fibroma

1. Arata MA, Peterson HA, Dahlin DC. Pathological fractures through non-ossifying fibromas. *J Bone Joint Surg* 1981;63A:980–988.
2. Bertoni F, Unni KK, McLeod RA, Sim FH. Xanthoma of bone. *Am J Pathol* 1988;90:377–384.
3. Blau RA, Zwick DL, Westphal RA. Multiple nonossifying fibromas. *J Bone Joint Surg* 1988;70A:299–304.
4. Brenner RJ, Hattner RS, Lilien DL. Scintigraphic features of nonosteogenic fibroma. *Radiology* 1979;131:727–730.
5. Caffey J. On fibrous defects in cortical walls of growing tubular bone: their radiologic appearance, structure prevalence, natural course and diagnostic significance. *Adv Pediatrics* 1955;7:13–51.
6. Cunningham BJ, Ackerman LV. Metaphyseal fibrous defects. *J Bone Joint Surg* 1956;38:797–808.

7. Dahlin DC, Unni KK.Bone Tumors. *General aspects and data on 8,542 cases,* 4th ed. Springfield, IL: Charles C Thomas, 1986.

8. Dunham WK, Marcus NW, Enneking WF, Haun C. Developmental defects of the distal femoral metaphysis. *J Bone Joint Surg* 1980;62A: 801–806.

9. Evans GA, Park WM. Familial multiple non-osteogenic fibromata. *J Bone Joint Surg* 1978;60B:416–419.

10. Friedland JA, Reinus WR, Fisher AJ, Wilson AJ. Quantitative analysis of the plain radiographic appearance of nonossifying fibroma. *Invest Radiol* 1995;30:474–479.

11. Greyson ND, Pang S. The variable bone scan appearances of nonosteogenic fibroma of bone. *Clin Nucl Med* 1981;6:242–245.

12. Hudson TM, Stiles RG, Monson DK. Fibrous lesions of bone. *Radiol Clin North Am* 1993;31:279–297.

13. Jaffe HL, Lichtenstein L. Non-osteogenic fibroma of bone. *Am J Pathol* 1942;18:205–221.

14. Jaffe HL. *Tumors and tumorous conditions of the bones and joints.* Philadelphia: Lea and Febiger, 1968.

15. Kumar R, Madewell JE, Lindell MM, Swischuk LE. Fibrous lesions of bones. *RadioGraphics* 1990;10:237–256.

16. Kumar R, Swischuk LE, Madewell JE. Benign cortical defect: site for an avulsion fracture. *Skeletal Radiol* 1986;15:553–555.

17. Mirra JM, Gold RH, Rand F. Disseminated nonossifying fibromas in association with café-au-lait spots (Jaffe-Campanacci syndrome). *Clin Orthop* 1982;168:192–205.

18. Moser RP Jr, Sweet DE, Haseman DB, Madewell JE. Multiple skeletal fibroxanthomas: radiologic-pathologic correlation of 72 cases. *Skeletal Radiol* 1987;16:353–359.

19. Ritschl P, Karnel F, Hajek PC. Fibrous metaphyseal defects—determination of their origin and natural history using a radiomorphological study. *Skeletal Radiol* 1988;17:8–15.

20. Ritschl P, Hajek PC, Pechmann U. Fibrous metaphyseal defects. Magnetic resonance imaging appearances. *Skeletal Radiol* 1989;18: 253–259.

21. Schajowicz F. Histological typing of bone tumors. *World Health Organization international histological classification of tumors.* Berlin: Springer-Verlag, 1993.

22. Schajowicz F. *Tumors and tumorlike lesions of bone: pathology, radiology, and treatment,* 2nd ed. Berlin: Springer-Verlag, 1994.

23. Schwartz AM, Ramos RM. Neurofibromatosis and multiple nonossifying fibroma. *Am J Roentgenol* 1980;135:617–619.

24. Selby S. Metaphyseal cortical defects in the tubular bones of growing children. *J Bone Joint Surg* 1961;43A:395–400.

25. Steiner GC. Fibrous cortical defect and non-ossifying fibroma of bone: a study of the ultrastructure. *Arch Pathol* 1974;97:205–210.

26. Unni KK. Fibrous and fibrohistiocytic lesions of bone. *Semin Orthop* 1991;6:177–186.

27. Wold LE. Fibrohistiocytic tumors of bone. In: Unni KK, ed. *Bone tumors.* New York: Churchill Livingstone, 1988;183–197.

Benign Fibrous Histiocytoma

28. Arii Y, Moritani M, Hirakoh H. A case of benign fibrous histiocytoma of the femur. *Orthop Surg (Seikeigeka)* 1991;42:1248–1250.

29. Bertoni F, Calderoni P, Bacchini P, Sudanese A. Benign fibrous histiocytoma of bone. *J Bone Joint Surg* 1986;68A:1225–1230.

30. Clarke BE, Xipell JM, Thomas DP. Benign fibrous histiocytoma of bone. *Am J Surg Pathol* 1985;9:806–815.

31. Dominok GW, Eisengarten W. Benignes fibroeses Histiozytom des Knochens. *Zentralbl Pathol* 1980;124:77–83.

32. Hamada T, Ito H, Araki Y, Fujii K, Inoue M, Ishida O. Benign fibrous histiocytoma of the femur: review of three cases. *Skeletal Radiol* 1996;25:25–29.

33. Huvos A. *Bone tumors: diagnosis, treatment and prognosis,* 2nd ed. Philadelphia: WB Saunders, 1991.

34. Matsuno T. Benign fibrous histiocytoma involving the ends of long bone. *Skeletal Radiol* 1990;19:561–566.

35. Mesiter P, Konrad E, Hohne N. Incidence and histological structure of the storiform pattern in benign and malignant fibrous histiocytomas. *Virchows Arch (A)* 1981;393:93–101.

36. Schajowicz F, Ackerman LV, Sissons HA. *Histological typing of bone tumors.* Geneva: World Health Organization, 1972.

37. Schajowicz F, Sissons HA, Sobin LH. The World Health Organizations histologic classification of bone tumors. A commentary on the second edition. *Cancer* 1995;75:1208–1214.

38. Spjut HJ, Dorfman HD, Fechner RE, Ackerman LV. Tumors of bone pathology. In: Firminger HI, ed. *Atlas of tumor pathology,* 2nd series, fascicle 5. Washington DC: Armed Forces Institute of Pathology, 1971.

39. Statz EM, Pochebit SM, Cooper A, Philipps E, Leslie BM. Case report 525. Benign fibrous histiocytoma (BFH) of thumb. *Skeletal Radiol* 1989;18:299–302.

Periosteal Desmoid

40. Barnes GR Jr, Gwinn JL. Distal irregularities of the femur simulating malignancy. *Am J Roentgenol* 1974;122:180–185.

41. Brower AC, Culver JE Jr, Keats TE. Histological nature of the cortical irregularity of the medial posterior distal femoral metaphysis in children. *Radiology* 1971;99:389–392.

42. Bufkin WJ. The avulsive cortical irregularity. *Am J Roentgenol* 1971; 112:487–492.

43. Burrows PE, Greenberg ID, Reed MH. The distal femoral defect: Technetium-99m pyrophosphate bone scan results. *J Can Assoc Radiol* 1982;33:91–93.

44. Kimmelstiel P, Rapp I. Cortical defect due to periosteal desmoids. *Bull Hosp Joint Dis* 1951;12:286–297.

45. Pennes DR, Braunstein EM, Glazer GM. Computed tomography of cortical desmoid. *Skeletal Radiol* 1984;12:40–42.

46. Resnick D, Greenway G. Distal femoral cortical defects, irregularities, and excavations: a critical review of the literature with the addition of histologic and paleopathologic data. *Radiology* 1982;143:345–354.

47. Velchik MG, Heyman S, Makler PT Jr, Goldstein HA, Alavi A. Bone scintigraphy: differentiating benign cortical irregularity of the distal femur from malignancy. *J Nucl Med* 1985;25:72–74.

48. Yamazaki T, Maruoka S, Takahashi S, Saito H, Takase K, Nakamura M, Sakamoto K. MR findings of avulsive cortical irregularity of the distal femur. *Skeletal Radiol* 1995;24:43–46.

Fibrous Dysplasia

49. Bullough PG. *Atlas of orthopaedic pathology with clinical and radiologic correlations* 2nd Ed. New York: Gower Medical Publishing, 1992.

50. Camilleri AE. Craniofacial fibrous dysplasia. *J Laryngol Otol* 1991; 105:662–666.

51. Creagh MF, Nunan TO. Positive gallium-67 citrate uptake in a patient with polyostotic fibrous dysplasia. *Clin Nucl Med* 1988;13:241–242.

52. Daffner RH, Kirks DR, Gehweiler JA Jr, Heaston DK. Computed tomography of fibrous dysplasia. *Am J Roentgenol* 1982;139:943–948.

53. Dahlin DC, Bertoni F, Beabout JW, Campanacci M. Fibrocartilaginous mesenchymoma with low grade malignancy. *Skeletal Radiol* 1984;12:263–269.

54. DeSmet AA, Travers H, Neff JR. Chondrosarcoma occuring in a patient with polyostotic fibrous dysplasia. *Skeletal Radiol* 1981; 7:197–201.

55. Dorfman HD, Ishida T, Tsuneyoshi M. Exophytic variant of fibrous dysplasia (fibrous dysplasia protuberans). *Hum Pathol* 1994;25: 1234–1237.

56. Drolshagen LF, Reynolds WA, Marcus NW. Fibrocartilaginous dysplasia of bone. *Radiology* 1985;156:32.

57. Fisher AJ, Totty WG, Kyriakos M. MR appearance of cystic fibrous dysplasia. Case report. *J Comput Assist Tomogr* 1994;18:315–318.

58. Gober GA, Nicholas RW. Case report 800. Skeletal fibrous dysplasia associated with intramuscular myxoma (Mazabraud's syndrome). *Skeletal Radiol* 1993;22:452–455.

59. Henry A. Monostotic fibrous dysplasia. *J Bone Joint Surg* 1969; 51B:300–306.

60. Hermann G, Klein M, Abdelwahab IF, Kenan S. Fibrocartilaginous dysplasia. *Skeletal Radiol* 1996;25:509–511.

61. Hoshi H, Futami S, Ohnishi T, Nagamachi S, Jinnouchi S, Murai N, Watanabe K. Gallium-67 uptake in fibrous dysplasia of the bone. *Ann Nucl Med* 1990;4:35–38.

62. Inamo Y, Hanawa Y, Kin H, Okuni M. Findings on magnetic resonance imaging of the spine and femur in a case of McCune-Albright syndrome. *Pediatr Radiol* 1993;23:15–18.

63. Ishida T, Dorfman HD. Massive chondroid differentiation in fibrous dysplasia of bone (fibrocartilaginous dysplasia). *Am J Surg Pathol* 1993;17:924–930.

64. Jee W-H, Choi K-H, Choe B-Y, Park J-M, Shinn K-S. Fibrous dys-

plasia: MR imaging characteristics with radiopathologic correlation. *Am J Roentgenol* 1996;167:1523–1527.

65. Kransdorf MJ, Moser RP, Gilkey FW. Fibrous dysplasia. *Radio-Graphics* 1990;10:519–537.

66. Lichtenstein L, Jaffe HL. Fibrous dysplasia of bone. *Arch Pathol* 1942;33:777–816.

67. Machida K, Makita K, Nishikawa J, Ohtake T, Ilio M. Scintigraphic manifestation of fibrous dysplasia. *Clin Nucl Med* 1986;11:426–429.

68. Mirra JM, Gold RH. Fibrous dysplasia. In: Mirra HM, Gold RH, Picci P, eds. *Bone tumors.* Philadelphia: Lea and Febiger 1989.

69. Mulder JD, Schütte HE, Kroon HM, Taconis WK. *Radiologic atlas of bone tumors.* Amsterdam: Elsevier, 1993;607–625.

70. Ragsdale BD. Polymorphic fibro-osseous lesions of bone: an almost site-specific diagnostic problem of the proximal femur. *Hum Pathol* 1993;24:505–512.

71. Riley GM, Greenspan A, Poirier VC. Fibrous dysplasia of a parietal bone. *J Comput Assist Tomogr* 1997;21:41–43.

72. Rodenberg J, Jensen OM, Keller J, Nielsen OS, Bünger C, Jurik AG. Fibrous dysplasia of the spine, costae and hemipelvis with sarcomatous transformation. *Skeletal Radiol* 1996;25:682–684.

73. Ruggieri P, Sim FH, Bond JA, Unni KK. Malignancies in fibrous dysplasia. *Cancer* 1994;73:1411–1424.

74. Schwartz DT, Alpert M. The malignant transformation of fibrous dysplasia. *Am J Med Sci* 1964;247:1–20.

75. Sissons HA, Malcolm AJ. Fibrous dysplasia of bone: case report with autopsy study 80 years after the original clinical recognition of the bone lesions. *Skeletal Radiol* 1997;26:177–183.

76. Sundaram M, McDonald DJ, Merenda G. Intramuscular myxoma: a rare but important association with fibrous dysplasia of bone. *Am J Roentgenol* 1989;153:107–108.

77. Utz JA, Kransdorf MJ, Jelinek JS, Moser RP, Berrey BH. MR appearance of fibrous dysplasia. *J Comput Assist Tomogr* 1989;13:845–851.

78. Yabut SM, Kenan S, Sissons HA, Lewis MM. Malignant transformation of fibrous dysplasia. *Clin Orthop* 1988;228:281–289.

Osteofibrous Dysplasia

79. Alguacil-Garcia A, Alonso A, Pettigrew NM. Osteofibrous dysplasia (ossifying fibroma) of the tibia and fibula and adamantinoma. *Am J Clin Pathol* 1984;82:470–474.

80. Campanacci M, Laus M. Osteofibrous dysplasia of the tibia and fibula. *J Bone Joint Surg* 1981;63A:367–375.

81. Campanacci M. Osteofibrous dysplasia of the long bones. A new clinical entity. *Ital J Orthop Traumatol* 1976;2:221–237.

82. Campbell CJ, Hawk T. A variant of fibrous dysplasia (osteofibrous dysplasia). *J Bone Joint Surg* 1982;64A:231–236.

83. Castelotte A, Garcia-Peña P, Lucaya J, Lorenzo J. Osteofibrous dysplasia. A report of two cases. *Skeletal Radiol* 1988;17:483–486.

84. Cohen DM, Dahlin DC, Pugh DG. Fibrous dysplasia associated with adamantinoma of the long bones. *Cancer* 1962;15:515–521.

85. Czerniak B, Rojas-Corona RR, Dorfman HD. Morphologic diversity of long bone adamantinoma. The concept of differentiated (regressing) adamantinoma and its relationship to osteofibrous dysplasia. *Cancer* 1989;64:2319–2334.

86. Keeney GL, Unni K, Beabout JW, Pritchard DJ. Adamantinoma of long bones. *Cancer* 1989;64:730–737.

87. Kempson RL. Ossifying fibroma of the long bones. A light and electron microscopic study. *Arch Pathol* 1966;82:218–233.

88. Markel SF. Ossifying fibroma of long bone. *Am J Clin Pathol* 1978;69:91–97.

89. Park Y, Unni KK, McLeod RA, Pritchard DJ. Osteofibrous dysplasia: clinicopathologic study of 80 cases. *Hum Pathol* 1993;24:1339–1347.

90. Sissons HA, Kancherla PL, Lehman WB. Ossifying fibroma of bone. Report of two cases. *Bull Hosp Joint Dis Orthop Inst* 1983;43:1–14.

91. Springfield DS, Rosenberg AE, Mankin HJ, Mindell ER. Relationship between osteofibrous dysplasia and adamantinoma. *Clin Orthop* 1994;309:234–244.

92. Sweet DE, Vinh TN, Devaney K. Cortical osteofibrous dysplasia of long bone and its relationship to adamantinoma. *Am J Surg Pathol* 1992;16:282–290.

93. Ueda Y, Blasius S, Edel G, Wuisman P, Bocker W, Roessner A. Os-

teofibrous dysplasia of long bones—a reactive process to adamantinomatous tissue. *J Cancer Clin Oncol* 1992;118:152–156.

94. Unni KK, Dahlin DC, Beabout JW, Ivins JC. Adamantinoma of long bones. *Cancer* 1974;34:1796–1805.

95. Wang J, Shih C, Chen W. Osteofibrous dysplasia (ossifying fibroms of long bones). *Clin Orthop* 1992;278:235–243.

96. Weiss SW, Dorfman HD. Adamantinoma of long bones. *Hum Pathol* 1977;8:141–153.

97. Zeanah WR, Hudson TM, Springfield DS. Computed tomography of ossifying fibroma of the tibia. *J Comput Assist Tomogr* 1983;7:688–691.

Desmoplastic Fibroma

98. Bertoni F, Calderoni P, Bacchini P, Campanacci M. Desmoplastic fibroma of bone: a report of six cases. *J Bone Joint Surg* 1984;66B:265–268.

99. Bridge JA, Rosenthal H, Sanger WG, Neff JR. Desmoplastic fibroma arising in fibrous dysplasia. Chromosomal analysis and review of the literature. *Clin Orthop Rel Res* 1989;247:272–278.

100. Crim JR, Gold RH, Mirra JM, Eckardt JJ, Bassett LW. Desmoplastic fibroma of bone: radiographic analysis. *Radiology* 1989;172:827–832.

101. Gebhardt MC, Campbell CJ, Schiller AL, Mankin HJ. Desmoplastic fibroma of bone. A report of eight cases and review of the literature. *J Bone Joint Surg* 1985;67A:732–747.

102. Greenspan A, Unni KK. Case report 787. Desmoplastic fibroma. *Skeletal Radiol* 1993;22:296–299.

103. Inwards CY, Unni KK, Beabout JW, Sim FH. Desmoplastic fibroma of bone. *Cancer* 1991;68:1978–1983.

104. Lichtman EA, Klein MJ. Case report 302. Desmoplastic fibroma of the proximal end of the left femur. *Skeletal Radiol* 1985;13:160–163.

105. Rabhan WN, Rosai J. Desmoplastic fibroma. Report of ten cases and review of the literature. *J Bone Joint Surg* 1968;50A:487–502.

106. Sugiura I. Desmoplastic fibroma. Case report and review of the literature. *J Bone Joint Surg* 1976;58A:126–130.

107. Taconis WK, Schütte HE, van der Heul RO. Desmoplastic fibroma of bone: a report of 18 cases. *Skeletal Radiol* 1994;23:283–288.

108. West R, Huvos AG, Lane JM. Desmoplastic fibroma of bone arising in fibrous dysplasia. *Am J Clin Pathol* 1983;79:630–633.

109. You JS, Lawrence S, Pathria M, Resnick D, Haghighi P. Desmoplastic fibroma of the calcaneus. *Skeletal Radiol* 1995;24:451–454.

110. Young JWR, Aisner SC, Levine AM, Resnik CS, Dorfman HD. Computed tomography of desmoid tumors of bone: Desmoplastic fibroma. *Skeletal Radiol* 1988;17:333–337.

Fibrosarcoma and Malignant Fibrous Histiocytoma

111. Aisen AM, Martel W, Braunstein EM, McMillin KI, Phillips WA, Kling TF. MRI and CT evaluation of primary bone and soft-tissue tumors. *Am J Roentgenol* 1986;146:749–756.

112. Bertoni F, Capanna R, Calderoni P, Bacchini P, Campanacci M. Primary central (medullary) fibrosarcoma of bone. *Semin Diagn Pathol* 1984;1:185–198.

113. Bloem JL, Taminiau AH, Eulderink F, Hermans J, Pauwels EK. Radiologic staging of primary bone sarcoma: MR imaging, scintigraphy, angiography, and CT correlated with pathologic examination. *Radiology* 1988;169:805–810.

114. Boland PJ, Huvos AG. Malignant fibrous histiocytoma of bone. *Clin Orthop* 1986;204:130–134.

115. Capanna R, Bertoni F, Bacchini P, Gacci G, Guerra A, Campanacci M. Malignant fibrous histiocytoma of bone: the experience at the Rizzoli Institute. Report of 90 cases. *Cancer* 1984;54:177–187.

116. Dahlin DC. Grading of bone tumors. In: Unni KK, ed. *Bone tumors.* New York: Churchill Livingstone, 1988;35–45.

117. Dahlin DC, Ivins JC. Fibrosarcoma of bone: a study of 114 cases. *Cancer* 1969;23:35–41.

118. Dahlin DC, Unni KK, Matsuno T. Malignant (fibrous) histiocytoma of bone—fact or fancy? *Cancer* 1977;39:1508–1516.

119. Dorfman HD, Norman A, Wolff H. Fibrosarcoma complicating bone

infarction in a caisson worker: case report. *J Bone Joint Surg* 1966; 48A:528–532.

120. Enzinger FM, Weiss SW. *Soft tissue tumors.* St Louis: CV Mosby, 1983.

121. Eyre-Brook AL, Price CHG. Fibrosarcoma of bone: review of 50 consecutive cases from the Bristol Bone Tumor Registry. *J Bone Joint Surg* 1969;51B:20–37.

122. Feldman F, Lattes R. Primary malignant fibrous histiocytoma (fibrous xanthoma) of bone. *Skeletal Radiol* 1977;1:145–160.

123. Feldman F, Norman D. Intra- and extraosseous malignant histiocytoma (malignant fibrous xanthoma). *Radiology* 1972;104:497–508.

124. Galli SJ, Weintraub HP, Proppe KH. Malignant fibrous histiocytoma and pleomorphic sarcoma in association with medullary bone infarcts. *Cancer* 1978;41:607–619.

125. Greenfield GB, Arrington JA. *Imaging of bone tumors. A multimodality approach.* Philadelphia, JB Lippincott, 1995.

126. Hudson TM, Hamlin DJ, Enneking WF, Pettersson H. Magnetic resonance imaging of bone and soft tissue tumors: early experience in 31 patients compared with computed tomography. *Skeletal Radiol* 1985; 13:134–146.

127. Huvos AG. Primary malignant fibrous histiocytoma of bone: clinicopathologic study of 18 patients. *NY State J Med* 1976;552–559.

128. Huvos AG, Heilweil M, Bretsky SS. The pathology of malignant fibrous histiocytoma of bone. A study of 130 patients. *Am J Surg Pathol* 1985;9:853–871.

129. Huvos AG, Higinbotham NL. Primary fibrosarcoma of bone: a clinico-pathologic study of 130 patients. *Cancer* 1975;35:837–847.

130. Huvos AG, Higinbotham NL, Miller TR. Bone sarcomas arising in fibrous dysplasia. *J Bone Joint Surg* 1972;64A:1047–1056.

131. Huvos AG, Woodard HQ, Heilweil M. Postrtiation malignant fibrous histiocytoma of bone: a clinicopathologic study of 20 patients. *Am J Surg Pathol* 1986;10:9–18.

132. Kahn LB, Webber B, Mills E, Anstey L, Heselson NG. Malignant fibrous histiocytoma (malignant fibrous xanthoma: xanthosarcoma) of bone. *Cancer* 1978;42:640–651.

133. Kempson RL, Kyriakos M. Fibroxanthosarcoma of the soft tissues. A type of malignant fibrous histiocytoma. *Cancer* 1972;29:961–976.

134. Lawson CW, Fisher C, Gatter KC. An immunohistochemical study of differentiation in malignant fibrous histiocytoma. *Histopathology* 1987;11:375–383.

135. Lin WY, Kao CH, Hsu CY, Liao SQ, Wang SH, Yeh SH. The role of Tc-99m MDP and Ga-67 imaging in the clinical evaluation of malignant fibrous histiocytoma. *Clin Nucl Med* 1994;19:996–1000.

136. McCarthy EF, Matsuno T, Dorfman HD. Malignant fibrous histiocytoma of bone: a study of 35 cases. *Hum Pathol* 1979;10:57–70.

137. Mirra JM, Bullough PG, Marcove RC, Jacobs B, Huvos AG. Malignant fibrous histiocytoma and osteosarcoma in association with bone infarcts. *J Bone Joint Surg* 1974;56A:932–940.

138. Mirra JM, Gold RH, Marafiote R. Malignant (fibrous) histiocytoma arising in association with a bone infarct in sickle-cell disease: coincidence or cause-and-effect? *Cancer* 1977;39:186–194.

139. Murphey MD, Gross TM, Rosenthal HG. Musculoskeletal malignant fibrous histiocytoma: radiologic-pathologic correlation. *RadioGraphics* 1994;14:807–826.

140. Nakashima Y, Morishita S, Kotoura Y, Yamamuro T, Tamura K, Onomura T, Sudo Y, Awaya G, Hamashima Y. Malignant fibrous histiocytoma of bone. *Cancer* 1985;55:2804–2811.

141. Pettersson H, Gillespy T, Hamlin DJ, Enneking WF, Springfield DS, Andrew ER, Spanier S, Slone R. Primary musculoskeletal tumors: examination with MR imaging compared with conventional modalities. *Radiology* 1987;164:237–241.

142. Pettersson H, Slone RM, Spanier S, Gillespy T III, Fitzsimmons JR, Scott KN. Musculoskeletal tumors: T1 and T2 relaxation times. *Radiology* 1988;167:783–785.

143. Pritchard DJ, Sim FH, Ivins JC, Soule EH, Dahlin DC. Fibrosarcoma of bone and soft tissues of the trunk and extremities. *Orthop Clin North Am* 1977;8:869–881.

144. Ros PR, Viamonte M Jr, Rywlin AM. Malignant fibrous histiocytoma: mesenchymal tumor of ubiquitous origin. *Am J Roentgenol* 1984;142: 753–759.

145. Seiss SW, Enzinger FM. Malignant fibrous histiocytoma: an analysis of 200 cases. *Cancer* 1978;41:2250–2260.

146. Smith J. Radiation-induced sarcoma of bone: clinical and radiographic findings in 43 patients irradiated for soft tissue neoplasms. *Clin Radiol* 1982;33:205–221.

147. Spanier SS, Enneking WF, Enriquez P. Primary malignant fibrous histiocytoma of bone. *Cancer* 1975;36:2084–2098.

148. Stout AP, Lattes R. Tumors of the soft tissues. In: *Atlas of tumor pathology,* 2nd fasicle series 1. Washington, DC: Armed Forces Institute of Pathology 1967.

149. Strauchen JA, Dimitriu-Bona A. Malignant fibrous histiocytoma: expression of monocyte-macrophage differentiation antigens detected with monoclonal antibodies. *Am J Pathol* 1986;124:303–309.

150. Sundaram M, McLeod RA. MR imaging of tumor and tumorlike lesions of bone and soft tissue. *Am J Roentgenol* 1990;155:817–824.

151. Taconis WK, Mulder JD. Fibrosarcoma and malignant fibrous histiocytoma of long bones: radiographic features and grading. *Skeletal Radiol* 1984;11:237–245.

152. Taconis WK, Van Rijssel TG. Fibrosarcoma of long bones: a study of the significance of areas of malignant fibrous histiocytoma. *J Bone Joint Surg* 1985;67B:111–116.

153. Unni KK. Osteosarcoma of bone. In: Unni KK, ed. *Bone tumors.* New York: Churchill Livingstone, 1988;107–133.

154. Wood GS, Beckstead JH, Turner RR, Hendrickson MR, Kempson RL, Warnke RA. Malignant fibrous histiocytoma tumor cells resemble fibroblasts. *Am J Surg Pathol* 1986;10:323–335.

155. Wood GS, Beckstead JH, Turner RR, Hendrickson MR, Kempson RL, Warnke RA. Malignant fibrous histiocytoma cells do not express the antigenic or enzyme histochemical features of cells of monocyte/macrophage lineage. *Lab Invest* 1985;52:78 (abstract).

156. Yuen WWH, Saw D. Malignant fibrous histiocytoma of bone. *J Bone Joint Surg* 1985;67A:482–486.

CHAPTER 5

Round Cell Lesions

BENIGN LESIONS
Langerhans Cell Granuloma (Eosinophilic
Granuloma)
MALIGNANT LESIONS
Ewing Sarcoma

Malignant Lymphoma
Non-Hodgkin lymphoma
Hodgkin lymphoma
Multiple Myeloma (Plasmacytoma)

BENIGN LESIONS

Langerhans Cell Granuloma (Eosinophilic Granuloma)

This is a tumor-like condition belonging to a group of disorders known as reticuloendothelioses. The incidence is estimated at 0.05 to 0.5 per 100,000 children per year in the United States, with a 2:1 male predominance (26,30). The disorder represents <1% of all biopsy-proven primary bone lesions (10,33). Lichtenstein (27,28) proposed the name *histiocytosis X* for the three conditions: eosinophilic granuloma (condition with bone lesions only); Hand-Schüller-Christian disease or xanthomatosis (characterized by the triad of bone lesions, diabetes insipidus, and exophthalmos); and Letterer-Siwe disease or nonlipid reticulosis (when disseminated disease is marked by wasting, lymphadenopathy, hepatosplenomegaly, and anemia). His rationale was the postulation that these lesions, being of unknown cause, appeared to represent an increasing spectrum of severity in which the common denominator was the presence of the histiocyte (6,48). Although this concept gained wide acceptance, the three diseases may, in fact, represent different entities (13). Schajowicz and Polak proposed the general term histiocytic granuloma for this group of disorders, which may appear without or with only isolated eosinophils or, more commonly, with many eosinophilic leukocytes, and may involve a single or several bones (44). Recently, histiocytosis X has been given the name of Langerhans cell histiocytosis (12,29,31) because it has been verified that the primary proliferative element in this disease is the Langerhans cell, a mononuclear cell of the dendritic type that is found in the epidermis but is derived from precursors in the bone marrow (39,40,43,46). Langerhans cell histiocytosis, although

causes and pathogenesis remain unsettled, is now considered a disorder of immune regulation rather than a neoplastic process. However, some laboratory studies have shown that certain lesions contain a clonal proliferation of cells, suggesting a neoplastic origin (49). The relationship of Langerhans cell histiocytosis to the immune system is supported by the observation that the severity of the disease is directly influenced by the immaturity of the immune system (46). In general, the younger the patient, the more severe the disease (33). The disorder exhibits a broad spectrum of clinical and radiologic abnormalities. It is characterized by an abnormal proliferation of histiocytes in various parts of the reticuloendothelial system such as bone, lungs, central nervous system, skin, and lymph nodes.

Clinical Presentation

Langerhans cell granuloma may manifest as a solitary lesion or as multiple lesions (18,32). It occurs most often during childhood, with a peak incidence between the ages of 5 and 10 years (50). It is slightly more common in males. The most commonly affected sites are the skull (calvaria, skull base, and facial bones), the ribs, the pelvis, the spine, and the long bones (Fig. 1). Epiphyseal lesions are relatively rare (46). Clinical manifestations include local pain, tenderness, and swelling, or a soft tissue mass adjacent to the site of the skeletal lesion (1). Fever, an elevated sedimentation rate, and leukocytosis may also be present (42). If a vertebra is affected, the patient may present with neurologic symptoms (10) resulting from a collapse of the vertebral body (19,24).

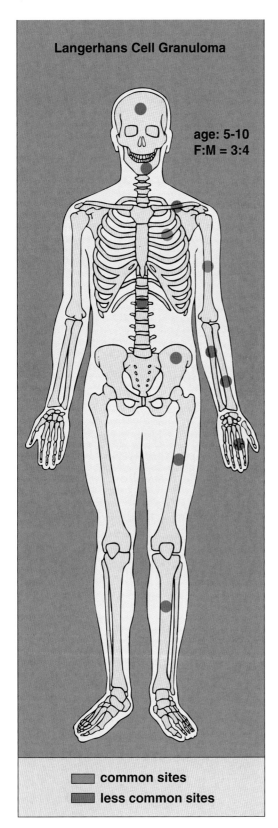

FIG. 1. Langerhans cell granuloma: skeletal sites of predilection, peak age range, and male-to-female ratio.

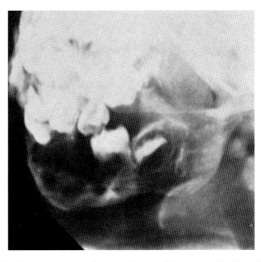

FIG. 2. Langerhans cell granuloma. A 3-year-old girl with extensive skeletal involvement had in addition a large destructive lesion in the mandible. Note the characteristic appearance of a floating tooth, which results from destruction of supportive alveolar bone.

Imaging

Plain radiography remains the most effective modality for the diagnosis of Langerhans cell granuloma. In the mandible, radiolucent lesions and "floating teeth" secondary to the destruction of the alveolar bone are characteristic (Fig. 2). In the skull, a beveled lytic lesion is typical (Fig. 3) (14). In the center of the lytic lesion there is sometimes a small sclerotic focus referred to as a button sequestrum (8) "cockade" image (in European literature) or "bull's eye" simulating an infectious process (10,27,42). In the spine, so-called vertebra plana (or coin-on-edge appearance) is a usual manifestation and results from a collapsed vertebral body (7) (Fig. 4). This finding was for a long time mistakenly considered an osteochondrosis of the vertebra and was (and in the European literature still is) named Calvé disease after its proposer.

In the long bones, Langerhans cell granuloma presents as a radiolucent destructive lesion, commonly associated with a lamellated periosteal reaction (Fig. 5) (16,17,43). This appearance may mimic that of a round cell malignant tumor, such as lymphoma or Ewing sarcoma. The lesion may have well-defined or poorly defined margins, with or without sclerotic borders (8). Occasionally, a cluster of partially overlapping lesions may be observed. In such instances, the superimposed areas of destruction have the appearance of a hole within a hole (36,37). A distinct and characteristic feature of many lesions is slanting or beveling of the edges (23). Sometimes the lesion is poorly demarcated and its indistinct borders gradually merge with the adjacent normal bone. The lesion may encroach on the endocortex, causing scalloping of the endosteal surface (Fig. 6). In later stages the lesion becomes more sclerotic, with dispersed radiolucencies (Fig. 7). The periosteal reaction is either absent or

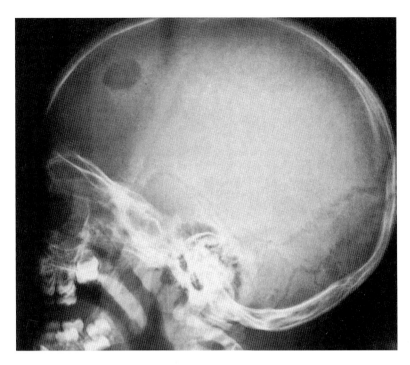

FIG. 3. Langerhans cell granuloma. Lateral radiograph of the skull of a 2½-year-old boy with disseminated process shows an osteolytic lesion in the frontal bone with a sharply outlined margin, giving it a punched-out appearance. Uneven involvement of the inner and outer tables results in its beveled presentation.

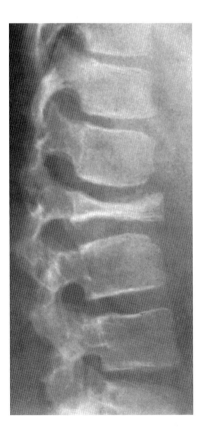

FIG. 4. Langerhans cell granuloma. Vertebra plana represents collapse of vertebral body secondary to destruction of bone by granulomatous lesion. Note the preservation of the intervertebral disk space.

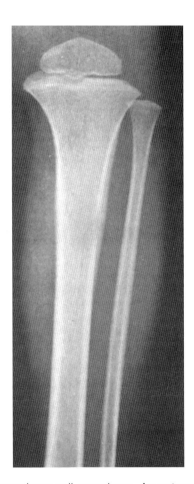

FIG. 5. Langerhans cell granuloma. An anteroposterior radiograph of the lower leg of a 4-year-old boy demonstrates a lesion in the diaphysis of the left tibia exhibiting a permeative type of bone destruction and a lamellated (onion-skin) type of periosteal reaction similar to that seen in osteomyelitis and Ewing sarcoma.

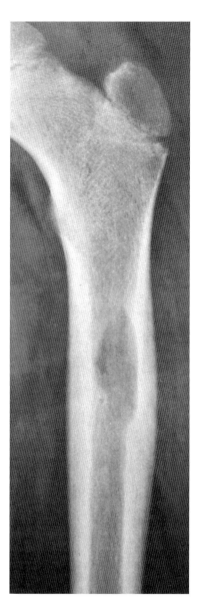

FIG. 6. Langerhans cell granuloma. An anteroposterior radiograph of the proximal femur of a 3-year-old boy with a limp and tenderness localized to the upper thigh shows an osteolytic lesion without sclerotic changes, causing scalloping of the lateral endocortex. There is fusiform thickening of the cortex and a solid uninterrupted type of periosteal reaction.

from Ewing sarcoma, which rarely has multiple foci (25,45). The study has its limitations, however, because approximately 35% of lesions show a normal uptake of the radiopharmaceutical tracer (22). Bone destruction may sometimes result in inadequate residual bone to produce uptake, and areas of photon deficiency are exhibited (2). Recent reports indicate the usefulness of thallium-201 scintigraphy, which proved to be positive in a lesion that exhibited photon deficiency on ^{99m}Tc-MDP scintigraphy (15).

Computed tomography (CT) may be useful if plain film radiography inadequately defines the extent of the process (34), particularly in cases of spine and pelvic involvement (21). This modality effectively demonstrates periosteal reaction, beveled edges, and reactive sclerosis (3).

There have been isolated reports of the usefulness of magnetic resonance imaging (MRI) in evaluating this condition (3). The MRI appearance varies and appears to correlate with the radiographic appearance (8). The MRI manifestations of Langerhans cell granuloma during the earlier stages are non-

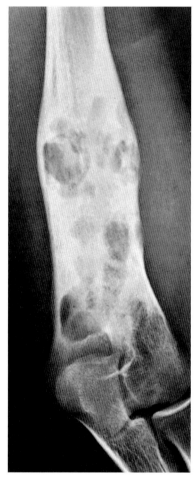

FIG. 7. Langerhans cell granuloma. The healing stage of the lesion, as seen here in the distal humerus of a 16-year-old girl, exhibits predominantly sclerotic changes with interspersed radiolucent foci, thickening of the cortex, and a well-organized periosteal reaction. In this stage, the lesion mimics chronic osteomyelitis.

more defined and appears nonaggressive. Vehlinger and later Mirra and Gold have distinguished three phases in the evolution of Langerhans cell granuloma: incipient, midphase, and late phase (33, 47). During the early phases the lesions tend to have aggressive patterns, with a lamellated periosteal reaction and poorly marginated or permeative lytic lesions. During the late phase the lesions tend to become more circumscribed (33).

The distribution of the lesion may be determined by radionuclide bone scan, which can aid in the detection of silent lesions and in differentiating Langerhans cell granuloma

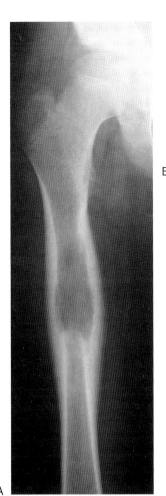
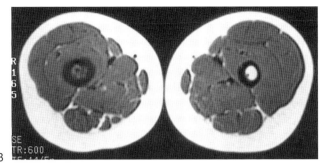
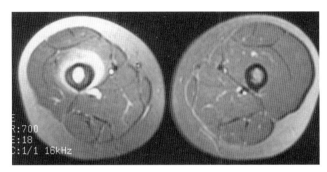
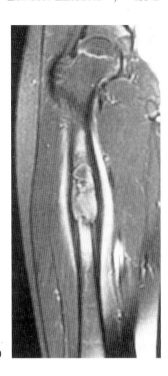

A

FIG. 5-8. Langerhans cell granuloma: magnetic resonance imaging. **A:** An anteroposterior radiograph of the right femur of a 13-year-old boy shows a radiolucent lesion in the proximal femoral diaphysis exhibiting a lamellated periosteal reaction. **B:** Axial T1-weighted (SE, TR 600, TE 14) MRI demonstrates the lesion to be of low signal intensity. The cortex is markedly thickened. **C:** Coronal T1-weighted (SE, TR 500, TE 15) MRI obtained after intravenous injection of gadolinium shows marked enhancement of the lesion and the soft tissues adjacent to the thickened femoral cortex. **D:** Axial T1-weighted (SE, TR 700, TE 18) MRI obtained after intravenous injection of gadolinium shows enhancement of both granuloma and perilesional edema.

specific and may simulate an aggressive lesion, such as osteomyelitis or Ewing sarcoma, and occasionally benign tumors, such as osteoid osteoma or chondroblastoma (3). After gadolinium-DTPA injection, the lesions show marked enhancement on T1-weighted images (11) (Fig. 8). Occasionally, MRI can demonstrate early bone marrow involvement in the absence of radiographic or scintigraphic abnormalities (26). In some studies on T1-weighted sequences, the lesions were isointense with adjacent structures (35,38). In the skull, lesions have been reported to show well-defined high-signal-intensity areas of marrow replacement on T2-weighted sequences. The most recent investigations have shown that the most common MRI appearance of Langerhans cell granuloma is that of a focal lesion, surrounded by an extensive, ill-defined signal from bone marrow and by soft tissue reaction with low signal intensity on T1-weighted images and high signal intensity on T2-weighted images, considered to represent bone marrow and soft tissue edema or the flare phenomenon (3, 17) (Fig. 9).

Histopathology

Histologically, Langerhans cell granuloma consists of agglomerates of more or less densely arranged large histiocytes

(Fig. 10). This pathognomonic cell was proved by electron microscopic observations to be identical to the Langerhans histiocyte seen in the skin (46,50). These cells are plump and pink, with a lightly granular cytoplasm. Their nuclei are translucent, ovoid, or kidney bean–shaped have distinct nuclear membranes; and may possess longitudinal grooves. Langerhans cells can be specifically identified in electron microscopy by the presence of racquet-shaped cytoplasmic organelles, known as Birbeck granules (4,46), also referred to as Langerhans cell granules or X granules (26). From Langerhans cells, giants cells are derived with five to seven nuclei. These cells react strongly with monoclonal antibodies Ia/HLA-DR and Leu M3 in frozen sections. Langerhans cells express a variety of surface antigens. The demonstration of S-100 protein by immunohistochemistry, identification of Birbeck granules by electron microscopy, and peanut agglutinin binding are the most useful markers for the Langerhans cells (20,23). Zones of necrosis are common. In older or multiple lesions, lipid-bearing foam cells can also be observed (44) (Fig. 11). Special stains can reveal abundant droplets of sudanophilic fat peripherally or in the middle of the giant cell cytoplasm (so-called Touton cells) (44). The granuloma develops during the first (incipient) phase (33,47).

During the second phase (midphase), more and more

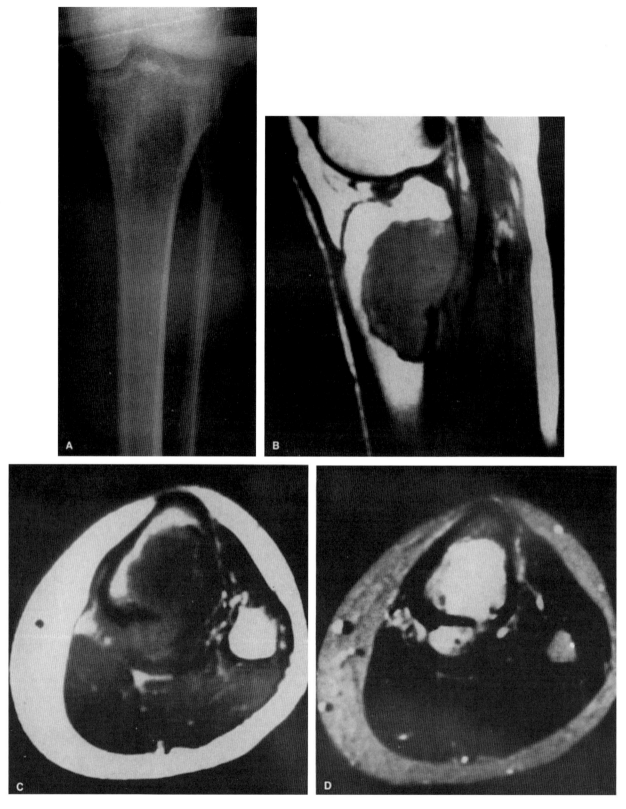

FIG. 9. Langerhans cell granuloma: magnetic resonance imaging. **A:** An anteroposterior radiograph of the left tibia of a 20-year-old woman shows an ill-defined osteolytic lesion in the proximal part of the bone. **B:** T1-weighted sagittal MRI shows a lobulated lesion exhibiting a low signal intensity. **C:** T1-weighted axial MRI shows that the lesion penetrated the posterior cortex and extended into the soft tissues. **D:** T2-weighted axial MRI shows high signal intensity of the lesion in and outside the tibia. In addition a high signal intensity soft tissue reaction surrounds the bone. (Reprinted with permission from Greenfield GB, Arrington JA. *Imaging of bone tumors: a multimodality approach.* Philadelphia: JB Lippincott, 1995;417.)

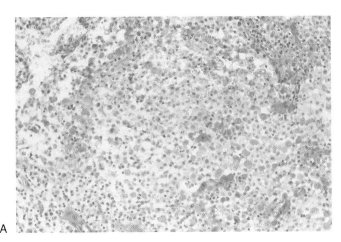 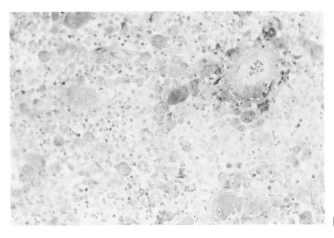

FIG. 10. Histopathology of Langerhans cell granuloma. **A:** Densely arranged large Langerhans cells are infiltrated by numerous eosinophilic granulocytes (hematoxylin and eosin, original magnification ×25). **B:** At higher magnification the complex structure of the granuloma formed of large pale histiocytes (Langerhans cells) and numerous roundish giant cells containing up to five nuclei (*upper half and right*) is clearly discernible. In addition, sparse lymphocytes are present (Giemsa, original magnification ×50).

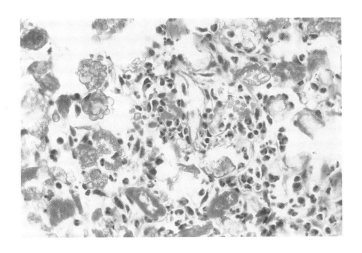

FIG. 11. Histopathology of Langerhans cell granuloma. Mulberry-like foam cells (*left and upper right*), eosinophilic granulocytes, and hyaline bodies prevail in this field of view (hematoxylin and eosin, original magnification ×50).

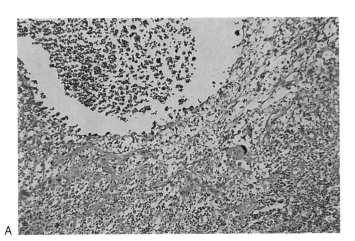 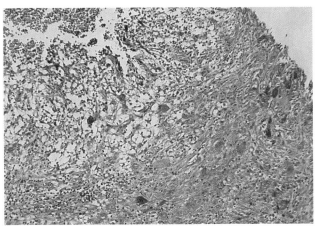

FIG. 12. Histopathology of Langerhans cell granuloma. **A:** In a later stage of development, nonspecific inflammatory cells, particularly lymphocytes, predominate. Some giant cells are also present. There is increased production of reticulin fibers (*lower half*) (Giemsa, original magnification ×25). **B:** In another field, fiber production is marked (*lower right*). Observe that numerous giant cells are still present and there is a dense accumulation of eosinophilic granulocytes (eosinophilic pseudoabscesses) (*upper left*) (Giemsa, original magnification ×25).

eosinophilic granulocytes containing lobulated nuclei and coarse eosinophilic granules infiltrate the granuloma, finally forming dense agglomerates, the so-called "eosinophilic pseudoabscesses" (Fig. 12). Sparse infiltrates of lymphocytes and plasma cells may be found, as well as giant cells and foci of hemorrhage. The phagocytic capacity of mononuclear and multinucleated histiocytic cells can be demonstrated by their ingestion of erythrocytes, eosinophils, and hemosiderin granules (23). The cytoplasm of the phagocytic cells often exhibits double-refractile neutral fat deposition (23). The eosinophilic granulocytes then progressively disappear. Some of these features are displayed to better advantage with methylene blue and Giemsa preparations. If the tissue of Langerhans cell granuloma has been overly decalcified, the eosinophilic cells become less readily identifiable. In areas where the eosinophilic leukocytes are undergoing fragmentation, proteinaceous crystalline structures, the so-called Charcot-Leyden crystals, are demonstrable (44).

In the third phase (late phase), fibroblasts, probably representing transformed histiocytes, produce collagen with concomitant reduction and final loss of histiocytes. The lesion then becomes indistinguishable from a focus of unspecific chronic fibroblastic osteomyelitis.

Differential Diagnosis

Radiology

The differential diagnosis depends on the site and extent of bony involvement, the phase of the disease, and the age of the patient (46). In a solitary lesion in long or flat bones, the main diagnostic considerations are *Ewing sarcoma* and *osteomyeli-*

tis (see Fig. 5). Both lesions may exhibit moth-eaten or permeative types of bone destruction and lamellated, onion-skin periosteal reaction. If a solitary lesion of Langerhans cell granuloma in a long tubular bone does not develop a periosteal reaction, a differential diagnosis of a *simple bone cyst* must be considered. However, the characteristic clinical features of Langerhans cell granuloma should always be taken into consideration: the so-called "tempo phenomenon" (23) is a useful sign, i.e., progression and disappearance of the bony lesion are very rapid. The differential diagnosis of a solitary skull lesion in a child or young adult should include *osteomyelitis, hemangioma,* and *fibrous dysplasia.* In an elderly patient, the considerations are the lytic phase of Paget disease (osteoporosis circumscripta), *myeloma,* and a metastasis. The beveled edge or double-contoured appearance of the lesion is always highly suggestive of Langerhans cell granuloma.

A lytic expansive lesion in the pelvis may mimic **f**ibrous *dysplasia, aneurysmal bone cyst, brown tumor of hyperparathyroidism,* or *hemophilic pseudotumor.* Disseminated osseous lesions must be distinguished from multifocal *osteomyelitis, leukemia, lymphoma, cystic angiomatosis,* fibrous dysplasia, brown tumors of hyperparathyroidism, and in older patients from *metastatic disease* and *multiple myeloma.*

Pathology

The major histologic differential diagnostic condition is infection because *osteomyelitis* is among the diseases capable of producing a polymorphous infiltrate of several inflammatory cell types. Moreover, there is an inflammatory reaction that simulates osteomyelitis, particularly during the

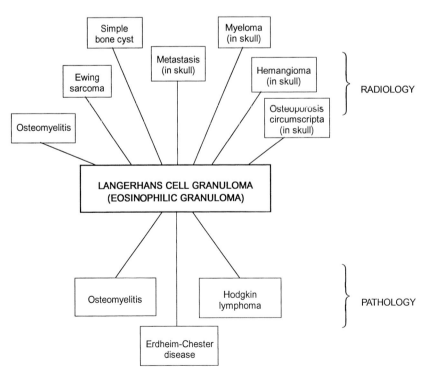

FIG. 13. Radiologic and pathologic differential diagnosis of Langerhans cell granuloma.

midphase of Langerhans cell granuloma, and it is therefore necessary to correlate histologic findings with the radiographic presentation before rendering a diagnosis. Furthermore, when histiocytes and eosinophils have disappeared in the late phase, chronic productive osteomyelitis cannot be differentiated by histologic means.

Another diagnostic consideration should be *Hodgkin lymphoma*, which can present as a solitary osseous defect with a mixed inflammatory infiltrate. The identification of Reed-Sternberg cells and the absence of Langerhans cells in the latter serve as positive diagnostic clues.

During the involutional stage of Langerhans cell granuloma, the eosinophils markedly diminish in number and disappear altogether as the lesion progresses (matures). The large mononucleated histiocytes may become lipid-laden in this stage. The presence of those foci of foam cells may lead to the mistaken diagnosis of the *Chester-Erdheim disease* (5,9).

The radiologic and pathologic differential diagnosis of Langerhans cell granuloma are depicted in Fig. 13.

MALIGNANT LESIONS

Round small-cell malignancies of bone form a heterogeneous group of neoplasms, distinguished from most other malignancies of bone by the fact that the tumors form a pure cellular growth without production of a tumor matrix (57). The common denominator is an undifferentiated, round cell, basophilic, cytoplasm-poor, stroma-poor, highly cellular tumor (95). These malignancies include primary bone tumors such as Ewing sarcoma, lymphoma, metastatic neuroblastoma, primitive neuroectodermal tumor, mesenchymal chondrosarcoma, myeloma, and some metastatic lesions (Table 1).

Ewing Sarcoma

Ewing sarcoma is considered to comprise a group of tumors, including conventional Ewing sarcoma, large-cell Ewing sarcoma, and primitive neuroectodermal tumor (PNET), that are closely related and often difficult to differentiate from each other.

Ewing sarcoma is the prototype of round, small-cell malignancies of bone. It is the sixth most common malignant tumor, comprising approximately 11% (91) to 12% (83) of all malignant tumors of bone, with a rather uniform histologic appearance. Conventional Ewing sarcoma is composed of densely packed small cells with round nuclei but without distinct cytoplasmic outlines (91). It exhibits no microscopic evidence of matrix production (64). Occasionally, similar tumors can arise as primary neoplasms of soft tissue. These are

TABLE 1. *Small round cell tumors of bone*

Tumor	Histopathologic features
Ewing sarcoma	Small, uniform sized cells with almost clear cytoplasm, round, slightly hyperchromatic nuclei. Cell borders indistinct.
Large-cell (atypical) Ewing sarcoma	Larger cells, with better delimited contours, more cytoplasm with eosinophilic "histiocytoid" appearance, nuclei may contain very prominent nucleoli; atypical variant merges into small-cell ES.
Primitive (peripheral) neuroectodermal (PNET) of bone	Similar to Ewing sarcoma. Focal Homer-Wright rosettes, often in tumor association with a fibrillary intercellular background. Reticulin fibers surrounding large groups of cells in a basket-like distribution.
Askin tumor of bone (thoracopulmonary of thoracospinal variant of PNET)	Similar to Ewing sarcoma. Focal of Homer-Wright rosettes. Compact sheets of cells with dark nuclei; nesting arrangement of cells with intervening fibrovascular stroma; serpiginous bands of cells with necrosis. May or may not display neural differentiation.
Malignant lymphoma	Aggregates of malignant lymphoid cells, typically mixture of small lymphocytic cells and large histiocytic cells. Cells are rounded, ovoid, and pleomorphic, displaying basophilic cytoplasm. Nuclei contain scanty chromatin, sometimes cleaved or horseshoe-shaped with prominent nucleoli.
Myeloma	Sheets of atypical plasmacytoid cells frequently bi- and trinucleated. Round nuclei possess dense, coarse chromatin with cartwheel-like distribution. Prominent nuclei eccentrically located in a strongly basophilic cytoplasm.
Small-cell osteosarcoma	Loose aggregations of small round cells with ovoid nuclei separated by collagenous bands of fine eosinophilic matrices. Occasional spindling of tumor cells. Focal production of osteoid or bone.
Mesenchymal chondrosarcoma	Small, round, uniform-sized cells with round or ovoid nuclei and scant cytoplasm, occasionally interspersed with spindle-shaped cells. Areas of well-differentiated cartilage containing foci of calcification.
Metastatic neuroblastoma	Very similar to PNET including Homer-Wright rosettes, a fibrillary intercellular background, long, thin tapering cytoplasmatic extensions creating appearance of a "pear" or "carrot" cells and higher degree of neural differentiation.
Metastatic primitive alveolar rhabdomyosarcoma	Similar to Ewing sarcoma. Alternating areas of cellularity and myxoid changes. Round or oval, occasionally spindled or tapered cells with scant eosinophilic cytoplasm.

Modified from Triche T., Cavazzana, A. Round cell tumors of bone. In: Unni KK, ed. *Bone tumors*, New York: Churchill Livingstone, 1988;199–223; from Meis-Kindblom JM, Stenman G, Kindblom L-G. Differential diagnosis of small round cell tumors. Seminars Diag Pathol 1996;13:213–214; and from Llombart-Bosch A, Contesso G, Peydro-Olaya A. Histology, immunohistochemistry, and electron microscopy of small round cell tumors of bone. Seminars Diag Pathol 1996;13:153–170.

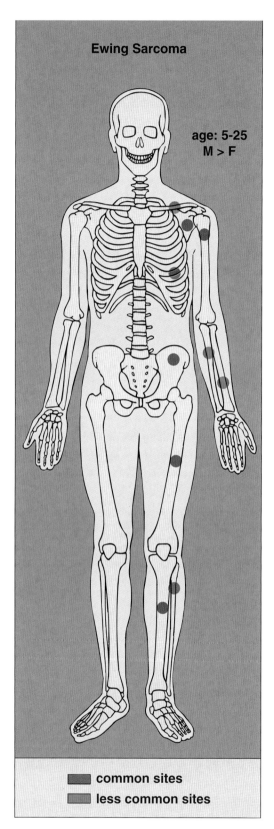

Ewing Sarcoma

age: 5-25
M > F

■ common sites
■ less common sites

FIG. 14. Ewing sarcoma: skeletal sites of predilection, peak age range, and male-to-female ratio.

referred to as extraskeletal or soft-tissue Ewing sarcomas (62). Even less commonly, Ewing sarcoma may exhibit periosteal location (51). There is also a rare form of Ewing sarcoma in which the cells are larger and more pleomorphic than those of conventional Ewing tumor. This form has been referred to as atypical Ewing sarcoma or large cell Ewing sarcoma (85). The clinical behavior and the prognosis in large-cell Ewing sarcoma appear similar to those of conventional tumor. Very rarely, Ewing sarcoma may be multifocal (55).

Clinical Presentation

Ewing sarcoma occurs primarily in young people, most commonly in the second decade. Approximately 90% of cases present before the age of 20 years, with a median age of about 13 years (86). The tumor has a decisively male predominance (3:2), and only exceptionally occurs in black individuals (91). Clinically, Ewing sarcoma may present as a localized, painful mass or with systemic symptoms such as fever, malaise, weight loss, leukocytosis, and increased erythrocyte sedimentation rate, a constellation of findings that may lead to an erroneous diagnosis of osteomyelitis. It has been speculated that the presence of systemic symptoms indicates dissemination of the tumor, with a consequently worsened prognosis (52). Diaphyses of the long bones (predominantly femur, tibia, and humerus), the ribs, and the flat bones, such as the scapula and the pelvis, are preferred sites (57,77) (Fig. 14). An epiphyseal location is rare (2%) (81, 91), and pathologic fractures are uncommon (64). Occasionally, Ewing sarcoma may metastasize to the other bones.

Imaging

In most cases, the radiographic presentation of Ewing sarcoma is quite characteristic. It consists of an ill-defined lesion with a permeative or moth-eaten pattern of bone destruction associated with a lamellated periosteal new bone formation that has an onion skin (or "onion peel") or, less commonly, a "sunburst" ("trimmed whiskers" effect) appearance (67), and a large soft tissue mass (Fig. 15). Ewing sarcoma occasionally presents as a large area of geographic bone destruction simulating any other type of bone sarcoma. At times the lesion in the bone is almost imperceptible, and the only prominent finding is a soft tissue mass (Fig. 16). The lesion sometimes creates a typical "saucerization" of the cortex, a feature once believed to be virtually pathognomonic for this tumor (Fig. 17). The saucerization may be related to the combination of destruction of the periosteal surface of bone by the tumor and an associated extrinsic pressure effect of the large soft tissue mass (87). This sign has recently been reported in other tumors and even in osteomyelitis. However, the presence of saucerization associated with a permeative lesion and a soft tissue mass favors the diagnosis of Ewing sarcoma. When the lesion exhibits a permeative appearance, it may be indistinguishable from osteomyelitis (Fig. 18). Because Ewing sarcoma does not pro-

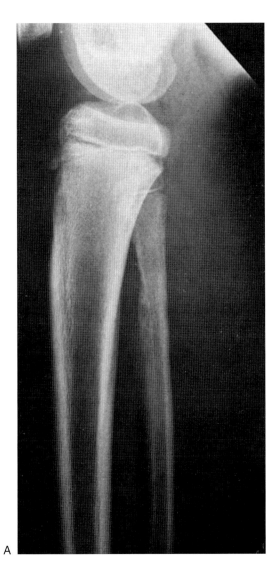

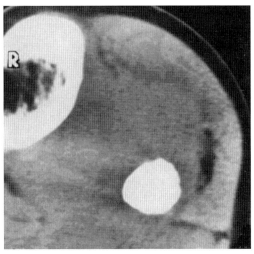

FIG. 15. Ewing sarcoma. **A:** A lateral radiograph of a 12-year-old boy shows the typical appearance of this malignancy in the diaphysis of the fibula. The poorly defined lesion exhibits a permeative bone destruction associated with an aggressive periosteal reaction. **B:** CT section through the tumor demonstrates a large soft tissue mass, not well depicted on the routine study. Note the complete obliteration of the marrow cavity by tumor.

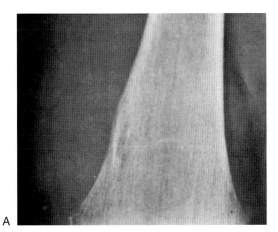

FIG. 16. Ewing sarcoma. **A:** Bone destruction is almost imperceptible on this magnification study of the distal femoral diaphysis of a 10-year-old girl. *Continued on page 258.*

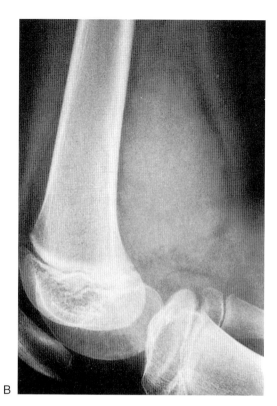

B

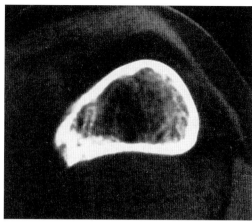

C

FIG. 16. *Continued.* **B:** Lateral radiograph of the distal femur, however, shows a large soft tissue mass. **C:** CT using a bone window demonstrates destruction of the medullary portion of the bone and invasion of the cortex.

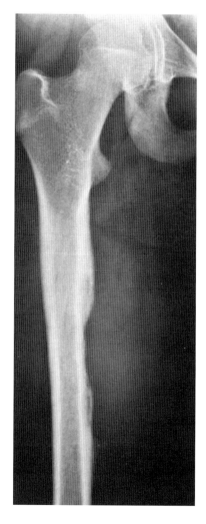

FIG. 17. Ewing sarcoma. An anteroposterior radiograph of the right femur of a 12-year-old girl shows saucerization of the medial cortex of the diaphysis, often seen in Ewing sarcoma.

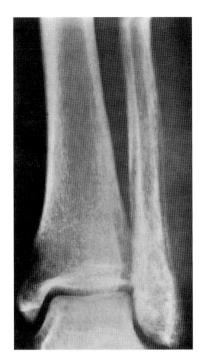

FIG. 18. Ewing sarcoma: differential diagnosis. A 24-year-old man presented with pain and swelling of the left ankle for eight weeks; he also had a fever. An anteroposterior radiograph of the ankle demonstrates a lesion of the distal fibula exhibiting a permeative type of bone destruction and a lamellated periosteal reaction. A soft tissue mass is also evident. The appearance is that of infection (osteomyelitis), but biopsy revealed Ewing sarcoma.

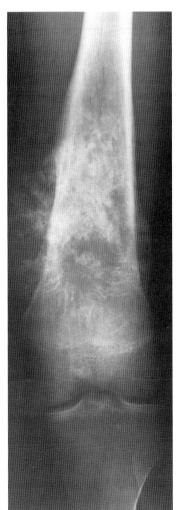

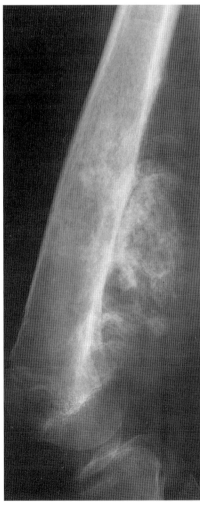

A

B

FIG. 19. Ewing sarcoma: differential diagnosis. (**A**) Anteroposterior and (**B**) lateral radiographs of the left femur of a 17-year-old boy, displaying a significant sclerosis of the tumor, that was originally interpreted as osteosarcoma.

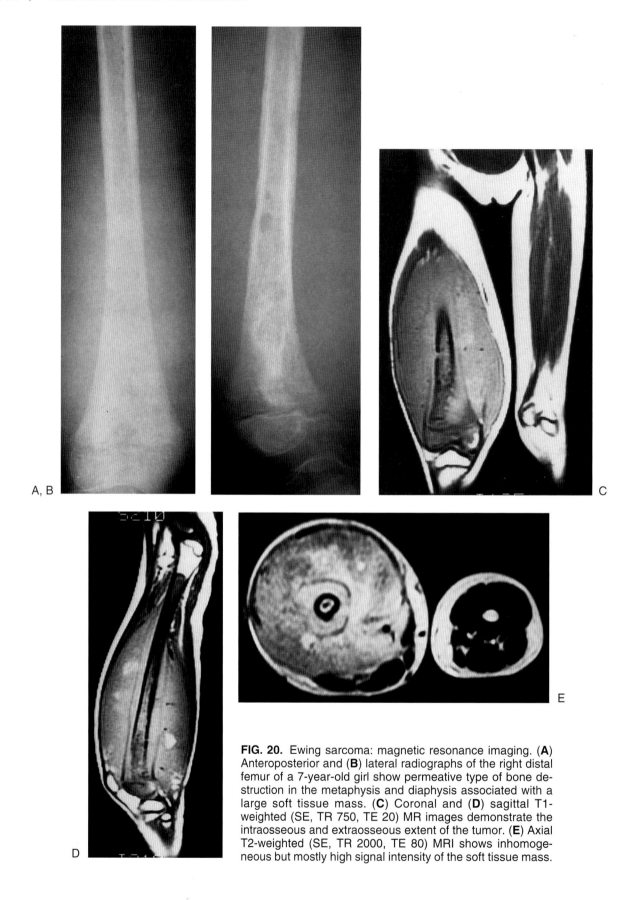

FIG. 20. Ewing sarcoma: magnetic resonance imaging. (**A**) Anteroposterior and (**B**) lateral radiographs of the right distal femur of a 7-year-old girl show permeative type of bone destruction in the metaphysis and diaphysis associated with a large soft tissue mass. (**C**) Coronal and (**D**) sagittal T1-weighted (SE, TR 750, TE 20) MR images demonstrate the intraosseous and extraosseous extent of the tumor. (**E**) Axial T2-weighted (SE, TR 2000, TE 80) MRI shows inhomogeneous but mostly high signal intensity of the soft tissue mass.

duce a matrix material, radiography reveals a lack of mineralization in the substance of the tumor. However, because there is often an abundant periosteal new bone formation, particularly in the flat bones, this appearance may mimic osteosarcoma, and differentiation between the two tumor types may be difficult (Fig. 19). Approximately one third of the cases affecting flat bones demonstrate a diffuse sclerosis. Unlike osteosarcoma, this sclerosis represents not a tumor bone but rather reactive bone to the tumor cell infiltration (92).

On radionuclide bone scan, Ewing sarcoma shows a very intense increase of technetium-99m methylene diphosphonate (^{99m}Tc-MDP) accumulation (84). Gallium-67-citrate (^{67}Ga-citrate) more readily identifies soft tissue tumor extension (61,63). Although scintigraphic findings are nonspecific, this technique provides reliable information concerning the presence of skeletal metastases (74,83).

CT reveals the pattern of bone destruction, and attenuation values (Hounsfield units) provide information about the medullary extension (61). In addition, CT may help to delineate extraosseous involvement (98) (see Fig. 15B).

MRI is essential for definite demonstration of the extent of intraosseous and extraosseous involvement by this tumor (Fig. 20) (53,99). In particular, MRI may effectively reveal extension through the epiphyseal plate (66). T1-weighted images show intermediate to low signal intensity, which becomes bright on T2 weighting. Hypocellular regions and areas of necrosis are of lesser intensity (61). Imaging after injection of gadolinium (Gd-DTPA) reveals signal enhancement of the tumor on T1-weighted sequences (66). Enhancement occurs only in the cellular areas, allowing differentiation of the tumor from the peritumoral edema.

Histopathology

The gross appearance of Ewing sarcoma may be misleading (101). Because the lesion does not produce any matrix,

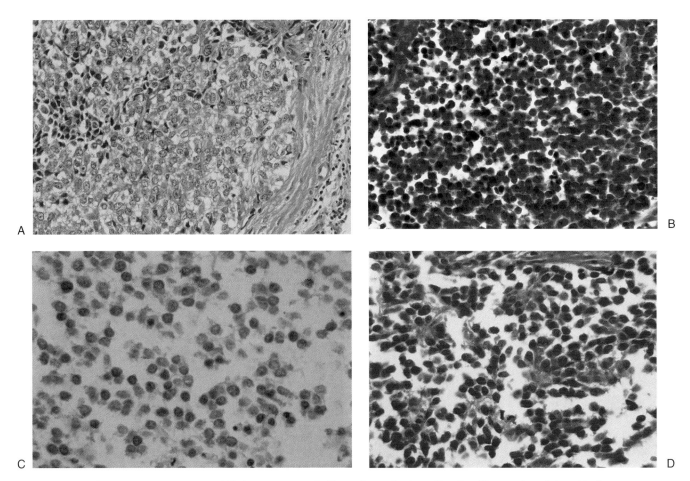

FIG. 21. Histopathology of Ewing sarcoma. **A:** Densely packed small cells with round nuclei and indistinct cell borders are characteristic for this tumor. To the right a prominent septum composed of fibrous connective tissue is visible (hematoxylin and eosin, original magnification ×50). **B:** At high magnification the uniform aspect of the round nuclei without clear cytoplasmic outlines is striking (hematoxylin and eosin, original magnification ×100). **C:** With Giemsa staining the cytoplasm is more distinct. The nuclei are darkly and homogeneously stained (Giemsa, original magnification ×100). **D:** With alcohol fixation, in this case there was better preservation of cell details (hematoxylin and eosin, original magnification ×100).

its appearance can range from a soft and fleshy but solid mass to an almost liquid consistency. When a tumor of the latter consistency is cut into at the time of surgery, it may actually run like pus. This can lead to a mistaken diagnosis of osteomyelitis, and the material may be sent for microbiologic culture rather than histopathologic examination, thus causing a delay in diagnosis (52).

The microscopic appearance of Ewing sarcoma is typical. At lower magnification, the tumor consists of small, uniform-sized cells characterized by an almost clear cytoplasm and nuclei that are round and slightly hyperchromatic. Prominent septa composed of fibrous connective tissue divide the tumor tissue into strands or lobules (91) (Fig. 21A). Because the cell borders are indistinct, it sometimes appears as if the tumor is composed of many nuclei floating in a sea of cytoplasm rather than being separated into discrete cells. The nucleoli are usually inconspicuous. Areas of necrosis and hemorrhage are often observed. At higher magnification, the nuclei appear round and uniform (Fig. 21B). Sometimes the cytoplasm contains a moderate amount of glycogen that can be demonstrated by periodic acid-Schiff (PAS) staining (Fig. 22) or, more specifically, with Best carmine stain. Mitotic figures are uncommon in classical Ewing sarcoma (91). Although no extracellular matrix is found between the tumor cells, reactive new bone formation may be observed, especially at the periphery. This reactive bone is sometimes difficult to distinguish from tumor bone formation, and small-cell osteosarcoma may therefore be erroneously diagnosed.

In extremely rare cases, Ewing sarcoma exhibits an epithelial differentiation (60,69,82,93). Other primary tumors of bone known to have epithelial features are adamantinoma of long bones (56), malignant fibrous histiocytoma (100), and osteosarcoma (58,76).

Electron microscopy of this lesion reveals highly characteristic ultrastructural features. The predominant or principal cell type is polygonal. The cytoplasm exhibits few organelles, with sparse rough endoplasm reticulum, and few mitochondria. However, a conspicuous Golgi complex is often present. The nuclei of these cells are round or oval. Typically, the chromatin is fine and evenly distributed, and there are single or multiple small nucleoli. The cytoplasm may contain many glycogen granules. In addition to the principal cell, there may be a small number of so-called dark cells (reflecting a darker cytoplasm) (91). It is still undetermined whether this cell is a precursor or a terminal form of the principal cell.

Differential Diagnosis

Radiology

On plain radiography, the most important differential consideration is to distinguish Ewing sarcoma from *osteomyelitis* and *Langerhans cell granuloma* because both of these entities may present with a similar aggressive moth-eaten or permeative pattern of bone destruction (see Fig. 18). It is not uncommon for all three conditions to appear identical. The clinical information, e.g., duration of the patient's symptoms, aids in radiographic differential diagnosis. In Langerhans cell granuloma, for example, the amount of bone destruction seen on radiography after 1 week of symptoms is usually the same as that seen after 4 to 6 weeks of symptoms in osteomyelitis and after 3 to 4 months in Ewing sarcoma (70). The other look-alike lesion to be distinguished is osteosarcoma. The latter tumor is usually metaphyseal in location (as opposed to the mostly diaphyseal location of Ewing sarcoma), more commonly than Ewing sarcoma exhibits sunburst and Codman triangle types of periosteal reaction, and displays (except for purely lytic lesions, such as telangiectatic or fibroblastic variants) bone formation within destructive lesions in the bone and within a soft tissue mass. It

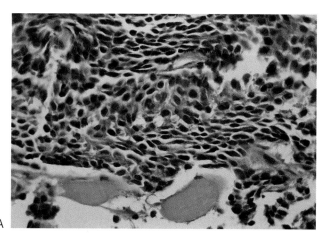 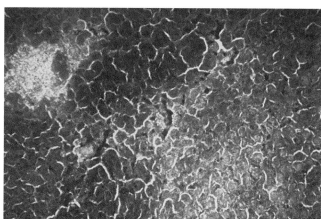

A   B

FIG. 22. Histopathology of Ewing sarcoma: periodic acid-Schiff (PAS) staining. **A:** Densely packed small cells with dark round nuclei infiltrate the muscle (*bottom*). The cells are somewhat artificially deformed. No glycogen has been preserved in the cells because of formaldehyde fixation (PAS, original magnification ×100). **B:** Fixed in ethanol, the glycogen granules in the cytoplasm of the tumor cells were stained red with PAS method (PAS, original magnification ×100).

should be stressed, however, that Ewing sarcoma may occasionally exhibit reactive sclerotic changes, thus mimicking bone-forming tumors (see Fig. 19).

Lymphoma must also be included in the differential diagnosis, although this lesion usually occurs in older age groups. The important radiologic difference is usually the absence of a soft-tissue mass in lymphoma, whereas in Ewing sarcoma a soft-tissue mass is almost invariably present, often being disproportionally large compared with the amount of bone destruction. The distinction between Ewing sarcoma and *primitive neuroectodermal tumor* (PNET) cannot be made on the basis of radiography (89,71), and differentiation between these two lesions must rely entirely on histologic examination (83). *Metastatic neuroblastoma,* which has a similar appearance on radiography and simulates Ewing sarcoma, invariably affects patients younger than 5 years of age.

Pathology

Differential diagnosis of so-called blue, round small-cell tumors by histopathologic examination is usually not possible without the use of additional methods, particularly immunohistochemistry and electron microscopy (83,87). For routine histologic diagnosis of these tumors, immunohistochemistry is now replacing electron microscopy (Table 2). Distinction between Ewing sarcoma, large-cell Ewing sarcoma, PNET, and other round small-cell tumors is now possible with a fair degree of accuracy (59,73). In immunohistochemistry, the markers HBA-71 and HNK-1 appear to be highly characteristic for the Ewing sarcoma group (Fig. 23). Recently, a marker termed MABO-13, which recognizes a product of the MIC-2 gene, was suggested to be specific for Ewing sarcoma and PNET (97,135). The absence of neuron-specific enolase (NSE) excludes PNET and other neuroectodermal tumors. On the other hand, the presence of NSE and

the electron microscopic finding of neuroendocrine granules are positive signs for PNET and other tumors of neuroectodermal origin (72). An additional distinguishing feature is the fact that in most cases the cytoplasm of Ewing sarcoma cells stains positively for glycogen, provided that the tumor tissue has been fixed in ethanol to prevent washing out of glycogen by aqueous solvents (see Fig. 22B). Schajowicz pointed out that PAS staining and Best carmine stain are positive in Ewing sarcoma but negative in most other round cell tumors (91). A specific proof for the presence of glycogen is the treatment of the slides with diastase washing out the glycogen by digestion.

On histologic examination, Ewing sarcoma should be differentiated from malignant *lymphoma.* In the latter tumor, the nuclei are larger and less uniform than those in Ewing sarcoma, with distinct indentations and lobulations. The tumor cells are positive for leukocyte common antigens (LCAs). A more or less dense net of reticulin fibers usually surrounds the cells. This is in contrast to Ewing sarcoma, in which the fibers are usually limited to the septa of fibrous tissue. As mentioned above, an additional distinguishing feature is the fact that the cytoplasm of the cell in Ewing sarcoma usually stains positively for glycogen. Schajowicz pointed out that PAS staining is positive in Ewing sarcoma but negative in malignant lymphoma (90). Immunoperoxidase reactions are seldom helpful in a positive manner because the only constant feature is the immunohistochemical reaction with antivimentin (78–80,95,96). A small number of Ewing sarcomas have been reported to stain with antikeratin (68). On the other hand, a negative reaction for LCA and neural protein antibodies is useful because these tests help to rule out lymphoma and PNET. Typical Ewing sarcoma cells are negative for LCA, surface immunoglobulins, lysosome, α_1-antitrypsin, α_1-anti-chymotrypsin, myosin, myoglobin, desmin, and factor VIII–related antigen (65,94).

The demonstration of glycogen, which formerly was con-

TABLE 2. *Small round cell tumors of bone and typical immunocytochemistry results*

Tumor	Keratin	Vimentin	Desmin	Neurofilament	HBA-71B (Mic 2)	Leu7 (CD 57)	NSE	LCA (CD 45)	κ or λ light chains
Ewing sarcoma	+/ᵃ	+	−	−/*	+	(+)	−	−	−
Primative neuroectodermal tumor of bone	−	+	−	(+)	+	(+)	+	−	−
Askin tumor	−	+	−	(+)	+	(+)	+	−	−
Malignant lymphoma	−	+	−	−	−	(+)	−	+	+/−
Myeloma	−	−/+	−	−	−	−	−	−/+	+
Small cell osteosarcoma	−	+	−	−	−	−	−	−	−
Mesenchymal chondrosarcoma	−	+	−	−	−	−	−	−	−
Metastatic neuroblastoma	−	−	−	+	−	(+)	+	−	−
Rhabdomyosarcoma	−	(+)	+	−	−	−	(+)	−	−
Synovial sarcoma	+	+	−	−	−	−	−	−	−

ᵃ Positive in single cases.
(+) Weak reaction.
Modified from Triche T, Cavazzana A. Round cell tumors of bone. In: Unni KK, ed. *Bone tumors.* New York: Churchill Livingstone, 1988;199–223.

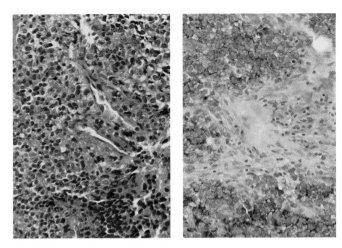

FIG. 23. Histopathology of Ewing sarcoma: immunohistochemistry. On the left the tumor shows typical small cells with dark, round nuclei (hematoxylin and eosin, original magnification ×50). On the right immunohistochemical reaction with HBA-71 marker is positive, confirming Ewing sarcoma (original magnification ×50).

sidered an absolutely distinctive marker for Ewing sarcoma (90), has fallen into disfavor because glycogen cannot be demonstrated in all cases of Ewing sarcoma. Moreover, malignant lymphoma, small cell osteosarcoma, rhabdomyosarcoma, and PNETs may sometimes contain glycogen (75,94). Since the advent of immunohistochemistry, lymphomas can usually be distinguished from Ewing sarcomas by the demonstration of LCA.

Neural tumors, unlike Ewing sarcoma, are marked by a positive reaction for NSE (Fig. 24) and are positive for neural filament proteins, and electron microscopy may demonstrate the presence of neurosecretory granules in tumors of neural origin. However, recent immunocytochemical analyses have suggested that Ewing sarcoma cells are derived from primitive pluripotential cells capable of differentiating into cells with mesenchymal, epithelial, and even neural features (82). Moreover, tissue culture studies of five Ewing

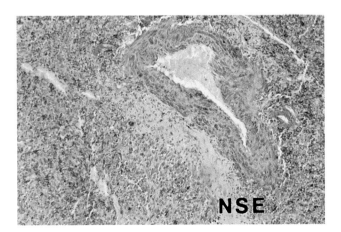

FIG. 24. Histopathology of Ewing sarcoma: immunohistochemistry. The absence of neuron-specific enolase in this preparation from Ewing sarcoma excludes neuroectodermal tumor (NSE marker, original magnification ×100).

sarcoma cell lines treated with cyclic adenosine monophosphate or phorbol-12-myristate-13-acetate showed that these treatments induced marked neural differentiation (54). These investigations led to the opinion that Ewing sarcoma may in fact be regarded as the most primitive form of a group of neural tumors that affect bone (see above).

In addition to malignant lymphoma, the differential diagnosis of Ewing sarcoma includes other small round cell malignancies, such as metastatic *neuroblastoma* and peripheral or *primitive neuroectodermal tumor* (PNET) (95,96). However, neuroblastomas usually occur in the first 3 years of life, whereas Ewing sarcoma is uncommon in patients younger than 5 years of age. Furthermore, most neuroblastomas are characterized by a neural filamentous material that is absent in Ewing sarcoma, and the former malignancy reveals elevated levels of urinary catecholamines. Among the light microscopic clues are the presence of Homer-Wright rosettes, a fibrillary intercellular background, and the tapering cytoplasmic processes that are present in metastatic neuroblastoma (64). On immunohistochemistry, neuroblastoma cells display a strong reaction for NSE, neurofilaments, synaptophysin, vimentin, and Leu7 (64). PNET, a relatively recent concept, suggests a primary small cell malignancy in bone or soft tissues that is related to the nervous system. Classically, NSE is positive in PNET. A diagnosis of PNET can be suspected if the tumor has a lobulated arrangement on low magnification and the tumor cells are arranged in a rosette fashion. A fibrillary background can usually be found in the center of the rosettes. However, these fibrils are not as clear-cut as those observed in classical metastatic neuroblastoma. Whether or not PNET forms a distinct small-cell malignancy of bone is still a matter of controversy. It appears that the NSE reaction may be positive in cases that are otherwise typical of Ewing sarcoma. Furthermore, the genetic abnormality associated with classical Ewing sarcoma, i.e., a translocation between chromo-

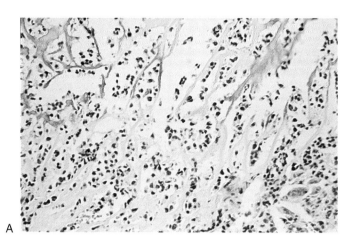
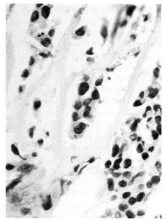
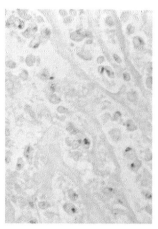

A   B

FIG. 25. Differential diagnosis of Ewing sarcoma: small-cell osteosarcoma. **A:** Loosely arranged tumor cells with hyperchromatic nuclei and some inconspicuous needle-like osteoid particles (*upper left and right*) make recognition of bone-forming tumor difficult (hematoxylin and eosin, original magnification ×50). **B:** On the left at higher magnification, the pleomorphism of the dark nuclei and the narrow cytoplasm seams betray the malignancy of the cells (hematoxylin and eosin, original magnification ×100). On the right, with reaction for osteonectin, most cells show a more or less distinct positivity (ochreous yellow) pointing to their malignant osteoblastic character (osteonectin, original magnification ×100). (Courtesy of Prof. Klaus Remberger, University of Saarland, Germany.)

somes 11 and 22, is also present in PNET. Some investigators believe that Ewing sarcoma is a neurally derived small cell malignancy and that PNET is a more differentiated form of Ewing sarcoma. Moreover, it appears that the management of Ewing sarcoma and PNET is the same.

Ewing sarcoma must also be differentiated from *Langerhans cell granuloma* and *osteomyelitis.* The former shows large, fairly clear cells of histiocytic origin arranged in granuloma form, the so-called Langerhans cells, which in immunohistochemistry react strongly with S-100 protein, and by electron microscopy exhibit the tennis racket-shaped, so-called Birbeck granules, which are specific. Furthermore, the Langerhans cells form various numbers of giant cells usually with up to five nuclei and with a typical roundish shape. The granuloma is infiltrated by small numbers of lymphocytes, plasma cells, and polymorphonuclear leukocytes. Only in the phase of maximal development of the granuloma are eosinophilic granulocytes present in large numbers, sometimes forming so-called eosinophilic (pseudo-) abscesses. The variegated histologic picture in contrast to the monomorphic tumor cells of Ewing sarcoma and the positivity of the granuloma cells for S-100 protein make the distinction easy.

In chronic osteomyelitis with a preponderance of plasma cells or of lymphocytes, there may be the chance of mistaking it for Ewing sarcoma. Again, the variegated histologic picture, with granulocytes and the possibility of demonstrating LCA positivity, should allow distinction.

Other entities to be differentiated from Ewing sarcoma are *small-cell osteosarcoma* and *mesenchymal chondrosarcoma.* The distinguishing feature of small-cell osteosarcoma is the presence of foci of osteoid (Fig. 25; **see also Fig. 2-71**). Furthermore, the positive markers for Ewing sarcoma should

help to differentiate the two entities. Mesenchymal chondrosarcoma is characterized by foci of cartilaginous matrix, although they may be scarce. In such instances, positivity for S-100 protein and negativity for the Ewing sarcoma markers is crucial.

Undifferentiated round cell areas of *synovial sarcoma* might also be mistaken for Ewing sarcoma, and because positivity for epithelial markers in the former is rarely present, this method is of no help in the differentiation. In *neuroblastoma,* the tumor cells usually have more cytoplasm and are often arranged in rosettes (83). Again, NSE is positive in this tumor, in contrast to Ewing sarcoma.

It is very possible for the large-cell variant of Ewing sarcoma to be mistaken for *large-cell lymphoma.* The presence of intracellular glycogen and the lack of reticulin fibers, except for those in the septa in Ewing sarcoma, the demonstration of LCA in lymphoma by immunohistochemistry, and the ultrastructural differences among the tumors mentioned above should help in making a secure diagnosis of Ewing sarcoma (64). The same is true for a *metastasis of seminoma,* which, only on the basis of histologic staining with hematoxylin and eosin (H&E), may be difficult to differentiate.

The radiologic and pathologic differential diagnosis of Ewing sarcoma is depicted in Fig. 26.

Malignant Lymphoma

The term malignant lymphoma refers to a group of neoplasms that are composed of lymphoid or histiocytic cells of different subtypes in various stages of maturation (83). Primary lymphoma of bone is very uncommon (119). Dahlin and Unni (57) have reported a prevalence of 7.2% for malignant lymphoma of bone (primary and secondary) in their se-

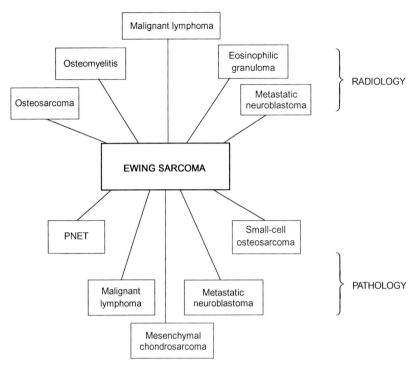

FIG. 26. Radiologic and pathologic differential diagnoses of Ewing sarcoma.

ries of 8542 primary malignant bone tumors, with only 3.1% of cases representing osseous involvement.

Lymphomas are subdivided into non-Hodgkin lymphoma and Hodgkin lymphoma. Although involvement of bones is relatively common in Hodgkin lymphoma (skeletal involvement is present in approximately 13% of patients who have Hodgkin disease), primary Hodgkin disease of bone is extremely rare (122). Similarly, a non-Hodgkin lymphoma may present as a primary bone neoplasm or may be part of a disseminated tumor process. A rare form of lymphoma seen predominantly in children in tropical Africa is known as Burkitt lymphoma. In this type of lymphoma involvement of the facial bones is particularly characteristic (137). Lesions affecting long tubular bones and flat bones are less common.

Non-Hodgkin Lymphoma

Primary lymphoma of bone is a rare tumor (comprising 3% to 4% of all malignant bone tumors). This lesion was formerly termed reticulum cell sarcoma or lymphosarcoma (103). Lymphomas are considered primary in bone only when a complete systemic workup reveals no evidence of extraosseous involvement. Moreover, some authorities consider that no evidence of extraosseous or nodal disease must be present for at least 6 months after the discovery of the osseous focus for lymphoma to be considered primary in the bone. It must be pointed out that the skeletal system may be secondarily involved in about 30% of malignant lymphomas

(111). Non-Hodgkin lymphomas encompass a heterogeneous spectrum of neoplasms that vary in their clinical and radiologic manifestations. The vast majority are large cell lymphomas (136). The classic reticulum cell sarcoma is a large cell lymphoma of B-cell origin (139).

Clinical Presentation

This malignancy occurs in the second to seventh decades, usually involving young and older adults, with a peak incidence between the ages of 35 and 45 years. As a whole, the patient population is distinctly older than the population with Ewing sarcoma, and there is a decisively male predominance, with a reported ratio ranging from 1.5:1, to 2:1, to 3:2 (23,57). Patients may present with local symptoms, such as pain and swelling, or with systemic symptoms, such as fever and weight loss, although some patients may be asymptomatic. The sites of predilection are the long bones (femur, tibia), the pelvis, the ribs, and the vertebrae (Fig. 27). Pathologic fractures are observed in approximately 25% of cases (57). Neurologic symptoms may be present in lesions localized in the vertebrae.

Imaging

The roentgenographic appearance of malignant lymphoma can vary widely (104). Lymphoma tends to involve a large portion of the affected bone and is usually localized

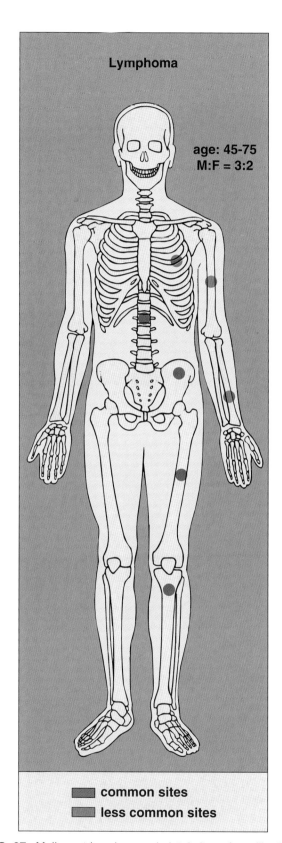

Lymphoma

age: 45-75
M:F = 3:2

common sites
less common sites

FIG. 27. Malignant lymphoma: skeletal sites of predilection, peak age range, and male-to-female ratio.

in the shaft. The lesion may be marked by a large area of geographic, lytic bone destruction (Fig. 28A) may exhibit a moth-eaten pattern (Fig. 28B) or may have a very subtle permeative pattern involving the medullary canal (Fig. 28C). In the latter case, plain radiographs may appear almost normal (17) (Fig. 29). As a rule, lymphoma rarely evokes any periosteal new bone formation and soft tissue mass, in distinct contrast to the presentation of Ewing sarcoma (116). A mixed pattern associated with a periosteal reaction may sometimes be observed. This lesion may also have an ivory bone appearance, a picture commonly seen in vertebrae (Fig. 30) or flat bones, although this presentation is not as common as in Hodgkin lymphoma. The radionuclide bone scan is usually positive (123,133), and the combination of a normal plain radiograph and positive scintigraphy should suggest the possibility of malignant lymphoma (52).

CT can reveal bone destruction and soft tissue involvement, often associated with osseous changes (114,125) (Figs. 31 and 32). It also can detect bony sequestra, which are estimated to occur in 11% of primary lymphomas of bone (129) (Fig. 33).

MRI may also be helpful in demonstrating the involvement of the bone marrow (110,112,138,140,170). On T1-weighted images, diffuse infiltration presents as an area of low signal intensity. On T2-weighted images, the affected areas are hyperintense compared with muscle but isointense compared with fat (118,130,132). On STIR images, with suppression of the normally bright marrow fat, the foci of lymphomatous infiltration exhibit a high signal intensity (117,141).

Histopathology

Malignant lymphoma of bone appears grossly similar to a lymphoma elsewhere in the body (e.g., in lymph nodes). Both lesions are soft and fleshy. Areas of necrosis are occasionally observed (134).

From the histologic standpoint, the appearance of lymphoma is also diverse (128). The lesion consists of aggregates of malignant lymphoid cells that fill the marrow spaces and induce resorption of cancellous bone trabeculae (Fig. 34). A diffuse growth pattern is invariably observed, typically exhibiting a mixture of small lymphocytic cells and a larger histiocytic component (57,64). The cells of this tumor are usually rounded, ovoid, and pleomorphic. The cytoplasm is basophilic and exhibits well-defined outlines (109). Unlike the case in Ewing sarcoma, the nuclei are rather large, contain relatively scanty chromatin, and are sometimes indented (cleaved) or horseshoe-shaped, with prominent nucleoli (Fig. 35). Cytoplasmatic glycogen is usually lacking, and reticulin fibers are usually present, forming a more or less uniformly distributed net around the tumor cells (91) (Fig. 36). A fibroblastic component is often prominent in intraosseous lymphomas and is sometimes associated with

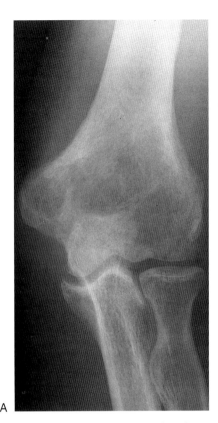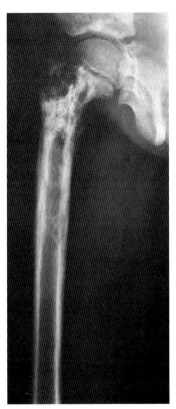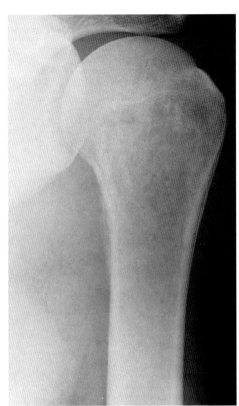

A   B, C

FIG. 28. Malignant lymphoma. **A:** An anteroposterior radiograph of the left elbow of a 42-year-old man shows a large osteolytic lesion in the distal humerus. **B:** An anteroposterior radiograph of the right femur of a 7-year-old girl who presented with pain in the upper thigh and a fever reveals a destructive lesion of the diaphysis extending to the growth plate. There is also a subtle lamellated periosteal reaction. **C:** An anteroposterior radiograph of the left shoulder in a 30-year-old man shows a permeative pattern of bone destruction in the proximal humerus accompanied by a lamellated periosteal reaction.

spindling of the neoplastic lymphoid cells (64). Non-Hodgkin lymphomas are made up of histiocytes or B or T lymphocytes. True histiocytic lymphoma is rare. Most lymphomas are composed of different subtypes of lymphoid cells that have been arrested at various stages of differentiation (83). Depending on the type of lymphoma, the infiltrate may be monomorphic or polymorphic. However, even in the polymorphic variant, the cells have a malignant rather than an inflammatory character. Mixed B-cell lymphomas and especially T-cell lymphomas tend to exhibit the largest admixture of cell types. In addition, T-cell lymphomas tend to be infiltrated by eosinophils (57). Electron microscopic studies may be helpful in distinguishing malignant lymphoma from Ewing sarcoma (65,88). The additional histologic differential diagnosis includes metastatic neuroblastoma and other small round cell tumors involving bone. Although the patient's age and the overall morphologic features usually are sufficient to categorize the tumor, the most important single procedure to distinguish lymphoma from all other major round cell tumors, as already mentioned, is the immunoreaction for LCA because lymphoid cells are the only cells that show positivity. Most lymphomas in bone present with large cells or a mixture of large and small cells. Skeletal lymphomas are difficult to classify by the same scheme as applied to nodal lymphomas. They are usually either of a diffuse mixed type or a diffuse large cell type. Quite often multinucleated cells or cells with clear cytoplasm are present, both suggesting a T-cell phenotype.

Special stains may be helpful in establishing the diagnosis of lymphoma of bone. As Schajowicz pointed out, PAS

FIG. 31. Malignant lymphoma: computed tomography. **A:** An anteroposterior radiograph of the lumbar spine of a 45-year-old man shows a destructive lesion of the L3 vertebra. The extent of the tumor can not be evaluated. **B:** CT section shows the full extent of the lesion in the bone and a large soft-tissue mass.

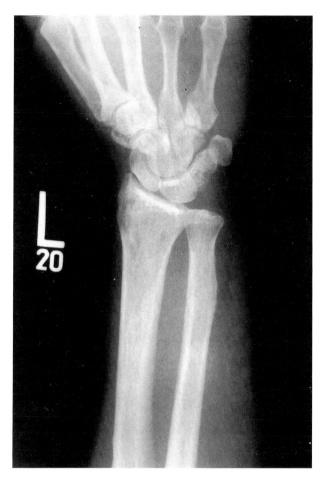

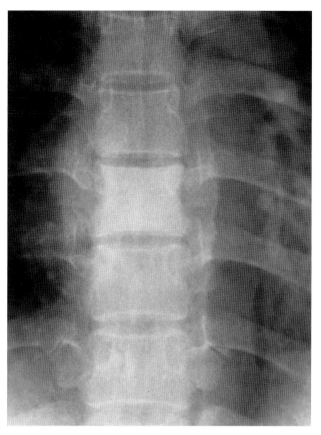

FIG. 30. Malignant lymphoma. An anteroposterior radiograph of the thoracic spine of a 32-year-old man shows sclerosis of Th 7 vertebra ("ivory vertebra"). Note bulging of the paraspinal line.

FIG. 29. Malignant lymphoma. An oblique radiograph of the left distal forearm and wrist in a 63-year-old woman shows almost imperceptible lesion in the distal radius. Note that there is no periosteal reaction present. (Reprinted with permission from Greenfield GB, Arrington JA. *Imaging of bone tumors: a multimodality approach.* Philadelphia: JB Lippincott, 1995;404.)

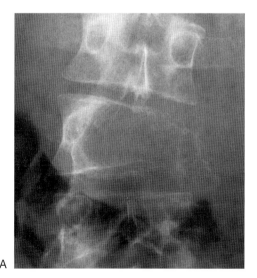

A

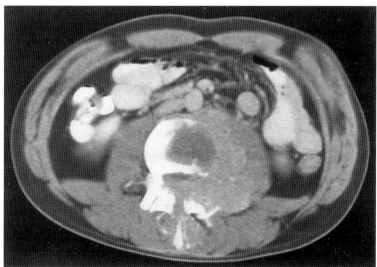

B

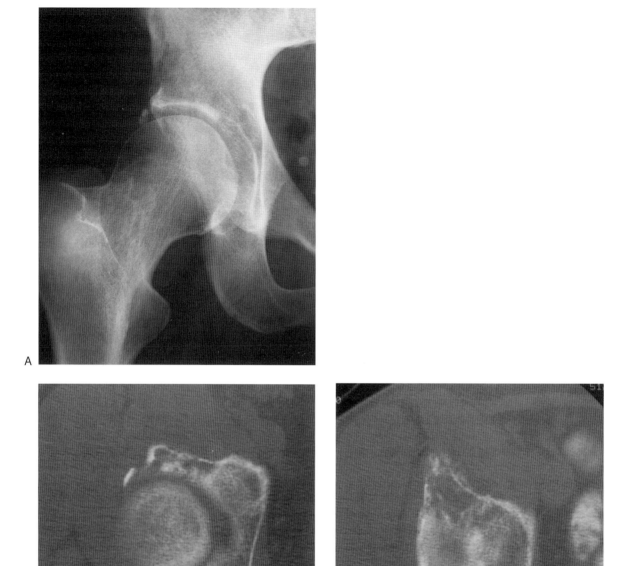

FIG. 32. Malignant lymphoma: computed tomography. **A:** An anteroposterior radiograph of the right hip of a 36-year-old man shows a very subtle osteolytic lesion of the acetabulum. **B,C:** Two CT sections demonstrate the involvement of the anterior column and roof of the acetabulum.

staining is usually but not invariably negative in this tumor (90) (Fig. 37). When a lymphoma of bone is suspected, all special studies usually done in lymphoma affecting lymph nodes should be performed.

Hodgkin Lymphoma

Hodgkin lymphoma, or Hodgkin disease, is a malignant tumor of the lymph nodes, constituting approximately 50%

of all malignant lymphomas. Males are more commonly affected than females and whites more often than blacks (113). Most cases of Hodgkin disease occur in patients aged 20 to 60 years, without an outstanding peak age (83). Secondary bone involvement is detected radiologically in 5% to 21% of patients (102,105). Primary Hodgkin lymphoma of bone is extremely rare (108,115) and usually involves the spine (131). The lower thoracic and upper lumbar vertebral bodies are favored (64) (Fig. 38). Therefore, when a biopsy speci-

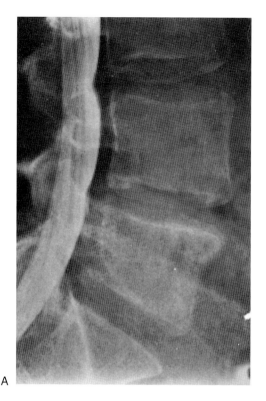

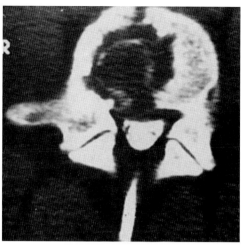

B

FIG. 33. Malignant lymphoma: computed tomography. A: A lateral myelogram in an 18-year-old woman, who presented with low back pain for several months with the clinical impression of herniated intervertebral disk, shows that the disk is normal, but the body of L5 vertebra exhibits a mottled appearance and its posterior border is indistinct. B: CT section demonstrates a large osteolytic lesion extending from the anterior to the posterior margins of the vertebral body. Note small sequestra within the lesion frequently seen in lymphomas.

A

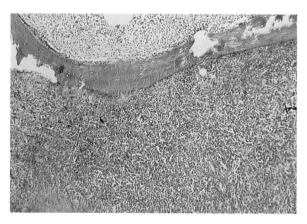

FIG. 34. Histopathology of malignant lymphoma. Pleomorphic round cells with well-defined cytoplasmic outline surround the bone trabecula (hematoxylin and eosin, original magnification ×100).

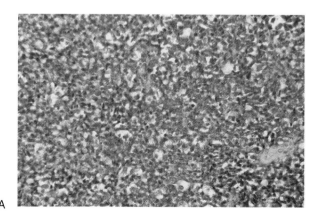

A

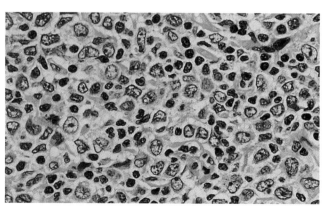

B

FIG. 35. Histopathology of malignant lymphoma. A: Densely arranged pleomorphic cells of medium size with roundish nuclei are present, some with a clear cytoplasm. The cells are larger and more pleomorphic than those in Ewing sarcoma (Giemsa, original magnification ×50). B: At high magnification the mixed cell population and the cleaved nuclei with prominent nucleoli mark the difference from Ewing sarcoma (hematoxylin and eosin, original magnification ×500). (From Bullough PG, *Atlas of orthopedic pathology,* 2nd ed. New York: Gower, 1992;17.15).

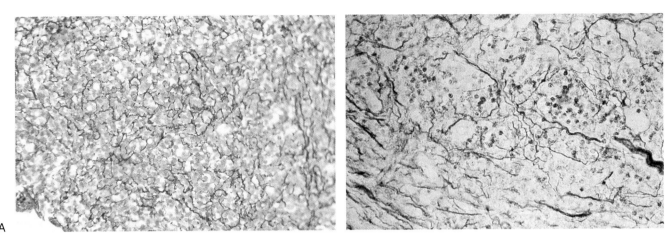

A   B

FIG. 36. Histopathology of malignant lymphoma: reticulin staining. **A:** With reticulin fiber staining, a fine black-appearing net surrounding individual cells is visible (Novotny, original magnification ×50). **B:** At high magnification abundant reticulin fibers form a dense network surrounding individual cells, or small groups of cells (Gomori silver stain, original magnification ×100).

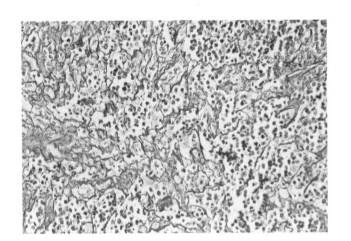

FIG. 37. Histopathology of malignant lymphoma: PAS staining. Small round cells are arranged in clusters separated by delicate reticulin fibers. Larger cells with small nuclei and clear cytoplasm create a "starry sky" appearance (*middle, upper and lower left*) characteristic of Burkitt lymphoma (PAS, original magnification ×50).

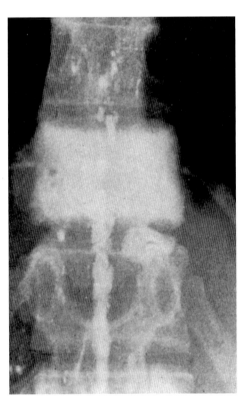

FIG. 38. Hodgkin lymphoma. Anteroposterior radiograph of the lower thoracic spine of a 35-year-old man shows sclerotic Th 10 vertebra ("ivory vertebra"). (From Bullough PG. *Atlas of orthopedic pathology,* 2nd ed. New York: Gower, 1992; 17.16.)

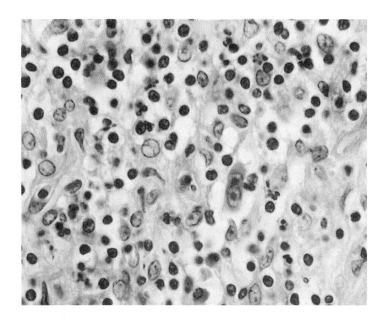

FIG. 39. Histopathology of Hodgkin lymphoma. Fibrous stroma with mixed cellular infiltrate of small round cells and large histiocytes is characteristic for this tumor (hematoxylin and eosin, original magnification ×400). (From Bullough PG. *Atlas of orthopedic pathology,* 2nd ed. New York: Gower, 1992;17.16.)

men from a spinal lesion suggests lymphoma, the possibility of Hodgkin disease should be included in the differential.

Symptoms include pain, often with an onset before the lesion becomes visible by radiography. Occasionally, a swelling over the affected bone can be noted (107). The majority of cases involve the spine and other bones with abundant red bone marrow, such as ribs, pelvic bones, and femur. The lesion is frequently sclerotic (e.g., ivory vertebra) (see Fig. 38) or mixed (lytic with sclerotic patches). A purely lytic geographic pattern is uncommon.

It is difficult to make a specific diagnosis of Hodgkin lymphoma of bone, largely because the histologic appearance may not be as classical as in cases involving the lymph nodes (121). In the latter, according to Rye's classification introduced by Lukes (124,126), four different stages are distinguished: (a) the lymphocyte-rich pattern; (b) the mixed-cell pattern (a reservoir for nonclassifiable cases); (c) the nodular sclerosis pattern; and (d) the diffuse fibrosis or lymphocyte depletion pattern. The prognostic significance of this histologic classification is not yet clear. The tumor cell (Hodgkin cell) is a large histiocytic cell with a large nucleus that possesses a conspicuous nucleolus. The histologic picture of Hodgkin lymphoma in the bone usually corresponds to the mixed-cell pattern, including lymphocytes, neutrophilic granulocytes, histiocytes, and plasma cells, in addition to the tumor cells (Fig. 39). Therefore, the differential diagnosis usually includes chronic osteomyelitis. It is noteworthy that patients with Hodgkin lymphoma of bone almost always have involvement of the lymph nodes, especially the retroperitoneal nodes.

Histologically, Hodgkin lymphoma is distinguished from other lymphomas by the presence of Reed-Sternberg cells. These are distinctive large cells with sharply delineated, abundant cytoplasm and a mirror-image double nucleus rich in chromatin, with a large, prominent, central eosinophilic nucleolus (106) (Fig. 40). These large nucleoli, almost the

size of a small lymphocyte, give the cell a conspicuous and almost specific "owl's eyes" appearance. Although pathognomonic Reed-Sternberg cells may be difficult to find, the immunochemical marker Leu-1 is useful for distinguishing them.

Differential Diagnosis

Radiology

The radiologic differential diagnosis must include other primary bone tumors. If the patient is an infant or a child (up to 10 years of age), *metastatic neuroblastoma* should be considered. Between the ages of 5 and 25 years, particularly if the lesion is osteolytic or has a moth-eaten or permeative pattern of bone destruction with lamellated or onion-skin periosteal reaction, *Ewing sarcoma* may be difficult to exclude (83). In more sclerotic lesions, particularly if the "sunburst" pattern of periosteal reaction is present, osteosarcoma is a serious consideration. If a sclerotic lesion extends into the articular end of bone, Paget disease should be considered (Fig. 41). In patients over the age of 40 or 50 years, *metastatic carcinoma* and *plasmacytoma* are differential possibilities. At any age, *osteomyelitis* should be a diagnostic consideration. In all of these differential possibilities, because the radiographic appearance of the lesion may be very similar, clinical and laboratory information must be taken into consideration.

Pathology

The main considerations are similarly appearing *Ewing sarcoma, metastatic neuroblastoma,* and *metastatic carcinoma.* Rarely, *osteomyelitis* with abundant lymphocytic

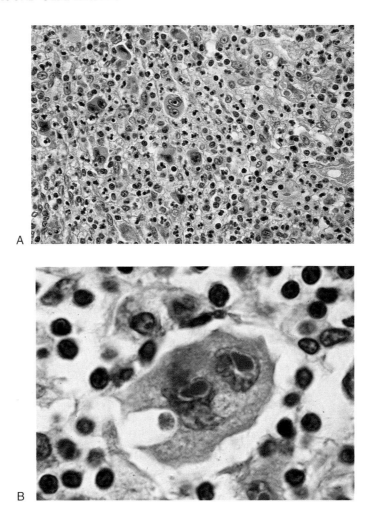

FIG. 40. Histopathology of Hodgkin lymphoma. **A:** Pleomorphic round cells are seen together with scattered Reed-Sternberg cells (hematoxylin and eosin, original magnification ×400). **B:** High-power photomicrograph demonstrates a binucleate Reed-Sternberg cell with prominent eosinophilic nucleoli (hematoxylin and eosin, original magnification ×1000). (From Bullough PG. *Atlas of orthopedic pathology,* 2nd ed. New York: Gower, 1992;17.16.)

cells is a differential possibility. The use of antibodies against LCA will almost invariably reveal the lymphoid character of lymphoma tumor cells (83).

Most lymphomas exhibit a variety of cytologic features within the lesion, making the histologic appearance that of a polymorphous growth. This is helpful in differentiating malignant lymphoma from Ewing sarcoma, which exhibits a growth of isomorphic small cells. The cells in lymphomas usually are less round than those in Ewing sarcoma, and they tend to have larger regular or even cleaved nuclei (see Fig. 35).

Another differential diagnostic consideration in a lesion suspected to be lymphoma of bone is a leukemic infiltrate of bone. However, all patients with chronic lymphocytic leukemia have peripheral blood abnormalities, and if the bones are affected the diagnosis should not be difficult. The same is true of patients with chronic myeloid (granulocytic) leukemia. Chronic and acute myeloic leukemia may present as a primary bone neoplasm, termed *myeloic (granulocytic)*

sarcoma or *chloroma.* The clinical and radiologic features of this condition may be similar to those of lymphoma. Biopsy specimens will exhibit sheets of large blast-like cells, although it is very difficult to make a specific diagnosis of granulocytic sarcoma from routine sections of bone. When this diagnosis is suspected, it is necessary to do immunohistochemical studies such as the reaction for lysozyme, which is considered the most helpful study because the blast cells will be positive. The acid chloracetate-esterase reaction is also helpful.

The histologic differential diagnosis of malignant lymphoma also includes benign conditions such as chronic osteomyelitis and other types of small cell malignancies such as metastatic carcinoma and Ewing sarcoma. Chronic osteomyelitis is usually characterized by a mixture of inflammatory cells and no evidence of cytologic atypia. There is also a proliferation of capillaries in the background, as well as fibrosis. It may be difficult to distinguish a large cell lymphoma from metastatic carcinoma. In these instances, spe-

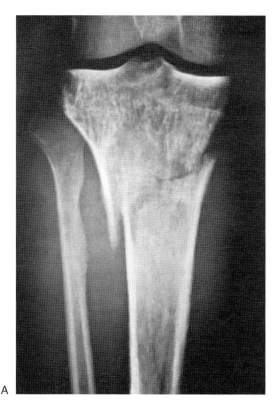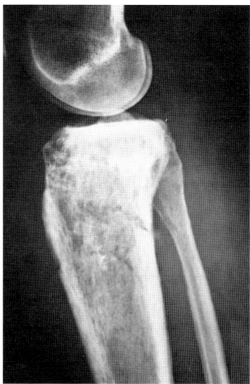

A   B

FIG. 41. Malignant lymphoma: differential diagnosis. (**A**) Anteroposterior and (**B**) lateral radiographs of the right knee of a 47-year-old woman show a mixed sclerotic and osteolytic lesion extending into the articular end of the tibia, associated with a pathologic fracture, originally diagnosed as Paget disease. Biopsy revealed a histiocytic lymphoma.

cial reactions using LCA and keratin antibodies may be helpful in making the distinction. Positivity of the undifferentiated cells for LCA is strong evidence for a malignant lymphoma, whereas positivity for anti-keratin suggests an epithelial origin.

Sometimes it is difficult to distinguish a lymphoma from a true sarcoma of bone. Lymphomas of bone may possess spindle cells that occasionally have a storiform pattern, suggesting the diagnosis of malignant fibrous histiocytoma. *Malignant fibrous histiocytomas* usually create large areas of bone destruction. If the lesion appears to be only permeative, i.e., it fills the marrow spaces and leaves behind normal bony trabeculae, the diagnosis of malignant lymphoma with spindling can be suspected. The immunoperoxidase reaction may be helpful in this instance because the spindle cells in malignant lymphoma react positively with LCA and negatively with lysozyme and α_1-antitrypsin, whereas the spindle cells of malignant fibrous histiocytoma exhibit the reverse pattern. However, it should be noted that bone biopsy specimens must not be decalcified because immunoperoxidase reaction may not work after the decalcification because certain antigenic determinants are denatured by acid decalcification.

Occasionally, the eosinophilic component and the histiocytes may be such prominent features of Hodgkin lymphoma

as to suggest the diagnosis of *Langerhans cell granuloma* (23). In this situation, the age of the patient is crucial: in a middle-aged or elderly patient, the diagnosis of Hodgkin lymphoma is much more likely and should be strongly considered (120).

The radiologic and pathologic differential diagnosis of malignant lymphoma are depicted in Fig. 42.

Multiple Myeloma (Plasmacytoma)

Myeloma, a tumor originating in the bone marrow (also known as multiple myeloma, plasma cell myeloma, or plasmacytoma), is the most common primary malignant tumor of bone and accounts for 27% of biopsied bone tumors (81). Most of these tumors are diagnosed by bone marrow biopsy. Myeloma is often associated with the presence of abnormal proteins in the blood and urine, and occasionally with the presence of amyloid in the tumor tissue or other organs (91,166). Solitary myeloma (or plasmacytoma) is a clinical variant (153) considered to represent an early stage of multiple myeloma (170), with stages of transition existing between the localized and the disseminated types (146,157, 171).

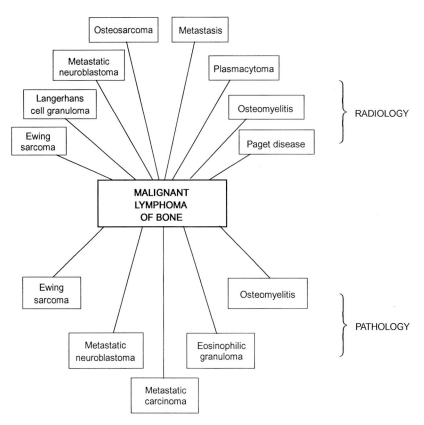

FIG. 42. Radiologic and pathologic differential diagnosis of malignant lymphoma of bone.

Clinical Presentation

Myeloma usually occurs in patients over 40 years of age and is most commonly seen between the fifth and seventh decades, with a median patient age at diagnosis of 64 years. Occurrence in the younger age group is exceptional (148,150,160,161,168) and is usually represented by cases of solitary myeloma (or plasmacytoma) (163). Males are affected more frequently than females (3:2 ratio). A clinical staging system based on the serum concentrations of hemoglobin, calcium, and paraprotein, urinary Bence-Jones protein excretion, and the number of skeletal lesions seen on radiographs has been proposed by Durie and Salmon (155). Myeloma arises primarily in bones that contain red marrow and therefore the axial skeleton is most commonly affected. However, no bone is exempt from involvement (Fig. 43). Skeletal involvement distal to the elbow and knee occurs in only 10% of cases (186). Pain, mild and transient, worse during the day, and enhanced by weight bearing and activity, may be the initial complaint and is present in about 75% of patients (154). Therefore, multiple myeloma may masquerade as sciatica or intercostal neuralgia in the stages before the diagnosis is established. Malaise, fatigue, weight loss, fever, and bone pain are other commonly encountered symptoms. Low-back pain or sciatic pain may sometimes be accompanied by neurologic symptoms. Rarely, a pathologic

fracture is the first sign of disease. Other common clinical features of multiple myeloma are related to a refractory, normocytic, normochromic anemia, resulting from bone marrow replacement by myeloma cells, to hypercalcemia resulting from widespread bone destruction, to renal dysfunction caused by renal tubule obstruction and damage by abnormal circulating proteins, and to decreased resistance to infection resulting from a deficiency of normal antibody production. Because the malignant cells represent a monoclonal proliferation of plasma cells, the tumor produces the specific immunoglobulin type associated with that particular neoplastic plasma cell. Characteristically, the ratio of serum albumin to globulins is reversed because of the high concentration of monoclonal immunoglobulin produced by the myeloma cells [most often IgG (65%), or IgA (20%), less frequently IgM and IgO]. Because the monoclonal immunoglobulin is of the same molecular weight and charge, during serum electrophoresis it moves to a single spot, and a concentrated narrow band, the so-called M component, appears as a peak when densitometry is performed on the electrophoretic strip. Immunoelectrophoresis of the serum predominantly shows a monoclonal heavy chain (83%) and a monoclonal light chain (8%) (167). Although the total immunoglobulin level is elevated because of the monoclonal protein, the normal serum immunoglobulin concentrations are markedly depressed, resulting in impaired humoral immunity. If light chains are

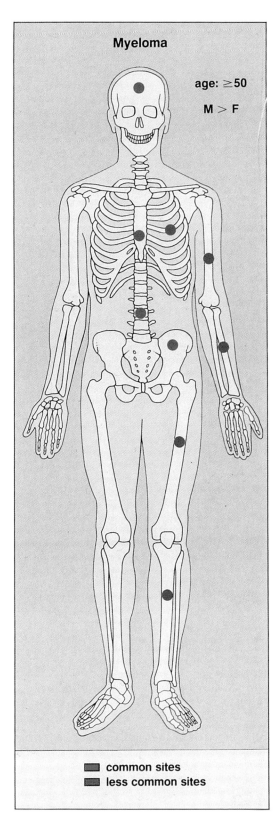

FIG. 43. Myeloma: skeletal sites of predilection, peak age range, and male-to-female ratio.

produced in excess, these pass into the renal tubules and are dimerized to form Bence-Jones protein in the urine (147).

Although myeloma is primarily a bone tumor, many other organs (including lymph nodes) may be affected (162).

Complications encountered with myeloma include pathologic fractures (of long bones, ribs, sternum, and vertebrae), amyloidosis (in about 15% of patients), increased incidence of infection, anemia, and a hyperviscosity syndrome. Most patients with solitary myeloma develop the systemic form of myeloma within 5 to 20 years (57).

Imaging

On radiography, multiple myeloma may present in a variety of patterns (Fig. 44). Most commonly it presents either as a lesion with a geographic type of bone destruction or as multiple small foci of bone destruction (Fig. 45). In the skull, characteristic roundish, punched-out areas of bone destruction, usually uniform in size, are observed (Fig. 46).

In the spine, multiple myeloma may present simply as osteoporosis, with no definitely identifiable lesions. A more common presentation, however, is the presence of multiple lytic lesions scattered throughout the vertebral column. Multiple compression fractures of the vertebral bodies may be seen in both forms.

In the ribs, lace-like areas of bone destruction and small osteolytic (punched-out) lesions accompanied by soft tissue masses are occasionally observed (173). In the flat and long bones, areas of medullary bone destruction are noted and, if these abut the cortex, endosteal scalloping of the inner cortical margin (so-called "rat bites") is seen (**see Fig. 45B**). Characteristically, there is no evidence of sclerosis and no periosteal reaction. Osteosclerotic lesions, even when mixed with lytic lesions, are rare in myeloma, and <1% of myelomas exhibit pure sclerotic lesions (sclerosing myelomatosis) (152).

Although scintigraphy in multiple myeloma is usually normal (145), increased uptake is occasionally demonstrated, presumably secondary to hyperemia, increased turnover in adjacent bone, and perhaps even to some osteoblastic activity (22,174). On some occasions, areas of decreased uptake (cold foci) are detected, presumably caused by a replacement of normal bone by myeloma tissue, which does not take up the tracer (187).

CT is better than plain film radiography for revealing the intraosseous extent of the tumor, cortical destruction, and extraosseous involvement. Some vertebral lesions that are not visible on plain radiography can also be demonstrated (182).

MRI is more sensitive than conventional imaging (plain radiography and CT) for detection of skeletal abnormalities in multiple myeloma (112,158,172,184). In particular, MRI is effective in demonstrating spinal lesions (169,183,185). The MRI changes may be either diffuse or focal. On T1-weighted images the lesions are visible as hypointense areas (usually of intermediate signal intensity), as contrasted with surrounding bone. On T2-weighted and STIR images, the le-

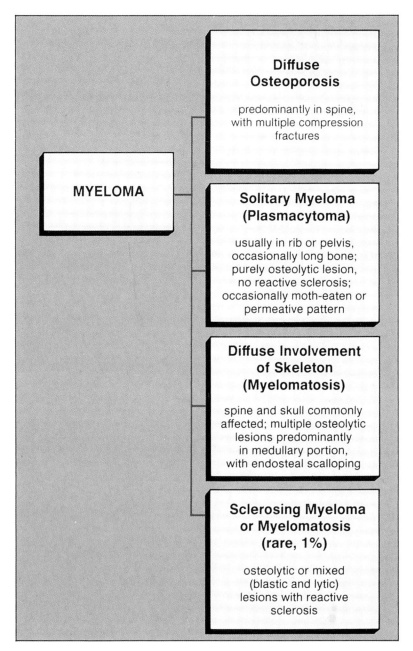

FIG. 44. Myeloma: variants in the radiographic presentation.

sions display homogeneously high signal intensity (143). The lesions show enhancement on turbo-FLASH (fast low-angle shot) images (175). On contrast-enhanced T1-weighted SE images, persistence of paramagnetic contrast agent is seen (175). Because the fatty tissue replacement that occurs within the vertebrae in older patients can mask the lesions, fat-suppressed MR images are of value for detecting myeloma (156,179).

It should be emphasized that the variable appearance of multiple myeloma on MRI is caused by a combination of factors. Although myeloma may involve the marrow dif-

fusely, the involvement is not necessarily homogeneous. The appearance of the bone marrow depends both on the extent of the disease and on the degree of fatty replacement, which varies considerably, and is greater in the older age group (169).

An interesting variant of sclerosing myeloma is the so-called POEMS syndrome, first described in 1968 (181) but gaining wide acceptance only more recently (151,159, 164,177,180). It consists of polyneuropathy (P); organomegaly (O), particularly of the liver and the spleen; endocrine disturbances (E), including amenorrhea, gynecomastia,

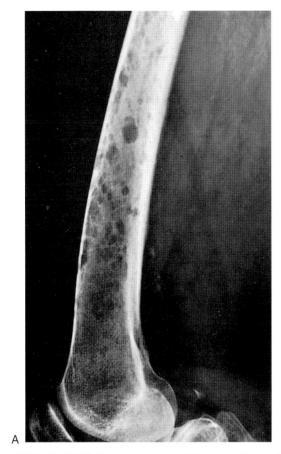
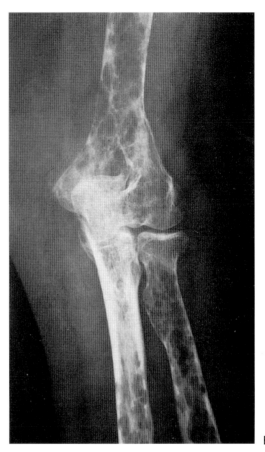

FIG. 45. Multiple myeloma. **A:** A lateral radiograph of the distal femur of a 65-year-old woman shows multiple osteolytic lesions. **B:** An anteroposterior radiograph of the left elbow in the same patient shows multiple osteolytic lesions and endosteal scalloping of the cortex typical of diffuse myelomatosis.

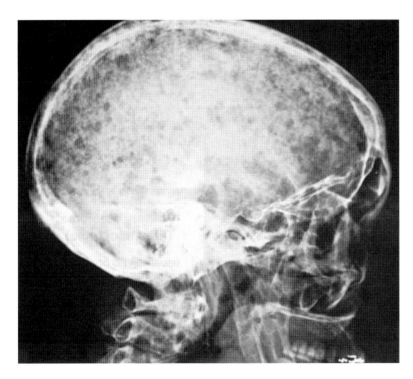

FIG. 46. Multiple myeloma. Involvement of the skull is a prominent feature of multiple myeloma of this 60-year-old woman. Note characteristic "punched-out," lytic lesions, most of which are uniform in size and lack sclerotic borders. Occasionally this pattern may be seen in metastatic disease.

impotence, diabetes mellitus, and hypothyroidism; monoclonal gammopathy (M), usually due to lambda light chains; and skin changes (S), such as hyperpigmentation and hirsutism. Additional associated abnormalities include papilledema, peripheral edema, ascites, and clubbing of the fingers (142). The exact pathogenesis of POEMS syndrome remains unsettled. It is still debatable whether the sclerotic changes are related to plasma cells that fail to secrete osteoclast-activating factor or perhaps are related to the secretion of an osteoblast-stimulating factor (144). Relatively few plasma cells are present in the marrow of patients with POEMS syndrome, and some investigators consider this entity a plasma cell dyscrasia rather than a true neoplasm (177). These patients do not have an increased incidence of amyloidosis and rarely have Bence-Jones proteinuria (151).

Certain radiologic findings concerning the lesions in POEMS syndrome have been emphasized by Resnick (177,178). These include irregular, spiculated, osseous proliferation involving multiple tendinous and ligamentous attachments (enthesopathy), especially of the posterior elements of the thoracic and lumbar spine, and lucent areas of bone destruction with a surrounding rim of sclerosis. Some authors describe sclerotic foci within the vertebral body ranging from very dense bone, resembling ivory vertebrae, to fine sclerotic lesions with irregular peripheral spiculations. Some of these sclerotic foci may even resemble bone islands. Positive bone scans in patients with POEMS syndrome appear to be exceptional. When positive, the accumulation of the radionuclide in the osseous foci is probably due to a sclerotic bone reaction and to the cortical expansion combined with a periosteal reaction that occurs in some cases (149,159).

Histopathology

The gross appearance of myeloma is that of either a fleshy white lesion, very similar to the appearance of lymphoma, or a grayish pink fleshy mass. However, the gross appearance alone is not diagnostic of myeloma.

The histologic appearance of myeloma is characteristic. The diagnosis is based on the presence of extended sheets of a population of atypical plasmacytoid cells that fill the trabecular bone marrow spaces and replace the normal fatty and hematopoietic marrow. The cytologic findings may vary. A high degree of differentiation is characterized by almost normal-appearing plasma cells (Fig. 47). Their round nuclei possess a dense, coarse chromatin that has a typical cartwheel-like distribution. The prominent nucleolus is excentrically located in a strongly basophilic cytoplasm that corresponds to the densely arranged rough endoplasmatic reticulum as revealed by electron microscopy and displays a perinuclear lighter halo that represents the well-developed Golgi apparatus. In addition, a wide variety of cytoplasmic inclusion bodies of crystallite form may be found in the cells. Increasing dedifferentiation is accompanied by an increasing pleomorphism of the cells and the nuclei, with loss of the regimented arrangement of the cell organelles. Furthermore,

there are increasing numbers of bi- and trinucleated cells (Fig. 48). Dedifferentiation is usually classified into three grades that are correlated with decreasing survival time for the patient (52,91,162). It may be difficult to differentiate a grade 3 myeloma from a lymphoma or from an undifferentiated carcinoma.

Although conventional myeloma is not associated with osteosclerosis, rare cases of myeloma are associated with this feature, known as sclerosing myeloma. These patients classically present with peripheral neuropathy. They also may have organomegaly, endocrine disturbances, monoclonal gammopathy, and skin lesions (POEMS syndrome; see above). They tend to be younger than patients with classical myeloma, and the disease progression is more indolent. The myeloma associated with peripheral neuropathy may be either localized or a part of multiple myeloma. The peripheral neuropathy may be arrested and may even improve with treatment of the underlying myeloma. Of all myelomas, 10% to 15% will exhibit the presence of amyloid within the tumor, in the form of eosinophilic hyaline masses or amyloid deposition within vascular walls. The amyloid may invoke a foreign body type of giant cell reaction. The presence of abundant amyloid may also obscure the underlying neoplasm. When amyloid is found in a bone biopsy specimen the pathologist should suspect a diagnosis of myeloma unless the patient has been receiving chronic hemodialysis because such patients may also deposit so-called amyloid tumors in the skeleton.

Differential Diagnosis

Radiology

When many osteolytic lesions in several bones are observed, the only alternative diagnosis is *metastatic disease*.

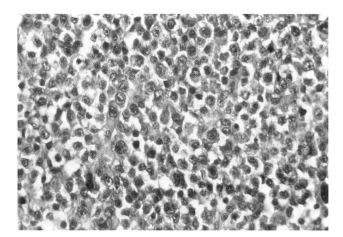

FIG. 47. Histopathology of multiple myeloma. In higher degree of differentiation, normal-appearing plasma cells are present mixed with a moderate number of cells with clearer and larger, slightly pleomorphic nuclei (grade 2). A small number of giant cells with two to three nuclei is also seen (Giemsa, original magnification ×100).

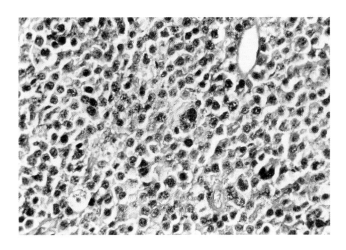

FIG. 48. Histopathology of multiple myeloma. In grade 3 tumor, between fewer than illustrated in Fig. 5-47 normal-appearing plasma cells noted are pleomorphic cells with clearer nuclei. Numerous giant cells with two and more nuclei are also present (Giemsa, original magnification ×100).

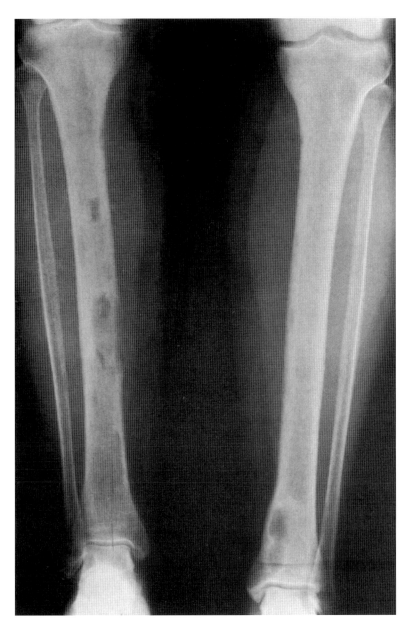

FIG. 49. Differential diagnosis of multiple myeloma: hyperparathyroidism. An anteroposterior radiograph of the lower legs of a 36-year-old woman with primary hyperparathyroidism shows multiple lytic lesions ("brown tumors") in both tibiae.

This is particularly true if the patient is older than 40 or 50 years. In younger patients, *brown tumors of hyperparathyroidism* (Fig. 49) and *Gaucher disease* (Fig. 50) should be considered. *Severe osteoporosis* may sometimes mimic the diffuse type of multiple myeloma. A valuable differential clue is the lack of endosteal scalloping in this condition, unlike multiple myeloma, in which scalloping is invariably present (see Fig. 45B). When the spine is involved, which occurs rather commonly, multiple myeloma must be differentiated from *metastatic carcinoma*. In this respect, the vertebral-pedicle sign identified by Murray and Jacobson may be helpful (173). These investigators contended that in the early stages of myeloma the pedicle, which does not contain as much red marrow as the vertebral body, is not initially involved, whereas in metastatic carcinoma the pedicle is af-

fected to the same extent as the vertebral body, even in the early stages (Fig. 51). In the late stages of multiple myeloma, however, the pedicle and the vertebral body are both affected. A more reliable distinction between these two processes is achieved with radionuclide bone scanning. Although the bone scan is invariably abnormal in cases of metastatic carcinoma, myeloma seldom produces an increased uptake of the radiopharmaceutical agent.

A solitary myeloma may create even more diagnostic problems. Because it is a purely radiolucent lesion, it may mimic other purely destructive processes such as *giant-cell tumor, brown tumor of hyperparathyroidism, fibrosarcoma, malignant fibrous histiocytoma,* and a *solitary metastatic focus* from a carcinoma of the kidney, lung, thyroid, or the gastrointestinal tract. Moreover, only a small percentage of solitary myelomas are associated with production of detectable monoclonal immunoglobulins.

Sclerosing myeloma with diffuse bone abnormalities should be differentiated from *sclerotic metastasis, mastocytosis, myelofibrosis,* and *renal osteodystrophy.* Focal sclerotic changes observed in myeloma should be differentiated from *tuberous sclerosis* and some sclerosing dysplasias (e.g., van Buchem disease; osteopoikilosis). Some myelomas with calcified amyloid depositions may be mistaken for *chondrosarcoma* (176). It must be pointed out that amyloidosis occurs in approximately 10% to 15% of cases of myeloma (165) and that calcifications are associated with both primary and secondary amyloidosis.

Pathology

The important differential diagnosis of myeloma includes a tumor and reactive forms of plasma cell proliferation, such as *plasmacytoid lymphoma, monoclonal gammopathy* of unknown significance (but only up to 5% plasmocytes in the bone marrow), *plasmacellular osteomyelitis,* and *rheumatoid arthritis* (up to 10% plasmocytes in bone marrow). The immunohistochemical demonstration of the monoclonal immunoglobulin produced by the myeloma cells allows a clearcut distinction between the tumor and the reactive form. The same is true for the differentiation of chronic plasmacellular osteomyelitis. In addition, the presence of other types of inflammatory cells and the formation of granulation tissue with proliferating capillaries in the latter condition provide aids to diagnosis. As mentioned above, distinguishing cases of undifferentiated myeloma or undifferentiated metastatic carcinoma from a lymphoma may be difficult, but the demonstration of the specific immunoglobulin in the former and of keratin markers in the latter will aid in making the diagnosis.

The radiologic and pathologic differential diagnosis of solitary plasmacytoma is depicted in Fig. 52, and differential diagnosis of multiple myeloma in Fig. 53.

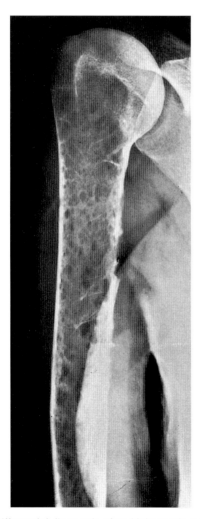

FIG. 50. Differential diagnosis of multiple myeloma: Gaucher disease. Destructive changes in Gaucher disease, seen here in the right humerus of a 52-year-old woman with the adult form of the disease, may assume a honeycombed appearance simulating multiple myeloma

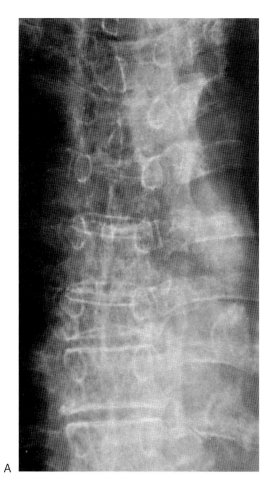

A

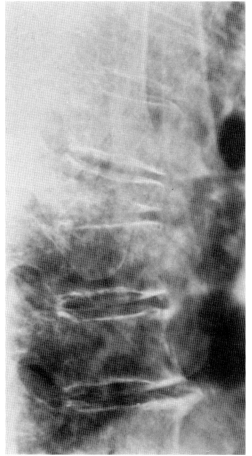

B

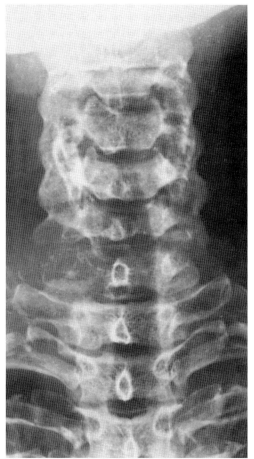

C

FIG. 51. Multiple myeloma: differential diagnosis. (**A**) Anteroposterior and (**B**) lateral radiographs of the spine of a 70-year-old man with multiple myeloma involving both the spine and appendicular skeleton show a compression fracture of the body of Th8 vertebra; several other vertebrae show only osteoporosis. The pedicles are preserved in contrast to metastatic disease of the spine (which usually also affects the pedicles), as seen on this anteroposterior radiograph of the cervical spine (**C**) in a 65-year-old man with colon carcinoma and multiple lytic metastases. Note the involvement of the right pedicle of C7 vertebra.

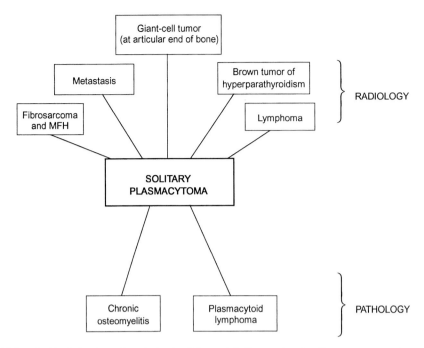

FIG. 52. Radiologic and pathologic differential diagnosis of solitary plasmacytoma.

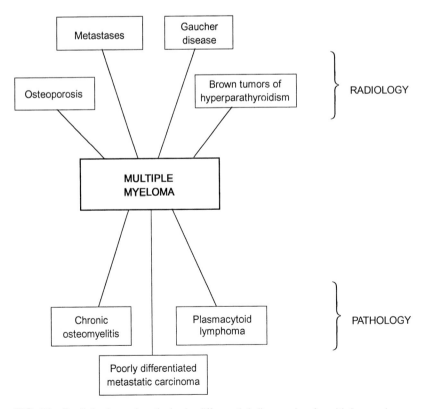

FIG. 53. Radiologic and pathologic differential diagnosis of multiple myeloma.

REFERENCES

Langerhans Cell Granuloma (Eosinophilic Granuloma)

1. Alexander JE, Seibert JJ, Berry DH, Glasier CM, Williamson SL, Murphy J. Prognostic factors for healing of bone lesions in histiocytosis X. *Pediatr Radiol* 1988;18:326–332.
2. Antonmattei S, Tetalman MR, Lloyd TV. The multiscan appearance of eosinophilic granuloma. *Clin Nucl Med* 1979;4:53–55.
3. Beltran J, Aparisi F, Marti Bonmati L, Rosenberg ZS, Present D, Steiner GS. Eosinophilic granuloma: MRI manifestations. *Skeletal Radiol* 1993;22:157–161.
4. Birbeck MS, Breathnach AS, Everall JD. An electron microscopic study of basal melanocytes and high-level clear cell (Langerhans cell) in vitiligo. *J Invest Dermatol* 1961;37:51–64.
5. Bohne WHO, Goldman AB, Bullough P. Case report 96. Chester-Erdheim disease (lipogranulomatosis). *Skeletal Radiol* 1979;4:164–167.
6. Cline MJ. Histiocytes and histiocytosis. *Blood* 1994;84:2840–2853.
7. Compere EL, Johnson WE, Coventry MB. Vertebra plana (Calvé's disease) due to eosinophilic granuloma. *J Bone Joint Surg* 1954;36:969–980.
8. Conway WF, Hayes CW. Miscellaneous lesions of bone. *Radiol Clin North Am* 1993;31:339–358.
9. Dalinka MK, Turner ML, Thompson JJ, Lee RE. Lipid granulomatosis of the ribs: focal Erdheim-Chester disease. *Radiology* 1982;142:297–299.
10. David R, Oria RA, Kumar R, Singelton EB, Lindell MM, Shirkhoda A, Madewell JE. Radiologic features of eosinophilic granuloma of bone. *Am J Roentgenol* 1989;153:1021–1026.
11. De Schepper AM, Ramon F, Van Marck E. MR imaging of eosinohilic granuloma: report of 11 cases. *Skeletal Radiol* 1993;22:163–166.
12. Favara BE. Langerhans cell histiocytosis—pathobiology and pathogenesis. *Semin Oncol* 1991;18:3–7.
13. Favara BE, McCarthy RC, Mierau GW. Histiocytosis X. *Hum Pathol* 1983;14:663–676.
14. Fisher AJ, Reinus WR, Friedland JA, Wilson AJ. Quantitative analysis of the plain radiographic appearance of eosinophilic granuloma. *Invest Radiol* 1995;30:466–473.
15. Flores LG II, Hiroaki H, Nagamachi S, Ohnishi T, Watanabe K, Fukijama J, Nao-i N, Sawada A. Thallium-201 uptake in eosinophilic granuloma of the frontal bone: comparison with technetium-99m-MDP imaging. *J Nucl Med* 1995;36:107–110.
16. Fowles JV, Bobechko WP. Solitary eosinophilic granuloma in bone. *J Bone Joint Surg* 1970;52B:238–243.
17. Greenfield GB, Arrington JA. *Imaging of Bone Tumors. A Multimodality Approach.* Philadelphia: JB Lippincott, 1995.
18. Grundy P, Ellis R. Histiocytosis X: a review of the etiology, pathology, staging, and therapy. *Med Pediatr Oncol* 1986;14:45–50.
19. Haggstrom JA, Brown JC, Marsh PW. Eosinophilic granuloma of the spine: MR demonstration. *J Comput Assist Tomogr* 1988;12:344–345.
20. Hajdu I, Zhang W, Gordon GB. Peanut agglutinin binding as a histochemical tool for diagnosis of eosinophilic granuloma. *Arch Pathol Lab Med* 1986;110:719–721.
21. Helms CA, Jeffrey RB, Wing VW. Computed tomography and plain film appearance of a bony sequestration: significance and differential diagnosis. *Skeletal Radiol* 1987;16:117–120.
22. Hudson TM. *Radiologic-Pathologic Correlation of Musculoskeletal Lesions.* Baltimore: Williams and Wilkins, 1987.
23. Huvos AG. *Bone tumors: diagnosis, treatment, and prognosis,* 2nd ed. Philadelphia: WB Saunders, 1991.
24. Kilpatrick SE, Wenger DF, Gilchrist GS, Shives TC, Wollan PC, Unni KK. Langerhans cell histiocytosis (histiocytosis X) of bone: a clinicopathologic analysis of 263 pediatric and adult cases. *Cancer* 1995;76:2471–2484.
25. Kumar R, Balachandran S. Relative roles of radionuclide scanning and radiographic imaging in eosinophilic granuloma. *Clin Nucl Med* 1980;5:538–542.
26. Leonidas JC. Langerhans cell histiocytosis. In: Taveras JM, Ferrucci JM, eds. *Radiology: diagnosis, imaging, intervention,* vol 5. Philadelphia: JB Lippincott, 1990;1–9.
27. Lichtenstein L. Histiocytosis X. I. Integration of eosinophilic granuloma of bone, Letterer-Siwe disease, and Schüller-Christian disease as related manifestations of single nosologic entity. *Arch Pathol* 1953;56:84–102.
28. Lichtenstein L. Histiocytosis X (eosinophilic granuloma of bone, Letterer-Siwe disease, and Schüller-Christian disease). *J Bone Joint Surg* 1964;46A:76–90.
29. Lieberman PH, Jones CR, Steinman RM, Erlandson RA, Smith J, Gee T, Huvosa et al. Langerhans cell (eosinophilic) granulomatosis. A clinicopathologic study encompassing 50 years. *Am J Surg Pathol* 1996;20:519–552.
30. Makley JT, Carter JR. Eosinophilic granuloma of bone. *Clin Orthop* 1986;204:37–44.
31. Meyer JS, Harty MP, Mahboubi S, Heyman S, Zimmerman RA, Womer RB, Dormans JP, D Angio GJ. Langerhans cells histiocytosis: Presentation and evolution of radiologic findings with clinical correlation. *RadioGraphics* 1995;15:1135–1146.
32. Mickelson MR, Bonfiglio M. Eosinophilic granuloma and its variations. *Orthop Clin North Am* 1977;8:933–945.
33. Mirra JM, Gold RH. Eosinophilic granuloma. In: Mirra JM, Gold RH, Picci P, eds. *Bone tumors: clinical, radiologic, and pathologic correlations.* Philadelphia: Lea and Febiger, 1989;1021–1039.
34. Mitnick JS, Pinto RS. Computed tomography in the diagnosis of eosinophilic granuloma. *J Comput Tomogr* 1980;4:791–793.
35. Moore JB, Kulkarni R, Crutcher DC, Bhimani S. MRI in multifocal eosinophilic granuloma: staging disease and monitoring reponse to therapy. *Am J Pediatr Hematol Oncol* 1989;11:174–177.
36. Moseley JE. *Bone changes in hematologic disorders (Roentgen aspects).* New York: Grune and Stratton, 1963;161–179.
37. Moseley JE. Patterns of bone change in the reticuloendothelioses. *J Mt Sinai Hosp* 1962;29:282–321.
38. Murayama S, Numaguchi Y, Robinson AE, Richardson DE. Magnetic resonance imaging of calvarial eosinophilic granuloma. *J Comput Tomogr* 1988;12:251–252.
39. Nezelof C, Basset F, Rousseau MF. Histiocytosis X: histogenetic arguments for a Langerhans cell origin. *Biomedicine* 1973;18:365–371.
40. Ostand ME. Histiocytosis X: Langerhans cell histiocytosis. *Hematol Oncol Clin North Am* 1987;1:737–751.
41. Resnick D. Lipidoses, histiocytoses, and hyperlipoproteinemias. In: Resnick D, ed. *Bone and joint imaging.* Philadelphia: WB Saunders, 1989;687–702.
42. Sartoris DJ, Parker BR. Histiocytosis X: rate and pattern of resolution of osseous lesions. *Radiology* 1984;152:679–684.
43. Siegelman SS. Taking the X out of histiocytosis X. *Radiol* 1997;204:322–324.
44. Schajowicz F. *Tumors and tumorlike lesions of bone: pathology, radiology, and treatment,* 2nd ed. Berlin: Springer-Verlag, 1994;552–566.
45. Schaub T, Ash JM, Gilday DL. Radionuclide imaging in histiocytosis X. *Pediatr Radiol* 1987;17:397–404.
46. Stull MA, Kransdorf MJ, Devaney KO. Langerhans cell histiocytosis of bone. *RadioGraphics* 1992;12:801–823.
47. Uhlinger E. Das eosinophile Knochengranulom. In: Heilmeyer L, Hittmair A, eds. *Handbuch der Gesamten Haematologie.* Munich: Urban and Schwartzenberg Verlag, 1963, Band IV/2;56.
48. Wester SM, Beabout JW, Unni KK, Dahlin DC. Langerhans cell granulomatosis (histiocytosis X) of bone in adults. *Am J Surg Pathol* 1982;6:413–426.
49. Willman CL. Detection of clonal histiocytes in Langerhans cell histiocytosis: biology and clinical significance. *Br J Cancer* 1994;70 (suppl 23):S29–S33.
50. Wilner D. *Radiology of bone tumors and allied disorders.* Philadelphia: Lea and Febiger, 1982.

Ewing Sarcoma

51. Bator SM, Bauer TW, Marks KE, Norris DG. Periosteal Ewing's sarcoma. *Cancer* 1986;58:1781–1784.
52. Bertoni F, Bacchini P, Ferruzzi A. Small round-cell malignancies of bone. Ewing's sarcoma, malignant lymphoma, and myeloma. *Semin Orthop* 1991;6:186–195.
53. Boyko OB, Cory DA, Cohen MD, Provisor A, Mirkin D, DeRosa GP. MR imaging of osteogenic and Ewing's sarcoma. *Am J Roentgenol* 1987;148:317–322.
54. Cavazzana AO, Miser JS, Jefferson J, Triche TJ. Experimental evidence for a neural origin of Ewing's sarcoma of bone. *Am J Pathol* 1987;127:507–518.
55. Coombs RJ, Zeiss J, McKann K, Phillips E. Multifocal Ewing's tumor of the skeletal system. *Skeletal Radiol* 1986;15:254–257.

56. Czerniak B, Rojas-Corona RR, Dorfman HD. Morphologic diversity of long bone adamantinoma. The concept of differentiated (regressing) adamantinoma and its relationship to osteofibrous dysplasia. *Cancer* 1989;64:2319–2334.

57. Dahlin DC, Unni KK. *Bone tumors. General aspects and data on 8,542 cases,* 4th ed. Springfield, IL: Charles C Thomas, 1986.

58. Dardick I, Schatz JE, Colgan TJ. Osteogenic sarcoma with epithelial differentiation. *Ultrastruct Pathol* 1992;16:463–474.

59. Dehner LP. Primitive neuroectodermal tumor and Ewing's sarcoma. *Am J Surg Pathol* 1993;17:1–13.

60. Dellagi K, Lipinski M, Paulin D, Portier MM, Lenoir GM, Brouet JC. Characterization of intermediate filaments expressed by Ewing tumor cell lines. *Cancer* 1987;47:1170–1173.

61. Eggli KD, Quiogue T, Moser RP. Ewing's sarcoma. *Radiol Clin North Am* 1993;31:325–337.

62. Enzinger FM, Weiss SW. *Soft tissue tumors.* St. Louis: CV Mosby, 1988;951–958.

63. Estes DN, Magill HL, Thompson EL, Hayes FA. Primary Ewing sarcoma: follow-up with Ga-67 scintigraphy. *Radiology* 1990;177:449–453.

64. Fechner RE, Mills SE. *Tumors of the bones and joints.* Washington, DC: Armed Forces Institute of Pathology, 1993.

65. Friedman B, Hanoaka H. Round cell sarcoma of bone. *J Bone Joint Surg* 1971;53A:1118–1136.

66. Frouge C, Vanel D, Coffre C, Couanet D, Contesso G, Sarrazin D. The role of magnetic resonance imaging in the evaluation of Ewing's sarcoma. A report of 27 cases. *Skeletal Radiol* 1988;17:387–392.

67. Garber CZ. Reactive bone formation in Ewing's sarcoma. *Cancer* 1951;4:839–845.

68. Gould VE, Moll, R, Berndt R, Roessner A, Franke WW, Lee I. Immunohistochemical analysis of Ewing's tumors. *Lab Invest* 1987;56:28 (Abstr).

69. Greco A, Steiner GC, Fazzini E. Ewing's sarcoma with epithelial differentiation. Fine structural and immunocytochemical study. *Ultrastruct Pathol* 1988;12:317–325.

70. Greenspan A. *Orthopedic radiology: a practical approach,* 2nd ed. New York: Gower, 1992;15.15.

71. Hindman BW, Gill HK, Zuppan CW. Primitive neuroectodermal tumor in a child with tuberous sclerosis. *Skeletal Radiol* 1997;26:184–187.

72. Isayama T, Iwasaki H, Kikuchi M, Yoh S, Takagishi N. Neuroectodermal tumor of bone. Evidence for neural differentiation in a cultured cell line. *Cancer* 1990;65:1771–1781.

73. Jaffe R, Santamaria M, Yunis EJ, Tannery NH, Agostini RM Jr, Medina J, Goodman M. The neuro-ectodermal tumor of bone. *Am J Surg* 1984;8:885–898.

74. Jones GR, Miller JH, White L, Lang WE, Shore NA. Improved detection of metastatic Ewing's sarcoma with the use of bone marrow scintigraphy. *Med Pediatr Oncol* 1987;15:78–81.

75. Kissane JM, Askin PB, Foulkes M, Stratton LB, Shirley SF. Ewing's sarcoma of bone. Clinicopathological aspects of 303 cases from the intergroup Ewing's sarcoma study. *Hum Pathol* 1983;14:773–779.

76. Kramer K, Hicks D, Palis J, Rosier RN, Oppenheimer J, Fallon MD, Cohen HJ. Epithelioid osteosarcoma of bone. Immunocytochemical evidence suggesting divergent epithelial and mesenchymal differentiation in a primary osseous neoplasm. *Cancer* 1993;71:2977–2982.

77. Levine E, Levine C. Ewing tumor of rib: Radiologic findings and computed tomography contribution. *Skeletal Radiol* 9:227–233, 1983.

78. Llombart-Bosch A, Contesso G, Henry-Amar M, Lacombe MJ, Oberlin O, Dubousset J, Rouesse J, Sarrazin D. Histopathological predictive factors in Ewing's sarcoma of bone and clinicopathologic correlations. A retrospective study of 261 cases. *Virchows Arch (A)* 1986;409:627–640 (erratum published in *Virchows Arch (A)* 1986;410:263).

79. Llombart-Bosch A, Lacombe MJ, Peydro-Olaya A, Perez-Bacete M, Contesso G. Malignant peripheral neuroectodermal tumors of bone other than Askin's neoplasm: characterization of 14 new cases with immunohistochemistry and electron microscopy. *Virchows Arch (A)* 1988;412:421–430.

80. Llombart-Bosch A, Terrier LMJ, Peydro-Olaya A, Contesso G. Peripheral neuroectodermal sarcoma of soft tissue (peripheral neuroepithelioma): a pathologic study of ten cases with differential diagnosis regarding other small, round cell sarcomas. *Hum Pathol* 1989;20:273–280.

81. Mirra JM, Picci P, Gold RH, eds. *Bone tumors: clinical, radiologic, and pathologic correlations.* Philadelphia: Lea and Febiger, 1989.

82. Moll R, Lee I, Gould V, Berndt R, Roessner A, Franke W. Immunocytochemical analysis of Ewing's tumors. Patterns of expression of intermediate filaments and desmosomal proteins indicate cell type heterogeneity and pluripotnetial differentiation. *Am J Pathol* 1987;127:288–303.

83. Mulder JD, Schütte HE, Kroon HM, Taconis WK. *Radiologic atlas of bone tumors.* Amsterdam: Elsevier, 1993.

84. Nair M. Bone scanning in Ewing's sarcoma. *J Nucl Med* 1985;26:349–352.

85. Nascimento AG, Unni KK, Cooper KL, Dahlin DC. A clinicopathologic study of 20 cases of large cell (atypical) Ewing's sarcoma of bone. *Am J Surg Pathol* 1980;4:29–36.

86. Nesbit ME Jr, Gehan EA, Burgert EO Jr, Vietti TJ, Cangir A, Tefft M, Evans R, Thomas P, Askin FB, Kissane JM, et al. Multimodal therapy for the management of primary, nonmetastatic Ewing's sarcoma of bone: a long-term follow-up of the First Intergroup study. *J Clin Oncol* 1990;8:1664–1674.

87. Reinus WR, Gilula LA. Ewing's sarcoma. In: Taveras JM, Ferruci JT, eds. *Radiology: diagnosis, imaging, intervention,* vol. 5. Philadelphia: JB Lippincott, 1987; Chap. 95.

88. Rice RW, Cabot A, Johnston A. The application of electron microscopy to the diagnostic differentiation of Ewing's sarcoma and reticulum cell sarcoma of bone. *Clin Orthop* 1973;97:174–184.

89. Rousselin B, Vanel D, Terrier-Lacombe MJ, Istria BJM, Spielman M, Masselot J. Clinical and radiologic analysis of 13 cases of primary neuro-ectodermal tumors of the bone. *Skeletal Radiol* 1989;18:115–120.

90. Schajowicz F. Ewing's sarcoma and reticulum cell sarcoma of bone: with special reference to the histochemical demonstration of glycogen as an aid to differential diagnosis. *J Bone Joint Surg* 1959;41A:349–356.

91. Schajowicz F. *Tumors and tumorlike lesions of bone,* 2nd ed. Berlin: Springer-Verlag, 1994.

92. Shirley SK, Gilula LA, Segal GP, Foulkes MA, Kissane JM, Askin FB. Roentgenographic-pathologic correlation of diffuse sclerosis in Ewing's sarcoma of bone. *Skeletal Radiol* 1984;12:69–78.

93. Steiner GC, Matano S, Present D. Ewing's sarcoma of humerus with epithelial differentiation. *Skeletal Radiol* 1995;24:379–382.

94. Steiner GC. Neuroectodermal tumor versus Ewing's sarcoma. Immunohistochemical and electron microscopic observations. *Curr Top Pathol* 1989;80:1–29.

95. Triche T, Cavazzana A. Round cell tumors of bone. In: Unni KK, ed. *Bone tumors.* New York: Churchill Livingstone, 1988;199–223.

96. Triche TJ, Askin FB, Kissane JM. Neuroblastoma, Ewing's sarcoma and the differential diagnosis of small, round blue cell tumors. In: Finegold M, ed. *Pathology of neoplasia in children and adolescents.* Philadelphia: WB Saunders, 1986;145–156.

97. Unni KK. *Dahlin's bone tumors: general aspects and data on 11,087 cases,* 5th ed. New York: Lippincott-Raven, 1996.

98. Vanel D, Contesso G, Couanet D, Piekarski JD, Sarrazin D, Masselot J. Computed tomography in the evaluation of 41 cases of Ewing's sarcoma. *Skeletal Radiol* 1982;9:8–13.

99. Vanel D, Couanet D, Leclerc J, Patte C. Early detection of bone metastases of Ewing's sarcoma by magnetic resonance imaging. *Diagn Imag Clin Med* 1986;55:381–383.

100. Weiss SW, Bratthauer GL, Morris PA. Post-radiation malignant fibrous histiocytoma expressing cytokeratin: implications for the immunodiagnosis of sarcomas. *Am J Surg Pathol* 1988;12:554–558.

101. Wilkins RM, Pritchard DJ, Burgert EO, Unni KK. Ewing's sarcoma of bone. Experience with 140 patients. *Cancer* 1986;58:2551–2555.

Malignant Lymphoma

102. Beackley MC, Lau BP, King ER. Bone involvement in Hodgkin's disease. *Am J* Roentgenol 1972;114:559–563.

103. Boston HC Jr, Dahlin DC, Ivins JC, Cupps RE. Malignant lymphoma (so-called reticulum cell sarcoma) of bone. *Cancer* 1974;34:1131–1137.

104. Bragg DG, Colby TV, Ward JH. New concepts in the non-Hodgkin lymphomas: radiologic implications. *Radiology* 1986;159:289–304.

105. Braunstein EM. Hodgkin's disease of bone: radiographic correlation with the histologic classification. *Radiology* 1980;137:643–646.

106. Bullough PG. *Atlas of orthopedic pathology with clinical and radiologic correlations,* 2nd ed. New York: Gower, 1992;17.1–17.29.

107. Castellino RA. Hodgkin disease: practical concepts for the diagnostic radiologist. *Radiology* 1986;159:305–310.
108. Chan K-W, Rosen G, Miller DR, Tan CTC. Hodgkin's disease in adolescents presenting as a primary bone lesion. A report of four cases and review of the literature. *Am J Pediatr Hematol Oncol* 1982; 4:11–17.
109. Clayton F, Butler JJ, Ayala AG, Ro JY, Zornoza J. Non-Hodgkin's lymphoma in bone: pathologic and radiologic features with clinical correlates. *Cancer* 1987;60:2494–2500.
110. Cohen MD, Klatte EC, Smith JA, Martin-Simmerman P, Carr B, Baehner R, Weetman R, Provisor A, Coates T, Berkow R. Magnetic resonance imaging of lymphomas in children. *Pediatr Radiol* 1985; 15:179–183.
111. Coles WC, Schultz MD. Bone involvement in malignant lymphoma. *Radiology* 1948;50:458–462.
112. Daffner RN, Lupetin AR, Dash N, Deeb ZL, Sefczek RJ, Shapiro RL. MRI in the detection of malignant infiltration of bone marrow. *Am J Roentgenol* 1986;146:353–358.
113. Fisher AMH, Kendall B, Van Leuven BD. Hodgkin's disease: a radiological survey. *Clin Radiol* 1962;13:115–127.
114. Fishman EK, Kuhlman JE, Jones RJ. CT of lymphoma: spectrum of disease. *RadioGraphics* 1991;11:647–669.
115. Gold RH, Mirra JM. Case report 101. Primary Hodgkin disease of humerus. *Skeletal Radiol* 1979;4:233–235.
116. Granger W, Whitaker R. Hodgkin's disease in bone, with special reference to periosteal reaction. *Br J Radiol* 1967;40:939–948.
117. Greco A, Jelliffe AM, Maher EJ, Leung AWL. MR imaging of lymphomas: impact on therapy. *J Comput Assist Tomogr* 1988;12: 785–791.
118. Hicks DG, Gokan T, O Keefe RJ, Totterman SM, Fultz PJ, Judkins AR, Meyers SP, Rubens DJ, Sickel JZ, Rosier RN. Primary lymphoma of bone. Correlation of MRI features with cytokine production by tumor cells. *Cancer* 1995;75:973–980.
119. Hillemanns M, McLeod RA, Unni KK. Malignant lymphoma. *Skeletal Radiol* 1996;25:73–75.
120. Jaffe HL. *Metabolic, degenerative, and inflammatory diseases of bones and joints.* Philadelphia: Lea and Febiger, 1972.
121. Kaplan H. *Hodgkin Disease*, 2nd ed. Cambridge, MA: Harvard University Press, 1980;85–92.
122. Klein MJ, Rudin BJ, Greenspan A, Posner M, Lewis MM. Hodgkin disease presenting as a lesion in the wrist. *J Bone Joint Surg* 1987; 69A:1246–1249.
123. Leeson MC, Makely JT, Carter JR, Krupco T. The use of radioisotope scans in the evaluation of primary lymphoma of bone. *Orthop Rev* 1989;18:410–416.
124. Lukes RJ, Buttler JJ. Pathology and nomenclature of Hodgkin disease. *Cancer Res* 1966;26:1063–2083.
125. Malloy PC, Fishman EK, Magid D. Lymphoma of bone, muscle, and skin: CT findings. *Am J Roentgenol* 1992;159:805–809.
126. Medeiros LJ, Jaffe ES. Pathology of non-Hodgkin's lymphomas and Hodgkin's disease. In: Wiernik PH, Canellos GP, Dutcher JP, Kyle RA, eds. *Neoplastic diseases of the blood*, 3rd ed. New York: Churchill Livingstone, 1996.
127. Melamed JW, Martinez S, Hoffman CJ. Imaging of primary multifocal osseous lymphoma. *Skeletal Radiol* 1997;26:35–41.
128. Mirra JM. Lymphoma and lymphoma-like disorders. In: Mirra JM, Picci P, Gold RH, eds. *Bone tumors: clinical, radiologic, and pathologic correlations.* Philadelphia: Lea and Febiger, 1989.
129. Mulligan ME, Kransdorf MJ. Sequestra in primary lymphoma of bone: prevalence and radiologic features. *Am J Roentgenol* 1993;160: 1245–1248.
130. Negendank W, Weissman D, Bey TM, de Planque MM, Karanes C, Smith MR, Ratanatharathorn V, Bishop CR, al-Katib AM, Sensenbrennen LL. Evidence for clonal disease by magnetic resonance imaging in patients with hypoplastic marrow disorders. *Blood* 1991;78: 2872–2879.
131. Newcomer LN, Silverstein MB, Cadman EC, Farber LR, Bertino JR, Prosnitz LR. Bone involvement in Hodgkin's disease. *Cancer* 1982; 49:338–342.
132. Olson DO, Shields AF, Scheurich JC, Porter BA, Moss AA. Magnetic resonance imaging of the bone marrow in patients with leukemia, aplastic anaemia and lymphoma. *Invest Radiol* 1986;21:540–546.
133. Orzel JA, Sawaf NW, Richardson ML. Lymphoma of the skeleton: scintigraphic evaluation. *Am J Roentgenol* 1988;150:1095–1099.
134. Ostrowski ML, Unni KK, Banks PM, Shives TC, Evans RG, O Connel

MJ, Taylor WF. Malignant lymphoma of bone. *Cancer* 1986;58: 2646–2655.
135. Perlman EJ, Dickman PS, Askin FB, Grier HE, Miser JS, Link MP. Ewing's sarcoma routine diagnostic utilization of MIC2 analysis: a Pediatric Oncology Group/Children's Cancer Group Intergroup Study. *Hum Pathol* 1994;25:304–307.
136. Pettit CK, Zukerberg LR, Gray MH, Ferry JA, Rosenberg AE, Harmon DC, Harris NL. Primary lymphoma of bone. A B-cell neoplasm with a high frequency of multilobated cells. *Am J Surg Pathol* 1990;14:329–334.
137. Resnick D, Haghighi P. Myeloproliferative disorders. In: Resnick D, ed. *Bone and joint imaging.* Philadelphia: WB Saunders, 1989; 703–714.
138. Salter M, Sollaccio RJ, Bernreuter WK, Weppelman B. Primary lymphoma of bone: the use of MRI in pretreatment evaluation. *Am J Clin Oncol* 1989;12:101–105.
139. Stein H, Kaiserling E, Lennert K. Evidence for B-cell origin of reticulum cell sarcoma. *Virchow's Arch (A)* 1974;A364:51–67.
140. Stiglbauer R, Augustin I, Kramer J, Schurawitzki H, Imhof H, Rodaszkiewicz T. MRI in the diagnosis of primary lymphoma of bone: correlation with histopathology. *J Comput Assist Tomogr* 1992; 16:248–253.
141. Vincent JM, NG YY, Norton AJ, Armstrong PA. Case report. Primary lymphoma of bone: MRI appearances with pathological correlation. *Clin Radiol* 1992;45:407–409.

Multiple Myeloma (Plasmacytoma)

142. Aggarwal S, Goulatia RK, Sood A, Prasad K, Ahuja GK, Mitchell M, Kumar A. POEMS syndrome: a rare variety of plasma cel dyscrasia. *Am J Roentgenol* 1990;155:339–341.
143. Avrahami E, Tadmor R, Kaplinsky N. The role of T2-weighted gradient echo in MRI demonstration of spinal multiple myeloma. *Spine* 1993;18:1812–1815.
144. Bardwick PA, Zvaifler NJ, Gill GN, Newman D, Greenway GD, Resnick D. Plasma-cell dyscrasia with polyneuropathy, organomegaly, endocrinopathy, M-protein and skin changes: the POEMS syndrome. Report on two cases and review of the literature. *Medicine* 1980;59:311–322.
145. Bataille R, Chevalier J, Ross M, Sany J. Bone scintigraphy in plasma-cell myeloma. *Radiology* 1982;145:801–804.
146. Bataille R, Sany J. Solitary myeloma: clinical and prognostic features of a review of 114 cases. *Cancer* 1981;48:845–851.
147. Bergsagel DE. Plasma cell myeloma. An interpretive review. *Cancer* 1972;30:1588–1594.
148. Bernstein SC, Perez-Atayde AR, Weinstein HJ. Multiple myeloma in a child. *Cancer* 1985;56:2143–2147.
149. Bessler W, Antonucci F, Stamm B, Stuckmann G, Vollrath T. Case report 646. POEMS syndrome. *Skeletal Radiol* 1991;20:212–215.
150. Bradwey TM, Murphy DA, Eyster RL, Cannon MW. Multiple myeloma in a 25-year-old woman. *Clin Orthop* 1993;294:290–293.
151. Brandon C, Martel W, Weatherbee L, Capek P. Case report 572. Osteosclerotic myeloma (POEMS syndrome). *Skeletal Radiol* 1989;18: 542–546.
152. Brown TS, Paterson CR. Osteosclerosis in myeloma. *J Bone Joint Surg* 1973;55B:621–623.
153. Campanacci M. Plasmacytoma. In: *Bone and soft tissue tumors.* New York: Springer-Verlag, 1990;560.
154. Dimopoulos MA, Moulopoulos A, Delasalle K, Alexanian R. Solitary plasmacytoma of bone and asymptomatic multiple myeloma. *Hematol Oncol Clin North Am* 1992;6:359–369.
155. Durie BGM, Salmon SE. A clinical staging system for multiple myeloma. *Cancer* 1975;36:842–854.
156. Dwyer AJ, Frank SL, Sank VJ, Reinig JW, Hickey AM, Doppman SL. Short TI inversion recovery pulse sequence: analysis and initial experience in cancer imaging. *Radiology* 1988;168:827–836.
157. Frassica DA, Frassica FJ, Schray MF, Sim FH, Kyle RA. Solitary plasmacytoma of bone: Mayo Clinic experience. *Int J Radiat Oncol Biol Phys* 1989;16:43–48.
158. Fruehwald FX, Tschalakoff D, Schwaighofer B, Wicke L, Neuhold A, Ludwig H, Hajek PC. Magnetic resonance imaging of the lower vertebral column in patients with multiple myeloma. *Invest Radiol* 1988; 23:193–199.

159. Hall FM, Gore SM. Osteosclerotic myeloma variant. *Skeletal Radiol* 1988;17:101–105.
160. Hermann H, Abdelwahab IF, Berson BD, Greenberg ML, Palestro CJ. Case report 621. Multiple myeloma (IgD) in a 28 year old woman. *Skeletal Radiol* 1990;19:379–381.
161. Hewell GM, Alexanian R. Multiple myeloma in young persons. *Ann Intern Med* 1976;84:441–443.
162. Hübner K. Pathologic anatomy of multiple myeloma. *Verh Dtsch Ges Path* 1983;671:423–439.
163. Ishida T, Dorfman HD. Plasma cell myeloma in unusually young patients: a report of two cases and review of the literature. *Skeletal Radiol* 1995;24:47–51.
164. Kelly JJ Jr, Kyle RA, Miles JM, Dyck PJ. Osteosclerotic myeloma and peripheral neuropathy. *Neurology* 1983;33:202–210.
165. Kyle RA, Bayrd ED. Amyloidosis: review of 236 cases. *Medicine* 1975;54:271–299.
166. Kyle RA. Diagnostic criteria of multiple myeloma. *Hematol Oncol Clin North Am* 1992;6:347–358.
167. Kyle RA. Multiple myeloma: review of 869 cases. *Mayo Clin Proc* 1975;50:29–40.
168. Lazarus HM, Kellermeyer RW, Aikaisa M, Herrig RH.: Multiple myeloma in young men: clinical course and electron microscopic studies of bone marrow plasma cells. *Cancer* 1980;46:1397–1400.
169. Lipshitz HI, Malthouse SR, Cunningham D, MacVicar AD, Husband JE. Multiple myeloma: appearance at MR imaging. *Radiology* 1992;182:833–837.
170. Meis JM, Butler JJ, Osborne BM, Ordonez NG. Solitary plasmacytomas of bone and extramedullary plasmacytomas. A clinicopathologic and immunohistochemical study. *Cancer* 1987;59:1475–1485.
171. Meyer JE, Schulz MD. Solitary myeloma of bone: a review of 12 cases. *Cancer* 1974;34:438–440.
172. Moulopoulos LA, Varma DGK, Dimopoulos MA, Leeds NE, Kim EE, Johnston DA, Alexanian R, Lipshitz HI. Multiple myeloma: spinal MR imaging in patients with untreated newly diagnosed disease. *Radiology* 1992;185:833–840.
173. Murray RO, Jacobson HG. *The radiology of bone diseases*, 2nd ed. New York: Churchill Livingstone, 1977.
174. Nilsson-Ehle H, Holmdahl C, Suurkula M, Westin J. Bone scintigraphy in the diagnosis of skeletal involvement and metastatic calcification in plasma cell-related dyscrasia. *Acta Med Scand* 1982;211:427–432.
175. Rahmouni A, Divine M, Mathieu D, Golli M, Dao TH, Jazaerli N, Anglade MC, Reyes F, Vasile N. Detection of multiple myeloma involving the spine: efficacy of fat-suppression and contrast-enhanced MR imaging. *Am J Roentgenol* 1993;160:1049–1052.
176. Reinus WR, Kyriakos M, Gilula LA, Brower AC, Merkel K. Plasma cell tumors with calcified amyloid deposition mistaken for chondrosarcoma. *Radiology* 1993;189:505–509.
177. Resnick D, Greenway GD, Bardwick PA, Zvaifler NJ, Gill GN, Newman DR. Plasma cell dyscrasia with polyneuropathy, organomegaly, endocrinopathy, M-protein, and skin changes: the POEMS syndrome. *Radiology* 1981;140:17–22.
178. Resnick D, Haghighi P, Guerra J Jr. Bone sclerosis and proliferaiton in a man with multisystem disease. *Invest Radiol* 1984;19:1–6.
179. Ricci C, Cova M, Kang YS, et al. Normal age-related patterns of cellular and fatty bone marrow distribution in the axial skeleton: MR imaging study. *Radiology* 1990;177:83–88.
180. Sartoris DJ, Pate D, Haghighi P, Greenway G, Resnick D. Plasma cell sclerosis of bone: a spectrum of disease. *Can Assoc Radiol J* 1986;37:25–34.
181. Shimpo S. Solitary myeloma causing polyneuritis and endocrine disorders. *Jpn J Clin Med* 1968;26:2444–2456.
182. Solomon A, Rahamani R, Seligsohn U, Ben-Artzi F. Multiple myeloma: early vertebral involvement assessed by computerized tomography. *Skeletal Radiol* 1984;11:258–261.
183. Stäbler A, Baur A, Bartl R, Munker R, Lamerz R, Reiser MF. Contrast enhancement and quantitative signal analysis in MR imaging of multiple myeloma: assessment of focal and diffuse growth patterns in marrow correlated with biopsies and survival rates. *Am J Roentgenol* 1996;167:1029–1036.
184. Steiner RM, Mitchell DG, Rao VM, Schweitzer ME. Magnetic resonance imaging of diffuse bone marrow disease. *Radiol Clin North Am* 1993;31:383–409.
185. Tertti R, Alanen A, Remes K. The value of magnetic resonance imaging in screening myeloma lesions of the lumbar spine. *Br J Haematol* 1995;91:658–660.
186. Wilner D. *Radiology of bone tumors and allied disorders.* Philadelphia: Lea and Febiger, 1982.
187. Woolfenden JM, Pitt MJ, Durie BGM, Moon TE. Comparison of bone scintigraphy and radiography in multiple myeloma. *Radiology* 1980;134:723–728.

CHAPTER 6

Vascular Lesions

BENIGN LESIONS
  Intraosseous Hemangioma
  Cystic Angiomatosis
  Lymphangioma and Lymphangiomatosis
  Glomus Tumor, Glomangioma, and
    Glomangiomyoma

MALIGNANT LESIONS
  Hemangioendothelioma
  Angiosarcoma
  Hemangiopericytoma

INTRODUCTION

Vascular lesions of bone constitute a spectrum of pathologic entities ranging from benign neoplasms (some of which may represent congenital vascular malformations, e.g., hemangioma) to highly malignant tumors that metastasize widely and have low survival rates (e.g., angiosarcoma) (82). Benign conditions, such as hemangioma, lymphangioma, lymphangiomatosis, hemangiomatosis, cystic angiomatosis, and even massive osteolysis or Gorham disease, are sometimes considered part of the spectrum of a single disease process despite attempts to identify features that would allow differentiation among these disorders (64,70). Benign vascular lesions are of either endothelial or pericytic origin. The first group includes hemangiomas and cystic angiomatosis. The second group includes glomus tumor and its variants, glomangioma and glomangiomyoma. The malignant and locally aggressive varieties are quite uncommon and they, too, are of either endothelial (hemangioendothelioma and angiosarcoma) or pericytic (hemangiopericytoma) origin.

BENIGN LESIONS

Intraosseous Hemangioma

Hemangioma is a benign lesion composed of newly formed blood vessels, often discovered incidentally on radiographs performed for other reasons. It composes approximately 2% of all benign and 0.8% of benign and malignant lesions of the skeletal system (60). Although its name suggests a neoplastic nature, the behavior of hemangioma is that of a vascular malformation (62). On the basis of their site of

origin, hemangiomas in general are classified as intraosseous, intracortical, periosteal, intraarticular (synovial), intramuscular, subcutaneous, or cutaneous. Depending on its vascular composition (i.e., the nature and size of the vessels predominating within the lesion), hemangioma is subclassified into capillary, cavernous, venous, arteriovenous, and mixed types (2). Capillary hemangiomas are composed of small vessels that consist merely of a flat endothelium, surrounded only by a basal membrane. In bone they most commonly occur in the vertebral body (70). Cavernous hemangiomas are composed of dilated, blood-filled spaces lined by the same flat endothelium with a basal membrane. Osseous cavernous hemangiomas most commonly involve the calvaria (24). Venous hemangiomas are composed of thick-walled vessels that possess a muscle layer. They frequently contain phleboliths. Arteriovenous hemangiomas are characterized by abnormal communications between arteries and veins (17). These are extremely rare in bone and almost exclusively involve the soft tissues (2).

The biologic classification of vascular anomalies has recently gained renewed attention (55). Based on a system by Mulliken and Glowacki (61), who advocate regarding hemangiomas as hamartomas rather than true neoplasms, this classification takes into consideration cellular turnover and histology, as well as natural history and physical findings. It clearly separates hemangiomas of infancy, with their early proliferative and later involutional stages, from vascular malformations, which are characterized as arterial, venous, capillary, lymphatic, or combined (55,61). However, epithelioid hemangiomas have been observed that apparently are true tumors (24).

Clinical Presentation

The incidence of intraosseous hemangiomas increases with age, and most patients present after their fourth decade. The majority of patients are asymptomatic and women are affected twice as often as men. The most common sites are vertebral bodies of the spine (particularly the thoracic segment) and the skull. Hemangiomas of the long bones (e.g., femur, humerus) and short tubular bones are less often encountered (22) (Fig. 1). Calvarial hemangiomas most commonly affect the frontal and parietal regions, and account for 20% of all intraosseous hemangiomas (57). These lesions arise in the diploic space and cause expansion that often involves the outer table to a great extent (63). Vertebral hemangiomas are very common and are observed in 11% of autopsied cases (40). They account for 28% of all skeletal hemangiomas (57). In this location the lesion typically involves the vertebral body, although it may extend into the lamina and, rarely, into the spinous process. Multiple vertebrae are sometimes affected. The majority of vertebral hemangiomas are asymptomatic and are discovered incidentally. Symptoms occur when the affected vertebra expands in the direction of the spinal cord and causes compression (27,54,70). This neurologic complication is most commonly associated with lesions in the midthoracic spine (34,47,58). Another mechanism considered responsible for compression of the cord, although less frequently, is a fracture of the involved vertebral body and the formation of a soft tissue mass or hematoma (5,8).

Imaging

On radiography, an osseous hemangioma in a long or short tubular bone is characterized by coarse striations or by multifocal lytic areas (48,77) (Fig. 2). Periosteal and cortical hemangiomas occur most commonly in the anterior tibial diaphysis. These lesions present as lytic, cortical erosions, occasionally accompanied by a periosteal reaction. In the vertebral body, hemangioma is characterized either by vertical striations or by multiloculated lytic foci (85). These are referred to as a corduroy cloth pattern (Fig. 3A) or honeycomb pattern (Fig. 3B), respectively, and are considered virtually pathognomonic for this lesion (48). A calvarial hemangioma commonly appears as a lytic lesion that exhibits a radiating configuration of thickened trabeculae, frequently arranged in a spoke-wheel or web-like pattern (63).

On CT scan, vertebral hemangioma characteristically exhibits a pattern of multiple dots (often referred to as the "polka-dot" appearance), representing a cross-section of reinforced trabeculae (Fig. 4).

On MRI, T1- and T2-weighted images usually reveal areas of a high-intensity signal that correspond to the vascular components (38,73) (Fig. 5). Areas of trabecular thickening exhibit a low signal intensity regardless of the pulse sequence used (63). Both computed tomography (CT) and magnetic resonance imaging (MRI) obtained after intra-

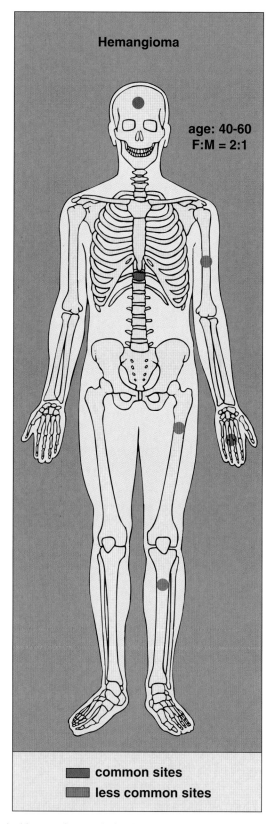

FIG. 1. Hemangioma: skeletal sites of predilection, peak age range, and male-to-female ratio.

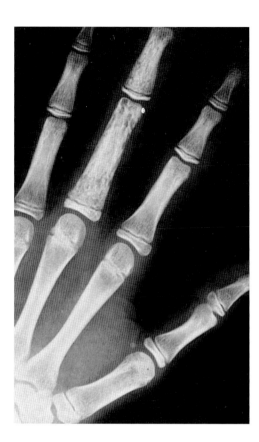

FIG. 2. Intraosseous hemangioma. Dorsovolar radiograph of the right hand of an 11-year-old girl with hemangioma involving the middle finger shows the lace-like pattern and honeycombing characteristic of this lesion.

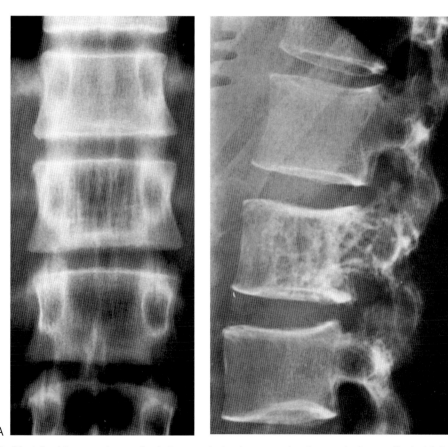

A   B

FIG. 3. Vertebral hemangioma. **A:** Anteroposterior tomography demonstrates vertical striations of hemangioma of L1 vertebra, referred to as a "corduroy cloth" pattern. **B:** Lateral radiograph of the lumbar spine demonstrates a "honeycomb" pattern of hemangioma of L2 vertebra.

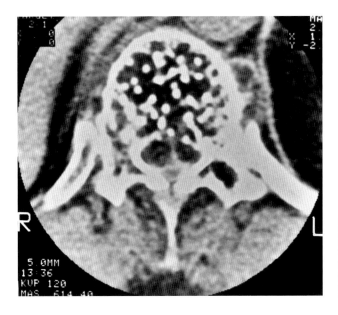

FIG. 4. Vertebral hemangioma: computed tomography. CT section of a T10 vertebra demonstrates coarse dots that indicate reinforced vertical trabeculae of the cancellous bone, characteristic of hemangioma.

venous administration of contrast material demonstrate a lesion enhancement (14,63,80).

On scintigraphy, the appearance of osseous hemangiomas ranges from photopenia (28) to a moderate increase in the uptake of radiopharmaceutical tracer (44,52,59). A recent study of single photon emission computed tomography (SPECT) imaging of vertebral hemangiomas and their correlation with

MRI showed that in most cases hemangiomas exhibited normal uptake on planar images. SPECT images were also normal, particularly if the lesions were <3 cm in diameter. This study also showed a disparity between SPECT images and MRI: there was no correlation between MRI signal intensity changes and patterns of uptake on bone imaging (37). Arteriography of the hemangioma is rarely indicated (49).

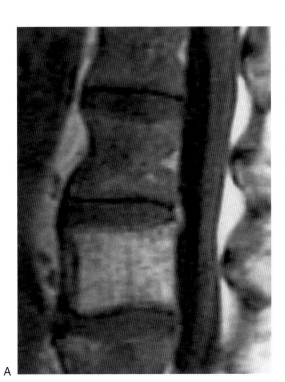
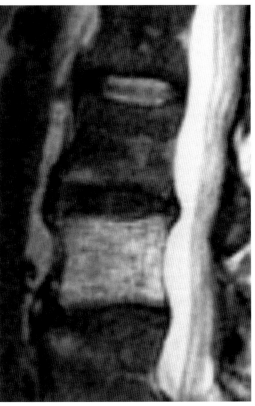

A   B

FIG. 5. Vertebral hemangioma: magnetic resonance imaging **(A)** Sagittal T1-weighted (SE, TR 517, TE 12) and **(B)** T2-weighted (SE, TR 2000, TE 80) MR images show high signal intensity of hemangioma of L4 vertebra.

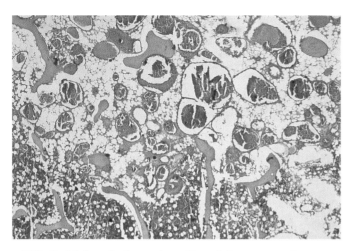

FIG. 6. Histopathology of capillary intraosseous hemangioma. Blood vessels of capillary character and partly of cavernous type lie between small bone trabeculae and border normal cancellous bone of the vertebrae containing hematopoietic marrow (*below*) (hematoxylin and eosin, original magnification ×25).

Histopathology

On histologic examination, most hemangiomas consist of simple channels formed by an endothelium-lined basal membrane, morphologically identical with normal capillaries (Fig. 6). The lining endothelial cells are small, flat, uniform, and inconspicuous (40). Mitotic figures are rarely seen (19). Some or all of the vascular channels may be enlarged and may have a sinusoidal appearance, in which case the lesion is referred to as cavernous type (Fig. 7), which incidentally is the most common, particularly in the calvaria (25). These lesions are composed of multiple large, thin-walled, dilated, blood-filled vascular spaces lined by endothelial cells (40). The hemangiomatous tissue often spreads between the preexisting bone trabeculae without distorting the

original bone pattern (60). Occasionally they are composed of larger, thick-walled arteries or veins and resemble arteriovenous malformations of the soft tissues (25,87).

Differential Diagnosis

Radiology

Solitary hemangioma in a small tubular bone, such as a metacarpal or metatarsal, may exhibit an expansive appearance, thus mimicking an *aneurysmal bone cyst* (18). In a long tubular bone, particularly when the lesion is predominantly radiolucent, a focus of *fibrous dysplasia* may be the consideration.

In a vertebra, the differential possibilities include *Paget disease, myeloma* (plasmacytoma), and *metastasis,* and in a younger patient hemangioma may mimic a *Langerhans cell granuloma.* In patients with a significant degree of *osteopenia,* the vertebrae sometimes exhibit vertical linear streaks, similar to the appearance of vertebral hemangioma (Fig. 8). In Paget disease, the vertebral body, unlike in hemangioma, is frequently enlarged, particularly dorsally, and the vertebral endplates are either indistinct or markedly sclerotic ("picture frame" appearance) (Fig. 9). If vertical striations are present, they are not so neatly arranged as in hemangioma (60). Myeloma and metastasis may exhibit lytic changes of the vertebral body, but there is no evidence of vertical striation. Conversely, hemangioma may present as a purely lytic lesion (Fig. 10). Langerhans cell granuloma usually presents as a collapsed vertebra (vertebra plana), whereas hemangiomas of the vertebra exhibit pathologic fractures only in exceptional cases.

Pathology

On microscopic examination, intraosseous hemangioma cannot be distinguished from *skeletal angiomatosis* (46). Differentiation is therefore based on the extensive nature of

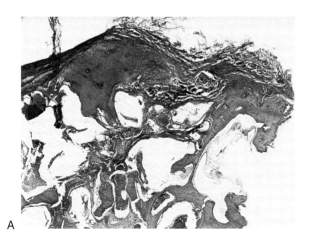
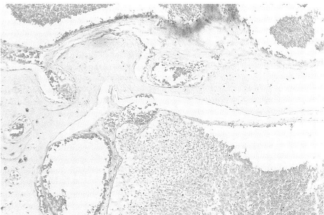

FIG. 7. Histopathology of cavernous intraosseous hemangioma. **A:** Cortical bone (*top*) and cancellous bone (*bottom*) stained red enclosing large, mostly empty vascular spaces (van Gieson, original magnification ×6). **B:** At higher magnification large vascular spaces filled with blood cells lie in the marrow spaces of cancellous bone. Surfaces of the trabeculae are lined with osteoblasts (hematoxylin and eosin, original magnification ×25).

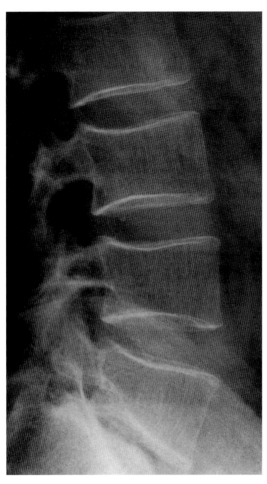

FIG. 8. Differential diagnosis of vertebral hemangioma: osteopenia. Vertical striations in the vertebral bodies secondary to osteopenia mimic hemangioma.

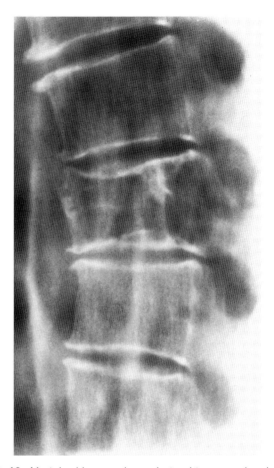

FIG. 10. Vertebral hemangioma. Lateral tomography shows a purely lytic hemangioma of the posterior part of vertebral body Th6. This presentation may be mistaken for metastasis or myeloma.

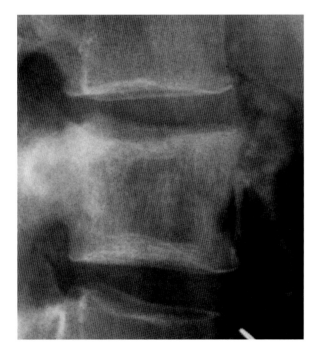

FIG. 9. Differential diagnosis of vertebral hemangioma: Paget disease. Vertebral body of L2 is enlarged, and the vertebral endplates are thickened, creating a "picture frame" appearance.

the latter (25). The differential diagnosis from *epithelioid hemangioendothelioma* and *angiosarcoma* should not create too much difficulty because flat, normal-appearing endothelial cells usually line the vascular spaces of hemangioma. There are, however, occasional cases in which, in addition to the conventional intraosseous hemangioma tissue, transitional forms of endothelial cells, similar to those seen in hemangioendothelioma, are present.

The radiologic and pathologic differential diagnosis of intraosseous hemangioma is depicted in Fig. 11.

Synovial Hemangioma

Synovial hemangioma is a rare benign lesion of the synovium that most commonly affects the knee articulation. This entity is discussed in Chapter 9.

Cystic Angiomatosis

Angiomatosis is defined as a diffuse involvement of bones by hemangiomatous lesions (12,24,31,32,36,56, 65,69), although some investigators also include under this rubric cases of lymphangiomatosis (24,25,70). The radiographic presentation of angiomatosis is that of lytic lesions, often with a honeycomb or lattice work ("hole-within-hole") appearance (11). When bone is extensively involved, the term cystic angiomatosis is applied (50,68). Some other terms used for this condition include diffuse skeletal

hemangiomatosis (56,84), cystic lymphangiectasia (39), and hamartous hemolymphangiomatosis (75). This is a rare bone disorder characterized by diffuse cystic lesions of bone, frequently (60% to 70% of cases) associated with visceral involvement (18,42). Schajowicz postulated that diffuse hemangiomatosis should be distinguished from cystic angiomatosis because of their different radiologic and macroscopic aspects (74). On histologic examination, cystic angiomatosis is characterized by cavernous angiomatous spaces, indistinguishable from benign hemangioma of bone.

Another condition that must be distinguished is so-called Gorham disease of bone (30), also known by the names massive osteolysis (81), disappearing bone disease, and phantom bone disease (16,29). This condition is characterized by progressive, localized bone resorption (43), probably caused by multiple or diffuse cavernous hemangiomas or lymphangiomas of bone or by a combination of both (74). The radiographic presentation of Gorham disease consists of radiolucent areas in the cancellous bone or concentric destruction of the cortex, giving rise to a sucked-candy appearance (25). Eventually, the entire medullary cavity and the cortex are destroyed (4,83). On histologic examination, a marked increase is observed in intraosseous capillaries, which form an anastomosing network of endothelium-lined channels that are usually filled with erythrocytes or serum (74). Although some investigators claim that there is no evidence of osteoclasts in areas of bone resorption (29), recent studies suggest that osteoclastic activity plays a role in pathogenesis of Gorham disease (78).

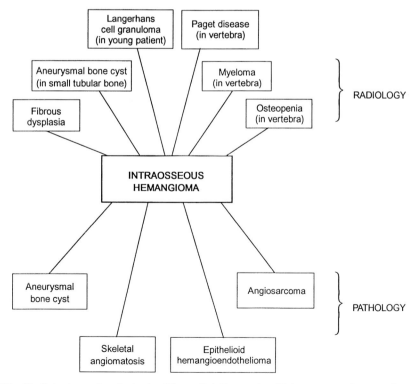

FIG. 11. Radiologic and pathologic differential diagnosis of intraosseous hemangioma.

Clinical Presentation

Patients with cystic angiomatosis usually present in the first three decades (63). There is 2:1 male to female predominance. The bones affected are most often those of the axial skeleton, as well as the femur, humerus, tibia, radius, and fibula (18,24,65) (Fig. 12). The bone-related symptoms are usually secondary to pathologic fractures through the cystic lesions. Most of the symptoms, however, are related to visceral involvement.

Imaging

On plain radiography, the osseous lesions are usually osteolytic (Fig. 13), occasionally with a honeycomb appearance (Fig. 14). They are well defined and surrounded by a rim of sclerosis, and they vary in size (13,51) (Fig. 15). Although medullary involvement predominates, cortical invasion, osseous expansion, and periosteal reaction can occur (18). Rarely, sclerotic lesions may be present (69), and in these instances the condition may mimic osteoblastic metastases (41). On MRI the lesions usually show an intermediate signal intensity on T1-weighted images, and T2-weighted images with fat saturation show a mixture of high, intermediate, and low signal intensities (7,66).

Histopathology

Whether cystic angiomatosis is truly of blood vessel origin or of lymphatic derivation, or even represents a mixture of the two, is difficult to decide in a given case (40). On gross examination, the lesions of cystic angiomatosis resemble simple bone cysts (18). They consist of large cavities lined by a dull yellowish gray membrane (69). Multiple communicating cysts, separated by thickened trabeculae of mature lamellar bone but without osteoblastic rimming (41), may also be present, producing a honeycomb appearance (71). In some cases osteoid and immature woven bone formation with rimming of active osteoblasts was reported (41). Histologically, the lesions are indistinguishable from those observed in capillary or cavernous hemangiomas (18). They contain multiple dilated, thin-walled vascular channels lined by flat endothelial cells.

Differential Diagnosis

Radiology

The predominant differential diagnosis must include *polyostotic fibrous dysplasia, enchondromatosis, Langerhans cell histiocytosis,* multiple *brown tumors of hyperparathyroidism,* and pseudotumors of hemophilia. In older patients, although the diagnosis of *metastatic disease* (33) or *multiple myeloma* must be considered, these conditions usually can be easily distinguished on the basis of both radiologic and clinical examinations. The osteosclerotic variant of cystic angiomatosis must be differentiated from *osteoblastic*

metastases (1, 15,41), *sclerosing variant of myeloma* (84), *lymphoma* (26), and *mastocytosis* (6). Careful interpretation of the radiographs may reveal the presence of mixed sclerotic and lytic lesions in cystic angiomatosis, a feature that is helpful in excluding some of the mentioned entities.

Pathology

Microscopically, the differential diagnosis of cystic angiomatosis should include *massive osteolysis* (Gorham disease). Because both lesions are pathologically almost identical, the diagnosis is based on clinical findings (25).

The radiologic and pathologic differential diagnosis of cystic angiomatosis is depicted in Fig. 16.

Lymphangioma and Lymphangiomatosis

Lymphangioma is a rare benign bone disorder, first described in 1947 by Bickel and Broders (9). The lesion is composed of sequestered, noncommunicating lymphoid tissue lined by lymphatic endothelium (24). The cause of this lesion is believed to be a congenital obstruction of lymphatic drainage. Lymphangiomas, similar to hemangiomas, are classified and subclassified, according to the size of the vessels, as capillary, cavernous, cystic, or mixed (20). The cystic variety is most common.

Clinical Presentation

There is no sex predilection and no hereditary tendency (53). The vast majority of these disorders are soft tissue lesions, with osseous involvement being rare (23,45). The most common sites of involvement are the diaphyses or metaphyses of the tibia and the humerus, as well as ilium, skull, mandible, and vertebrae (35,79). These lesions are usually discovered at birth (50% to 65% of cases) or at least within the first 2 years of life (90%) (10,63). The lesion may be solitary or multifocal (72). When the lesions are multiple, the term lymphangiomatosis is applied (79,86).

Imaging

On radiography, these lesions are indistinguishable from hemangiomas and hemangiomatosis (see above), exhibiting a multiple or multilocular expansive osteolytic appearance (3,21). In some cases the margin may have a "soap-bubble" appearance, whereas in others it may be quite poorly defined, with a moth-eaten pattern of bone destruction (76) (Fig. 17).

A CT scan can be useful in demonstrating the relative sparing of the medullary cavity in preference to the cortex (35,53). MRI demonstrates bone lacunae displaying a hypointense signal on T1-weighted and a hyperintense signal on T2-weighted images, which indicates the presence of a liquid-filled lesion. There is no enhancement after gadolinium injection (53). Lymphography is very effective for

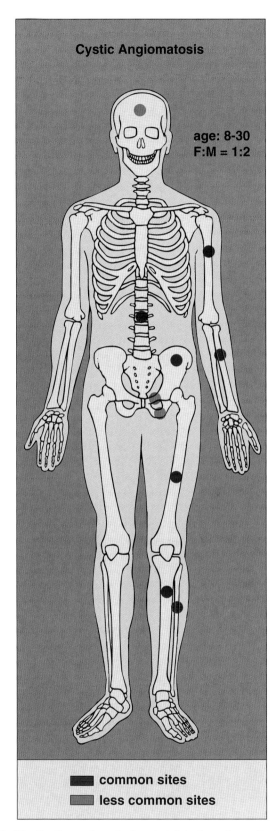

FIG. 12. Cystic angiomatosis: skeletal sites of predilection, peak age range, and male-to-female ratio.

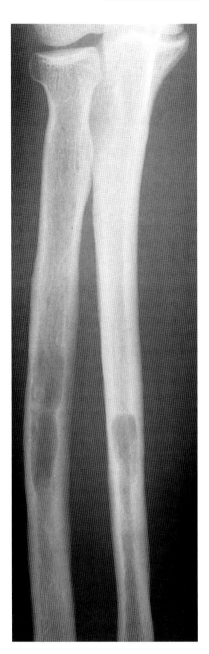

FIG. 13. Cystic angiomatosis. Several osteolytic lesions affect the shafts of the radius and ulna in this 25-year-old man.

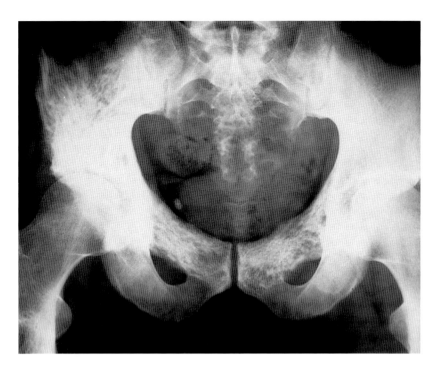

FIG. 14. Cystic angiomatosis. A 28-year-old man with honeycomb pattern seen in the right ilium and both pubic bones.

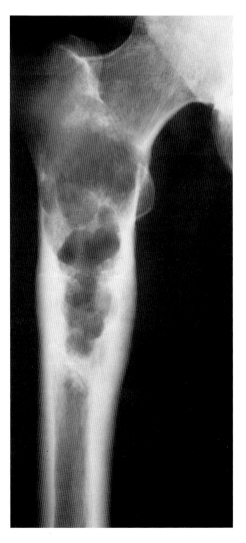

FIG. 15. Cystic angiomatosis. Several confluent lesions with peripheral sclerosis and cortical thickening are seen in the right femur of a 20-year-old man.

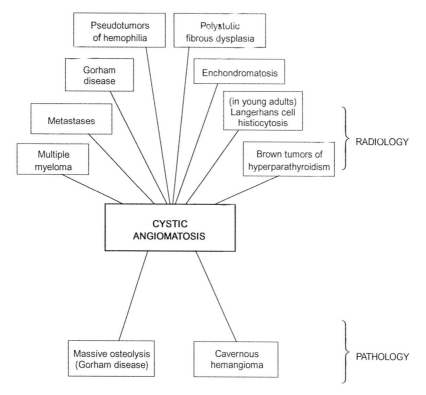

FIG. 16. Radiologic and pathologic differential diagnosis of cystic angiomatosis.

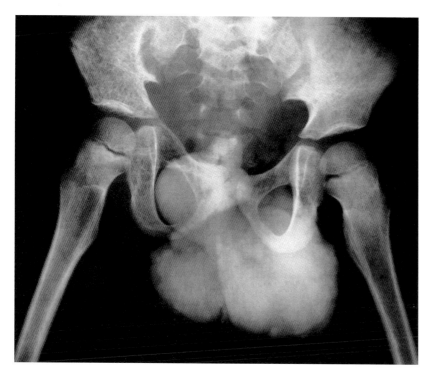

FIG. 17. Skeletal lymphangiomatosis. A 2-year-old boy presented with multiple bony lesions, particularly affecting the pelvis and proximal femora. Note honeycomb and moth-eaten pattern of bone destruction. In addition to skeletal involvement, lymphangiomas were also present in the soft tissues.

demonstration of abnormal and dilated lymphatic channels filling the cystic bone lesions (67).

Histopathology

The histopathology of lymphangioma is essentially the same as that of hemangioma. The most common is the cystic capillary form.

Differential Diagnosis

Radiology

Based on the radiographic appearance, the differential diagnosis must include *lymphoma, plasmacytoma,* and *fibrosarcoma* when the lesion is solitary, and *metastatic neuroblastoma, hemangiomatosis, Langerhans cell histiocytosis, polyostotic fibrous dysplasia, congenital fibromatosis,* and *Gaucher disease* when there is polyostotic involvement.

Pathology

Because the wall of a lymphatic vessel is structurally identical in histology to that of a blood capillary (see above), most investigators base their differential diagnosis on the presence or absence of erythrocytes in the lumen. Nevertheless, it is possible that an erythrocyte may be found in a lumen of a lymphatic vessel because of artificial translocation during the histologic preparation of the tissue. Therefore, this finding does not constitute an absolute proof of whether the vessel is lymphatic or not. The differential diagnosis is therefore the same as for hemangioma (see above).

Glomus Tumor, Glomangioma, and Glomangiomyoma

Glomus tumor and its variants, glomangioma and glomangiomyoma, are extremely rare benign lesions of bone composed of rounded uniform cells often arranged in a brick-work-like manner. They are intimately associated with vascular structures and are derived from the neuromyoarterial glomus (24). Of the three, the glomus tumor is most common, whereas the other two are very rare. The occurrence of a glomus tumor primarily arising in the bone (only about 100 published cases), rather than originating in the adjacent soft tissues and eroding bone secondarily, is extremely rare (40). At one time this tumor was considered to derive from the above-mentioned neuromyoarterial glomus, a neurovascular structure. At present, however, the smooth muscle cells of this lesion are considered to be the stem cells.

Clinical Presentation

The vast majority of intraosseous glomus tumors occur at the fingertips (89), arising in the distal phalanges (88). Very rarely they affect the coccyx. Patients are adults in the third to fifth decade, with a female predilection. The main clinical symptoms include localized pain and exquisite point tenderness (92). Exposure to cold or minimal trauma may induce severe paroxysmal attacks of pain (70).

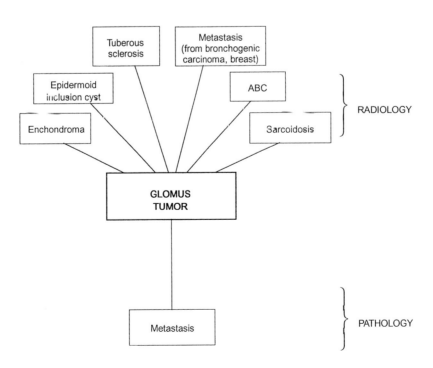

FIG. 18. Radiologic and pathologic differential diagnosis of glomus tumor.

Imaging

On radiography, glomus tumor presents as a small, lytic bony defect with sharply marginated edges, usually located at the dorsal aspect of the distal phalanx. If the lesion arises primarily in the soft tissue and erodes bone secondarily, an adjacent soft tissue mass is present (63). On CT examination, a nonspecific subungual mass is demonstrated, with an attenuation value similar to that of other soft tissue lesions. On T2-weighted MR images the lesion exhibits a homogeneous high signal intensity (63,91).

Histopathology

Histologically, the lesion is composed of lobules, strands, and broad sheets of rounded, uniform glomus cells, often arranged in the above-mentioned brick-work-like manner, with indistinct capillaries in the walls of the surrounding large blood vessels (22,24). In glomangioma, the larger blood vessels are more conspicuous, with the tumor cells arranged in smaller areas within their walls. In glomangiomyoma, spindle cells resembling smooth muscle cells are found in variable numbers (25).

Differential Diagnosis

Radiology

On plain radiography the lesion closely resembles an *enchondroma* (90). Other lesions that should be included in the differential diagnosis are e*pidermal inclusion cyst, metastasis* (particularly from a bronchogenic carcinoma), *aneurysmal bone cyst, sarcoidosis,* and *tuberous sclerosis* (88).

Pathology

The differentiation of this tumor from other entities is usually easy because of its conspicuous clinical behavior. Histologically, a *metastasis* from a small cell epithelial or mesenchymal tumor must be taken into account. The very regular arrangement of the glomus tumor cells and their connection with the walls of larger vessels are helpful in making the distinction.

The radiologic and pathologic differential diagnosis of glomus tumor is depicted in Fig. 18.

MALIGNANT LESIONS

The existing nomenclature used to describe malignant vascular tumors is not uniform and therefore can be confusing. Different terms, including hemangiosarcoma (angiosarcoma), hemangioendothelioma, and hemangioendothelial sarcoma, have been used as synonyms, or the tumors have been classified into different grades, from grade I hemangioendothelioma (well-differentiated) to grade III hemangiosarcoma (poorly differentiated) (74). Because of the confusion that still prevails, the World Health Organization (WHO) classification system, although recently revised, continues to classify these lesions as intermediate or indeterminate (including hemangioendothelioma and hemangiopericytoma) and clearly malignant (angiosarcoma). However, an unequivocal distinction among these tumors is sometimes difficult (74).

Hemangioendothelioma

A lesion in which the vascular channels are densely arranged with multiple communications and in which the endothelial cells are somewhat plump and atypical is uncommon. When such areas predominate in a vascular tumor, the lesion is referred to as hemangioendothelioma. The synonyms used for hemangioendothelioma, most notably hemangioendothelial sarcoma and low-grade angiosarcoma, reflect the uncertainty of pathologists in predicting their biologic behavior. More recently, the term epithelioid hemangioendothelioma has been preferred by most investigators (74,113,119,124,125). Hemangioendotheliomas are considered true neoplasms rather than malformations because of their independent growth potential, because of the nuclear atypia that is frequently present, accompanied by occasional mitotic activity, and because they not uncommonly recur after inadequate local excision (100). Some of these lesions may appear to behave in a benign fashion. In general, however, the biologic behavior of hemangioendothelioma cannot be predicted, and it is therefore regarded as a bone tumor of low-grade malignancy (97). Characteristic for this tumor is the formation of irregular, anastomosing vascular channels that are lined with atypical endothelial cells that have an anaplastic and immature appearance (107). Hemangioendotheliomas constitute <1% of all the primary malignant tumors of bone (64,126).

Clinical Presentation

Hemangioendothelioma can occur at any age within a range of 10 to 75 years. The lesion may be solitary or multicentric (98). There is a slightly more common predilection for males in the second and third decades (63). Patients affected by multifocal disease are, on average, 10 years younger than those with a solitary lesion. Osseous hemangioendotheliomas most commonly affect the calvaria, spine, and bones of the lower extremities. They may occur in any part of a bone, and it is not unusual to see multiple lesions in contiguous anatomic sites (e.g., in several carpal or tarsal bones).

Hemangioendothelioma usually causes dull local pain and tenderness; some swelling may also be observed, and hemorrhagic joint effusion sometimes occurs (74). A vertebral location for this tumor is characterized by radiculopathy. Symptoms are quite variable in their duration, ranging from a few weeks to many years (average 5 months) (107). A soft tissue mass or a pathologic fracture is only rarely the presenting symptom.

Imaging

On radiography, hemangioendothelioma exhibits an osteolytic appearance; it may be well circumscribed or may have a wide zone of transition. There may be variable degrees of peripheral sclerosis, sharply demarcating the lesion. Frequently a soap-bubble appearance with expansion of bone is observed, with occasional extension into the soft tissues (25). However, unless there is an associated pathologic fracture, a soft tissue mass is usually not present. Scintigraphy shows an increased uptake of the radiopharmaceutical tracer (95,110). On MRI the tumor shows a mixed signal on T1-weighted images with moderate increase in the signal intensity on T2 weighting (116,120) (Fig. 19).

Histopathology

On histologic examination, hemangioendothelioma reveals endothelial cells with abundant faintly eosinophilic or amphophilic cytoplasm (121). The interanastomosing vascular channels, often arranged in an antler-like pattern, are delimited by a basal membrane (Fig. 20). Markedly pleomorphic endothelial cells, with hyperchromatic nuclei and prominent nucleoli, are attached to this membrane (107). Individual cells may exhibit intracytoplasmic lumina of variable size, whose diameters often approximate that of an entrapped erythrocyte. Larger lumina appear to be formed as the result of fusion of their smaller intracytoplasmic counterparts. A residual strand of attenuated cytoplasm frequently bridges the opening. Although mitotic figures may be absent, one or two figures per 10 high-power fields are usually seen. An inflammatory infiltrate is often present, consisting of various percentages of eosinophils, lymphocytes, and plasma cells. Rarely, eosinophils predominate and other inflammatory elements are virtually absent. Small foci of hemorrhage or necrosis may be observed (129). The stroma typically varies from fibrous to myxoid, and may appear more hyalinized, thus resembling a hyaline cartilage-like matrix (25). That the cells composing these tumors are differentiated is evident from their frequent positive immunohistochemical staining for Factor VIII and for the lectin *Ulex europaeus.*

Weiss et al. emphasized four major patterns, often characterized by transitional zones. These include (a) plump, polygonal, or elongated cells possessing large vacuoles that resemble signet ring cells; (b) aggregates of the above cells arranged into elongated cords or clusters; (c) formation of vascular lumina, which may be interconnected and may also contain erythrocytes; and (d) solid or spindle cell areas that sometimes contain nests of cells (128). The first three patterns are usually seen in association with a myxoid or chondromyxoid stromal background. The former pattern is sometimes called myxoid angioblastoma (25).

Criteria for the grading of hemangioendothelioma include mitotic rate, degree of atypia, presence of necrosis, and the morphologic features of their vascular spaces.

Certain hemangioendotheliomas can be classified as the epithelioid (histiocytoid) subtype when the endothelial cells have an epithelioid appearance (93,109,114,124). These are considered to be borderline or low-grade malignancies and consist of endothelial cells with a conspicuous cytoplasm that imparts an epithelioid (histiocytoid) appearance (25). The stroma is scant but may assume a myxoid character. The term "epithelioid" or "histiocytoid" was chosen because of the resemblance to the lesion originally described by Rosai et al. and named histiocytoid hemangioma (117).

Spindle-cell hemangioendothelioma is a recently described rare tumor of borderline malignancy, exhibiting histologic features of both cavernous hemangioma and Kaposi sarcoma (105,128).

Differential Diagnosis

Radiology

On radiologic studies it is very difficult to differentiate hemangioendothelioma from other vascular lesions, both benign and malignant. A solitary osteolytic lesion may mimic a *metastasis, fibrosarcoma, MFH, plasmacytoma,* or *lymphoma.* Lesions with a sclerotic border may resemble a *Brodie abscess, intraosseous ganglion, enchondroma,* or *chondroblastoma,* and those extending to the articular end of bone can be mistaken for a *giant-cell tumor.* A multicentric presentation should be differentiated from other polyostotic conditions, such as *brown tumors of hyperparathyroidism, pseudotumors of hemophilia, metastatic disease,* and *multiple myeloma.* When lytic lesions are seen predominantly in the cortex, the metastatic disease is a strong consideration (33,104). Because the radiologic presentation of hemangioendothelioma is usually nonspecific, clinical information may be helpful in narrowing the differential diagnosis.

Pathology

The differential diagnosis of epithelioid hemangioendothelioma includes metastatic adenocarcinoma, adamantinoma of the long bones, angiosarcoma ("malignant hemangioendothelioma"), myxoid chondrosarcoma, telangiectatic osteosarcoma, and melanoma. The differentiation between hemangioendothelioma and *angiosarcoma* is in many cases an arbitrary one, as a clear distinction is not possible because areas with the characteristics of the first tumor may merge into areas with the picture of the latter (see below). Only the clinical follow-up, particularly the development of recurrences and metastases, can provide the key to correct diagnosis. The vascular, often antler-like arrangement, as described above, is characteristic of a hemangioendothelial tumor and not for *carcinoma* or *melanoma.* Monoclonal antibodies directed against keratins of various molecular weights will identify the presence of carcinoma cells,

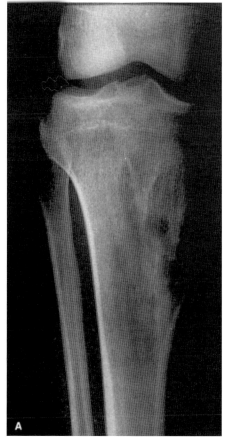

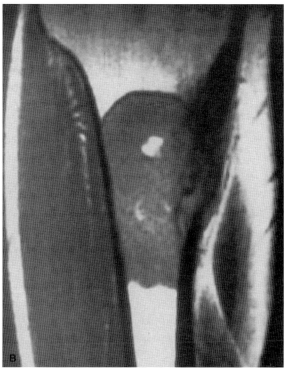

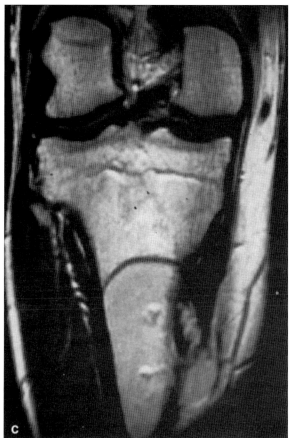

FIG. 19. Hemangioendothelioma: magnetic resonance imaging. **A:** An anteroposterior radiograph of the proximal tibia shows a radiolucent destructive lesion affecting mainly the medial aspect of the bone. The cortex is destroyed. **B:** Coronal T1-weighted MRI shows a low-signal-intensity tumor replacing bone marrow. Small foci of high signal represent hemorrhagic areas. **C:** Coronal T2-weighted MRI demonstrates an increase in the signal intensity of the tumor, which exhibits nonhomogeneous appearance. (Reprinted with permission from Greenfield GB, Arrington JA. *Imaging of bone tumors.* Philadelphia: JB Lippincott, 1995;161.)

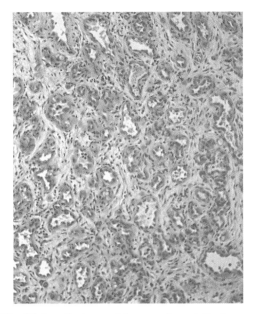

FIG. 20. Histopathology of hemangioendothelioma. A fibrous stroma is filled with proliferating vascular channels that are lined with plump endothelial cells that lack obvious pleomorphism or significant mitotic activity (hematoxylin and eosin, original magnification ×40). (From Bullough PG. *Atlas of orthopedic pathology,* 2nd ed. New York: Gower, 1992; 17.9.)

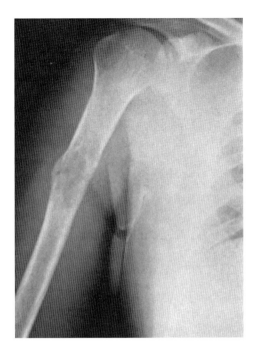

FIG. 21. Angiosarcoma. An osteolytic lesion with a wide zone of transition is present in the proximal humerus of a 42-year-old man. Note a pathologic fracture through the tumor. A soft tissue mass is not well demonstrated on this study.

whereas vascular tumor cells exhibit no such immune reaction (102,107). Conversely, Factor VIII-AG or *Ulex europaeus* immunoperoxidase staining methods demonstrate a positive cytoplasmic reaction of the vascular tumor cells or a heightened cytoplasmic binding around the microscopic lumen formations (102,107,115).

Telangiectatic osteosarcoma may have areas that strongly resemble hemangioendothelioma. However, the presence of osteoid formation in the former is diagnostic.

Myxoid chondrosarcoma may exhibit the nodular arrangement and epithelioid appearance of the tumor cells (103). However, the myxoid background and the positive staining for S-100 protein are not features of hemangioendothelioma.

Adamantinoma exhibits a characteristic biphasic pattern consisting of epithelial strands intimately admixed with a fibrous stroma. In this tumor, however, the epithelial component is usually scant and is often difficult to discern, in contrast to hemangioendothelioma, in which the rather large epithelioid cells are conspicuous in size and number.

Angiosarcoma

Angiosarcoma of bone represents the most malignant end of the spectrum of vascular tumors. This is an aggressive malignancy, characterized by frequent local recurrence and distant metastases (63,99).

Clinical Presentation

Angiosarcomas most commonly involve the skin (33%) and soft tissues (24%), with bone being involved in only 6% of cases (101). These lesions occur during the second to the seventh decade, although the peak is during the third to fifth decade (18). Males are affected twice as frequently as females. The most common osseous locations are the long bones (approximately 60% of cases), particularly the tibia (23%), femur (18%), and humerus (13%), as well as pelvis (7%) (63,70). The two most common symptoms are local pain and swelling. Metastases to the lungs and other parenchymal organs are found in about 66% of cases.

Imaging

On radiologic studies it is impossible to distinguish among hemangioendothelioma, hemangiopericytoma, and angiosarcoma. Angiosarcomas have radiographic features similar to those of hemangioendotheliomas. However, they are usually solitary lesions and almost invariably there is a wide transitional zone between tumor and uninvolved bone. Soft tissue masses are common. Angiosarcomas are predominantly lytic and sometimes they exhibit a honeycomb or hole-within-hole pattern, similar to the appearance of hemangioma. More aggressive features include osseous expansion, cortical permeation, and an associated soft tissue mass (63) (Fig. 21). Multifocal involvement is common. Skeletal scintigraphy is invariably positive, revealing increased tracer

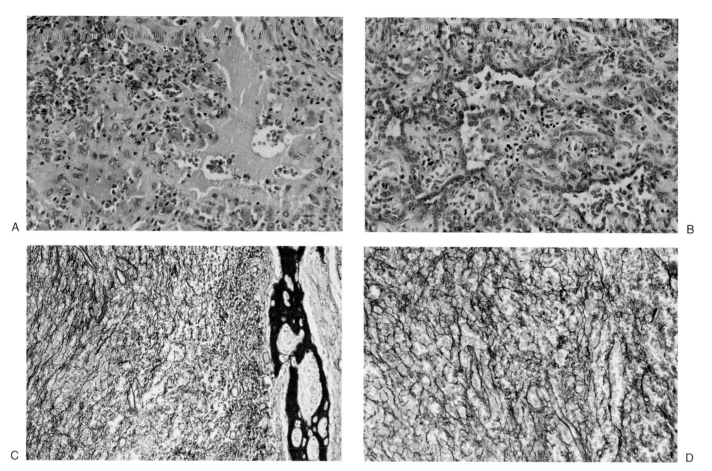

FIG. 22. Histopathology of angiosarcoma. **A:** Clusters of very large polygonal cells with large pleomorphic and hyperchromatic nuclei border blood-filled vascular spaces. The solid areas of the tumor resemble large cell metastatic cancer (hematoxylin and eosin, original magnification ×50). **B:** In another field of view the vascular spaces are larger and better visible. The vascular character of the tumor is obvious (hematoxylin and eosin, original magnification ×50). **C:** Reticulin fiber stain shows that the tumor cells lie corona-like within the rims of reticulin fibers (*black*). Note newly formed cortex made up of trabecular woven bone (Novotny, original magnification ×25). **D:** At higher magnification the interconnected network of vascular spaces each bound by a rim of reticulin fibers (*black*) is seen, surrounding a seam of large tumor cells (Novotny's, original magnification ×50).

uptake (95). The CT and MRI appearances of these lesions are decidedly nonspecific (18).

Histopathology

Histologically, angiosarcomas are composed of poorly formed blood vessels that exhibit complicated infolding and irregular anastomoses. The endothelial cells lining these blood vessels display features of frank malignancy, with the presence of often plump intraluminal cells resembling hobnails, frequent and atypical mitoses, and nuclear hyperchromatism (Fig. 22). Solid areas of the tumor may contain spindle cells and epithelioid cells. Spontaneous necrosis is often present. According to Stout (121), two fundamental histologic criteria are necessary for diagnosing an angiosarcoma: (a) formation of greater number of atypical endothelial cells than would be necessary to line vessels with a simple endo-

thelial membrane, and (b) formation of vascular tubes and channels that exhibit a framework of reticulin fibers and that usually anastomose. Markers for Factor VIII and *Ulex europaeus* yield inconsistent and sometimes negative results, reflecting poor tumor differentiation.

Differential Diagnosis

Radiology

Because the radiologic characteristics of angiosarcoma are not specific, several possibilities should be considered in the differential diagnosis, including *metastasis, plasmacytoma, lymphoma, fibrosarcoma,* and MFH. As always in such situations, the radiologist should rely on clinical information.

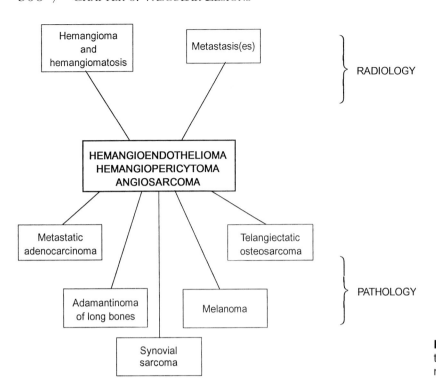

FIG. 23. Radiologic and pathologic differential diagnosis of hemangioendothelioma, hemangiopericytoma, and angiosarcoma.

Pathology

As in the case of other vascular tumors, differential diagnosis must include *hemangioendothelioma* and *hemangiopericytoma*. Because it is usually difficult to determine the tumor's vascular pattern, staining for reticulin fibers should always be utilized to identify the basal membrane in the vessel wall (60). In angiosarcoma, the tumor cells lie within the basal membrane whereas in hemangiopericytoma they lie outside. Some poorly differentiated but extremely vascular sarcomas may strongly resemble angiosarcoma. Telangiectatic osteosarcoma and metastases from renal cell carcinoma may contain areas that strongly resemble a vascular tumor. In such cases, marking with the Factor VIII–related antigen may be helpful for demonstration of the endothelial nature of tumor cells in the solid regions of an angiosarcoma (60).

The radiologic and pathologic differential diagnosis of hemangioendothelioma, hemangiopericytoma, and angiosarcoma is depicted in Fig. 23.

Hemangiopericytoma

Hemangiopericytoma arises from the cells of Zimmerman that are located around vessels (122). This is a tumor of intermediate aggressiveness that has both benign and malignant potential (63).

Clinical Presentation

Hemangiopericytoma has been reported in patients ranging from 15 to 48 years of age (107). The tumor commonly affects the lower extremities (35%), particularly the soft tissues of the thigh and pelvis. Primary osseous lesions are rare (101). Symptoms consist primarily of pain or swelling, or a combination of both, with a duration of 1 month to 1 year (25,112). Occasionally there is associated hypophosphatemic osteomalacia (111).

Imaging

The radiographic features of hemangiopericytoma are nonspecific. Approximately 70% of these tumors are purely lytic (Fig. 24), whereas various degrees of sclerosis are present in about 30% of cases (130). When sclerosis predominates, bony trabeculae become prominent, giving the lesion a honeycomb appearance similar to that of a hemangioma (18). Although the cortex may be expanded, a periosteal reaction is rare. Wold et al. reported a correlation between the histologic malignancy and the radiographic aggressiveness of this tumor, although they found it very difficult, if not impossible, to distinguish benign from malignant lesions on the basis of radiographic appearance alone (130). Thus far, CT and MRI have also failed to facilitate this distinction (18,94). Angiography does not provide additional information (131).

Histopathology

Histologically, hemangiopericytomas are composed of vascular channels lined at their inner side by normal endothelial cells not belonging to the tumor and surrounded by spindly, round, or oval cells individually enclosed by a basket of reticulum fibrils, which are the pericytes of Zimmer-

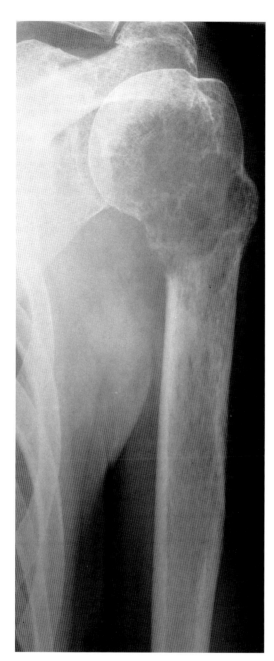

FIG. 24. Hemangiopericytoma. An anteroposterior radiograph of the right humerus in a 30-year-old man shows an osteolytic lesion with wide zone of transition. (From Bullough PG. *Atlas of orthopedic pathology,* 2nd ed. New York: Gower, 1992;17.10.)

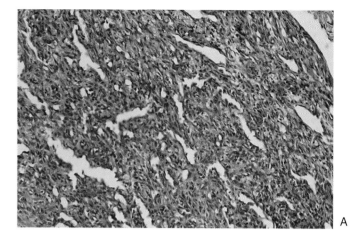

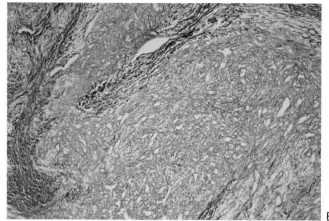

FIG. 25. Histopathology of hemangiopericytoma. **A:** Solid tumor tissue containing interconnected small blood vessel lumina are surrounded by polygonal cells of medium size. The blood vessels show a seam of flat endothelium different from the other cells (hematoxylin and eosin, original magnification ×50). **B:** With reticulin fiber staining, the numerous capillary lumina containing a seam of normal endothelia and being surrounded by a sharp narrow band corresponding to the basal membrane become distinct. The tumor cells lie outside the basal membrane (Novotny, original magnification ×25).

man and which represent the stem cells of the tumor (106) (Fig. 25A). The perivascular pattern of these tumors can be best recognized in reticulin preparations (118). Silver reticulin staining of the basal membrane of the vessel reveals that the tumor cells (pericytes) lie outside this membrane (82) (Fig. 25B). The proliferation of pericytes outside the vascular spaces distinguishes hemangiopericytoma from endothelial lesions in which the cells line the inner surface of the basal membrane of the vascular spaces (123). The tumor

may be of low-grade malignancy or of a high grade, with anaplasia and multiple mitoses (107).

Differential Diagnosis

Radiology

Like hemangioendothelioma, hemangiopericytoma is also difficult to distinguish from other vascular lesions. If the lesions exhibit osteolytic features, the same differential diagnoses apply as for hemangioendothelioma. An expansive solitary lesion may mimic *aneurysmal bone cysts,* and lesions that extend to the articular end of bone should be differentiated from *giant-cell tumor.* Sclerotic lesions may mimic *sclerosing hemangiomas* and even o*steoblastic metastases.*

Pathology

Hemangiopericytoma can be microscopically confused with a monophasic type of *synovial sarcoma*, when the latter exhibits a prominent hemangiopericytomatous histologic growth pattern (25). However, the typical features of synovial sarcoma include glandular and pseudoglandular patterns, and the lesion actually arises in soft tissues with only secondary involvement of bone, both of which features are helpful in the differentiation (107).

Hemangiopericytoma may also mimic *glomus tumor*, but it lacks the spindle cells derived from muscle cells, which are characteristic of the latter lesion. It should be pointed out that small foci of tissue closely resembling hemangiopericytoma can be found in a variety of tumors, including osteosarcoma, fibrosarcoma, and mesenchymal chondrosarcoma. Therefore, meticulous examination of the entire specimen is crucial. If the cell pattern characteristic of hemangiopericytoma is found throughout the tumor, the other diagnoses can be excluded (60).

REFERENCES

Intraosseous Hemangioma, Cystic Angiomatosis, Lymphangioma and Lymphangiomatosis

1. Abdelwahab IF. Sclerosing hemangiomatosis: a case report and review of the literature. *Br J Radiol* 1991;64:894–897.
2. Allen PW, Enzinger FM. Hemangioma of skeletal muscle: an analysis of 89 cases. *Cancer* 1972;29:8–22.
3. Asch MJ, Cohen AH, Moore TC. Hepatic and splenic lymphangiomatosis with skeletal involvement. Report of a case and review of the literature. *Surgery* 1974;76:334–339.
4. Assoun J, Richardi G, Railhac JJ, Le Guennec P, Caulier M, Dromer C, Sixou L, Fournie B, Mansat M, Durroux D. CT and MRI of massive osteolysis of Gorham. *J Comput Assist Tomogr* 1994;18:981–984.
5. Baker ND, Greenspan A, Neuwirth M. Symptomatic vertebral hemangiomas: a report of four cases. *Skeletal Radiol* 1986;15:458–463.
6. Barer M, Peterson LFA, Dahlin DC, Winkelmann RK, Stewart JR. Mastocytosis with osseous lesions resembling metastatic malignant lesions in bone. *J Bone Joint Surg* 1968;50A:142–152.
7. Bergman AG, Rogero GW, Hellman B, Lones MA. Case report 841. Skeletal cystic angiomatosis. *Skeletal Radiol* 1994;23:303–305.
8. Bergstrand A, Hook O, Lidvall H. Vertebral haemangiomas compressing the spinal cord. *Acta Neurol Scand* 1963;39:59–66.
9. Bickel WH, Broders AC. Primary lymphangioma of the ilium: report of a case. *J Bone Joint Surg* 1947;29:517–522.
10. Bill AH, Sumner DS. A unified concept of lymphangioma and cystic hygroma. *Surg Gynecol Obstet* 1965;120:79–86.
11. Boyle WJ. Cystic angiomatosis of bone. *J Bone Joint Surg* 1972;54B:626–636.
12. Brower AC, Culver JE Jr, Keats TE. Diffuse cystic angiomatosis of bone. Report of 2 cases. *Am J Roentgenol Radium Ther Nucl Med* 1973;118:456–463.
13. Brower AC, Culver JE, Keats TE. Diffuse cystic angiomatosis of bone: report of two cases. *Am J Roentgenol* 1973;118:456–463.
14. Buetow PC, Kransdorf MJ, Moser RP Jr, Jelinek JS, Berrey BH. Radiologic appearance of intramuscular hemangioma with emphasis on MR imaging. *Am J Roentgenol* 1990;154:563–567.
15. Bullough PG. *Atlas of orthopedic pathology with clinical and radiologic correlation,* 2nd ed. New York: Gower, 1992;15.12–15.14.
16. Choma ND, Biscotti CV, Bauer TW, Betho AC, Licata AA. Gorham's syndrome: a case report and review of the literature. *Am J Med* 1987;83:1151–1156.
17. Cohen JW, Weinreb JC, Redman HC. Arteriovenous malformations of the extremities: MR imaging. *Radiology* 1986;158:475–479.
18. Conway WF, Hayes CW. Miscellaneous lesions of bone. *Radiol Clin North Am* 1993;31:339–358.
19. Cooper PH. Is histiocytoid hemangioma a specific pathologic entity? *Am J Surg Pathol* 1988;12:815–817.
20. Cutillo DP, Swayne LC, Cucco J, Dougan H. CT and MRI imaging in cystic abdominal lymphangiomatosis. *J Comput Assist Tomogr* 1989;13:534–536.
21. Daoud S, Lefort G, Munzer M, Behar S, Bouche-Pillon MA, Lefebvre F, Gomès H. Lymphangiomatose osseuse disséminée, à propos de six observations. *Chir Pédiatr* 1988;29:342–348.
22. Dorfman HD, Steiner GC, Jaffe HL. Vascular tumors of bone. *Hum Pathol* 1971;2:349–376.
23. Ellis GL, Brannon RB. Intraosseous lymphangiomas of the mandible. *Skeletal Radiol* 1980;5:253–256.
24. Enzinger FM, Weiss SW. Benign tumors and tumorlike lesions of blood vessels. In: Enzinger FM, Weiss SW, eds. *Soft tissue tumors,* 3rd ed. St Louis: CV Mosby, 1995.
25. Fechner RE, Mills SE. *Tumors of the bones and joints.* Washington, DC: Armed Forces Institute of Pathology, 1993.
26. Foley WD, Baum JK, Wheeler RH. Diffuse osteosclerosis with lymphocytic lymphoma. A case report. *Radiology* 1975;117:553–554.
27. Friedman DP. Symptomatic vertebral hemangiomas: MR findings. *Am J Roentgenol* 1996;167:359–364.
28. Gerard PS, Wilck E. Spinal hemangioma. An unusual photopenic presentation on bone scan. *Spine* 1992;17:607–610.
29. Gorham LW, Stout AP. Massive osteolysis (acute spontaneous absorption of bone, phantom bone, disappearing bone): its relation to haemangiomatosis. *J Bone Joint Surg* 1955;37A:985–1004.
30. Gorham LW, Wright AW, Shultz HH, Mexon FC Jr. Disappearing bones: a rare form of massive osteolysis. *Am J Med* 1954;17:674–682.
31. Graham DY, Gonzales J, Kothari SM. Diffuse skeletal angiomatosis. *Skeletal Radiol* 1978;3:131–135.
32. Gramiak R, Ruiz G, Campeti FL. Cystic angiomatosis of bone. *Radiology* 1957;69:347–353.
33. Greenspan A, Norman A. Osteolytic cortical destruction: an unusual pattern of skeletal metastases. *Skeletal Radiol* 1988;17:402–406.
34. Greenspan A, Klein MJ, Bennett AJ, Lewis MM, Neuwirth M, Camins MB. Case report 242. Hemangioma of the T6 vertebra with a compression fracture, extradural block and spinal cord compression. *Skeletal Radiol* 1978;10:183–188.
35. Griffin GK, Tatu WF, Fischer LM, Keats TE, Tegtmeyer CJ. Fechner RE. Systemic lymphangiomatosis: a combined diagnostic approach of lymphangiography and computed tomography. *J Comput Assist Tomogr* 1986;10:335–339.
36. Gutierrez RM, Spjut HJ. Skeletal angiomatosis: report of three cases and review of the literature. *Clin Orthop* 1972;85:82–97.
37. Han BK, Ryu J-S, Moon DH, Shin MJ, Kim YT, Lee HK. Bone SPECT imaging of vertebral hemangioma. Correlations with MR imaging and symptoms. *Clin Nucl Med* 1995;20:916–921.
38. Hawnaur JM, Whitehouse RW, Jenkins JPR, Isherwood I. Musculoskeletal haemangiomas: comparison of MRI with CT. *Skeletal Radiol* 1990;19:251–258.
39. Hayes JT, Brody GL. Cystic lymphangiectasis of bone. A case report. *J Bone Joint Surg* 1961;43A:107–117.
40. Huvos AG. Hemangioma, lymphangioma, angiomatosis/lymphangiomatosis, glomus tumor. In: Huvos AG, ed. *Bone tumors: diagnosis, treatment and prognosis,* 2nd ed. Philadelphia: WB Saunders, 1991.
41. Ishida T, Dorfman HD, Steiner GC, Norman A. Cystic angiomatosis of bone with sclerotic changes mimicking osteoblastic metastases. *Skeletal Radiol* 1994;23:247–252.
42. Jacobs JE, Kimmelstiel P. Cystic angiomatosis of the skeletal system. *J Bone Joint Surg* 1953;35A:409–420.
43. Johnson PM, McClure JG. Observations on massive osteolysis: a review of the literature and report of a case. *Radiology* 1958;71:28–42.
44. Joseph UA, Jhingran SG. Technetium-99m labeled red blood cells in the evaluation of hemangioma. *Clin Nucl Med* 1987;12:845–847.
45. Jumbelic M, Feuerstein IM, Dorfman HD. Solitary intraosseous lymphangioma: a case report. *J Bone Joint Surg* 1984;66A:1479–1480.
46. Karlin CA, Brower AC. Multiple primary hemangiomas of bone. *Am J Roentgenol* 1977;129:162–164.
47. Laredo JD, Assouline E, Gelbert F, Wybier M, Merland JJ, Tubiana JM. Vertebral hemangiomas: fat content as a sign of aggressiveness. *Radiology* 1990;177:467–472.

48. Laredo JD, Reizine D, Bard M, Merland JJ. Vertebral hemangiomas: radiologic evaluation. *Radiology* 1986;161;183–189.
49. Levin DC, Gordon DH, McSweeney J. Arteriography of peripheral hemangiomas. *Radiology* 1976;121:625–630.
50. Levey DS, MacCormack LM, Sartoris DJ, Haghighi P, Resnick D, Thorne R. Cystic angiomatosis: Case report and review of the literature. *Skeletal Radiol* 1996;25:287–293.
51. Lomasney LM, Martinez S, Demos TC, Harrelson JM. Multifocal vascular lesions of bone: imaging characteristics. *Skeletal Radiol* 1996;25:255–261.
52. Makhija M, Bofill ER. Hemangioma: a rare cause of photopenic lesion on skeletal imaging. *Clin Nucl Med* 1988; 13:661–662.
53. Martinat P, Cotten A, Singer B, Petyt L, Chastanet P. Solitary cystic lymphangioma. *Skeletal Radiol* 1995;24:556–558.
54. Marymont JV, Shapiro WM. Vertebral hemangioma associated with spinal cord compression. *South Med J* 1988;81:1586–1587.
55. Meyer JS, Hoffer FA, Barnes PD, Mulliken JB. Biological classification of soft-tissue vascular anomalies: MR correlation. *Am J Roentgenol* 1991;157:559–564.
56. Mirra JM, Arnold WD. Skeletal hemangiomatosis in association with hereditary hemorrhagic telangiectasia. *J Bone Joint Surg* 1973; 55A:850–854.
57. Mirra JM. Vascular tumors. In: Mirra JM, ed. *Bone tumors: clinical, radiologic, and pathologic considerations.* Philadelphia: Lea & Febiger, 1989.
58. Mohan V, Gupta SK, Tuli SM, Sanyal B. Symptomatic vertebral hemangiomas. *Clin Radiol* 1980;31:575–579.
59. Moreno AJ, Reeves TA, Turnbull GL. Hemangioma of bone. *Clin Nucl Med* 1988;13:668–669.
60. Mulder JD, Kroon HM, Schütte HE, Taconis WK. *Radiologic atlas of bone tumors.* Elsevier: Amsterdam, 1993;241–254;507–516.
61. Mulliken JB, Glowacki J. Hemangiomas and vascular malformations in infants and children: a classification based on endothelial characteristics. *Plast Reconstr Surg* 1982;69:412–420.
62. Mulliken JB, Zetter BR, Folkman J. In vitro characteristics of endothelium from hemangiomas and vascular malformations. *Surgery* 1982;92:348–353.
63. Murphey MD, Fairbairn KJ, Parman LM, Baxter KG, Parsa MB, Smith WS. Musculoskeletal angiomatous lesions: radiologic-pathologic correlation. *RadioGraphics* 1995;15:893–917.
64. Netherlands Committee on Bone Tumors. *Radiological atlas of bone tumors,* vol 1. Baltimore: Williams & Wilkins, 1966.
65. Paley D, Evans DC. Angiomatous involvement of an extremity: a spectrum of syndromes. *Clin Orthop Rel Res* 1986;206:215–218.
66. Pearce WH, Rutherford RB, Whitehill TA, Davis K. Nuclear magnetic resonance imaging: its diagnostic value in patients with congenital vascular malformations of the limbs. *J Vasc Surg* 1988;8:64–70.
67. Peh WCG, Ngan H. Lymphography still useful in the diagnosis of lymphangiomatosis. *Br J Radiol* 1993;66:28–31.
68. Reid AB, Reid IL, Johnson G, Hamonic M, Major P. Familial diffuse cystic angiomatosis of bone. *Clin Orthop Rel Res* 1989;238:211–218.
69. Resnick D, Niwayama G. *Diagnosis of bone and joint disorders,* 2nd ed. Philadelphia: WB Saunders, 1988.
70. Resnick D, Kyriakos M, Greenway GD. Tumors and tumor-like lesions of bone: imaging and pathology of specific lesions. In: Resnick D, ed. *Diagnosis of bone and joints disorders,* 3rd ed. Philadelphia: WB Saunders, 1995;3628–3938.
71. Ritchie G, Zeier FG. Hemangiomatosis of the skeleton and the spleen. *J Bone Joint Surg* 1956;38A:115–122.
72. Rosenquist CJ, Wolfe DC. Lymphangioma of bone. *J Bone Joint Surg* 1978;50:158–162.
73. Ross JS, Masaryk TJ, Modic MT, Carter JR, Mapstone T, Dengel FH. Vertebral hemangioma: MR imaging. *Radiology* 1987;165:165–169.
74. Schajowicz F. *Tumors and tumorlike lesions of bone. Pathology, radiology, and treatment,* 2nd ed. Berlin: Springer-Verlag, 1994.
75. Schajowicz F, Aiello CL, Francone MV, Giannini RE. Cystic angiomatosis (hamartous haemolymphangiomatosis) of bone. *J Bone Joint Surg* 1978;60B:100–106.
76. Schopfner CE, Allen RP. Lymphangioma of bone. *Radiology* 1961; 76:449–453.
77. Sherman RS, Wilner D. The roentgen diagnosis of hemangioma of bone. *Am J Roentgenol* 1961;86:1146–1159.
78. Spieth ME, Greenspan A, Forrester DM, Ansari AN, Kimura RL, Gleason-Jordan I. Gorham's disease of the radius: radiographic, scin-tigraphic, and MRI findings with pathologic correlation. *Skeletal Radiol* 1997. In press
79. Steiner GM, Farman J, Lawson JP. Lymphangiomatosis of bone. *Radiology* 1969;93:1093–1098.
80. Suh JS, Hwang G, Hahn SB. Soft tissue hemangiomas: MR manifestations in 23 patients. *Skeletal Radiol* 1994;23:621–625.
81. Torg JS, Steel HH. Sequential roentgenographic changes occurring in massive osteolysis. *J Bone Joint Surg* 1969;51A:1649–1655.
82. Unni KK. *Dahlin's bone tumors. General aspects and data on 11,087 cases,* 5th ed. New York: Lippincott-Raven, 1996.
83. Vinee P, Tanyu O, Havenstein KH, Sigmund G, Stover B, Adler CP. CT and MRI of Gorham syndrome. *J Comput Assist Tomogr* 1994;18:985–989.
84. Waldron RT, Zeller JA. Diffuse skeletal hemangiomatosis with visceral involvement. *J Can Assoc Radiol* 1969;20:119–123.
85. Williams AG Jr, Mettler FA Jr. Vertebral hemangioma. Radionuclide, radiographic, and CT correlation. *Clin Nucl Med* 1985;10:598.
86. Winterberger AR. Radiographic diagnosis of lymphangiomatosis of bone. *Radiology* 1972;102:321–324.
87. Wold LE, Swee RG, Sim FH. Vascular lesions of bone. *Pathol Annu* 1985;20/2:101–137.

Glomus Tumor, Gliomangioma, and Glomangiomyoma

88. Bjorkengren AG, Resnick D, Haghighi P, Sartoris DJ. Intraosseous glomus tumor: report of a case and review of the literature. *Am J Roentgenol* 1986;147:739–741.
89. Fornage BD. Glomus tumor in the fingers: diagnosis with US. *Radiology* 1988;167:183–185.
90. Greenfield GB, Arrington JA. *Imaging of bone tumors. A multimodality approach.* Philadelphia: JB Lippincott, 1995.
91. Kneeland JB, Middleton WD, Matloub HS, Jesmanowicz A, Froncisz W, Hyde JS. High resolution MR imaging of glomus tumor. *J Comput Assist Tomogr* 1987;11:351–352.
92. Sugiura I. Intra-osseous glomus tumor: a case report. *J Bone Joint Surg* 1976;58B:245–247.

Hemangioendothelioma, Angiosarcoma, and Hemangiopericytoma

93. Abrahams TG, Bula W, Jones M. Epithelioid hemangioendothelioma of bone. *Skeletal Radiol* 1992;21:509–513.
94. Alpern MB, Thorsen MK, Kellman GM, Pojunas K, Lawson TL. CT appearance of hemangiopericytoma. *J Comput Assist Tomogr* 1986;10:264–267.
95. Anez LF, Gupta SM, Berger D, Spera J, Johns WD. Scintigraphic evaluation of multifocal hemangioendothelioma of bone. *Clin Nucl Med* 1993;18:840–843.
96. Armstrong SJ, Watt I. Lipoma arborescens of the knee. *Br J Radiol* 1989;62:178–180.
97. Boutin RD, Spaeth HJ, Mangalik A, Sell JJ. Epithelioid hemangioendothelioma of bone. *Skeletal Radiol* 1996;25:391–395.
98. Campanacci M, Boriani S, Giunti A. Hemangioendothelioma of bone: a study of 29 cases. *Cancer* 1980;46:804–814.
99. Coldwell DM, Baron RL, Charnsangavej C. Angiosarcoma: diagnosis and clinical course. *Acta Radiol* 1989;30:627–631.
100. Enzinger FM, Weiss SW. Hemangioendothelioma: vascular tumors of intermediate malignancy. In: Enzinger FM, Weiss SW, eds. *Soft tissue tumors,* 3rd ed. St Louis: CV Mosby, 1995.
101. Enzinger FM, Weiss SW. Malignant vascular tumors. In: Enzinger FM, Weiss SW, eds. *Soft tissue tumors,* 3rd ed. St Louis: CV Mosby, 1995.
102. Fulling KH, Gersell DJ. Neoplastic angioendotheliomatosis. Histologic, immunohistochemical, and ultrastructural findings in two cases. *Cancer* 1983;51:1107–1118.
103. Greenspan A, Unni KK, Blake L, Rab G. Extraskeletal myxoid chondrosarcoma: an unusual tumor in a 6-year-old boy. *Can Assoc Radiol J* 1994;45:62–65.
104. Hendrix RW, Rogers LF, Davis TM. Cortical bone metastases. *Radiology* 1991;181:409–413.
105. Hisaoka M, Aoki T, Kouho H, Chosa H, Hashimoto H. Maffucci's

syndrome associated with spindle cell hemangioendothelioma. *Skeletal Radiol* 1997;126:191–194.

106. Hudson TM. *Radiologic-pathologic correlation of musculoskeletal lesions.* Baltimore: Williams & Wilkins, 1987.

107. Huvos AG. Angiosarcoma of bone (epithelioid hemangioendothelioma, malignant hemangioendothelioma). In: Huvos AG, ed. *Bone tumors: diagnosis, treatment and prognosis,* 2nd ed. Philadelphia: WB Saunders, 1991.

108. Kida T, Hujita Y, Munaka S, Sasaki M, Inoue J. Malignant hemangioendothelioma demonstrated by thalium imaging. *Clin Nucl Med* 1987;11:886–887.

109. Kleer CG, Unni KK, McLeod RA. Epithelioid hemangioendothelioma of bone. *Am J Surg Pathol* 1996;20:1301–1311.

110. Lee KS, Rossleigh MA, Fernandes VB, Morris JG. Scintigraphic features of malignant epithelioid hemangioendothelioma. *Clin Nucl Med* 1989;14:501–503.

111. Linovitz RJ, Resnick D, Keissling P, Kondon JJ, Sehler B, Nejdl RJ, Rowe JH, Deftos LJ. Tumor-induced osteomalcia and rickets: a surgically curable syndrome. Report of two cases. *J Bone Joint Surg* 1976; 58A:419–423.

112. Lorigan JG, David CL, Evans HL, Wallace S. The clinical and radiologic manifestations of hemangiopericytoma. *Am J Roentgenol* 1989; 153:345–349.

113. Maruyama N, Kumagai Y, Ishida Y, Sato H, Sugano I, Nagao K, Kondo Y. Epithelioid hemangioendothelioma of the bone tissue. *Virchows Arch (A)* 1985;407:159–165.

114. O'Connell JX, Kattapuram SV, Mankin HJ, Bhan AK, Rosenberg AE. Epithelioid hemangioma of bone. A tumor often mistaken for low-grade angiosarcoma or malignant hemangioendothelioma. *Am J Surg Pathol* 1993;17:610–617.

115. Ordonez NG, Batsakis JG. Comparison of *Ulex europaeus* I lecting and factor VIII-related antigen in vascular lesions. *Arch Pathol Lab Med* 1984;108:129–132.

116. Rong Y, Sato K, Yamamura S, Sugiura H, Katagiri H, Iwata H. Malignant hemangioendothelioma of the left calcaneus associated with fever and hematological abnormalities. *Skeletal Radiol* 1997;26: 64–66.

117. Rosai J, Gold J, Landy R. The histiocytoid hemangiomas. A unifying concept embracing several previously described entities of skin, soft tissue, large vessels, bone, and heart. *Hum Pathol* 1979;10:707–730.

118. Sahin, Akyar G, Fitöz S, Akpolat I, Saglik Y, Erekul S. Primary hemangiopericytoma of bone located in the tibia. *Skeletal Radiol* 1997; 26:47–50.

119. Shin MS, Carpenter JT, Ho KJ. Epithelioid hemangioendothelioma: CT manifestations and possible linkage to vinyl chloride exposure. *J Comput Assist Tomogr* 1991;15:505–507.

120. Steinbach LS, Ominsky SH, Shpall S, Perkocha LA. MR imaging of spindle cell hemangioendothelioma. *J Comput Assist Tomogr* 1991; 15:155–157.

121. Stout AP. Hemangioendothelioma: a tumor of blood vessels featuring vascular endothelial cells. *Ann Surg* 1943;118:445–464.

122. Stout AP, Murray MR. Hemangiopericytoma: a vascular tumor featuring Zimmermann's pericytes. *Ann Surg* 1942;116:26–33.

123. Tang JS, Gold RH, Mirra JM, Eckardt J. Hemangiopericytoma of bone. *Cancer* 1988;62:848–859.

124. Tsang WY, Chan JK. The family of epithelioid vascular tumors. *Histol Histopathol* 1993;8:187–212.

125. Tsuneyoshi M, Dorfman HD, Bauer TW. Epitheloid hemangioendothelioma of bone. A clinicopathologic, ultrastructural, and immunohistochemical study. *Am J Surg Pathol* 1986;10:754–764.

126. Unni KK, Ivins JC, Beabout JW, Dahlin DC. Hemangioma, hemangiopericytoma, and hemangioendothelioma (angiosarcoma) of bone. *Cancer* 1971;27:1403–1414.

127. Weiss SW, Enzinger FM. Epitheloid hemangioendothelioma: a vascular tumor often mistaken for a carcinoma. *Cancer* 1982;50: 970–981.

128. Weiss SW, Enzinger FM. Spindle cell hemangioendothelioma. A low-grade angiosarcoma resembling a cavernous hemangioma and Kaposi's sarcoma. *Am J Surg Pathol* 1986;10:521–530.

129. Weiss SW, Ishak KG, Dail DH, Sweet DE, Enzinger FM. Epithelioid hemangioendothelioma and related lesions. *Semin Diagn Pathol* 1986;3:259–287.

130. Wold LE, Unni KK, Beabout JW, Ivins JC, Bruckman JE, Dahlin DC. Hemangioendothelial sarcoma of bone. *Am J Surg Pathol* 1982; 6:59–70.

131. Wold LE, Unni KK, Cooper KL, Sim FH, Dahlin DC. Hemangiopericytoma of bone. *Am J Surg Pathol* 1982;6:53–58.

132. Yagmai I. Angiographic features of soft-tissue and osseous hemangiopericytomas. *Radiology* 1978;126:653–659.

CHAPTER 7

Miscellaneous Tumors and Tumor-like Lesions

BENIGN LESIONS
  Giant-Cell Tumor
  Simple Bone Cyst
  Aneurysmal Bone Cyst
  Intraosseous Lipoma

Fibrocartilaginous Mesenchymoma
MALIGNANT LESIONS
  Adamantinoma of Long Bones
  Chordoma
  Leiomyosarcoma of Bone

BENIGN LESIONS

Giant-Cell Tumor

Giant-cell tumor (GCT) is a locally aggressive neoplasm characterized by richly vascularized tissue containing proliferating mononuclear stromal cells and many osteoclast-like, multinucleated giant cells randomly but evenly distributed throughout (20,67). GCT represents approximately 5% (75) to 8.6% (67) of all primary bone tumors and about 22.7% of benign bone tumors (75), and is the sixth most common primary osseous neoplasm (24).

Clinical Presentation

GCT occurs almost exclusively after skeletal maturity, when the growth plates are obliterated, and patients are usually between the ages of 20 and 40 years, with a female preponderance (2:1). At least 60% of cases arise in long bones and almost all extend to the articular end (23). Those unusual cases with presentation in the metaphysis are seen in skeletally immature patients (37,58). The most common skeletal sites are the distal femur, the proximal tibia, the distal radius, the proximal humerus, and the sacrum (20). Rarely, the tumor arises in other sites, such as the bones of hands and feet, the vertebral bodies, the ribs (13,33,75), the scapula (3), and the ischium (68) (Fig. 1). Very uncommonly, GCT may be multifocal (57,69,77), with a reported frequency of 0.04% to 1% (18,19,47,73). The majority of multifocal GCTs are associated with Paget disease of bone (25,32,60), and most have a predilection for the skull, face (34), and ilium (67). Multifocal GCTs in patients who do not exhibit Paget disease usually occur in the bones of the hand (5,6,17) and characteristically affect a slightly younger age group (15,79).

The symptoms most commonly reported include pain of increasing intensity, with local swelling and tenderness of the affected area. Limitation of motion of the adjacent joint is also present in many patients (67). Only in exceptional cases is a pathologic fracture the first sign of a GCT. Although a histologic grading system exists, the clinical behavior of GCT cannot be accurately predicted on the basis of histologic, clinical, or radiologic features (8,9,11,22). Recurrences after surgical curettage and bone grafting are common [reported recurrence rates range from 12% to 50% (31)].

Imaging

The characteristic radiographic features of GCT are those of a purely destructive lesion with a geographic type of bone destruction (40). The lesion is radiolucent, frequently expansive, and eccentrically located, without marginal sclerosis but usually with well-defined borders (Figs. 2 and 3). Internal trabeculations or pseudotrabeculations are occasionally present (67) (Fig. 4), most likely representing a nonuniform growth of the tumor (51). There is usually no periosteal reaction. Attempts have been made to assess the aggressiveness of GCT on the basis of radiologic criteria. According to some investigators (49), nonaggressive tumors exhibit a prominent trabeculation and no cortical expansion or soft tissue mass. Conversely, aggressive tumors exhibit a lack of trabeculation, and expansion or destruction of the cortex and soft-tissue mass are present (Fig. 5).

Conventional tomography, particularly trispiral or hypocycloidal tomography, reveals the osseous margins of the lesion and the status of the cortex more definitely than plain radiographs. Arthrotomography is effective for the evaluation of tumor invasion through the subchondral plate and articular cartilage (30). When a soft-tissue mass is present,

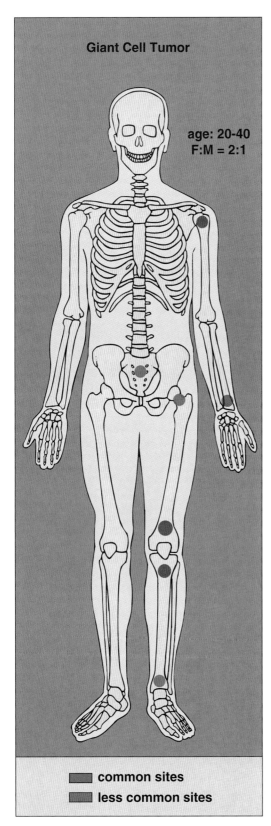

FIG. 1. Giant-cell tumor: skeletal sites of predilection, peak age range, and male-to-female ratio.

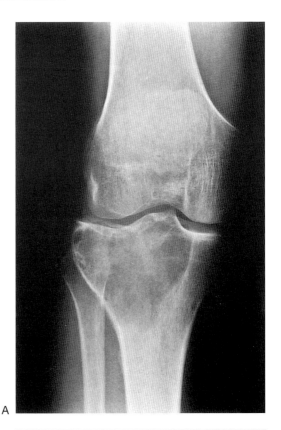

A

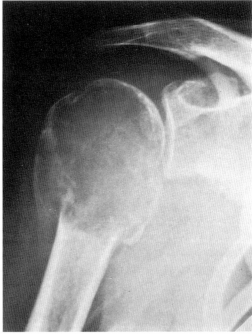

B

FIG. 2. Giant-cell tumor. A: An anteroposterior radiograph of the right knee of a 30-year-old woman shows an osteolytic lesion eccentrically located in the proximal tibia and extending into the articular end of bone. B: A radiolucent lesion in a 27-year-old woman affects almost entire proximal end of the humerus. Note a pathologic fracture at the distal extent of the tumor.

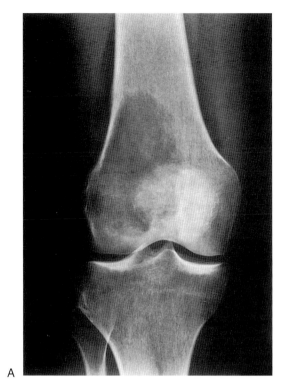

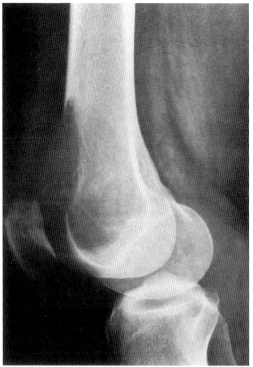

A

B

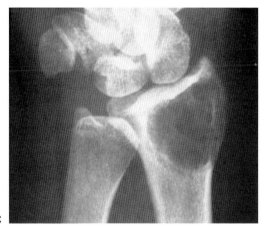

C

FIG. 3. Giant-cell tumor. (**A**) Anteroposterior and (**B**) lateral radiographs of the right knee of a 32-year-old man show a purely osteolytic lesion in the distal end of the femur. Note its eccentric location, the absence of reactive sclerosis, and the extension of the tumor into the articular end of the bone. (**C**) In another patient, an eccentric osteolytic lesion extends into the articular end of the distal radius.

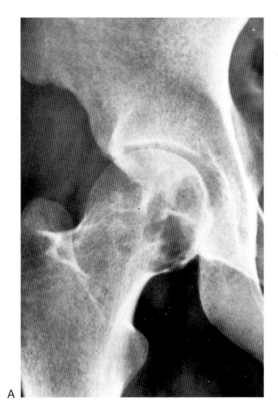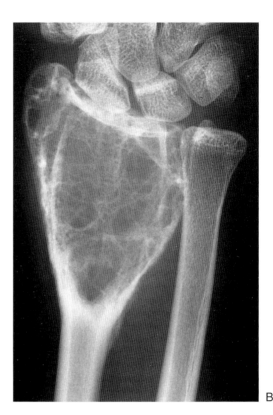

A

B

FIG. 4. Giant-cell tumor. **A:** An anteroposterior radiograph of the right hip of a 27-year-old woman shows a radiolucent lesion with internal trabeculations in the femoral head. **B:** An anteroposterior radiograph of the left wrist of a 36-year-old woman shows a trabeculated lesion in the distal radius.

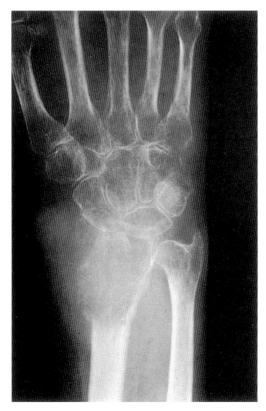

FIG. 5. Giant-cell tumor. Dorsovolar radiograph of the left wrist of a 56-year-old woman shows an osteolytic lesion in the distal radius that has destroyed the cortex and that extends into the soft tissues.

CT or MRI examination may be particularly helpful (46,61,72). CT may outline the tumor extent and better delineate areas of cortical destruction (Fig. 6). The attenuation coefficient of unenhanced GCT averaged 44 Hounsfield units, similar to measurements of other noncalcified bone lesions (30). However, enhancement after infusion of a contrast agent is striking according to Hudson (30). Conversely, deSantos and Murray did not observe a significant contrast enhancement (21).

Fluid levels in the tumor have been reported (36,61) and are considered by some investigators to be secondary to an aneurysmal bone cyst (ABC) component (30,36). Like most bone tumors, GCT exhibits a low to intermediate signal intensity on T1-weighted MRI images, and a high signal on T2-weighted sequences (Fig. 7). The intramedullary portion of tumor is best seen on T1 weighting, whereas its extraosseous component is more clearly observed on T2-weighted images (10,29) (Fig. 8). Some reports in the literature indicate that certain instances of GCT containing large amounts of hemosiderin may show different MRI characteristics (2). Aoki et al. (1) found in these instances a markedly decreased signal on both T1- and T2-weighted sequences and, in one case, the extraosseous tumor extension appeared as a signal void area on MR imaging. MRI is also effective in demonstrating subchondral breakthrough and extension of tumor into the adjacent joint (29).

Radionuclide bone scan rarely provides additional information because the degree of tracer uptake does not correlate with the histologic grade of the tumor (30,44,56,76). However, scintigraphy may help in detection of multiple foci if a multicentric GCT is clinically suspected. In a study by Hudson et al., these investigators found in 49% of cases an abnormal uptake pattern resembling a doughnut: intense uptake around the periphery with relatively little activity in the central portion of the tumor (30). They contended that this appearance was due to uptake of the bone-seeking radiopharmaceutical agents predominantly by reactive new bone or by hyperemic bone around the tumor, with the tumor tissue retaining little tracer. Occasionally, an increased tracer activity can be detected across the adjacent joint (39). This phenomenon may be due to increased blood flow and to increased bone turnover secondary to disuse osteoporosis (70).

Although 5% to 10% of GCT undergo malignant degeneration (or are malignant from their inception), malignant GCT is unaccompanied by additional or specific radiologic characteristics and therefore cannot be diagnosed radiographically.

The radiographic presentation of GCT complicating Paget disease is usually that of an expansive lytic lesion, frequently accompanied by a soft tissue mass (44,53,66).

Histopathology

The histologic features of GCT consist of a dual population of mononuclear stromal cells (which are considered to form the characteristic tissue of the tumor) and of giant cells that are usually uniformly distributed throughout the tumor (Fig. 9). Morphologically, the giant cells bear some resemblance to osteoclasts and, like all resorptive giant cells, they exhibit marked acid phosphatase activity (4). However, they are much larger than true osteoclasts, and are not apposed to bone surfaces, hence do not possess a ruffled border (71). Therefore, they do not appear to participate actively in bone resorption. The cells are round, oval, or fusiform, and they

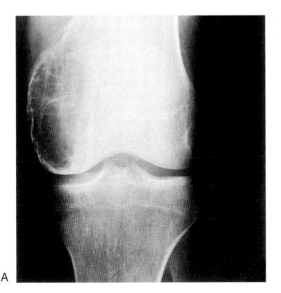 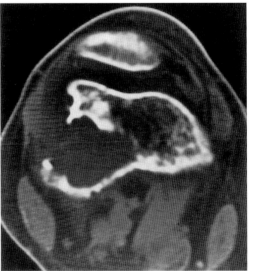

A   B

FIG. 6. Giant-cell tumor: computed tomography. **A:** Anteroposterior radiograph of the left knee of a 33-year-old woman shows an osteolytic lesion in the medial femoral condyle. There is no definite evidence of cortical break-through. **B:** Axial CT section through the tumor demonstrates destruction of the cortex and the presence of a soft tissue mass.

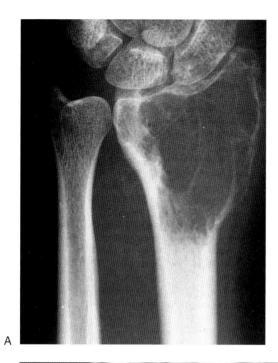

A

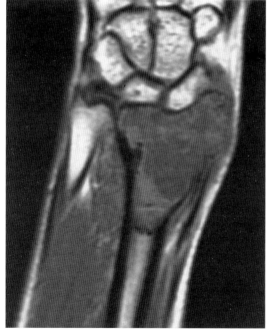

B

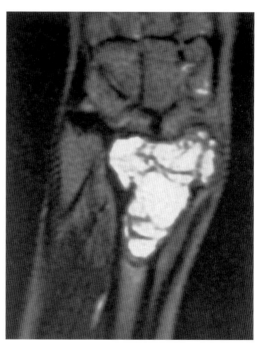

C

FIG. 7. Giant-cell tumor: magnetic resonance imaging. **A:** A dorsovolar radiograph of the right wrist of a 36-year-old woman shows an osteolytic lesion in the distal radius. **B:** Coronal T1-weighted (SE, TR 500, TE 20) MR image shows the tumor to be of low signal intensity. **C:** On coronal T2-weighted (SE, TR 2000, TE 80) MRI the lesion becomes bright, displaying low-signal septations.

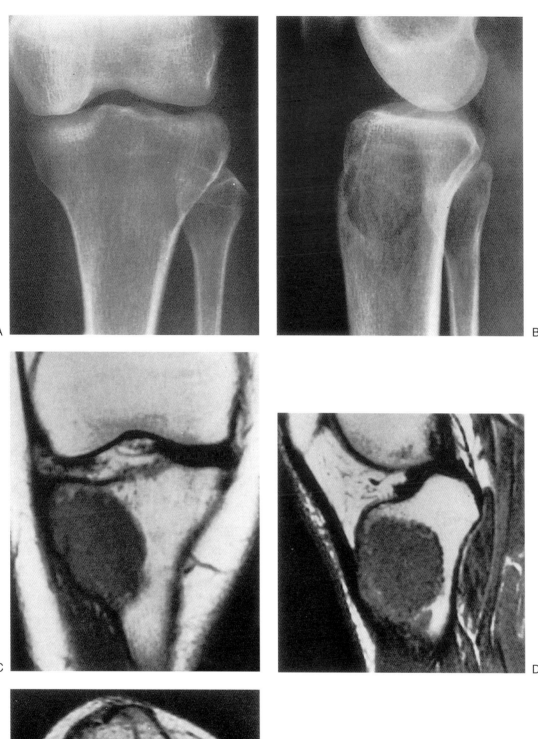

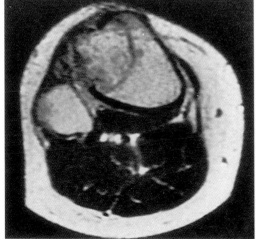

FIG. 8. Giant-cell tumor: magnetic resonance imaging. **(A)** Anteroposterior and **(B)** lateral radiographs of the left knee of a 45-year-old woman show a radiolucent lesion in the proximal tibia, but its full intraosseous extent can not be properly assessed. **(C)** Coronal and **(D)** sagittal T1-weighted (SE, TR 600, TE 20) MR images accurately outline the tumor, which displays intermediate signal intensity. **(E)** Axial T2-weighted (SE, TR 2000, TE 80) image reveals that the lesion, now displaying nonhomogeneous high signal, has penetrated the cortex and extends laterally into the soft tissues.

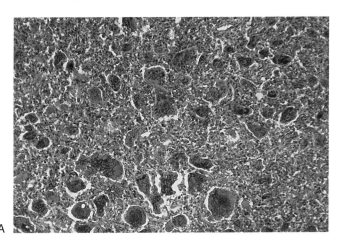
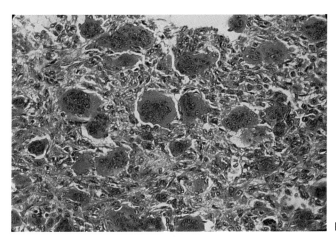

A   B

FIG. 9. Histopathology of a giant-cell tumor. **A:** Densely arranged tumor tissue consists of mononuclear cells intermixed with numerous uniformly distributed large giant cells containing up to 50 and more nuclei, much larger than those observed in other tumors (hematoxylin and eosin, original magnification ×100.) **B:** At higher magnification the characteristic appearance of giant cells is better appreciated (hematoxylin and eosin, original magnification ×250).

vary considerably in shape owing to their capacity for amoeboid motility. In general, they possess large nuclei with little chromatin and a very few inconspicuous nucleoli (67). The number of nuclei varies considerably, but usually there are more than 20. Although some of the giant cells resemble osteoclasts, their nuclei never exhibit mitotic activity. For this reason, the formerly used term "osteoclastoma" for giant cell tumor is inappropriate. Frequently, areas of hemorrhage and occasionally groups of foam cells and of hemosiderin-laden macrophages are present (24).

The matrix of the tumor contains variable amounts of collagen. On histologic study, silver staining reveals a dense network of reticulin fibers surrounding the individual cells but without penetrating the giant cells (67). The tumor is rich in newly formed blood vessels of the capillary type, with walls composed of only a single endothelial layer. Occasionally the vascular channels appear to be directly lined with tumor cells (67). Bone or osteoid formation can be seen at sites of previous pathologic fracture or curettage and, occasionally, surrounding a focus of recurrent tumor in the soft tissue.

Because mitotic activity is regularly seen in the mononuclear stromal cells and because the nuclei of the giant cells may resemble those of the stromal cells, it was long believed that the giant cells represent a fusion product of the stromal cells. Studies by Burmester and colleagues and by Ling and associates confirmed the monocytic nature of the stromal cells and the probable derivation of the giant cells from these mononuclear cells (12,41). Mitoses do not indicate malignancy in GCT.

A fibroxanthomatous pattern is sometimes observed in GCT with only a few scattered giant cells. The presence of these lipoid-bearing foam cells, particularly in the vicinity of necrotic foci and with association of fibrous tissue, may indicate spontaneous regression and healing of the tumor (34) or, as others have suggested, a less aggressive type of tumor (67). When this pattern predominates, the GCT may be misdiagnosed as benign fibrous histiocytoma. Some authorities, however, consider the latter lesion to represent merely the end stage of a burned-out GCT (45).

Attempts to correlate the histologic appearance of the tumor with its biologic behavior have proven unreliable and have now been abandoned (15,27). Histologic classification of GCT tumor into three grades, corresponding to the number and size of giant cells and the degree of pleomorphism of the mononuclear cells (grade III being frankly malignant histologically), has been attempted in the past (35). In this classification, grade I tumor is characterized by a dense layer of huge giant cells with up to 100 or more nuclei, almost covering the tumor tissue proper of mononuclear cells. Grade II tumor exhibits a considerable reduction in the size and number of giant cells, and the mononuclear cells may be pleomorphic to some degree. In grade III tumors, the giant cells are further reduced in number and there is an increase in pleomorphic mononuclear cells. All three grades may be characterized by extended fields with spindle cells and practically no giant cells. Moreover, some reactive bone formation may be observed. As a part of this grading system, some investigators also include the mitotic rate, vascular invasion, infiltration of soft tissue, and occurrence of a peritumoral zone of reactive tissue formation (43). Dahlin (19) categorizes GCT only as benign or malignant, and he does not find grading of benign tumors to be helpful in predicting the local recurrence or sarcomatous transformation, which is why this classification has now been abandoned (15,27). Therefore, most investigators agree that grading of GCT is without practical value because prediction of the evolution of a giant-cell tumor based on its histologic features is impossible (67), and histologic grading has not been shown to correlate with local recurrence rate or the incidence of pulmonary metastases (14,27,43).

Malignant Giant-Cell Tumor

Although GCT is usually benign, malignant tumors have been reported (52,63). However, one must be very cautious in making the diagnosis of malignant GCT. Several reported cases of "primary" malignant GCT later proved to be sarcomas rich in multinucleated giant cells of the osteoclast type, such as telangiectatic osteosarcomas, giant cell–rich osteosarcomas, fibrosarcomas, or malignant fibrohistiocytomas (67). Dahlin and Unni (75) believe that primary malignant GCT is extremely unusual and that most of these cases actually represent another type of malignancy arising within GCT. Nevertheless, malignant transformation may occur spontaneously, after surgery (81), or after radiation therapy. McGrath (48) divided malignant GCT into three types: (a) primary , in which the tumor was malignant from the onset (de novo); (b) evolutionary, in which there was malignant transformation of originally benign GCT spontaneously or after multiple surgical resections for recurrent lesions, or after a long latency period; and (c) secondary, developing as a result of malignant transformation of an initially benign tumor after radiation therapy. In the latter group, the majority of sarcomas that occur are fibrosarcomas, malignant fibrous histiocytomas, or osteosarcomas (67). Exceedingly rare cases represent the so-called dedifferentiated GCT, in which there is the concomitant presence of a typical GCT of bone juxtaposed to a sarcoma [such as a malignant fibrous histiocytoma (50)]. The diagnosis of malignant GCT requires either a frankly sarcomatous change in the lesion or a sarcoma arising in the previous site of a treated GCT (75). The histologic diagnosis of malignant GCT is established only when the stromal cells are frankly sarcomatous, as indicated by pleomorphism, atypia, and high mitotic activity (65,81). In addition, areas of typical benign GCT should be present in the tumor at the time of diagnosis or in tissues taken previously from the same lesion (32,75). Histologic grading of GCT in an attempt to predict local recurrence and clinical prognosis has generally met with little success. Moreover, there are reports of completely benign-appearing GCT that were followed by distant metastases to the lung, having the histologic characteristics of classic GCT (38,43,54,62, 74,75,80).

Differential Diagnosis

Radiology

Various lesions may be mistaken for GCT and, conversely, GCT can mimic other lesions that affect the articular end of a bone. Primary aneurysmal bone cyst rarely affects the articular end of a bone and occurs in a younger age group. However, after obliteration of the growth plate at skeletal maturity, this lesion may extend into the subarticular region of a long bone, becoming indistinguishable from a GCT. Occasionally, if the fluid-fluid level is demonstrated

either on CT or MRI examination, this feature is more consistent with aneurysmal bone cyst (61). However, it should be noted that aneurysmal bone cyst may sometimes coexist with other lesions, among them the giant-cell tumor. The so-called solid aneurysmal bone cyst, or a giant-cell reparative granuloma at the articular end, may have the same radiologic characteristics as a conventional GCT (7,55). Benign fibrous histiocytoma, because of its frequent location at the end of a long bone, may appear identical to a GCT. However, as mentioned earlier, some investigators consider benign fibrous histiocytoma to be an end stage of a "burned-out" GCT (45). Brown tumor of hyperparathyroidism is yet another lesion that radiologically can mimic GCT. However, the former lesion is usually accompanied by other skeletal manifestations of hyperparathyroidism, such as osteopenia, cortical or subperiosteal resorption, resorptive changes at the distal phalangeal tufts, or loss of the lamina dura of the teeth (44). Occasionally, an unusually large intraosseous ganglion may be mistaken for GCT, although the former lesion invariably exhibits a sclerotic border (Fig. 10A). Some malignant lesions, such as chondrosarcoma, may extend into the articular end of bone and, particularly without radiographically identified calcifications, may closely mimic GCT. Myeloma and a lytic metastasis occupying subchondral segments of bone can usually be distinguished from GCT without much difficulty (the older age group in which the latter malignancies usually occur is a helpful hint), although at times the radiographic differences between the lesions may not be so obvious (Figs. 10B, C). Finally, on rare occasions, fibrosarcoma, malignant fibrous histiocytoma, or fibroblastic osteosarcoma because of their purely lytic radiographic presentation, may exhibit some similarities to GCT.

Multicentric giant-cell tumor should be differentiated from osteolytic metastases, myeloma, brown tumor of hyperparathyroidism, and multicentric giant cell reparative granulomas (16,26,28,42,58).

Pathology

Diagnosis of a grade I GCT with its typical histology and cytology of giant cells, usually does not create a problem. The characteristic radiologic picture of an expansile, eccentric lytic lesion in the articular end of a long tubular bone adds to the security of the histologic diagnosis. For a grade II or III tumor, diagnosis has been and is still difficult. In such cases several lesions must be considered in the differential diagnosis. In the epiphysis, chondroblastoma has in the past been considered as a cartilage-containing giant-cell tumor. However, it can now be easily differentiated from GCT by the presence of cartilage islands that are not observed in GCT. Another giant cell–containing epiphyseal lesion, benign fibrous histiocytoma, which some authors consider to be a burned-out GCT (45) may create diagnostic difficulties because GCT may contain areas of storiform and cellular fibrous tissue intermingled with a few giant cells in a pattern exactly like that of benign fibrous histiocytoma.

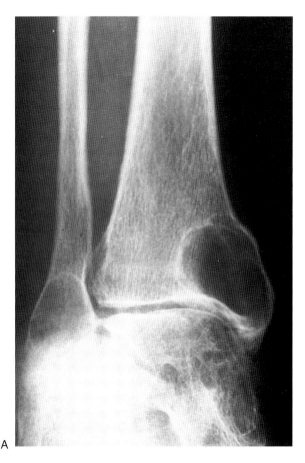

A

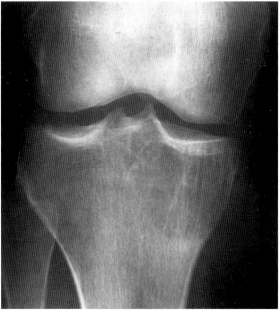

B

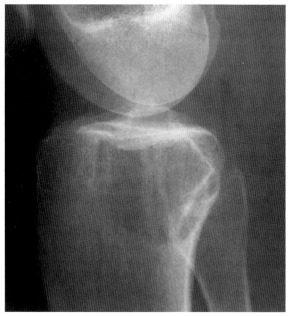

C

FIG. 10. Differential diagnosis of giant-cell tumor. **A:** A large lytic eccentric lesion extending into the articular end of distal tibia of a 40-year-old man was originally thought to represent a giant-cell tumor. The biopsy revealed an intraosseous ganglion. Note a distinct sclerotic border, rarely present in giant-cell tumors. **B, C:** An osteolytic metastasis from a renal cell carcinoma into the articular end of the tibia in this 42-year-old woman has an appearance of a giant-cell tumor.

However, the latter tumor does not exhibit broad sheets of polygonal mononuclear cells with heavy interspersal of giant cells, which is a pattern diagnostic of GCT. It is possible for certain epiphyseal lesions to be arbitrarily diagnosed as GCT or as benign fibrous histiocytoma (24). Matsuno reclassified three of five epiphyseal lesions with the latter diagnosis as

being GCT (45). *Clear-cell chondrosarcoma* is fairly easy to distinguish from GCT because it contains clusters of large clear cells (see Chapter 3).

If the giant cell–containing lesion is located in the metaphysis and the growth plate is still open, there are several possibilities in the differential diagnosis. *Nonossifying fi-*

broma and, with a lower probability, *fibrous cortical defect* can be considered, but because of their giant cells arranged in small groups and exhibiting a resorption activity, and the more or less marked cartwheel-like pattern of the spindle cell stroma, the histiocytic character of these lesions becomes obvious. Both lesions may be characterized by groups of foam cells. Microscopic fields within GCT may contain spindle cells, fibrosis, and clumps of foamy macrophages that cannot be histologically distinguished from nonossifying fibroma (24). In most cases these changes are only focal and the typical GCT pattern predominates. *Aneurysmal bone cyst* can be differentiated because of its more or less large spaces bordered by flat undifferentiated cells and containing blood, as well as the presence of smaller and not evenly distributed giant cells, whereas in a true GCT the giant cells are larger and contain more nuclei (Fig. 11). However, it should be kept in mind that GCT, like many other tumors, may be associated with secondary aneurysmal bone cyst formation, so that constituents of both lesions may be found. Differentiation is particularly difficult in so-called solid aneurysmal bone cyst or *giant-cell reparative granuloma* (7,78). This tumor contains giant cells, often in large numbers, and has a solid component that resembles the spindle cell variant of GCT. Its smaller size and the clustered arrangement of the giant cells may assist in the differential diagnosis. The tissue of GCT usually contains less fibrosis and is largely composed of sheets of characteristic mononuclear cells (24). Giant-cell reparative granuloma, on the other hand, is more fibrotic, and hemorrhage and hemosiderin deposition are more prominent. Both lesions may exhibit foci of reactive bone formation, but this is more commonly seen in giant-cell reparative granuloma (24). *Chondromyxoid fibroma* is usually not a diagnostic problem because large areas of the tumor possess typical myxoid characteristics. *Brown tumor of hyperparathyroidism* contains numerous giant cells,

but these are smaller than in GCT and, instead of being uniformly distributed, are usually arranged in groups (Fig. 12).

The differential diagnosis must also consider giant cell–containing malignant tumors. A particular problem is that of *osteosarcoma* with prominent giant cells (so-called giant cell–rich osteosarcoma), which emphasizes the fact that giant cell tumor is frequently a diagnosis of exclusion. The histologic examination of some osteosarcomas reveals that they consist predominantly of large sheets of giant cells, many or most of which are histologically bland. Production of osteoid may be minimal, detectable only by high-power microscopy as fine strands that surround a population of pleomorphic, mononuclear stromal cells. These cells may be undetectable at low power. However, on higher power examination the tissue consists of scattered hyperchromatic cells exhibiting many atypical mitotic figures. When radiographic studies suggest the presence of matrix production, a permeative growth pattern, a lesion not extending to the articular cartilage, or a lesion in a bone with an active growthplate, giant cell–rich osteosarcoma should be suspected and a very careful histologic examination is warranted (24). By the same token, the giant cell–rich variant of *malignant fibrous histiocytoma* should be included in the differential diagnosis, particularly when irregular arrangement of the usually smaller giant cells and the pleomorphism and the hyperchromasia of their nuclei is present. *Telangiectatic osteosarcoma* may be difficult to exclude unless special consideration is given to the conspicuous pleomorphism of the tumor tissue and the high number of blood-filled spaces. In all three of these malignant tumors, the usual location in the metaphysis may be of help in differentiation from GCT, which is usually located in the articular end of bone.

Giant-cell tumor may occasionally be confused with *metastatic carcinoma* containing giant cells. These lesions

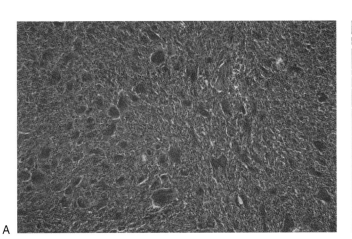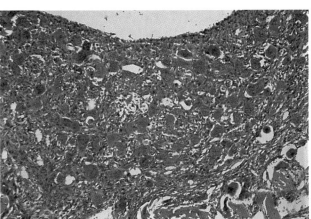

A B

FIG. 11. Giant-cell tumor: differential diagnosis. **A:** True giant-cell tumor is characterized by spindle cell tissue containing numerous giant cells which are usually larger and contain more nuclei than in aneurysmal bone cyst (hematoxylin and eosin, original magnification ×50). **B:** In a solid area of an aneurysmal bone cyst the giant cells are smaller and are not evenly distributed, but instead arranged in groups. In addition the presence of osteoid (*bottom right*) and vascular spaces (*top*) makes the distinction obvious (hematoxylin and eosin, original magnification ×100).

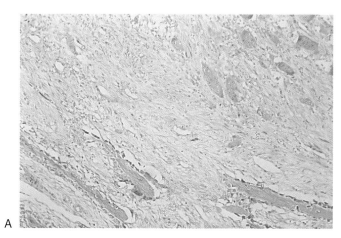
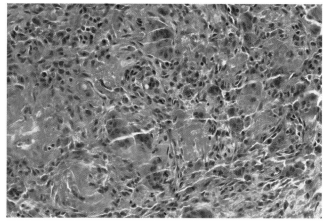

A

B

FIG. 12. Differential diagnosis of giant-cell tumor: brown tumor of hyperparathyroidism. **A:** The loose connective tissue with a group of osteoclasts (*upper right corner*) is bordered by immature bone trabeculae made up of woven bone and lined by dense seams of osteoblasts (*bottom*) (hematoxylin and eosin, original magnification ×25). **B:** At high magnification there is an obvious difference between these giant osteoclasts seen in hyperparathyroidism and giant cells of a giant-cell tumor (compare with Fig. 11A) (hematoxylin and eosin, original magnification ×250).

may contain large numbers of giant cells, indistinguishable from those of GCT. The thyroid, breast, and pancreas (64) are the most common primary sites for these giant cell–rich metastatic lesions. Immunohistochemistry should demonstrate the epithelial quality of the mononuclear carcinoma cells and, in the case of thyroid carcinoma, may show evidence of thyroglobulin production.

As can be seen from this discussion, tumors and tumor-like lesions containing considerable numbers of giant cells are quite common (Table 1). Each of these must be taken into account and must be differentiated from true giant-cell tumor when a giant cell–containing lesion is under investigation. As shown in Table 1, the giant cells are considered to have different functions. However, with the exception of tumor giant cells, which are formed by and belong to the tumor tissue proper, all are derived from the monohistiocytic branch of hematogenic stem cells and are very close relatives, with

corresponding enzymatic pathways involved in their resorptive activity.

The radiologic and pathologic differential diagnosis of giant cell tumor is depicted in Fig. 13.

Simple Bone Cyst

The simple bone cyst (SBC), also called unicameral bone cyst, is a tumor-like lesion of unknown cause, attributed to a local disturbance of bone growth (88,92,100,120). Although the pathogenesis is still unknown (109), the lesion appears to be reactive or developmental rather than to represent a true neoplasm (24). Simple bone cyst consists of a solitary cavity lined by a membrane of variable thickness and filled with a clear yellow fluid (83). It represents approximately 3% of all primary bone lesions (89).

TABLE 1. *Giant-cell tumor and lesions containing different forms of giant cells (GC)*

Tumor or tumor-like lesion	Type of giant cells
Giant-cell tumor of bone	Osteoclast-like gigantic GC
Osteoid osteoma	Osteoclast GC
Osteoblastoma	Osteoclast GC
Aneurysmal bone cyst	Osteoclast and resorptive GC
Giant-cell reparative granuloma	Osteoclast and resorptive GC
Simple bone cyst	Osteoclast and resorptive GC
Chondroblastoma	"Chondroclast" GC
Chondromyxoid fibroma	"Chondroclast" GC
Clear-cell chondrosarcoma	Osteoclast GC
Giant cell–rich osteosarcoma	Tumor and osteoclast GC
Telangiectatic osteosarcoma	Tumor GC
Nonossifying fibroma (fibrous cortical defect)	Resorptive GC
Malignant fibrous histiocytoma (giant cell–rich variant)	Tumor GC
Brown tumor of hyperparathyroidism	Osteoclast GC
Langerhans cell granuloma	Histiocytic GC
Paget disease	Osteoclast GC

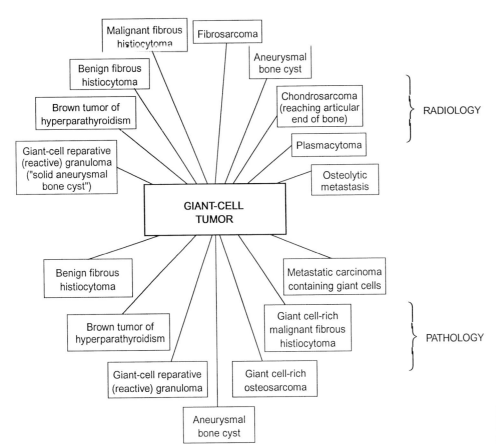

FIG. 13. Radiologic and pathologic differential diagnosis of giant cell tumor.

Clinical Presentation

The SBC is more common in males (3:1) and is usually detected during the first two decades of life (94). About 65% of these cysts occur in teenagers, and an additional 20% in the first decade of life (24,113). The vast majority of SBC are located in the proximal diaphysis of the humerus and the femur, especially when they occur in patients younger than 17 years (100,112). The symptoms include pain, swelling, or stiffness at the nearest joint (87). A pathologic fracture is often the first sign of the lesion (93,98). In fact, this is the most common complication of SBC and occurs in about 66% of cases. In older patients, the incidence of involvement of atypical sites, such as the calcaneus, talus, and ilium, rises significantly (95,113) (Fig. 14). In these sites the lesion is usually asymptomatic and is discovered by accident.

Imaging

Radiographically, the appearance of an SBC is that of a centrally located, well-circumscribed, radiolucent lesion with sclerotic margins. The lesion is located within the metaphysis or diaphysis of a long bone, abutting or being remote from the cartilaginous growth plate (Fig. 15). Epiphyseal extension is unusual (90,96).

The cortex is frequently thinned and cortical expansion may be present, but, unlike the aneurysmal bone cyst, the width of the SBC does not exceed the width of the neighboring growth plate (94). A periosteal reaction is absent unless there has been a pathologic fracture, and this feature distinguishes it from aneurysmal bone cyst, in which there is almost invariably some degree of periosteal response. Diagnosis is best based on plain film radiographs; conventional tomography and computed tomography (CT) are used only exceptionally in equivocal cases.

Occasionally (in 20% of cases in the experience of Struhl et al.), one can identify a characteristic "fallen fragment" sign (106, 118). This represents a piece of fractured cortex that is displaced into the interior of the lesion, indicating that the lesion is either hollow or is filled with fluid, as most SBCs are (Fig. 16). A variant of this phenomenon is the "trap door" sign (94) [also called a "forme fruste" of the fallen fragment by Reynolds (115)], in which the fragment remains attached to the periosteum but folds inward at the fracture site and floats in the fluid. It is important to obtain multiple views of the cyst to accurately identify this sign because a pathologic fracture through a solid lesion can also produce fragments that appear intramedullary on one view but are in fact adjacent to the outer cortex or are located in the soft tissue. Plain radiographs taken in both the erect and the recumbent position (111), or the observation of a movement of the fallen fragment under fluoroscopy, may demonstrate the free movement of the fragments within the cyst. These signs permit differentiation of SBC from radiographically similar ra-

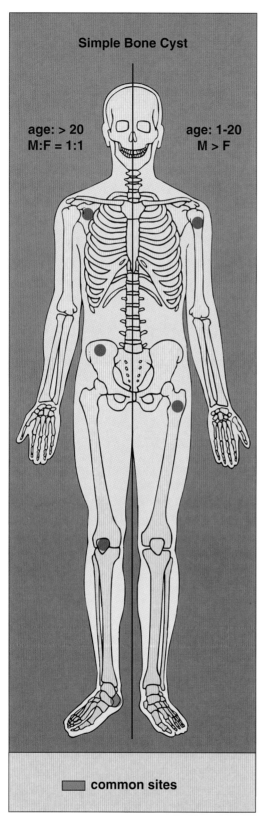

FIG. 14. Simple bone cyst: skeletal sites of predilection, peak age range, and male-to-female ratio. The left half of the skeleton shows sites of occurrence seen in an older patient population.

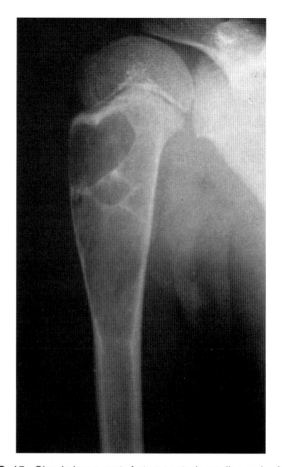

FIG. 15. Simple bone cyst. Anteroposterior radiograph of the right shoulder in a 6-year-old boy shows the typical appearance of this lesion. Its location in the metaphysis and the proximal diaphysis of the humerus is also characteristic. The radiolucent lesion is centrally located and shows pseudosepta. Note the slight thinning of the cortex and lack of periosteal reaction.

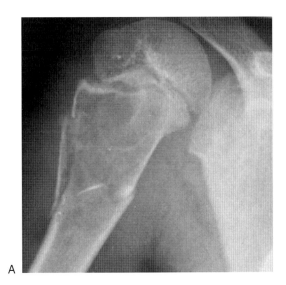

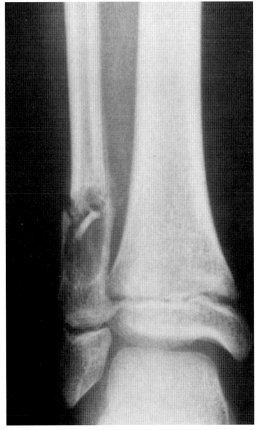

FIG. 16. Simple bone cyst: "fallen fragment" sign. **A:** One of the most common complications of simple bone cyst is pathologic fracture, as seen here in the proximal humeral diaphysis of a 6-year-old boy. The presence of the "fallen fragment" sign is characteristic for this lesion. **B:** Anteroposterior radiograph of the right ankle of a 5-year-old boy shows a radiolucent lesion in the distal diaphysis of the fibula. There is a pathologic fracture through the lesion and the associated periosteal reaction. A radiodense cortical fragment in the center of the lesion represents the "fallen fragment" sign, identifying this lesion as a simple bone cyst.

diolucent lesions containing solid fibrous or cartilaginous tissue, such as aneurysmal bone cyst, fibrous dysplasia, nonossifying fibroma, and enchondroma.

CT may be helpful when the appearance of an SBC is atypical or when the lesion is located in the pelvis. This modality may also assist in the identification of a fallen fragment sign (118). Attenuation values of 15 to 20 Hounsfield units have been reported in the center of fluid-filled cysts (86,95). Bone scintigraphy may demonstrate an increased peripheral uptake around the cyst and a decreased central activity, although this appearance is not specific for the SBC (98). Some cysts may be scintigraphically normal. Magnetic resonance imaging (MRI) of a cyst shows the signal characteristics of fluid: a low to intermediate signal on T1-weighted images and a bright, homogeneous signal on T2 weighting (94) (Fig. 17).

Histopathology

Histologically, SBC is a diagnosis of exclusion. A vigorous surgical curettage, if the lesion is not simply injected, yields almost no solid tissue, but the walls of the cavity may show remnants of fibrous tissue or, occasionally, a flattened single-cell lining (Fig. 18). Granulation tissue, containing hemosiderin deposits and small lymphocyte infiltrates, is often present, along with scattered osteoclasts (24). Chemi-

cal examination of the fluid usually identifies an elevated alkaline phosphatase level (116). Furthermore, a cloudy-appearing, cell-free material is often found in the loose connective tissue surrounding the cysts (99). With stains for collagen, such as van Gieson stain, the material stains strongly and reveals loose and irregularly arranged fibers. It therefore cannot be fibrin, which it is considered by some authors to represent on the basis of H&E staining (Fig. 19).

Differential Diagnosis

Radiology

In a long bone, the main differential diagnosis is an *aneurysmal bone cyst*. The primary differences are that SBC is a centric solitary lesion, with minimal expansion, invariably lacks periosteal reaction, and never extends into the soft tissues. In contrast, an aneurysmal bone cyst is almost invariably an eccentric lesion, with a significant blown-up appearance, and is always accompanied by a solid periosteal reaction (usually in form of a buttress) (see Figs. 25 and 26).

Fibrous dysplasia may mimic an SBC, but usually it lacks trabeculation and exhibits a ground-glass, smoky appearance. If a pathologic fracture occurs and the fallen fragment sign can be demonstrated, a diagnosis of a SBC is usually confirmed.

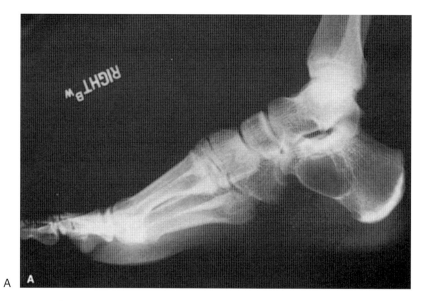

A

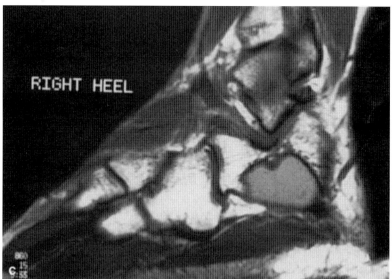

RIGHT HEEL

B

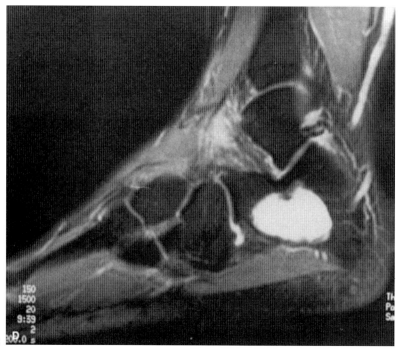

C

FIG. 17. Simple bone cyst: magnetic resonance imaging. **A:** The lateral radiograph of the foot of an 18-year-old man shows a radiolucent lesion in the calcaneus with slightly sclerotic border. **B:** Sagittal T1-weighted (SE, TR 850, TE 15) MRI demonstrates homogenous intermediate signal intensity within the lesion, rimmed by low-signal intensity sclerotic margin. **C:** Sagittal STIR MR image shows that the lesion now is of homogeneous high signal intensity. (From Greenfield GB, Arrington JA. *Imaging of bone tumors,* Philadelphia: JB Lippincott, 1995;217, 218.)

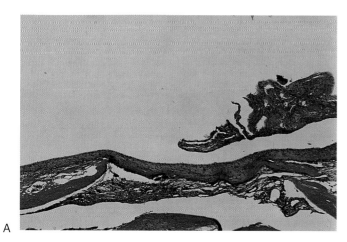
A

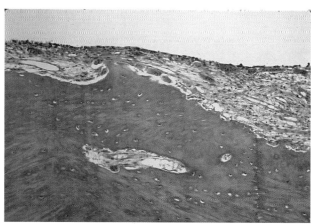
B

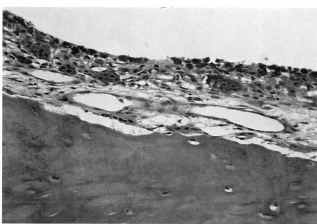
C

FIG. 18. Histopathology of simple bone cyst. **A:** Flattened fibrous lining contains a few bone trabeculae (hematoxylin and eosin, original magnification ×25). **B:** At higher magnification within a fibrous lining several giant cells are present (hematoxylin and eosin, original magnification ×100). **C:** High magnification photomicrograph shows more clearly the flat fibrous lining with scattered giant cells (hematoxylin and eosin, original magnification ×250).

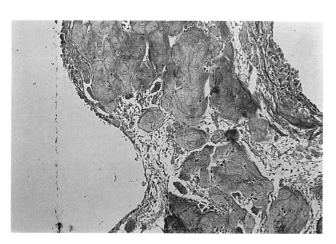

FIG. 19. Histopathology of simple bone cyst. The cyst cavity (*left*) is bordered by an undifferentiated flat cell layer. In the loose connective tissue of the cyst wall there are extended areas of a "cloudy," loose, collagen-positive material bordered by some giant cells. Because of its collagenous characteristics the material cannot be fibrin (van Gieson, original magnification ×25).

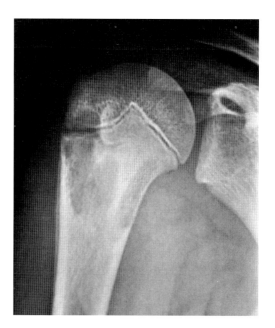

FIG. 20. Differential diagnosis of simple bone cyst. A bone abscess may mimic a simple bone cyst, as seen here in the proximal humerus of a 12-year-old boy. The periosteal reaction in the absence of pathologic fracture and the extension of the lesion into the epiphysis favors the diagnosis of bone abscess.

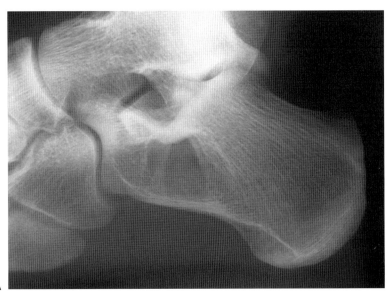

A

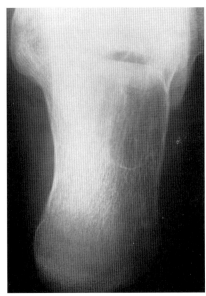

B

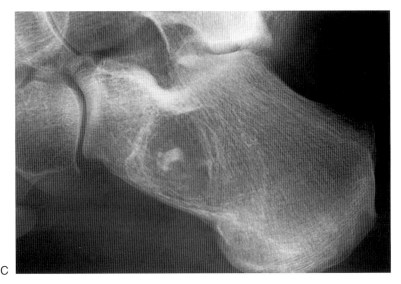

C

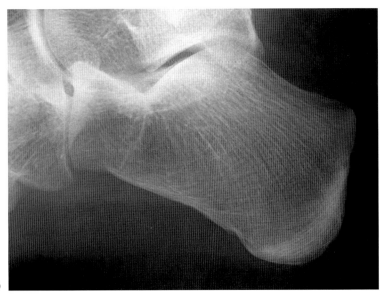

D

FIG. 21. Differential diagnosis of simple bone cyst. (**A**) Lateral and (**B**) axial views of the ankle in a 32-year-old man show a simple bone cyst in the calcaneus. Typically, bone cysts occurring at this site are located in the anterolateral aspect of the bone. (**C**) A bone infarct in the region of Ward triangle exhibits central calcification. (**D**) A pseudotumor in the region of Ward triangle exhibits no sharp margination unlike the simple bone cyst, and in addition shows some bone trabeculae traversing the radiolucent area.

Nonossifying fibroma can usually be distinguished by its eccentric location and its well-defined, usually thick, sclerotic margin.

Brown tumor of hyperparathyroidism may at times appear similar to SBC, particularly if it is located in the proximal humerus or proximal femur. In this situation, one should look for other features of hyperparathyroidism, such as osteopenia and subcortical resorption. *Bone abscess* likewise may occasionally mimic SBC, particularly when it is located in sites of SBC predilection such as the proximal humerus or the proximal femur. However, the presence of a periosteal reaction and the frequent extension of the former lesion beyond the boundaries of a growth plate are important features indicating a bone abscess (Fig. 20).

In the calcaneus, SBC is characteristically located at the base of the calcaneal neck on the lateral aspect of the bone, within a particular anatomic structure poor in trabeculae called Ward triangle. Most of the "cysts" in this location have a characteristic shape: the anterior margin is usually straight and vertically oriented, and the posterior border is typically curvilinear, paralleling the trabeculae in the posterior portion of the bone (82) (Fig. 21A, B). In this location, SBC must be differentiated from a bone infarct, an aneurysmal bone cyst, and several other benign bone tumors (84,114). Here are some helpful hints.

A *bone infarct* often exhibits central calcifications, which are never present in an SBC (Fig. 21C).

Aneurysmal bone cyst of the calcaneus is more expansive than SBC. The margin may be either poorly defined or sharp and thinly sclerotic (103), and is usually located toward the plantar and posterior aspect of the bone (85,97), although occasionally it may be found within Ward's triangle. In the latter location it probably develops secondary to other lesions, such as bone infarct or an intraosseous hemorrhage.

Chondroblastoma of the calcaneus is usually a subarticular lesion and is located in the subtalar region. It may exhibit a sclerotic, lobulated margin. Seven percent of chondroblastomas located in the calcaneus present with punctate calcifications (104).

It is important to remember that Ward triangle normally contains fatty marrow, and this feature has been interpreted as an intraosseous lipoma by several authors (91,102,107). These pseudotumors are usually found by serendipity, as they are not symptomatic (101,117,119) (Fig. 21D).

Pathology

SBC is a diagnosis of exclusion, and pathologists must rely on the radiologic examination. In a long tubular bone the diagnosis is usually readily made. Most problems occur when the lesion is located in the calcaneus. In this instance, a *bone infarct* must be included in the differential diagnosis (105). The presence of characteristic microscopic features of dead bone marrow is diagnostic for the latter (Fig. 22).

If the membrane of the SBC contains giant cells of the osteoclastic type, *aneurysmal bone cyst* may be a considera-

tion. However, fairly characteristic of SBC is the finding of focal deposits of the amorphous, fibrillar, cloudy eosinophilic material that stains strongly for collagen with special stains. This material resembles osteoid and may undergo calcification or even ossification (110).

The radiologic and pathologic differential diagnosis of simple bone cyst is depicted in Fig. 23.

Aneurysmal Bone Cyst

The term aneurysmal bone cyst (ABC) was first used by Jaffe and Lichtenstein to describe two examples of blood-filled cysts in which tissue from the cyst wall contained conspicuous spaces, areas of hemosiderin deposition, giant cells, and occasional bone trabeculae (100). In a subsequent publication, Jaffe chose the designation aneurysmal bone cyst as a descriptive term for this lesion to emphasize the blown-out appearance (145). Although the cause of this lesion is unknown (131), alterations in local hemodynamics related to venous obstruction or arteriovenous fistula are believed to play an important role (127,159). Some investigators believe that the lesion is caused by a trauma (108,132,157,160). Dahlin and McLeod believe that it may be similar to and related to other reactive nonneoplastic processes, such as giant-cell reparative granuloma or traumatic reactions observed in periosteum and bone (134). ABC constitutes approximately 6% of the primary lesions of bone (144). The lesion may arise *de novo* in bone, in which case no recognizable preexisting lesion can be demonstrated in the tissue, or it may be associated with various benign (e.g., giant-cell tumor, osteoblastoma, chondroblastoma, chondromyxoid fibroma, fibrous dysplasia) and malignant (e.g., osteosarcoma, fibrosarcoma, or chondrosarcoma) lesions (128,146,153). The concept of ABC as a secondary phenomenon occurring in a preexisting lesion has been validated by several investigators (147,149,

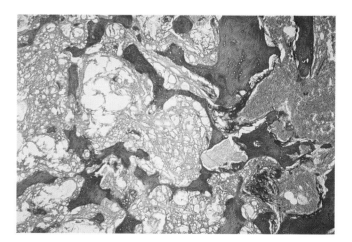

FIG. 22. Differential diagnosis of simple bone cyst: histopathology of bone infarct. Necrotic remnants of fatty marrow with "oil lakes" (*center and left*) are seen in addition to bone trabeculae with empty osteocyte lacunae. A cell-rich and fiber-rich reparative connective tissue is growing in (right) (van Gieson, original magnification ×12).

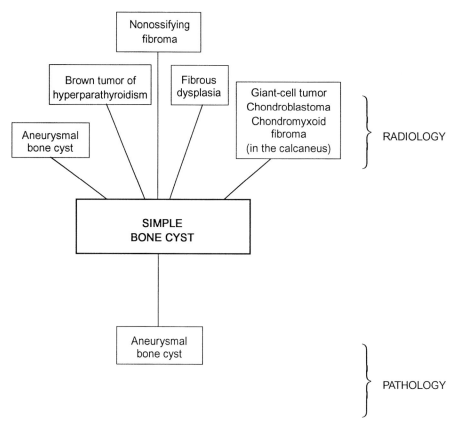

FIG. 23. Radiologic and pathologic differential diagnosis of simple bone cyst.

154,155). Some investigators, however, regard ABC as a reparative process, probably the result of trauma or tumor-induced anomalous vascular process (138,156). The typical ABC affects the medullary portion of a long bone (151). ABC localized to the cortex or in a subperiosteal location are unusual (130,164). Malignant transformation of ABC is extremely rare (148) and it is still a controversial issue.

Clinical Presentation

ABC is seen predominantly in childhood, and 76% of cases occur in patients younger than 20 years of age (173). There is a slight female preponderance (162,171). The metaphysis of the long bones is the site of predilection, although the diaphysis, the flat bones, the short tubular bones (124), and even the spine may be involved (145) (Fig. 24). The pelvis accounts for about 50% of all flat bone lesions (174). When the spine is affected, the lesion is usually situated in the posterior elements (neural arch) (134,145,150), but the vertebral body may also be affected (171). In this location, ABC may occasionally cross the intervertebral disk to involve more than one vertebra (144). Lesions in a spinal location often produce clinical symptoms by compression of adjacent structures (the spinal cord or nerve roots) or as a result of a pathologic fracture (158,159). The most common

symptoms in lesions located in the long tubular bones include pain and local swelling (133,158).

Imaging

The radiographic hallmark of ABC is a multicystic, eccentric expansion (blow-out) of the bone, with a buttress or thin shell of periosteal response (Fig. 25). In the short tubular bones the lesion may appear more central, destroying the entire shaft of the bone (137,141). The lesion exhibits a geographic type of bone destruction with a narrow zone of transition and often a sclerotic margin (136,167) (Fig. 26). Sometimes ridges or trabeculations are observed within the lesion (Fig. 27). Rarely, internal calcifications may be present (166). A soft-tissue extension is produced by bulging of the periosteum. This periosteal envelope may or may not be visible on plain radiographs. The outer shell of bone may be partially absent (141) but, if seen, the diagnosis can frequently be ascertained. In the vertebral column the posterior elements are usually affected. Although plain radiographs are usually sufficient to evaluate the lesion, other modalities, such as conventional tomography, radionuclide bone scan, CT, and MRI can be of further assistance (Fig. 28).

CT is superior to plain radiography in defining these lesions, particularly in areas in which bony anatomy is complex (e.g., the pelvis). The cortical or periosteal shell sur-

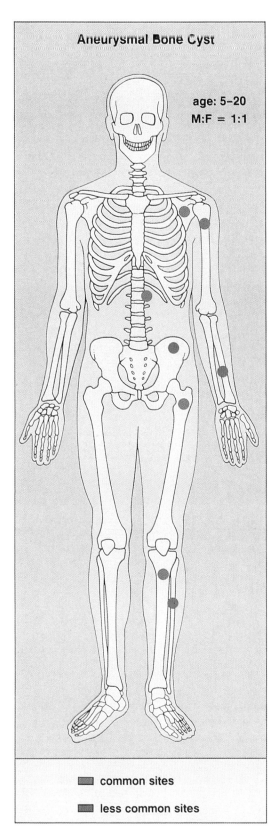

FIG. 24. Aneurysmal bone cyst: skeletal sites of predilection, peak age range, and male-to-female ratio.

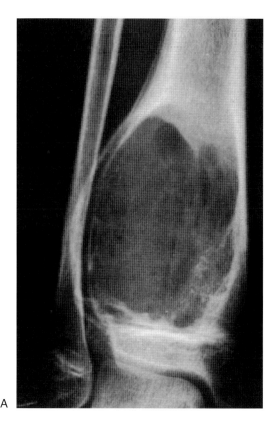

A

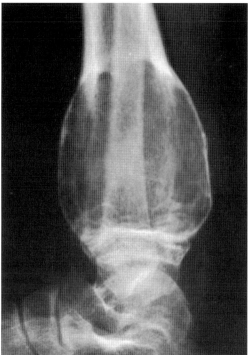

B

FIG. 25. Aneurysmal bone cyst. (A) Anteroposterior and (B) lateral radiographs of the right lower leg in an 8-year-old girl show an expansive radiolucent lesion in the metaphysis of the distal tibia, extending into the diaphysis. Note its eccentric location in the bone and the buttress of periosteal reaction at the proximal aspect of the lesion.

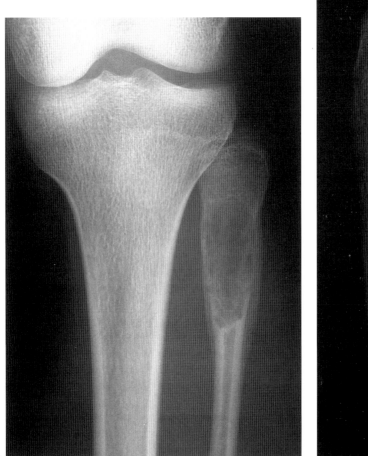
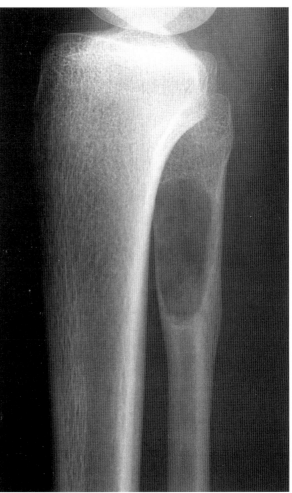

A
B

FIG. 26. Aneurysmal bone cyst. **(A)** Anteroposterior and **(B)** lateral radiographs of the left upper leg of a 17-year-old girl show a radiolucent lesion in the proximal fibula exhibiting a narrow zone of transition, a sclerotic margin, and a well-organized periosteal reaction.

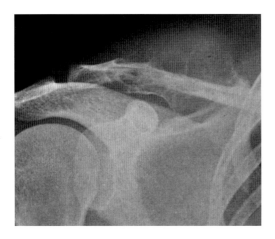

FIG. 27. Aneurysmal bone cyst. An anteroposterior radiograph of the right shoulder of a 19-year-old woman shows an expansive, trabeculated lesion in the right clavicle. Note also a soft-tissue extension.

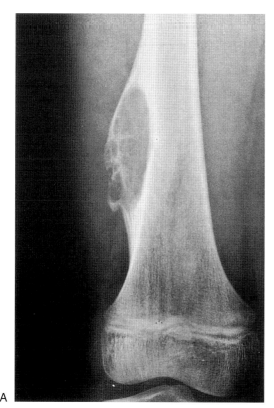

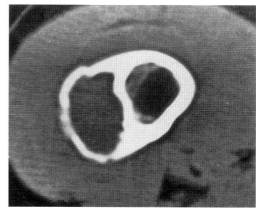

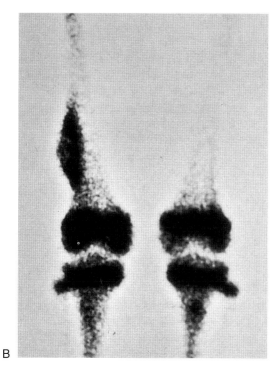

FIG. 28. Aneurysmal bone cyst: scintigraphy and computed tomography. **A:** Plain radiograph of the distal femur of an 8-year-old boy with a six-month history of pain in the lower right thigh shows a radiolucent expansive lesion located eccentrically in the femur and buttressed proximally and distally by a solid periosteal reaction. **B:** Radionuclide bone scan obtained after injection of 10 mCi (375 MBq) of technetium-99m-labeled diphosphorate (MDP) demonstrates increased uptake of radiopharmaceutical tracer by the lesion. **C:** CT section shows intracortical location of the lesion, which balloons out from the lateral aspect of the femur but is contained within an uninterrupted shell of periosteal new bone.

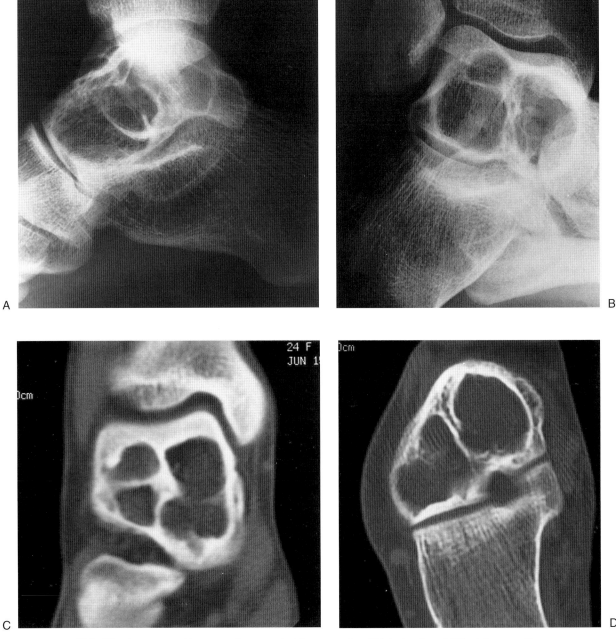

FIG. 29. Aneurysmal bone cyst: computed tomography. **(A)** Lateral and **(B)** oblique radiographs of the right ankle of a 24-year-old woman show a radiolucent, trabeculated lesion in the talus. **(C)** Coronal and **(D)** axial CT sections demonstrate the internal ridges to better advantage.

rounding ABC and its soft tissue extension, as well as the sharp interface between the extraosseous mass and the adjacent tissue planes, are well demonstrated with this technique (141,165). CT may also show ridges in the bony walls, described on plain radiographs as trabeculation or septation (141), and corresponding to the ridges found pathologically (Fig. 29). Attenuation coefficient values (Hounsfield units) range from 20 to 78. Fluid-fluid levels can also be demonstrated (97,140,142,143). These fluid levels are believed to represent the sedimentation of red blood cells and serum within the cystic cavities (125,172). To demonstrate this phenomenon, the patient must remain motionless for at least 10 min before scanning, and imaging must be performed in a plane perpendicular to the fluid levels.

Skeletal scintigraphy may occasionally be helpful because it reflects the vascular nature of the lesion (142,147). Some investigators have described an increased uptake in a ring-like pattern around the periphery of an ABC (139,142, 152,168). Although this phenomenon is not specific for the lesion, because it can also be observed in simple bone cyst, bone infarct, and other lesions (170), the scintigraphic findings corroborate the radiographic presentation. Hudson found no correlation between the histologic features of the lesion, the amount and type of fluid contained within the cyst and the scintigraphic pattern or intensity of uptake in his experience with 25 patients with ABC who underwent skeletal scintigraphy using ^{99m}Tc-MDP and ^{99m}Tc-pyrophosphate (142).

MRI findings are rather characteristic and usually allow a specific diagnosis of ABC (176). These include a well-defined lesion, often with lobulated contours (159) (Fig. 30), cystic cavities with fluid-fluid levels of varying intensity, multiple internal septations, and an intact rim of low-inten-

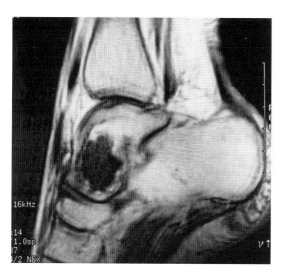

FIG. 30. Aneurysmal bone cyst: magnetic resonance imaging. A sagittal T1-weighted (SE, TR 600, TE 16) MRI (same patient as in Fig. 29) demonstrates a lobulated low-signal-intensity lesion in the talus. Unlike on CT examination, the septa are not well delineated.

sity signal surrounding the lesion (125). This rim has been described as an indicator of a benign process (175). Occasionally, small diverticulum-like projections arising in the walls of the cyst have been observed. The wide range of signal intensities within the cyst on both T1- and T2-weighted sequences is probably due to settling of degraded blood products and reflects intracystic hemorrhages of different ages (125) (Fig. 31).

Histopathology

Histologically, the lesion consists of multiple blood-filled spaces alternating with more solid areas (134,169) (Fig. 32). These spaces are lined by a single layer of flat undifferentiated cells which react negatively with all endothelial markers (123). An endothelial lining and other blood vessel components are rarely identified (122,134). The solid tissue surrounding these spaces is composed of fibrous, richly vascular connective tissue, the blood vessels exhibiting a progression from small to large caliber (75). Mitotic figures may be observed in the fibroblasts (121,158). The fibrous lining contains many giant cells, usually in clusters (Fig. 33). Furthermore, lamellae of primitive woven bone may be present in the lining of the cyst as well as deeper in the connective tissue (Fig. 34). Deposits of iron pigment are a common finding (158).

Differential Diagnosis

Radiology

The conditions that should always be included in the differential diagnosis at any age are *simple bone cyst* (SBC) and *chondromyxoid fibroma* and, after skeletal maturity, when the lesion extends into the articular end of bone, *giant-cell tumor* (150). The most critical points in differentiation of ABC from SBC are that the former is an eccentric, expansive lesion, invariably associated with some degree of periosteal reaction (usually a solid layer or solid buttress), whereas the latter is a centrally located lesion, showing little if any expansion, and exhibiting periosteal reaction only when a pathologic fracture has occurred. In thin bones, such as the ulna, fibula, metacarpals, or metatarsals, the characteristic eccentricity of ABC may be lost and, conversely, SBC may demonstrate expansive features. Because the former contains solid tissue, whereas SBC is a hollow structure filled with fluid, a fallen fragment sign (if present) is a good differential feature, pointing to the latter diagnosis. *Chondromyxoid fibroma* may be indistinguishable from ABC because both lesions are eccentric, expansive, and usually affect the metaphysis, exhibiting a reactive sclerotic rim and the above-mentioned solid periosteal reaction (usually in the form of a buttress). CT and MRI are sometimes effective in making this distinction if it identifies fluid-fluid levels, a phenomenon that points to the diagnosis of ABC because chondromyxoid fibroma is a solid lesion. In the mature

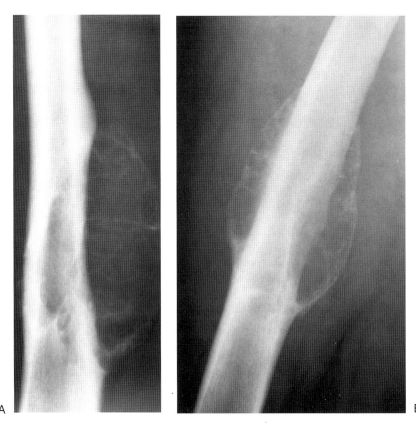

A

B

FIG. 31. Aneurysmal bone cyst: magnetic resonance imaging. (**A**) Anteroposterior and (**B**) lateral radiographs of the midshaft of right femur of a 15-year-old girl show an expansive lesion arising eccentrically from the medial aspect of the bone. Note a thin shell of periosteal bone covering the lesion and a buttress of periosteal reaction at its proximal and distal extent. (**C, D**) Coronal T1-weighted (SE, TR 600, TE 20) MR images demonstrate inhomogeneity of the lesion and internal septations. (**E**) Axial T2-weighted (SE, TR 2000, TE 90) MRI shows the lesion to exhibit a high signal intensity. A fluid-fluid level, frequently seen in aneurysmal bone cyst, is well demonstrated.

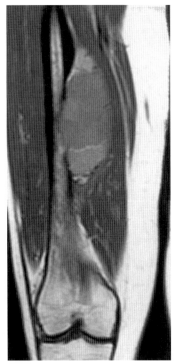

C

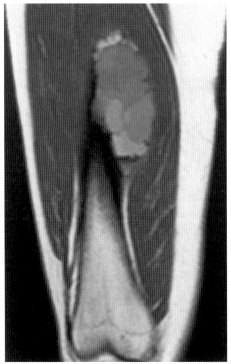

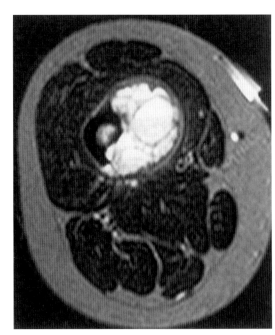

D

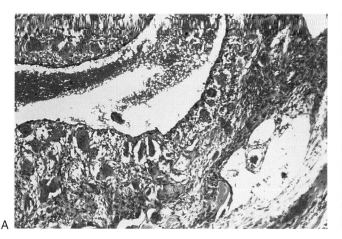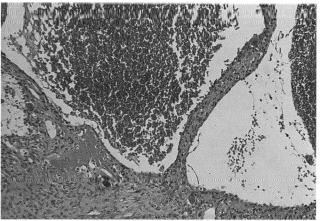

A

B

FIG. 32. Histopathology of aneurysmal bone cyst. **A:** Vascular spaces are bordered with solid tissue containing spindle cells and giant cells (hematoxylin and eosin, original magnification ×100). **B:** In another area blood-filled spaces are separated by narrow septae containing spindle fibroblasts bordering the vascular spaces with flat undifferentiated cells but without any blood vessel structures. Newly formed osteoid is also present (*lower left*) (hematoxylin and eosin, original magnification ×50).

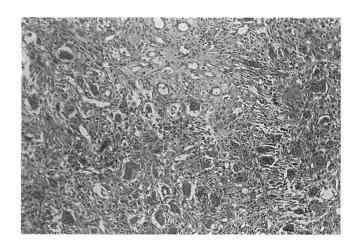

FIG. 33. Histopathology of aneurysmal bone cyst. Solid areas with densely arranged capillaries contain fairly large numbers of the giant-cells osteoclast type, similar to those of a giant-cell tumor. Here, however, they are grouped in clusters, are smaller, and less numerous than in the true giant-cell tumor (hematoxylin and eosin, original magnification ×50).

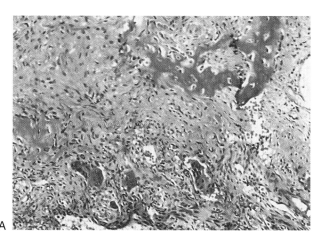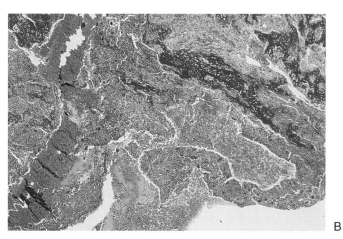

A

B

FIG. 34. Histopathology of aneurysmal bone cyst. **A:** Blood cyst (*bottom*) lined by a seam of flat undifferentiated cells and randomly scattered small giant cells. Above noted is formation of considerable amounts of primitive woven bone lined by osteoblasts. (hematoxylin and eosin, original magnification ×40). **B:** Typical lamellar structure (*lower right*) is surrounded by fresh blood. Fairly extended trabeculae of primitive woven bone (*red*) are seen close to the surface of the cyst (*upper right*) (van Gieson, original magnification ×12).

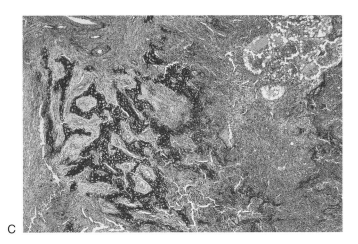

C

FIG. 34. (*Continued.*) **C:** Solid areas are made up of fibrous tissue with large amount of bone formation (*red*) and some small cysts (*upper right corner*). Significant fresh bleeding is present (van Gieson, original magnification ×12).

skeleton, giant cell tumor may closely mimic ABC, although it usually is not associated with a periosteal reaction and rarely exhibits a zone of reactive sclerosis.

Giant-cell reparative granuloma (so-called solid aneurysmal bone cyst) may be indistinguishable from the solid parts of the conventional ABC (28, 129). This lesion, however, unlike true ABC, usually involves the short tubular bones of the hands and feet (26,58,78,161). The cortex is thin but is characteristically intact (135). Extension into the surrounding soft tissues is distinctly uncommon, and the periosteal reaction is usually absent (26).

Nonossifying fibroma, if it is predominantly radiolucent and is associated with a cortical expansion (a rare occurrence) (Fig. 35), may resemble ABC (**see also Fig. 4-8**). However, the former lesion never exhibits a periosteal reaction (unless a pathologic fracture has already occurred).

In smaller bones, such as the fibula, metacarpals, or metatarsals, ABC due to expansive growth may destroy the cortex, mimicking an aggressive tumor such as *osteosarcoma.*

Pathology

In pathologic differential diagnosis of ABC, an essential point to be kept in mind is the fact that, with the exception of SBC, all other entities to be differentiated may in fact contain some elements of ABC (secondary aneurysmal bone cyst engrafted on the other lesions) (Fig. 36). The most critical issue, however, is to distinguish ABC from *telangiectatic osteosarcoma* and from osteosarcoma with engrafted secondary aneurysmal bone cyst. In both of these lesions the presence of pleomorphism and of anaplastic cells is diagnostic. In telangiectatic osteosarcoma it is crucial to recognize pleomorphic tumor tissue immediately bordering the blood-

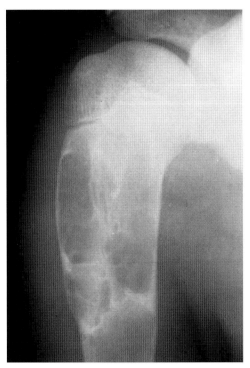

FIG. 35. Differential diagnosis of aneurysmal bone cyst: nonossifying fibroma. In this 12-year-old boy a radiolucent trabeculated lesion in the proximal diaphysis of the right humerus abutting the growth plate was thought to represent either a simple bone cyst or an aneurysmal bone cyst. Note, however, lesion's eccentric location (bulging of the lateral cortex) that speaks against SBC, and lack of periosteal reaction that militate against ABC. On biopsy the lesion proved to be a nonossifying fibroma.

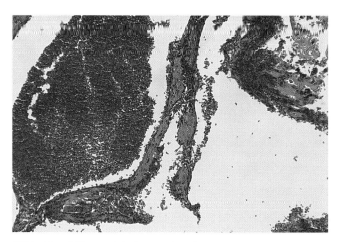

FIG. 36. Differential diagnosis of aneurysmal bone cyst: osteoblastoma with secondary aneurysmal bone cyst. In the center of the lesion of osteoblastoma large blood-filled spaces are bordered by narrow septae of fibrous tissue with some bone formation (hematoxylin and eosin, original magnification ×25).

filled cavity. In osteosarcoma with coexisting ABC, the benign connective tissue bordering the cavity of ABC must be distinguished from the pleomorphic tumor tissue of osteosarcoma. Atypical mitotic figures are often present in both entities and the osteoid, unlike that in ABC, has a more irregular, closely packed pattern (135).

So-called solid aneurysmal bone cyst should also be considered in the differential diagnosis. The term, coined by Sanerkin et al. in 1983, represents in fact a *giant-cell reparative granuloma* (55,134,163). Histologically, this is a predominantly spindle-cell lesion with a plump fibroblastic proliferation and occasional mitotic figures (144). The lesion contains a characteristic reticulated, lacy, chondroid-like material, similar to that seen in conventional ABC but without the typical cyst-like cavities (147). Giant cells are numerous but are smaller and are clustered rather than being in a randomly even distribution, a characteristic feature of giant-cell tumor (28). Fibrous cell proliferation is often associated with strands of irregular islands of osteoid or bone (126). The exact nature of solid aneurysmal bone cyst and its relationship to the solid areas of a true ABC still remain unsettled (135).

Differentiation from *SBC* may be a major problem if only small fragments of the wall are available for histopathologic diagnosis. The presence of cloudy collagenous material suggests SBC, whereas the presence of multiple blood-filled spaces suggests ABC. A *giant-cell tumor* can usually be excluded by the lack of the characteristic findings for this neoplasm, i.e., the dual population of cells: mononuclear stromal cells and evenly distributed giant cells with a much greater number of nuclei (see above). One must remember, however, that there are cases of ABC containing unusually large numbers of giant cells with a greater number of nuclei (Fig. 37), and in such a situation there may be a problem in the histologic differentiation of these two entities.

The radiologic and pathologic differential diagnosis of aneurysmal bone cyst is depicted in Fig. 38.

Intraosseous Lipoma

Lipomas can be categorized according to their location in the bone as intraosseous, cortical, or parosteal lesions (206,207). In the older (183) as well as in more recent (67) publications, intraosseous lipoma is considered to be an extremely rare tumor, in spite of the fact that the normal fatty tissue is so abundant in bone. Most cases of so-called intraosseous lipomas were considered to represent a simple hyperplasia of fat tissue rather than a true tumor (209). Particularly so-called vertebral lipomas, which have been found in 0.6% of a large series of autopsy material, are considered to represent merely foci of fatty marrow (189,209). Also in the current literature intraosseous lipoma is considered to be extremely rare with an incidence of <1 in 1,000 primary bone tumors (67,181). Fewer than 100 cases have been reported (199,211).

In the recent years, an increasing number of reports of intraosseous lipoma have appeared, particularly located in the intertrochanteric and subtrochanteric regions of the femur and in the calcaneus (91,102,105,180,199,203). The authors of these publications apparently do not take into account the fact that, describing the lesions in areas scanty of bone trabeculae but rich in fatty tissue they are dealing with normal bone structures of the particular regions, known as Ward triangle in the anatomical (186), and in the radiologic literature (101,179,187,190,193,210). The calcified lipomas and bone cysts which have been described, particularly located in the calcaneus, are lesions secondary to an infarct (67) and probably developing because of the special anatomic arrangement of the vascular supply in and around the calcaneus (114,191); they do not represent true tumors.

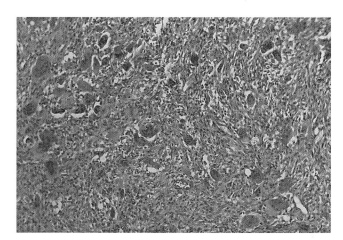

FIG. 37. Histopathology of aneurysmal bone cyst: differential diagnosis. Solid part of the aneurysmal bone cyst contains large giant cells of osteoclast type similar to the presentation of a grade 2 giant-cell tumor. Distinction is based on group arrangement of the giant cells and their smaller size, as well as on the presence of blood-filled spaces (hematoxylin and eosin, original magnification ×50).

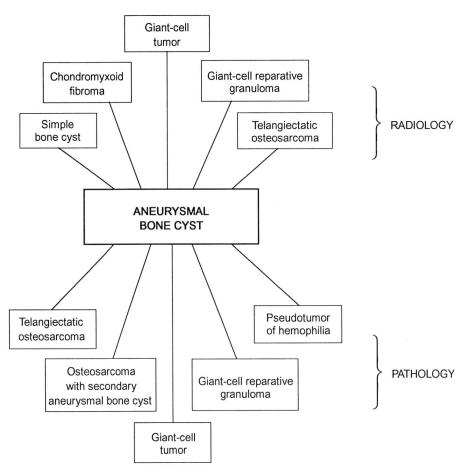

FIG. 38. Radiologic and pathologic differential diagnosis of aneurysmal bone cyst.

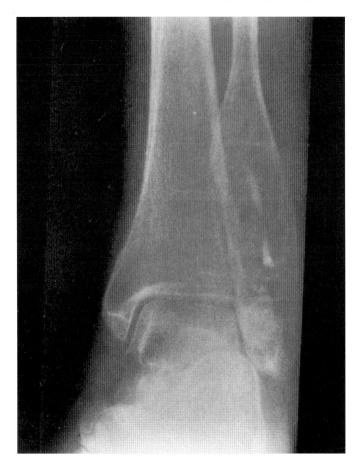

FIG. 39. Intraosseous lipoma. Anteroposterior radiograph of the left ankle shows a radiolucent lesion in the distal fibula exhibiting expansive character, thinning of the cortex, and central calcifications. (Reprinted from Bullough PG. *Atlas of orthopedic pathology,* 2nd ed. New York: Gower, 1992;16.20.)

Clinical Presentation

The tumor has no sex predilection and occurs in the wide range of age from 5 to 75 years (84,199). It is usually an asymptomatic lesion, found on radiographic examinations performed for other reasons (200). Some investigators report a higher incidence of symptomatic patients (204), however, even when a patient is symptomatic, the symptoms are not necessarily related to the lesion. In the largest series to date of 61 intraosseous lipomas (199), the most common site was the inter- and subtrochanteric region of the femur, followed by the calcaneus, ilium, proximal tibia, and sacrum (212). As it is clear from the above discussion, because the intertrochanteric area and Ward triangle in the calcaneus are inherited sites of a prominent amount of fatty tissue, the presence of interosseous lipomas at these sites must be questioned.

Imaging

Intraosseous lipoma has a rather characteristic plain film radiography appearance. It is invariably a nonaggressive ra-

diolucent lesion with sharply defined borders, associated with thinning and bulging of the cortex particularly in thin bones such as fibula or rib (182,183,185,188) (Fig. 39). The central calcifications and ossifications described in a very large numbers of cases (194) invariably represent a sign of fat necrosis that is seen in an infarct of the fatty marrow. CT may be helpful in the diagnosis of these lesions since the Hounsfield units are consistent with fat (202,204). Magnetic resonance imaging (MRI) shows on T1- and T2-weighted images lesion to have a signal similar to subcutaneous fat (178,197) (Fig. 40). After administration of intravenous gadolinium there is no enhancement of the lesion (198). MRI is very effective in demonstrating the exact intraosseous extension of the lesion.

Histopathology

Histologically, intraosseous lipomas are composed of lobules of mature adipose tissue and are characterized by the presence of mature lipocytes, which are slightly larger than nonneoplastic fat cells, in a background of fibroblasts with

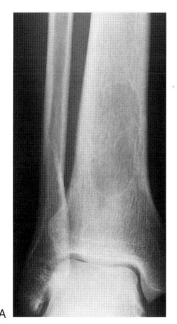
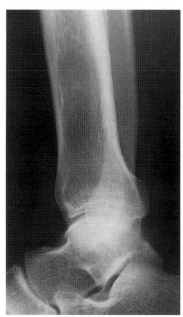
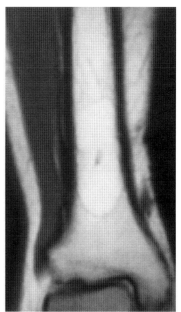

A

B, C

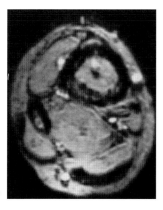

D

FIG. 40. Intraosseous lipoma: magnetic resonance imaging. **A:** Anteroposterior radiographs of the right ankle in a 42-year-old man shows a radiolucent lesion in the distal tibia sharply delineated by a thin sclerotic margin. **B:** On the lateral radiograph there is a suggestion of a faint calcific body in the center of a radiolucent lesion. **C:** Coronal T1-weighted (SE, TR 685, TE 20) MRI demonstrates the lesion to be of a high signal intensity paralleling that of a subcutaneous fat. A small focus of low signal is present within the lesion. **D:** Axial T2-weighted (SE, TR 2000, TE 70) MRI shows that the lesion becomes of lower intensity, again paralleling the signal of subcutaneous fat.

occasional foci of fat necrosis (195, 204). A capsule may occasionally encompass all or part of the tumor mass (196), and in most cases reported, atrophic bone trabeculae are found throughout the lesion. In the nontumorous fatty marrow contained in the above-mentioned segments in the femur and the calcaneus, infarcts may arise for yet unknown reasons although some investigators believe that circulatory abnormalities are the last link in the pathogenetic chain (205). The necrotic fat cells may calcify, and then ossify, and secondary bone cysts may form in the necrotic region (201). Usually, the calcifications exhibit a birch-broom-like picture, but dense aggregates of calcification can exhibit a Liesegang ring–like configuration (185).

Differential Diagnosis

Radiology

Because the MRI appearance of intraosseous lipoma is so characteristic, with this technique there is essentially no possibility to make a mistake in rendering this diagnosis (184). The same is true if the fatty marrow becomes necrotic such as in *medullary bone infarct*. In the latter lesion, however, the necrotic tissue exhibits a characteristic peripheral rim of fibrosis, separating the lesion from the viable bone. Occasionally, however, a secondary cyst may develop in the medullary bone infarct (201) that may mimic an intraosseous lipoma (Fig. 41). So-called intraosseous lipomas of the calcaneus usually represent bone infarction, simple bone cyst, aneurysmal bone cyst, or pseudocyst in the fatty marrow of the normally radiolucent Ward triangle (114).

Pathology

Similar to the radiologic appearance, histopathology of intraosseous lipoma is almost specific. The differential diagnosis becomes more complex if there is a necrosis of the marrow presenting as a *bone infarct*, in which case the lesions characteristically exhibit necrotic marrow and empty osteocyte lacunae.

Another differential possibility is *intraosseous liposarcoma*. This extremely rare lesion is characterized by the pleomorphic appearance of the neoplastic cells with varying degrees of lipogenic differentiation. Signet ring cells are usually present (177,192), with a large, single globule of lipid filling the cytoplasm (185). Evidence of malignancy is the finding of lipoblasts which show a rather broad seam of cytoplasm with numerous fat vacuoles and an indented somewhat hyperchromatic nucleus.

The other entities that may be considered in the differential diagnosis are either primary or secondary *aneurysmal bone cyst* and *simple bone cyst*. If an aneurysmal bone cyst or a simple bone cyst develops in the area of bone infarction (201), the primary necrosis of the bone marrow may be covered by the secondary lesion.

The radiologic and pathologic differential diagnosis of intraosseous lipoma is depicted in Fig. 42.

Fibrocartilaginous Mesenchymoma

Fibrocartilaginous mesenchymoma is an extremely rare tumor composed of two distinct tissues, one benign and cartilaginous, resembling an active growth plate, and the other resembling a low-grade fibrosarcoma (215). Mirra et al. classify this lesion as desmoid tumor with enchondroma-like nodules (218). The number of reported cases is probably <20, although there may exist several unpublished cases (Remagen, personal communication).

Clinical Presentation

Fibrocartilaginous mesenchymoma has been reported in patients ranging from 9 to 23 years of age (mean age 13

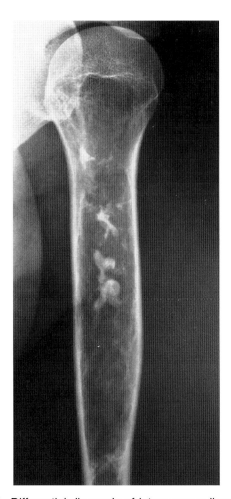

FIG. 41. Differential diagnosis of intraosseous lipoma: cyst formation in bone infarction. Anteroposterior radiograph of the left humerus in a 31-year-old woman shows an expansive radiolucent lesion in the proximal shaft with central calcifications typical for bone infarction and a rim of reactive sclerosis. (Courtesy Dr. Alex Norman, Valhalla, New York.)

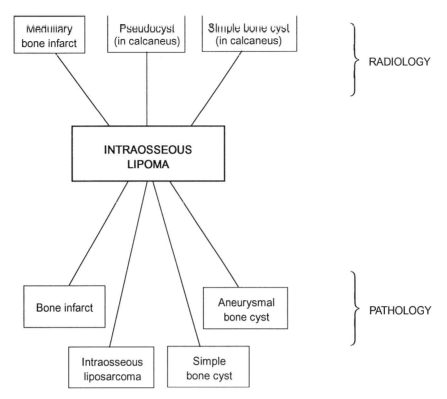

FIG. 42. Radiologic and pathologic differential diagnosis of intraosseous lipoma.

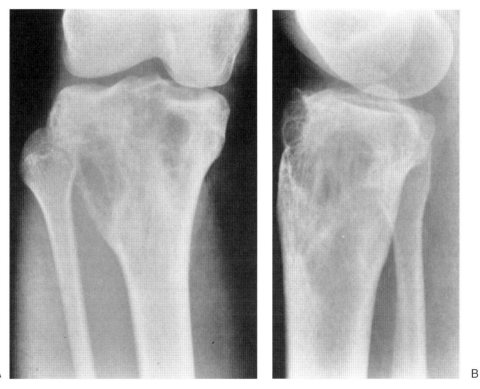

A   B

FIG. 43. Fibrocartilaginous mesenchymoma. (**A**) Anteroposterior and (**B**) lateral radiographs of the right knee of a 23-year-old man show a radiolucent trabeculated lesion in the proximal tibia, bulging the anterolateral cortex and extending into the articular end of bone.

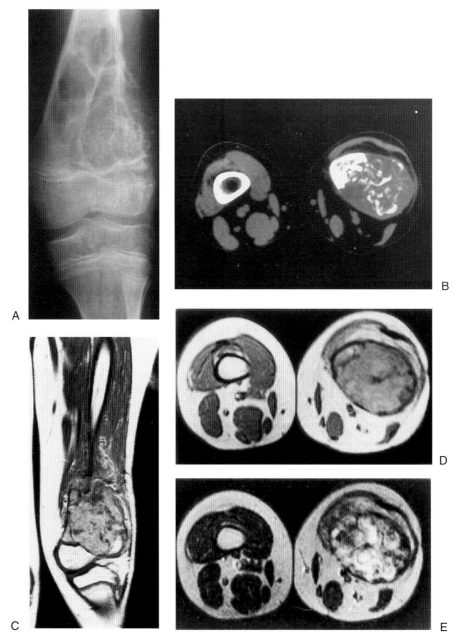

FIG. 44. Fibrocartilaginous mesenchymoma: computed tomography and magnetic resonance imaging. **A:** An oblique radiograph of the left knee of a 14-year-old boy shows an osteolytic trabeculated lesion in the distal femur abutting the growth plate. The lateral cortex is destroyed. **B:** CT section through the tumor shows destruction of the posterolateral cortex and a large soft tissue mass containing calcifications. **C:** Coronal T1-weighted MRI shows nonhomogeneous signal of the tumor that violated the growth plate and extended into the distal femoral epiphysis. **D:** Axial T1-weighted MRI shows destruction of the cortex and a large soft tissue mass of intermediate signal. Calcifications within the mass display a low signal intensity. **E:** On axial T2-weighted MR image the tumor becomes of high signal intensity. Pseudoseptation of the mass and nonhomogeneous character is well demonstrated.

years). Males were more frequently affected. The lesion is located usually in the epiphysis of a long bone, such as the fibula or humerus. The symptoms usually indicate a slow-growing tumor. They consist of slight discomfort and tenderness at the site of the lesion, and occasionally a palpable mass.

Imaging

On radiography, the lesion is radiolucent with scalloped borders, extending to or abutting the growth plate. After skeletal maturity the lesion may extend into the articular end of bone (Fig. 43). Occasionally the cortex is expanded and thinned. The cortex may be invaded, and in these cases the lesion extends into the soft tissues (Fig. 44). This can be effectively demonstrated with CT and MRI. Although a periosteal reaction is usually absent, when present it is sparse and of benign appearance. The tumor may contain visible calcifications typical of cartilaginous matrix (see Fig. 44B).

Histopathology

By microscopy, the lesion is composed of a tissue made up of intersecting bundles of spindle cells and collagen fibers. The tissue is fairly cellular, the nuclei are plump, and there is evidence of pleomorphism and hyperchromatism, with occasional mitotic figures (215). Superimposed on this background are well-defined islands of obviously benign cartilage, varying in density from case to case, from a cartilage island here and there to densely packed, bowed bands of cartilage that resemble the epiphyseal growth plate, with

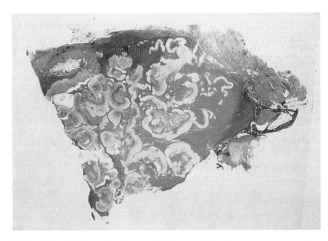

FIG. 46. Histopathology of fibrocartilaginous mesenchymoma. Numerous curved cartilage particles lie in scanty spindle cell tissue, giving the tumor a "shrimp cocktail" appearance (hematoxylin and eosin, original magnification ×0.2).

characteristic gradual columnation, cellular hypertrophy, and endochondral ossification (215) (Fig. 45). On hematoxylin-eosin staining, this gives the tumor a very typical "shrimp cocktail" appearance, with the white cartilage ("shrimps") lying in the red spindle cell tumor ("sauce") (Fig. 46). In other cases, the cartilage more closely resembles the islands of an enchondroma. Furthermore, variable amounts of detached trabeculae of woven bone similar to fibrous dysplasia may be found (Fig. 47). Therefore these cases are considered to be an entity of its own, related to fibrous dysplasia and called "fibrocartilaginous dysplasia" (213,217). However, we have observed at least one case where fibrous dysplasia-like structures were combined with the presence of epiphyseal plate-like cartilage, not allowing that distinction (Remagen, unpublished observations). In its first description the tumor was named fibrocartilaginous mesenchymoma with low-grade malignancy (216). However, because metastases have never been observed thus far, the group at the Mayo Clinic later deleted that addition (214), calling it, simply, fibrocartilaginous mesenchymoma.

Differential Diagnosis

Radiology

Because the lesion is metaphyseal and often arises in a growing skeleton, benign lesions such as *aneurysmal bone cyst* and *chondromyxoid fibroma* should be included in the differential diagnosis. After obliteration of the growth plate, *giant-cell tumor* and *chondrosarcoma* must be considered. Other tumors that may have a similar appearance include *desmoplastic fibroma, fibrosarcoma, malignant fibrous histiocytoma*, and *osteosarcoma*.

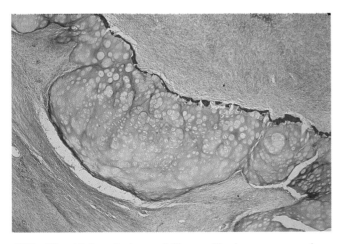

FIG. 45. Histopathology of fibrocartilaginous mesenchymoma. Typical aspect of the tumor consists of two components: cartilage structured similar to the growth plate, and surrounding spindle cell tissue exhibiting subtle to moderate pleomorphism and some collagen formation (van Gieson, original magnification ×12).

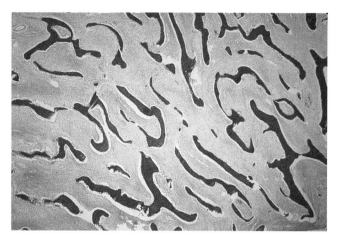

FIG. 47. Histopathology of fibrocartilaginous mesenchymoma. In the areas free of cartilage the tumor resembles fibrous dysplasia because of formation of deformed Chinese character-like immature bone trabeculae (van Gieson, original magnification ×12).

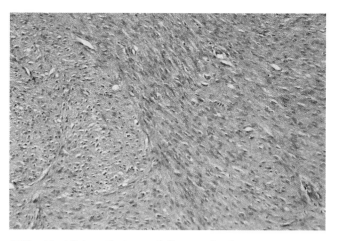

FIG. 48. Histopathology of fibrocartilaginous mesenchymoma. In the areas free of cartilage and bone the tumor clearly resembles a desmoplastic fibroma, however, the pleomorphism of the cells and nuclei is more pronounced (hematoxylin and eosin, original magnification ×10).

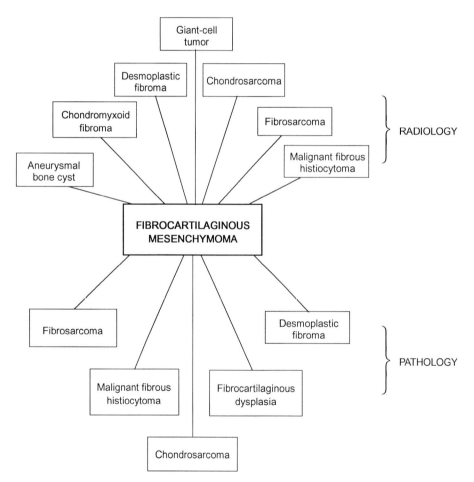

FIG. 49. Radiologic and pathologic differential diagnosis of fibrocartilaginous mesenchymoma.

Pathology

The histologic differential diagnosis must include *fibrosarcoma, chondrosarcoma,* particularly mesenchymal and dedifferentiated variants, *fibrocartilaginous dysplasia* (fibrous dysplasia with cartilaginous metaplasia), and *desmoplastic fibroma* (Fig. 48).

The presence of the benign cartilaginous component allows differentiation from fibrosarcoma. This is also true for chondrosarcoma and the listed variants. In fibrous dysplasia, the spindle cell stroma has a benign aspect and the cartilaginous component resembles an enchondroma, in contrast to fibrocartilaginous mesenchymoma, where the cartilaginous component resembles the growth plate.

The radiologic and pathologic differential diagnosis of fibrocartilaginous mesenchymoma is depicted in Fig. 49.

MALIGNANT LESIONS

Adamantinoma of Long Bones

Adamantinoma is a rare malignant tumor characterized by the formation of apparently epithelial cells surrounded by a spindle cell fibrous tissue (67). The tumor owes its name (given by Fischer in 1913) to its close morphologic resemblance to adamantinoma of the jaw (226). The histogenesis of adamantinoma has long been debated. A number of authors have advocated an endothelial (227,232) or an epithelial (237, 245) derivation. However, recent advances in electron microscopy and immunohistochemistry have provided good evidence in support of an epithelial origin (229,243).

Clinical Presentation

Adamantinoma occurs with equal frequency in males and females between the second and fifth decades, and has a predilection for the tibia in 90% of cases (221). Rarely, it can involve the humerus or the ulna (Fig. 50). The lesion is usually confined to the middle or distal third of the tibia, but a simultaneous occurrence in tibia and fibula has occasionally been reported (223,245). A history of trauma is obtained in approximately two thirds of cases (243,245). The most common presenting complaint is localized swelling or enlargement of the affected bone (67,234,235). Pain is mild at onset and becomes more severe as the size of the lesion increases. Physical examination notes a firm, tender mass or swelling, usually affixed to the underlying bone (236).

Imaging

The radiographic appearance of adamantinoma is that of well-delineated, elongated osteolytic defects of various sizes, separated by areas of sclerotic bone, occasionally having a soap-bubble appearance (Fig. 51A). A saw-toothed area of cortical destruction, when present, is quite distinctive

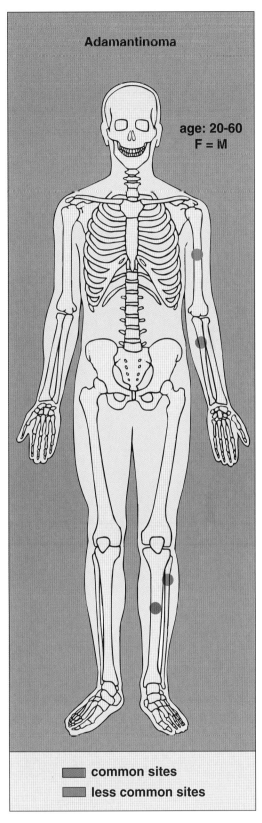

FIG. 50. Adamantinoma: skeletal sites of predilections, peak age range, and male-to-female ratio.

for this tumor (Fig. 51B). One study noted that 80% of all lesions were >5 cm in length (230). At times, the entire bone is involved by multiple satellite lesions. Some long-standing lesions may exhibit a more sclerotic, ground-glass appearance and therefore can be confused with fibrous dysplasia (Fig. 52). Occasionally, adamantinoma manifests as a single, large lytic lesion in the cortex, which expands and destroys the cortex and produces a soft tissue mass (94).

On MRI examination, a hypointense (compared to the normal bone marrow) signal on T1-weighted images and a hyperintense signal on T2-weighted images is noted. After intravenous administration of Gd-DTPA, no significant enhancement of the lesion is seen (248). The main purpose of MRI is not to diagnose the tumor but to determine the extent of intraosseous and extraosseous involvement (94).

Scintigraphy invariably reveals an increased uptake of the radiopharmaceutical tracer (243) (Fig. 53).

Histopathology

Histologically, the tumor is biphasic and consists of an epithelial component intimately admixed in various proportions with a fibrous component (Fig. 54) (240,246). The epithelial component, usually consisting of islands of polyhedral cells in pavemented nests or in gland-like spaces, exhibits peripheral nuclear palisading and a looser, myxoid inner zone that resembles the stellate reticulum of odontogenic tissue. The palisading and columnar arrangement of the peripheral cells, accompanied by stellate central cells, somewhat resembles an ameloblastoma of the jaw (219). Epithelium-like cells may have a variety of patterns. There are four basic forms, found in a variety of combinations: tubular, spindle, squamous, and basaloid (94). The cells of adamantinoma are strongly marked by antigens to keratin, an immunohistochemical property that helps to distinguish this tumor from other similar-appearing lesions, such as fibrous dysplasia or nonossifying fibroma (229). Squamous metaplasia is sometimes present and, if it is extensive, the lesion may be erroneously interpreted as a squamous cell carcinoma. The fibrous component consists of spindle cells, which usually exhibit only slight atypias. The epithelial spaces and stroma may sometimes become highly vascularized, and the lesion may resemble a vascular neoplasm. However, ultrastructural and immunohistochemical evidence points towards an epithelial derivation (225,231,237,238,247). A positive reaction of the epithelial cells for α-smooth muscle actin has been described in some cases (229). Despite all these findings, it is still difficult to conceive how an epithelial neoplasm can arise as a primary in bone. The lesion may contain spicules of bone and may exhibit cystic cavities that contain either blood or a straw-colored fluid (94).

A relationship of adamantinoma with osteofibrous dysplasia (Kempson-Campanacci lesion) and fibrous dysplasia has been suggested by some investigators (228,244). Although this remains a controversial matter (233), adamantinoma may contain a fibro-osseous component that on pathologic examination resembles both fibrous and osteofibrous dysplasias (242) (see also discussion in Chapter 4).

Differential Diagnosis

Radiology

The main differential diagnosis includes fibrous dysplasia, osteofibrous dysplasia, and osteomyelitis. *Fibrous dysplasia* is less aggressive looking and, unlike adamantinoma that predominantly involves the anterior cortex, the former is more centric in location. Moreover, osteolytic cortical defects are almost never encountered in fibrous dysplasia.

Osteofibrous dysplasia is a lesion of infancy and childhood, whereas adamantinoma (with a few exceptions (248)) is never seen before skeletal maturity. The lesion of osteofibrous dysplasia is usually well defined, without the destructive features of adamantinoma, although, albeit rarely, larger lesions may destroy the cortical bone and invade the medullary cavity.

Osteomyelitis of the tibia may at times be difficult to distinguish from adamantinoma. The presence of a periosteal reaction and sequestra in the former may point to the correct diagnosis.

Nonossifying fibroma is a lobulated, well-demarcated lesion with a sclerotic border, showing no evidence of cortical invasion, whereas a fibrous cortical defect, when it reaches the zone of metaphyseal diminution, may mimic a small focus of adamantinoma.

Desmoplastic fibroma may present as an aggressive lesion. It frequently exhibits internal septation or trabeculation, features not typical of adamantinoma.

Very small intracortical lesions may occasionally mimic a *Brodie abscess, osteoid osteoma*, or even a *stress fracture* (248).

Pathology

The most important point is to distinguish this lesion from *osteofibrous dysplasia* (222). The latter lesion does not possess the epithelial component within the fibro-osseous stroma that is characteristic of adamantinoma. Immunohistochemically, osteofibrous dysplasia, in contrast to adamantinoma, does not show any keratin-positive cells. However, more problems are encountered in distinguishing so-called osteofibrous dysplasia-like adamantinoma from conventional osteofibrous dysplasia (241). Moreover, in recent years, patients have presented with lesions that contained foci of epithelial tissue corresponding to adamantinoma within areas of osteofibrous dysplasia (220,224). Czerniak et al. have termed such lesions "differentiated (regressing) adamantinomas" (224). According to these authors, features characteristic of differentiated adamantinomas include onset during the first two decades of life, an exclusively intracortical location, uniform predominance of osteofibrous dyspla-

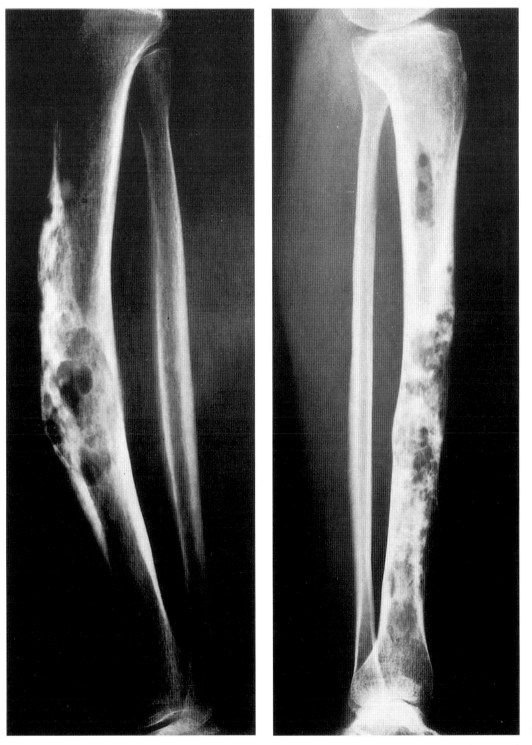

A

B

FIG. 51. Adamantinoma. **A:** A lateral radiograph of the left leg in a 64-year-old woman shows a destructive lesion in the midshaft of tibia. The lesion is multiloculated and slightly expansive, with mixed osteolytic and sclerotic areas creating a soap bubble appearance. **B:** A lateral radiograph of the right leg of a 28-year-old woman shows multiple, confluent lytic lesions involving almost the entire tibia. The articular ends are spared. The anterior cortex exhibits a predominantly saw-tooth type of destruction.

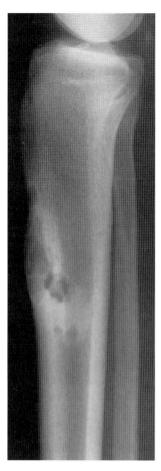

FIG. 52. Adamantinoma. A single, predominantly sclerotic lesion in the midshaft of tibia of this 20-year-old man was thought to represent fibrous dysplasia. A biopsy revealed adamantinoma.

sia, and scattered foci of cytokeratin-positive epithelial elements that are identical to those observed in classic adamantinoma (94). This suggests that a single disease entity may exhibit a spectrum of manifestations with benign osteofibrous dysplasia at one end of the spectrum and malignant adamantinoma at the other end. Lesions that contain both histologic patterns would be characterized by intermediate malignant potential (94) (Fig. 55).

Fibrous dysplasia and *nonossifying fibroma* can usually be excluded by the immunohistochemical demonstration of the epithelial component of adamantinoma, which may consist of a very few epithelial cells or very small islands looking like blood vessels, but which are positive for keratin markers (239).

If squamous metaplasia is present, and particularly if it is extensive, adamantinoma may be mistaken for *squamous cell carcinoma*. This is the only differential in which the epithelial and keratin markers are not helpful. In such cases, the age of the patient and radiologic differences should be considered.

The radiologic and pathologic differential diagnosis of adamantinoma is depicted in Fig. 56).

Chordoma

Chordoma is a rare malignant bone tumor that arises from developmental embryonic remnants of the notochord (which disappears during the second month of embryonal life) (288). This tumor is characterized by a lobular arrangement of the tissue with vacuolated so-called physaliphorous cells and mucoid intercellular material (271). Chordoma accounts for about 1% of all malignant bone tumors. The tumor occurs only at sites in which notochordal remnants are not normally present. Therefore, although it is a midline lesion of the axial skeleton, it never occurs in the nuclei pulposi.

Clinical Presentation

The lesion is most frequently discovered between the fifth and seventh decades (mean age 56 years) and males are more commonly affected (M/F ratio 2:1). The predilection of chordoma for the spinal axis is well documented (259–261). The three most common sites for this tumor are the sacro-coccygeal area (55%), the spheno-occipital area, mainly the clivus (35%) (272), and the second cervical vertebra (8%) (Fig. 57). Chordoma is a locally aggressive lesion (250, 267). In most series reported, metastases occurred only rarely, usually late in the course of the disease (251). Because chordoma usually grows slowly, often the symptoms have been present for a year or more (269). The symptoms are closely related to the location of the lesion. The usual presenting complaint is sharp or dull pain affecting the lower back or the cervical spine, sacrum, or coccyx (252). Spheno-occipital lesions give rise to headache, cranial nerve palsies, and signs of endocrine dysfunction caused by the compression of the pituitary gland (282). Lesions of the cervical vertebrae usually cause cord compression. Lesions of the sacro-coccyx produce increasing lower back pain, anorectal or bladder dysfunction, and paresthesias (263,283). The incidence of reported distant metastases ranges from 10% to 43% (270).

Imaging

The radiographic appearance of chordoma is that of a highly destructive, expansive lytic lesion, with irregular scalloped borders and occasionally with matrix calcifications, which are probably caused by extensive tumor necrosis (285) (Fig. 58). Sclerosis of the tumor edges may be observed and a pathologic fracture is often present (280). Soft tissue masses are commonly associated with the lesion (264).

Although conventional radiography, including tomography, delineates the tumor well, CT and MRI are important to demonstrate the soft tissue extension, and myelography of-

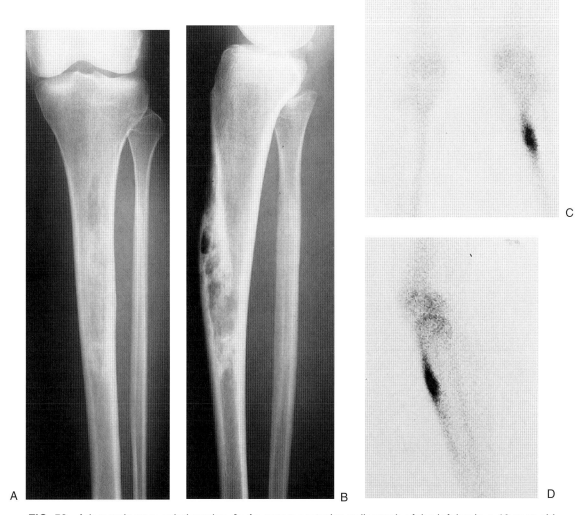

A

B

C

D

FIG. 53. Adamantinoma: scintigraphy. **A:** An anteroposterior radiograph of the left leg in a 46-year-old woman shows multiple radiolucent lesions in the midshaft of the tibia. The lateral cortex is slightly thickened. **B:** A lateral radiograph shows mixed sclerotic and osteolytic lesion predominantly affecting anterior tibial cortex. **(C)** Frontal and **(D)** lateral radionuclide bone scan obtained after injection of 20 mCi (740 MBq) of ^{99m}Tc-labeled methylene diphosphonate (MDP) show markedly increased uptake of radiopharmaceutical tracer in the lesion.

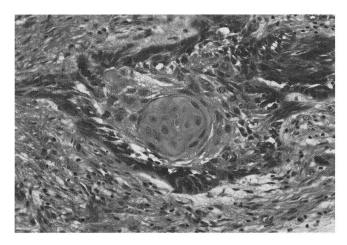

FIG. 54. Histopathology of adamantinoma. Within a spindle cell fibrous stroma admixed is an island of small epithelial cells containing an extended area of squamous cell metaplasia (hematoxylin and eosin, original magnification ×50).

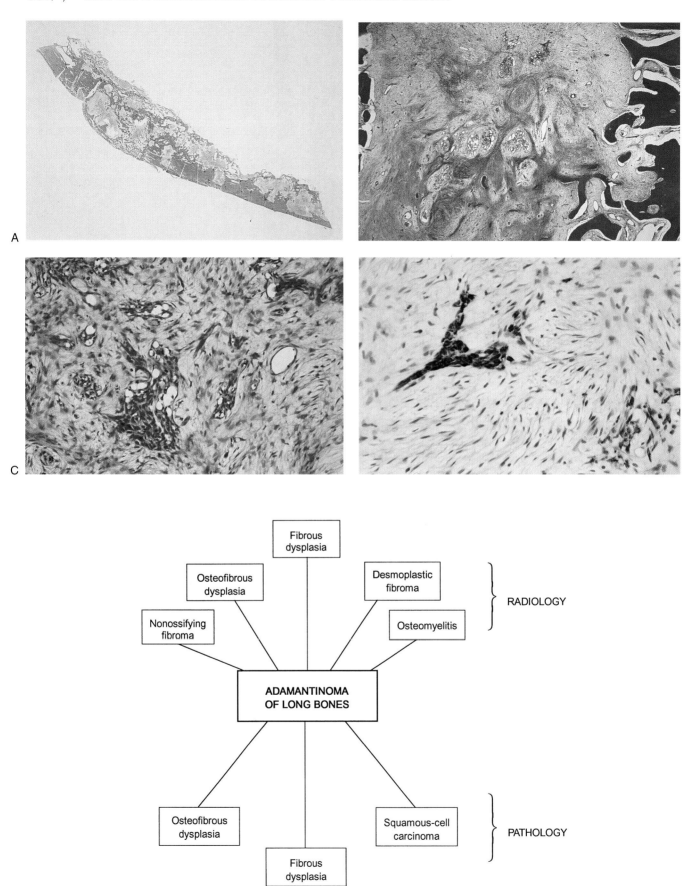

FIG. 56. Radiologic and pathologic differential diagnosis of adamantinoma.

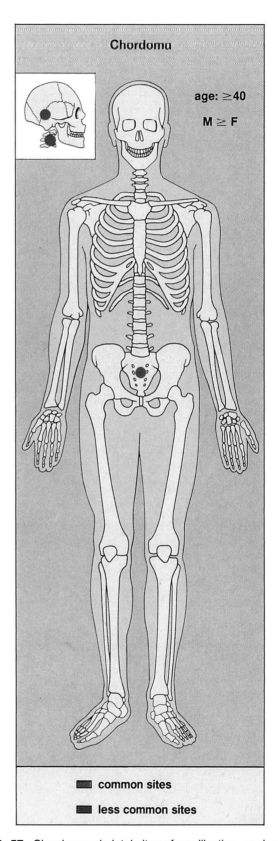

FIG. 55. Histopathology of adamantinoma coexisting with osteofibrous dysplasia. **A:** Resected fragment of the anterior tibia shows irregular thickening and thinning of the cortex associated with metaplastic new bone formation (hematoxylin and eosin, reduced scale). **B:** Fibrous tissue of various density contains an island of adamantinoma (*middle third*). Metaplastic new bone formation (*lower right*) is seen and the inner limit of cortical bone with signs of remodeling (*right*) (hematoxylin and eosin, original magnification ×12). **C:** At higher magnification the tubular and solid structures of epithelial cells are conspicuous. Slight hyperchromatism and pleomorphism of the nuclei is present. Some capillaries (*right middle and top*) have to be differentiated from the epithelial structures (hematoxylin and eosin, original magnification ×50). **D:** Immunocytochemical marking of epithelial cells (*brown*) with a panepithelial marker displays single positive cells laying in the fibrous tissue (*lower right*) (Lu5 marker, original magnification ×100).

FIG. 57. Chordoma: skeletal sites of predilection, peak age range, and male-to-female ratio.

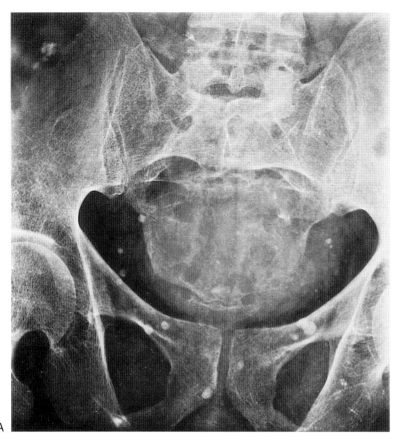
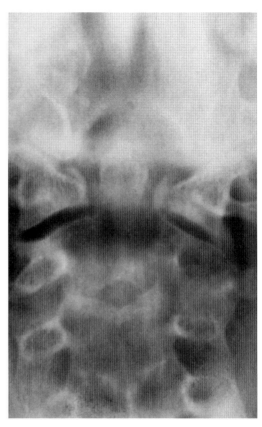

A   B

FIG. 58. Chordoma. **A:** A destructive osteolytic lesion in the lower sacrum with scalloped borders and the amorphous calcifications in the tumor matrix is seen in this 60-year-old woman. **B:** Open-mouth anteroposterior tomography of the cervical spine of a 52-year-old man demonstrates an osteolytic lesion in the body of C2 vertebra, destroying the left pedicle.

ten demonstrates an invasion of the spinal canal (293). CT can reveal the extent of bone destruction, the presence of a soft tissue mass, growth within the spinal canal, and invasion of adjacent structures (273,278). The MRI characteristics (287), which include a low or intermediate signal intensity on T1-weighted images and a high signal on T2-weighted images (256), are not specific for chordoma (280,284). However, a very high signal intensity on T2 weighting, combined with a lobulated appearance of the tumor, suggests the diagnosis of chordoma (Fig. 59).

Scintigraphy reveals an increased uptake of radiopharmaceutical tracer around the periphery of the tumor. Areas of abnormally decreased activity due to complete replacement of bone by the tumor may also be observed (270). Lack of uptake of the tracer within the tumor itself is probably secondary to the absence of vascularity and the lack of ossification (270).

Histopathology

Chordoma may demonstrate considerable variations in its histologic appearance (255). Apart from the degree of differ-

entiation, the histology is also determined by the extent of anaplasia. At present, on the basis of microscopic appearance, the tumor is divided into three subtypes: conventional, chondroid, and dedifferentiated (263).

Conventional chordoma microscopically resembles the fetal notochord. The tumor consists of cord-like arrays and lobules of large polyhedral cells with a vacuolated cytoplasm and vesicular nuclei (Fig. 60), referred to as physaliphorous (from Greek for "bubble-bearing") (266). The vacuoles contain a mucinous substance with neutral mucopolysaccharides (249,280) and a mixture of weakly sulfated and carboxylated glycoproteins (291). The mucinous material is either secreted into the intercellular space or freed upon the death of cells. In addition, cells of the signet ring type, in which the nucleus is displaced to one side by one or two vacuoles, are also observed (271). Some cells have an eosinophilic, nonvacuolated cytoplasm (263). Nuclear pleomorphism is usually mild and mitotic figures are rarely discerned, predominantly seen in the most cellular areas. The fibrous septa contain the vascular channels and occasionally are infiltrated by lymphocytes (289).

Chondroid chordoma, originally described by Falconer

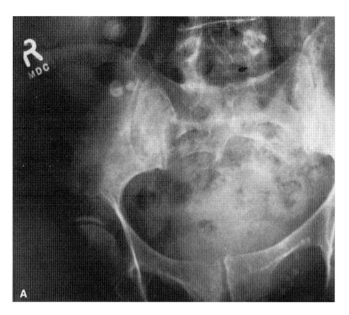

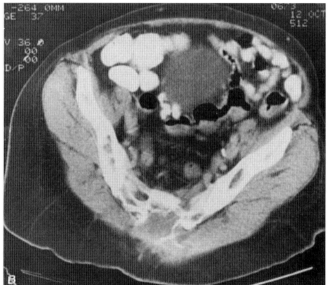

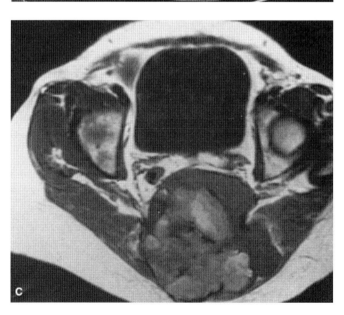

FIG. 59. Chordoma: computed tomography and magnetic resonance imaging. **A:** An anteroposterior radiograph of the pelvis of a 68-year-old woman shows destructive lesion in the middle and lower part of the sacrum associated with a soft tissue mass. **B:** CT section demonstrates the low-attenuation tumor destroying the sacral bone. **C:** Axial T1-weighted (SE, TR 600, TE 20) MRI shows a large, nonhomogeneous tumor mass displaying intermediate signal intensity with areas of higher signal probably representing hemorrhage.

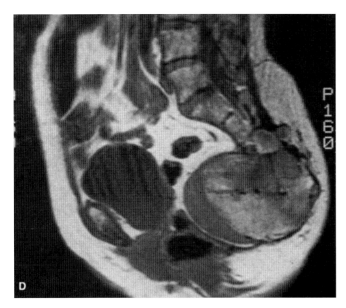
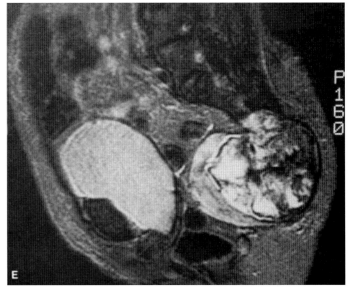

FIG. 59. *Continued* **D:** Sagittal T1-weighted (SE, TR 650, TE 20) MRI shows the extraosseous extension of the tumor mass. **E:** On the sagittal T2-weighted (SE, TR 2000, TE 90) image the lobulated tumor displays a high signal and shows great deal of heterogeneity. (Reprinted from Greenfield GB, Arrington JA. *Imaging of bone tumors.* Philadelphia: JB Lippincott, 1995;149–150.)

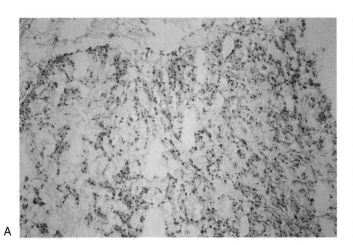
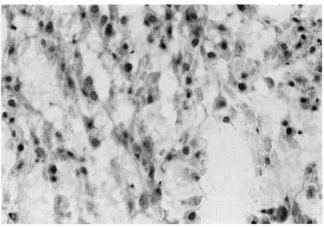

A

B

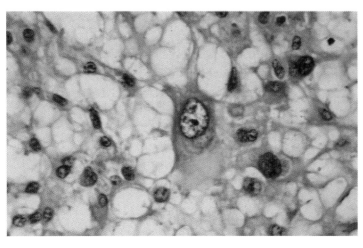

C

FIG. 60. Histopathology of chordoma. **A:** Cords and clusters of large polymorphous cells contain an eosinophilic cytoplasm and large roundish slightly pleomorphic nuclei. Between the cells a faintly pale amorphous mass represents mucus extruded by the cells (hematoxylin and eosin, original magnification ×50). **B:** At higher magnification some of the large cells show vacuoles giving the typical physaliphorous appearance (*center*). The pleomorphism of the large dark nuclei is obvious (hematoxylin and eosin, original magnification ×100). **C:** High magnification photomicrograph shows the large variegated and vacuolated physaliphorous cells characteristic of chordoma (hematoxylin and eosin, original magnification ×400). (Reprinted from Bullough PG. *Atlas of orthopedic pathology,* 2nd ed. New York: Gower, 1992;16.28.)

and associates, is a slowly growing variant of conventional chordoma (254,262). It is characterized by a substantial chondroid component, which resembles either chondroma or chondrosarcoma, intermixed with foci more characteristic of conventional chordoma. The cartilaginous tissue possesses cells within lacunae, separated by a matrix of hyaline cartilage (263).

Dedifferentiated chordoma, in addition to features of conventional chordoma, exhibits features that resemble malignant fibrous histiocytoma, fibrosarcoma, osteosarcoma, or high-grade chondrosarcoma (252,274,277,279,286).

Differential Diagnosis

Radiology

The main radiologic considerations in differential diagnosis, when the tumor involves the sacral bone, are *chondrosarcoma* and *metastasis* (253). Both lesions may very closely mimic chordoma, and vice versa, although metastasis rarely is accompanied by a soft tissue mass (290). The purely lytic lesion may closely resemble *plasmacytoma.* In doubtful instances, positive scintigraphy is highly suggestive of chordoma (265). *Osteomyelitis* and *lymphoma* are two additional considerations. Because the radiologic appearance of these entities is very similar to that of chordoma, detailed clinical information may be a helpful aid in differential diagnosis.

Pathology

Metastatic adenocarcinoma of the rectosigmoid colon, especially of the mucinous type, is an occasional consideration in differential diagnosis. This is particularly true when the chordoma possesses many cells with single cytoplasmic vacuoles (263). Furthermore, both of these lesions may contain glycogen, mucin, cytokeratins, and epithelial membrane antigen (EMA). In addition, both tumors may be positive for S-100 protein (280). The keys to the correct diagnosis are examination of several histologic sections and careful evaluation of the clinical details (271). The points to be stressed are that gland formation does not occur in chordomas and that physaliphorous cells are absent in adenocarcinomas. When necessary, mucin staining can be performed, as chordoma contains acid-sulfated mucin that is positive for colloidal iron and resistant to predigestion with hyaluronidase (257,263). The mucin in signet ring adenocarcinomas is of the neutral, epithelial type that stains with periodic acid-Schiff (PAS).

Myxoid chondrosarcoma is another diagnostic possibility because of its lobular architecture, cord-like arrangement of cells, and myxoid matrix. This lesion is occasionally termed chordoid sarcoma because of its histologic similarity to chordoma (275,276,292). Helpful in the differential diagnosis is the fact that myxoid chondrosarcomas are extremely rare in the spine. They do not contain physaliphorous cells, and the cells are negative for cytokeratin and epithelial membrane antigen but positive for lysozyme (281).

An interesting tumor to distinguish from chordoma is so-called *parachordoma,* first described by Dabska (258). This tumor exhibits a cytoplasmic vacuolization of the cells, which thus resemble the physaliphorous cells of chordoma. Parachordoma also contains fibrous septa similar to the latter tumor. This rare peripheral tumor is lobular and pseudo-encapsulated, and it frequently occurs adjacent to tendons, synovium, and osseous structures. Occasionally it may arise

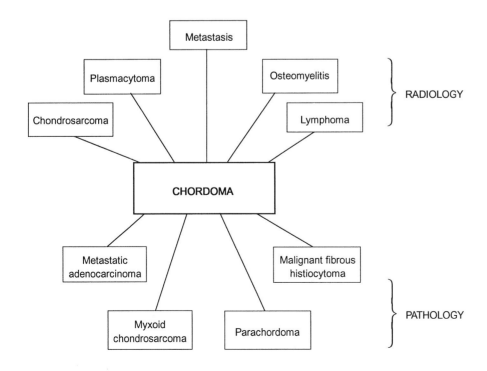

FIG. 61. Radiologic and pathologic differential diagnosis of chordoma.

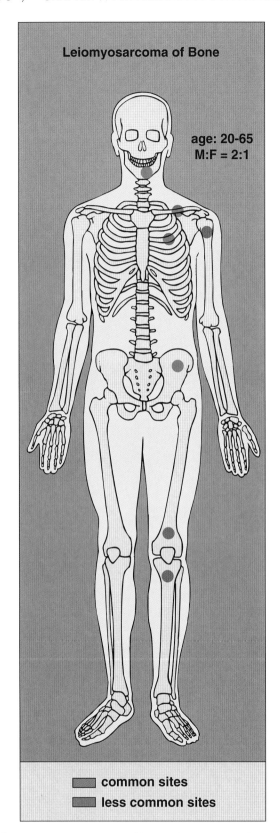

FIG. 62. Leiomyosarcoma of bone: skeletal sites of predilection, peak age range, and male-to-female ratio.

in bone. Parachordoma is still a controversial entity and has not been accepted by all authorities.

The radiologic and pathologic differential diagnosis of chordoma is depicted in Fig. 61.

Leiomyosarcoma of Bone

Primary leiomyosarcomas of bone are very rare malignancies, with about 50 cases thus far reported (298,300–304, 306–309). Berlin et al. reported 16 cases and suggested that this tumor may be more common than previously recognized (297). Recently, a single case report described a radiation-induced leiomyosarcoma (295). It is a malignant, predominantly spindle cell neoplasm exhibiting smooth muscle differentiation (263).

Clinical Presentation

The reported patients ranged from 9 to 80 years of age (mean 44 years). However, occurrence before the age of 20 is uncommon. Males are affected about twice as often as females. The usual presentation is pain of variable intensity and duration (294). A soft tissue mass is occasionally encountered (296). The most common sites are the distal femur, proximal tibia (263), and proximal humerus (303). Other bones that may be affected include the pelvis, clavicle, ribs, and mandible (300) (Fig. 62).

Imaging

Although there are no characteristic radiographic features of leiomyosarcoma in the reported cases the tumor most often presented either as a lytic area of geographic bone destruction or with aggressive-looking, ill-defined borders (Fig. 63). Some lesions exhibited an aggressive permeative and moth-eaten pattern. A periosteal reaction was present in about 50% of cases (297).

Histopathology

Microscopy reveals interlacing fascicles of spindle-shaped cells that resemble leiomyosarcoma of the soft tissues (299,308). Cellularity varies from case to case. Most cellular areas exhibit little intervening stroma (303). Less cellular foci contain variably abundant intercellular collagen (Fig. 64). Rarely, a storiform-like pattern, reminiscent of malignant fibrous histiocytoma, is seen (303). The spindle cells have oval or elongated cigar-shaped nuclei and an eosinophilic (picrinophilic) cytoplasm, occasionally having a fibrillary pattern. The nuclei quite often exhibit a depression on both ends, caused by a clear vacuole. Giant cells are rarely encountered. When present, they contain multiple hyperchromatic nuclei, prominent nucleoli, and indistinct cytoplasmic borders. Mitotic figures are frequently observed.

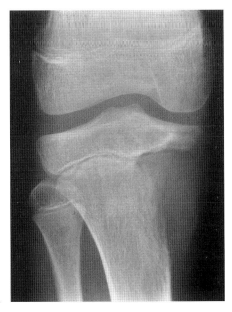
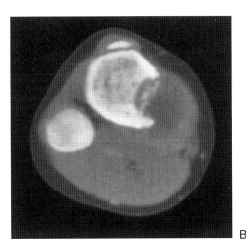

A

B

FIG. 63. Leiomyosarcoma of bone. **A:** Anteroposterior radiograph of the right knee of a 12-year-old boy shows an osteolytic lesion in the proximal tibial metaphysis destroying the medial cortex and extending into the soft tissues. **B:** CT section shows destruction of the medial aspect of the tibia and an associated soft tissue mass.

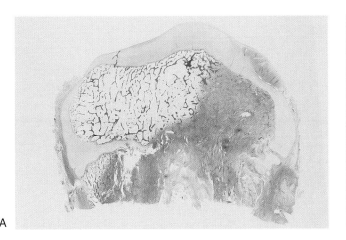
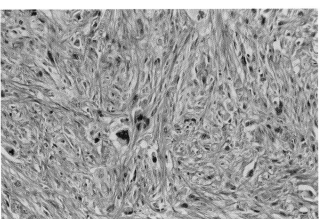

A

B

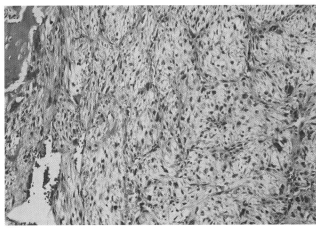

C

FIG. 64. Histopathology of leiomyosarcoma of bone. **A:** The tumor located in the metaphysis of the tibia destroyed the medial part of the growth plate and extended into the epiphysis infiltrating the cancellous bone (hematoxylin and eosin, original magnification ×1/5). **B:** Irregular bundles of elongated spindle cells producing intracellular collagen (*red*) show marked pleomorphism of the nuclei. Some tumor giant cells are present (*center*). Differentiation from high grade fibrosarcoma is almost impossible and should be done with immunohistochemical markers (van Gieson, original magnification ×50). **C:** In another area the pseudoepithelial clear cell aspect of the tumor—a typical variant—helps in differentiation from fibrosarcoma (hematoxylin and eosin, original magnification ×25).

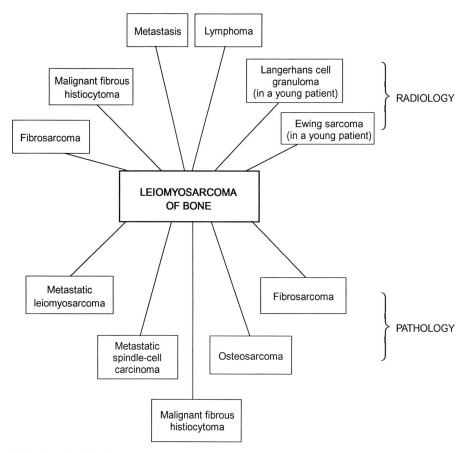

FIG. 65. Radiologic and pathologic differential diagnosis of leiomyosarcoma of bone.

Immunoreaction for muscle-specific actin is invariably positive, and desmin marking also may be positive. Some cases exhibit positive keratin marking.

Ultrastructurally, most leiomyosarcoma cells are elongated; however, a few cells are round to polygonal (303). Nuclei often exhibit corrugate profiles. Most cells contain many intermediate smooth muscle filaments in their cytoplasm, with dense bodies along their course. They also display subplasmalemmal densities, and pinocytotic vesicles are present (303).

Differential Diagnosis

Radiology

Leiomyosarcoma of bone does not have a characteristic radiologic presentation. Therefore, several possibilities should be considered in the differential diagnosis. Because of the frequently aggressive type of bone destruction exhibited by this tumor, *fibrosarcoma, malignant fibrous histiocytoma,* and *lymphoma* are primary considerations. Solitary metastasis in older patients is always a possibility. In younger patients, *Ewing sarcoma* and *Langerhans cell granuloma* must be considered.

Pathology

The most important differentiation is from a *metastasis of an extraskeletal leiomyosarcoma,* particularly from the uterus. Therefore, the diagnosis of a primary skeletal leiomyosarcoma is a diagnosis of exclusion, and clinical information about the case is crucial. *Fibrosarcoma* and *malignant fibrous histiocytoma* should be considered, particularly if areas of a herring-bone arrangement or a storiform pattern are present (305). *Osteosarcoma* must be a consideration because occasionally broad bands of hyalinized collagen may mimic osteoid. Because the histologic differentiation of leiomyosarcoma from these tumors with a reasonable degree of probability is almost impossible, immunocytochemical demonstration of a characterizing pattern of several smooth muscle cell markers in tumor cells is always mandatory (300).

The radiologic and pathologic differential diagnosis of leiomyosarcoma of bone is depicted in Fig. 65.

REFERENCES

Giant-Cell Tumor

1. Aoki J, Moriya K, Yamashita K, Fujioka F, Ishii K, Karakida O, Imai S, Sakai F, Imai Y, Sone S. Giant cell tumors of bone containing large amounts of hemosiderin: MR-pathologic correlation. *J Comput Assist Tomogr* 1991;15:1024–1027.

2. Aoki J, Tanikawa H, Ishii K, Seo GS, Kurakida O, Sone S, Ichikawa T, Kachi K. MR findings indicative of hemosiderin in giant-cell tumor of bone: frequency, cause, and diagnostic significance. *Am J Roentgenol* 1996;166:145–148.

3. Aoki J, Moser RP Jr, Vinh TN. Giant cell tumor of the scapula. A review of 13 cases. *Skeletal Radiol* 1989;18:427–434.

4. Athanasou NA, Bliss E, Gatter KC, Heryet A, Woods CG, McGee JO. An immunohistological study of giant-cell tumor of bone: evidence for an osteoclast origin of the giant cells. *J Pathol* 1985;147:153–158.

5. Averill R, Smith R, Campbell CJ. Giant cell tumors of the bones of the hand. *J Hand Surg* 1980;5:39–50.

6. Bacchini P, Bertoni F, Ruggieri P, Campanacci M. Multicentric giant cell tumor of skeleton. *Skeletal Radiol* 1995; 24:371–374.

7. Bertheussen KJ, Holck S, Schiodt T. Giant cell lesion of bone of the hand with particular emphasis on giant cell reparative granuloma. *J Hand Surg (Am)* 1983;8:46–49.

8. Bertoni F, Present D, Enneking WF. Giant cell tumor of bone with pulmonary metastases. *J Bone Joint Surg* 1985;67A:890–900.

9. Bertoni F, Present D, Sudanese A, Baldini N, Bacchini P, Campanacci M. Giant cell tumor of bone with pulmonary metastases: Six case reports and a review of the literature. *Clin Orthop* 1988;237:275–285.

10. Brady TJ, Gebhardt MC, Pykett IL, Buonanno FS, Newhouse JH, Burt CT, Smith RJ, Mankin HJ. NMR imaging of forearms in healthy volunteers and patients with giant-cell tumor of bone. *Radiology* 1982; 144:549–552.

11. Bridge JA, Neff JR, Bhatia PS, Sanger WG, Murphey MD. Cytogenetic findings and biologic behavior of giant cell tumors of bone. *Cancer* 1990;65:2697–2703.

12. Burmester GR, Winchester RJ, Dimitriu-Bona A, Klein MJ, Steiner G, Sissons HA. Delineation of four cell types comprising the giant cell tumor of bone. *J Clin Invest* 71:1633–1648, 1983.

13. Campanacci M, Baldini N, Boriani S, Sudanese A. Giant cell tumor of bone. *J Bone Joint Surg* 1987;69A:106–114.

14. Campanacci M, Giunti A, Olmi R. Giant-cell tumors of bone: a study of 209 cases with long-term follow-up in 130. *Ital J Orthop Traumatol* 1975;1:249–277.

15. Carrasco CH, Murray JA. Giant cell tumors. *Orthop Clin North Am* 1989;20:395–405.

16. Caskey PM, Wolf MD, Fechner RE. Multicentric giant cell reparative granuloma of the small bones of the hand. A case report and review of the literature. *Clin Orthop* 1985;193:199–205.

17. Dahlin DC. Giant cell bearing lesions of bone of the hands. *Hand Clin* 1987;3:291–297.

18. Dahlin DC. Giant cell tumor of bone: Highlights of 407 cases. *Am J Roentgenol* 1985;144:955–960.

19. Dahlin DC, Unni KK. *Bone tumors: several aspects and data on 8,542 cases,* 4th ed. Springfield, IL: Charles C Thomas, 1986.

20. Dahlin DC, Cupps RE, Johnson EW Jr. Giant-cell tumor: a study of 195 cases. *Cancer* 1970;25:1061–1070.

21. deSantos LA, Murray JA. Evaluation of giant cell tumor by computerized tomography. *Skeletal Radiol* 1978;2:205–212.

22. Duncan CP, Morton KS, Arthur JS. Giant cell tumor of bone: Its aggressiveness and potential for malignant change. *Can J Surg* 1983;26:475–476.

23. Eckhardt JJ, Grogan TJ. Giant cell tumor of bone. *Clin Orthop* 1986; 204:45–58.

24. Fechner RE, Mills SE. *Tumors of the bones and joints.* Washington, DC: Armed Forces Institute of Pathology, 1993;173–186.

25. Francis R, Lewis E. CT demonstration of giant cell tumor complicating Paget disease. *J Comput Assist Tomogr* 1983;7:917–918.

26. Glass TA, Mills SE, Fechner RE, Dyer R, Martin W, Armstrong P. Giant-cell reparative granuloma of the hands and feet. *Radiology* 1983; 149:65–68.

27. Goldenberg RR, Campbell CJ, Bonfiglio M. Giant-cell tumor of bone. An analysis of two hundred and eighteen cases. *J Bone Joint Surg* 1970;52A:619–664.

28. Hermann G, Abdelwahab IF, Klein MJ, Berson BD, Lewis MM. Case report 603. Giant cell reparative granuloma of the distal end of right femur. *Skeletal Radiol* 1990;19:367–369.

29. Herman SD, Mesgarzadeh M, Bonakdarpour A, Dalinka MK. The role of magnetic resonance imaging in giant cell tumor of bone. *Skeletal Radiol* 1987;16:635–643.

30. Hudson TM, Schiebler M, Springfield DS, Enneking WF, Hawkins IF Jr, Spanier SS. Radiology of giant cell tumors of bone: computed tomography, arthrotomography, and scintigraphy. *Skeletal Radiol* 1984; 11:85–95.

31. Hudson TM. *Radiologic-pathologic correlation of musculoskeletal lesions.* Baltimore: Williams and Wilkins, 1987;209–237.

32. Hutter RVP, Worcester JN Jr, Francis KC, Foote FW Jr, Stewart FW. Benign and malignant giant cell tumors of bone. A clinicopathological analysis of the natural history of the disease. *Cancer* 1962;15:653–690.

33. Huvos AG. *Bone tumors: diagnosis, treatment, and prognosis,* 2nd ed. Philadelphia: WB Saunders, 1991.

34. Jaffe HL. *Tumors and tumorous conditions of the bones and joints.* Philadelphia: Lea and Febiger, 1958.

35. Jaffe HL, Lichtenstein L, Portis RB. Giant cell tumor of bone. Its pathologic appearance, grading, supposed variants and treatment. *Arch Pathol* 1940;30:993–1031.

36. Kaplan PA, Murphy M, Greenway G, Resnick D, Sartoris DJ, Harms S. Fluid-fluid levels in giant cell tumors of bone: report of two cases. *Computed Tomogr* 1987;11:151–155.

37. Kransdorf MJ, Sweet DE, Buetow PC, Giudici MA, Moser RP Jr. Giant cell tumor in skeletally immature patients. *Radiology* 1992;184:233–237.

38. Ladanyi M, Traganos F, Huvos AG. Benign metastasizing giant cell tumors of bone: a DNA flow cytometric study. *Cancer* 1989;64:1521–1526.

39. Levine E, DeSmet AA, Neff JR, Martin NL. Scintigraphic evaluation of giant cell tumor of bone. *Am J Roentgenol* 1984;143:343–348.

40. Levine E, DeSmet AA, Neff JR. Role of radiologic imaging in management planning of giant cell tumor of bone. *Skeletal Radiol* 1984; 12:79–89.

41. Ling L, Klein MJ, Sissons HA, Steiner GC, Winchester RJ. Expression of Ia and monocyte-macrophage lineage antigens in giant cell tumor of bone and related lesions. *Arch Pathol* Lab Med 1988;112:65–69.

42. Lorenzo JC, Dorfman HD. Giant-cell reparative granuloma of short tubular bones of the hands and feet. *Am J Surg Pathol* 1980;4:551–563.

43. Maloney WJ, Vaughan LM, Jones HH, Ross J, Nagel DA. Benign metastasizing giant-cell tumor of bone. Report of three cases and review of the literature. *Clin Orthop* 1989;243:208–215.

44. Manaster BJ, Doyle AJ. Giant cell tumor of bone. *Radiol Clin* North Am 1993;31:299–323.

45. Matsuno T. Benign fibrous histiocytoma involving the ends of long bone. *Skeletal Radiol* 1990;19:561–566.

46. May DA, Good RB, Smith DK, Parsons TW. MR imaging of musculoskeletal tumors and tumor mimickers with intravenous gadolinium: experience with 242 patients. *Skeletal Radiol* 1997;26:2–15.

47. McDonald DJ, Sim FH, McLeod RA, Dahlin DC. Giant cell tumor of bone. *J Bone Joint Surg* 1986;68A:235–242.

48. McGrath J. Giant-cell tumour of bone: an analysis of fifty–two cases. *J Bone Joint Surg* 1972;54B:216–229.

49. McInerney DP, Middlemis JH. Giant-cell tumors of bone. *Skeletal Radiol* 1978;2:195–204.

50. Meis JM, Dorfman HD, Nathanson SD, Haggar AM, Wu KK. Primary malignant giant cell tumor of bone: dedifferentiated giant cell tumor. *Mod Pathol* 1989;2:541–546.

51. Moser RP Jr, Kransdorf MJ, Gilkey FW, Manaster BJ. Giant cell tumor of the upper extremity. *RadioGraphics* 1990;10:83–102.

52. Nascimento AG, Huvos AG, Marcove RC. Primary malignant giant cell tumor of bone: a study of eight cases and review of the literature. *Cancer* 1979;44:1393–1402.

53. Nusbacher N, Sclafani SJ, Birla SR. Case report 155. Polyostotic Paget disease complicated by benign giant cell tumor of left clavicle. *Skeletal Radiol* 1981;6:233–235.

54. Nojima T, Takeda N, Matsuno T, Inoue K, Nagashima K. Case report 869. Benign metastasizing giant cell tumor of bone. *Skeletal Radiol* 1994;23:583–585.

55. Oda Y, Tsuneyoshi M, Shinohara N. Solid variant of aneurysmal bone cyst (extragnatic giant cell reparative granuloma) in the axial skeleton and long bones: a study of its morphologic spectrum and distinction from allied giant cell lesions. *Cancer* 1992;70:2642–2649.

56. O' Reilly M, Chew FS. The scintigraphic features of giant-cell tumors in relation to other imaging modalities. *Clin Nucl Med* 1996;21:43–48.

57. Peimer CA, Schiller AL, Mankin HJ, Smith RJ. Multicentric giant cell tumor of bone. *J Bone Joint Surg* 1980;62A:652–656.

58. Picci P, Baldini N, Sudanese A, Boriani S, Campanacci M. Giant cell reparative granuloma and other giant cell lesions of the bones of the hand and feet. *Skeletal Radiol* 1986;15:415–421.

59. Picci P, Manfrini M, Zucchi V, Gherlinzoni F, Rock M, Bertoni F, Neff JR. Giant cell tumor bone in skeletally immature patients. *J Bone Joint Surg* 1983;65A:486–490.

60. Potter HG, Schneider R, Ghelman B, Healey JH, Lane JM. Multiple giant cell tumors and Paget disease of bone: Radiographic and clinical correlations. *Radiology* 1991;180:261–264.

61. Resnik CS, Steffe JW, Wang SE. Case report 353. Giant cell tumor of distal end of the femur, containing a fluid level as demonstrated by computed tomography. *Skeletal Radiol* 1986;15:175–177.

62. Rock MG, Pritchard DJ, Unni KK. Metastases from histologically be-nign giant-cell tumor of bone. *J Bone Joint Surg* 1984;66:269–274.

63. Rock MG, Sim FH, Unni KK, Witrak GA, Frassica FJ, Schray MF, Beabout JW, Dahlin DC. Secondary malignant giant-cell tumor of bone. Clinicopathological assessment of nineteen patients. *J Bone Joint Surg* 1986;68A:1073–1079.

64. Rosai J. Carcinoma of pancreas simulating giant cell tumor of bone. Electron-microscopic evidence of its acinar cell origin. *Cancer* 1968; 22:333–344.

65. Sanerkin NG. Malignancy, aggressiveness and recurrence in giant cell tumor of bone. *Cancer* 1980;46:1641–1649.

66. Schajowicz F, Slullitel J. Giant cell tumor associated with Paget's dis-ease of bone. *J Bone Joint Surg* 1966;48A:1340–1349.

67. Schajowicz F. *Tumors and tumorlike lesions of bone: pathology, ra-diology, and treatment*, 2nd ed. Berlin: Springer-Verlag, 1994; 257–299.

68. Shankman S, Greenspan A, Klein MJ, Lewis MM. Giant cell tumor of the ischium. A report of two cases and review of the literature. *Skele-tal Radiol* 1988;17:46–51.

69. Sim FH, Dahlin DC, Beabout JW. Multicentric giant cell tumors of bone. *J Bone Joint Surg* 1977;59A:1052–1060.

70. Simon MA, Kirchner PT. Scintigraphic evaluation of primary bone tu-mors. *J Bone Joint Surg* 1980;62A:758–764.

71. Steiner GC, Ghosh L, Dorfman HD. Ultrastructure of giant cell tumor of bone. *Hum Pathol* 1972;3:569–586.

72. Tehranzadeh J, Murphy BJ, Mnaymneh W. Giant cell tumor of the proximal tibia: MR and CT appearance. *J Comput Assist Tomogr* 1989;13:282–286.

73. Tornberg DN, Dick HM, Johnston AD. Multicentric giant-cell tumors in the long bones. A case report. *J Bone Joint Surg* 1975; 57A:420–422.

74. Tubbs WS, Brown LR, Beabout JW, Rock MG, Unni KK. Benign gi-ant-cell tumor of bone with pulmonary metastases: clinical findings and radiologic appearance of metastases in 13 cases. *Am J Roentgenol* 1992;158:331–334.

75. Unni KK. *Dahlin's bone tumors: general aspects and data on 11,087 cases*, 5th ed. New York: Lippincott-Raven, 1996.

76. Van Nostrand D, Madewell JE, McNiesh LM, Kyle RW, Sweet D. Ra-dionuclide bone scanning in giant cell tumor. *J Nucl Med* 1986;27: 329–338.

77. Williams HT. Multicentric giant cell tumor of bone. *Clin Nucl Med* 1989;14:631–633.

78. Wold LE, Dobyns JH, Swee RG, Dahlin DC. Giant cell reaction (gi-ant cell reparative granuloma) of the small bones of the hands and feet. *Am J Surg Pathol* 1986;10:491–496.

79. Wold LE, Swee RG. Giant cell tumor of the small bones of the hand and feet. *Semin Diagn Pathol* 1984;1:173–184.

80. Wray CC, MacDonald AW, Richardson RA. Benign giant-cell tumor with metastases to bone and lung. *J Bone Joint Surg* 1990; 72B:486–489.

81. Zhu X, Steiner GC. Malignant giant cell tumor of bone: malignant transformation of a benign giant cell tumor treated by surgery. *Bull Hosp Joint Dis Orthop Inst* 1990;50:169–176.

Simple Bone Cyst

82. Abdelwahab IF, Lewis MM, Klein MJ, Barbera C. Case report 515. Simple (solitary) bone cysts of the calcaneus. *Skeletal Radiol* 1989;17: 607–610.

83. Baker DM. Benign unicameral bone cyst. *Clin Orthop* 1970;71: 140–151.

84. Barcelo M, Pathria MN, Abdul-Karim FW. Intraosseous lipoma. A clinicopathologic study of four cases. *Arch Pathol Lab Med* 1992;116: 947–950.

85. Berlin SJ. A review of 2,720 lesions of the foot. *J Am Podiatr Assoc* 1980;70:318–324.

86. Blumberg ML. CT of iliac unicameral bone cysts. *Am J Roentgenol* 1981;136:1231–1232.

87. Boseker EH, Bickel WH, Dahlin DC. A clinicopathologic study of simple unicameral bone cysts. *Surg Gynecol Obstet* 1968;127: 550–560.

88. Broder HM. Possible precursor of unicameral bone cysts. *J Bone Joint Surg* 1968;50A:503–507.

89. Campanacci M, Capanna R, Picci P. Unicameral and aneurysmal bone cysts. *Clin Orthop* 1986;204:25–36.

90. Capanna R, Van Horn J, Ruggieri P, Biagini R. Epiphyseal involve-ment in unicameral bone cysts. *Skeletal Radiol* 1986;15:428–432.

91. Chow LT, Lee K. Intraosseous lipoma. A clinicopathological study of nine cases. *Am J Surg Pathol* 1992;16:401–410.

92. Cohen J. Etiology of simple bone cyst. *J Bone Joint Surg* 1970; 52A:1493–1497.

93. Cohen J. Unicameral bone cysts: a current synthesis of reported cases. *Orthop Clin North Am* 1977;8:715–726.

94. Conway WF, Hayes CW. Miscellaneous lesions of bone. *Radiol Clin North Am* 1993;31:339–358.

95. Goldberg RP, Genant HK. Case report 67. Solitary bone cyst of the right ilium. *Skeletal Radiol* 1978;3:118–121.

96. Haims AH, Desai P, Present D, Beltran J. Epiphyseal extension of a unicameral bone cyst. *Skeletal Radiol* 1997;26:51–54.

97. Hertzanu Y, Mendelsohn DB, Gottschalk F. Aneurysmal bone cyst of the calcaneus. *Radiology* 1984;151:51–52.

98. Hudson TM. *Radiologic-Pathologic correlation of musculoskeletal lesions*. Baltimore: Williams and Wilkins, 1987;249–252.

99. Huvos AG. *Bone tumors: diagnosis, treatment, and prognosis*, 2nd ed. Philadelphia: WB Saunders, 1991;713–726.

100. Jaffe HL, Lichtenstein L. Solitary unicameral bone cyst with empha-sis on the roentgen picture, the pathologic apearance, and the patho-genesis. *Arch Surg* 1942;44:1004–1025.

101. Keats TE. *Atlas of normal roentgen variants that may simulate dis-ease*, 4th ed. Chicago: Year Book, 1988;699–700.

102. Ketyer S, Braunstein S, Cholankeril J. CT diagnosis of intraosseous lipoma of the calcaneus. *J Comput Assist Tomogr* 1983;7:546–547.

103. Kricun ME. Tumors of the foot. In: Kricun ME, ed. *Imaging of bone tumors*. Philadelphia: WB Saunders, 1993;221–225.

104. Kricun ME, Kricun R, Haskin ME. Chondroblastoma of the calca-neus: radiographic features with emphasis on location. *Am J Roentgenol* 1977;128:613–616.

105. Lagier R. Calcaneus lipoma with bone infarct. *Fortschr Röentgenstr* 1985;142:472–474.

106. McGlynn FJ, Mickelson MR, El-Khoury GY. The fallen fragment sign in unicameral bone cyst. *Clin Orthop* 1981;156:157–159.

107. Milgram JW. Intraosseous lipomas. A clinicopathological study of 66 cases. *Clin Orthop* 1988;231:277–302.

108. Moore TE, King AR, Travis RC, Allen BC. Post-traumatic cysts and cyst-like lesions of bone. *Skeletal Radiol* 1989;18:93–97.

109. Morton KS. The pathogenesis of unicameral bone cyst. *Can J Surg* 1964;7:140–150.

110. Mulder JD, Kroon HM, Schütte HE, Taconis WK. *Radiologic atlas of bone tumors*. Amsterdam: Elsevier, 1993;579–590.

111. Murray RO, Jacobson HG. *The radiology of skeletal disorders*, 2nd ed. New York: Churchill Livingstone, 1977.

112. Neer CS II, Francis KC, Marcove RC, Tertz J, Carbonara PN. Treat-ment of unicameral bone cyst. A follow-up study of one hundred sev-enty-five cases. *J Bone Joint Surg* 1966;48A:731–745.

113. Norman A, Schiffman M. Simple bone cyst: factors of age depen-dency. *Radiology* 1977;124:779–782.

114. Remagen W, Lampérth BE, Jundt G, Schildt R. Das sogenannte oste-olytische Dreieck des Calcaneus. Radiologische und pathoanatomis-che Befunde. *Osteologie* 1994;3:275–283.

115. Reynolds J. The fallen fragment sign in the diagnosis of unicameral bone cysts. *Radiology* 1969;92:949–953.
116. Schajowicz F. *Tumors and Tumorlike Lesions of Bone and Joints,* 2nd ed. New York: Springer-Verlag, 1994;505–514.
117. Smith RW, Smith CF. Solitary unicameral bone cyst of the calcaneus. A review of 20 cases. *J Bone Joint Surg* 1974;56A:49–56.
118. Struhl S, Edelson C, Pritzker H, Seimon LP, Dorfman HD. Solitary (unicameral) bone cyst. The fallen fragment sign revisited. *Skeletal Radiol* 1989;18:261–265.
119. Van Linthoudt D, Lagier R. Calcaneal cysts: a radiological and anatomical-pathological study. *Acta Orthop Scand* 1978;49:310–316.
120. Weisel A, Hecht HL. Development of a unicameral bone cyst. *J Bone Joint Surg* 1980;62A:664–666.

Aneurysmal Bone Cyst

121. Aho HJ, Aho AJ, Einola S. Aneurysmal bone cyst, a study of ultrastructure and malignant transformation. *Virchows Arch (A)* 1982;395:169–179.
122. Aho HJ, Aho AJ, Pellineimi LJ, Ekfors TO, Foidart JM. Endothelium in aneurysmal bone cyst. *Histopathology* 1985;9:381–387.
123. Alles JU, Schulz A. Immunohistochemical markers (endothelial and histiocytic) and ultrastructure of primary aneurysmal bone cysts. *Hum Pathol* 1986;17:39–45.
124. Apaydin A, Özkaynak C, Yilmaz S, Akyildiz F, Sindel T, Aydin AT, Karpuzoglu G, Lüleci E. Aneurysmal bone cyst of metacarpal. *Skeletal Radiol* 1996;25:76–78.
125. Beltran J, Simon DC, Levy M, Herman L, Weis L, Mueller CF. Aneurysmal bone cysts: MR imaging at 1.5 T. *Radiology* 1986;158:689–690.
126. Bertoni F, Bacchini P, Capanna R, Ruggieri P, Biagini R, Feruzzi A, Bettelli G, Picci P, Campanacci M. Solid variant of aneurysmal bone cyst. *Cancer* 1993;71:729–734.
127. Biesecker JL, Marcove RC, Huvos AG, Miké V. Aneurysmal bone cysts. A clinicopathologic study of 66 cases. *Cancer* 1970;26:615–625.
128. Bonakdarpour A, Levy WM, Aegerter E. Primary and secondary aneurysmal bone cysts: a radiological study of 75 cases. *Radiology* 1978;126:75–83.
129. Buirski G, Watt I. The radiological features of solid aneurysmal bone cysts. *Br J Radiol* 1984;57:1057–1065.
130. Burnstein MI, De Smet AA, Hafez GR, Heiner JP. Case report 611. Subperiosteal aneurysmal bone cyst of tibia. *Skeletal Radiol* 1990;4:294–297.
131. Clough JR, Price CH. Aneurysmal bone cyst: pathogenesis and long term results of treatment. *Clin Orthop* 1973;97:52–63.
132. Dabezies EJ, D Ambrosia RD, Chuinard RG, Ferguson AB Jr. Aneurysmal bone cyst after fracture. A report of three cases. *J Bone Joint Surg* 1982;64A:617–621.
133. Dabska M, Buraczewski J. Aneurysmal bone cyst. Pathology, clinical course and radiologic appearances. *Cancer* 1969;23:371–389.
134. Dahlin DC, McLeod RA. Aneurysmal bone cyst and other nonneoplastic conditions. *Skeletal Radiol* 1982;8:243–250.
135. Fechner RE, Mills SE. *Tumors of the bones and joints.* Washington, DC: Armed Forces Institute of Pathology, 1993;181–184, 253–258.
136. Freeby JA, Reinus WR, Wilson AJ. Quantitative analysis of the plain radiographic appearance of aneurysmal bone cyst. *Invest Radiol* 1995;30:433–439.
137. Fush SE, Herndon JH. Aneurysmal bone cyst involving the hand: a review and report of two cases. *J Hand Surg* 1979;4A:152–159.
138. Godfry LW, Gresham GA. The natural history of aneurysmal bone cyst. *Proc R Soc Med* 1959;52:900–905.
139. Heyman S, Treves S. Scintigraphy in pediatric bone tumors. In: Jaffe N, ed. *Bone tumors in children.* Littleton, MA: Wright, 1979;79–96.
140. Hudson TM. Fluid levels in aneurysmal bone cysts: a CT feature. *Am J Roentgenol* 1984;141:1001–1004.
141. Hudson TM. *Radiologic-pathologic correlation of musculoskeletal lesions.* Baltimore: Williams and Wilkins, 1987;261–265.
142. Hudson TM. Scintigraphy of aneurysmal bone cysts. *Am J Roentgenol* 1984;142:761–765.
143. Hudson TM, Hamlin DJ, Fitzimmons JR. Magnetic resonance imaging of fluid levels in an aneurysmal bone cyst and in anticoagulated human blood. *Skeletal Radiol* 1985;13:267–270.
144. Huvos AG. *Bone tumors: diagnosis, treatment, and prognosis,* 2nd ed.

Philadelphia: WB Saunders, 1991,727–743.
145. Jaffe HL. Aneurysmal bone cyst. *Bull Hosp Joint Dis* 1950,11.3–19.
146. Kinley S, Wiseman F, Wertheimer SJ. Giant cell tumor of the talus with secondary aneurysmal bone cyst. *J Foot Ankle Surg* 1993;32:38–46.
147. Kransdorf MJ, Sweet DE. Aneurysmal bone cyst: concept, controversy, clinical presentation, and imaging. *Am J Roentgenol* 1995;164:573–580.
148. Kyriakos M, Hardy D. Malignant transformation of aneurysmal bone cyst, with an analysis of the literature. *Cancer* 1991;68:1770–1780.
149. Levy WM, Miller AS, Bonakdarpour A, Aegerter E. Aneurysmal bone cyst secondary to other osseous lesions. Report of 57 cases. *Am J Clin Pathol* 1975;63:1–8.
150. Lichtenstein L. Aneurysmal bone cyst. A pathological entity commonly mistaken for giant cell tumor and occasionally for hemangioma and osteogenic sarcoma. *Cancer* 1950;3:279–289.
151. Lichtenstein L. Aneurysmal bone cyst. Observations on fifty cases. *J Bone Joint Surg* 1957;39A:873–882.
152. Makhija MC. Bone scanning in aneurysmal bone cyst. *Clin Nucl Med* 1981;6:500–501.
153. Martinez V, Sissons HA. Aneurysmal bone cyst. A review of 123 cases including primary lesions and those secondary to other bone pathology. *Cancer* 1988;61:2291–2304.
154. McCarthy EF, Dorfman HD. Vascular and cartilaginous hamartoma of the ribs in infancy with secondary aneurysmal bone cyst formation. *Am J Surg Pathol* 1980;4:247–253.
155. Mintz MC, Dalinka MK, Schmidt R. Aneurysmal bone cyst arising in fibrous dysplasia during pregnancy. *Radiology* 1987;165:549–550.
156. Mirra JM. *Bone tumors: clinical, radiologic, and pathologic correlations.* Philadelphia: Lea and Febiger, 1989;1267–1311.
157. Moore TE, King AR, Travis RC, Allen BC. Post-traumatic cysts and cyst-like lesions of bone. *Skeletal Radiol* 1989;18:93–97.
158. Mulder JD, Kroon HM, Schütte HE, Taconis WK. *Radiologic atlas of bone tumors.* Amsterdam: Elsevier, 1993;557–578.
159. Munk PL, Helms CA, Holt RG, Johnston J, Steinbach L, Neumann C. MR imaging of aneurysmal bone cysts. *Am J Roentgenol* 1989;153:99–101.
160. Ratcliffe PJ, Grimmer RJ. Aneurysmal bone cyst arising after tibial fracture. A case report. *J Bone Joint Surg* 1993;75A:1225–1227.
161. Ratner V, Dorfman HD. Giant-cell reparative granuloma of the hand and foot bones. *Clin Orthop* 1990;260:251–258.
162. Ruiter DJ, van Rijssel TG, van der Velde EA. Aneurysmal bone cysts. A clinicopathological study of 105 cases. *Cancer* 1977;39:2231–2239.
163. Sanerkin NG, Mott MG, Roylance J. An unusual intraosseous lesion with fibromyxoid elements: solid variant of aneurysmal bone cyst. *Cancer* 1983;51:2278–2286.
164. Schoedel K, Shankman S, Desai P. Intracortical and subperiosteal aneurysmal bone cysts: a report of three cases. *Skeletal Radiol* 1996;25:455–459.
165. Scully SP, Temple HT, O Keefe RJ, Gebhardt MC. Case report 830. Aneurysmal bone cyst. *Skeletal Radiol* 1994;23:157–160.
166. Sharma P, Elangovan S, Ratnakar C. Case report: calcification within aneurysmal bone cyst. *Br J Radiol* 1994;67:306–308.
167. Sherman RS, Soong KY. Aneurysmal bone cyst: its roentgen diagnosis. *Radiology* 1957;68:54–64.
168. Simon MA, Kirchner PT. Scintigraphic evaluation of primary bone tumors. *J Bone Joint Surg* 1980;62A:758–764.
169. Spjut HJ, Dorfman HD, Fechner RE, Ackerman LV. *Tumors of bone and cartilage.* Washington, DC: Armed Forces Institute of Pathology, 1971.
170. Thrall JH, Geslien GE, Corcoron RJ, Johnson MC. Abnormal radionuclide deposition patterns adjacent to focal skeletal lesions. *Radiology* 1975;115:659–663.
171. Tillman BP, Dahlin DC, Lipscomb PR, Stewart JR. Aneurysmal bone cyst: an analysis of ninety-five cases. *Mayo Clin Proc* 1968;43:478–495.
172. Tsai JC, Dalinka MK, Fallon MD, Zlatkin MB, Kressel HY. Fluid-fluid level: a nonspecific finding in tumors of bone and soft tissue. *Radiology* 1990;175:779–782.
173. Unni KK. *Dahlin's bone tumors: general aspects and data on 11,087 cases,* 5th ed. New York: Lippincott-Raven, 1996.
174. Vergel De Dios AM, Bond JR, Shives TC, McLeod RA, Unni KK. Aneurysmal bone cyst. A clinicopathologic study of 238 cases. *Cancer* 1992;69:2921–2931.

175. Zimmer WD, Berquist TH, McLeod RA, Sim FH, Pritchard DJ, Shives TC, Wold LE, May GR. Bone tumors: magnetic resonance imaging versus computed tomography. *Radiology* 1985;155:709–718.
176. Zimmer WD, Berquist TH, Sim FH, Wold LE, Pritchard DJ, Shives TC, McLeod RA. Magnetic resonance imaging of aneurysmal bone cyst. *Mayo Clin Proc* 1984;59:633–636.

Intraosseous Lipoma

177. Addison AK, Payne SR. Primary liposarcoma of bone. Case report. *J Bone Joint Surg* 1982;64A:301–304.
178. Blacksin MF, Ende N, Benevenia J. Magnetic resonance imaging of intraosseous lipomas: a radiologic-pathologic correlation. *Skeletal Radiol* 1995;24:37–41.
179. Bonnet J, Garreta L, Ducloux J-M. Les lacunes calcanéennes. (Calcaneal lacunae.) *Ann Radiol* 1968;11:171–184.
180. Bruni L. The cockade image: a diagnostic sign of calcaneum intraosseous lipoma. *Rays* 1986;11:51–54.
181. Dahlin DC, Unni KK. *Bone tumors: general aspects and data on 8,542 cases,* 4th ed. Springfield IL: Charles C Thomas, 1986;181–185.
182. DeLee JC. Intraosseous lipoma of the proximal part of the femur: case report. *J Bone Joint Surg* 1979;61A:601–603.
183. Dominok GW, Knoch HG. *Knochengeschwülste und Geschwulstähnliche Knochenerkrankungen,* 3rd ed., Jena: VEB Gustav Fischer Verl, 1971;267–275.
184. Dooms GC, Hricak H, Sollitto RA, Higgins CB. Lipomatous tumors and tumors with fatty component: MR imaging potential and comparison of MR and CT results. *Radiology* 1985;157:479–483.
185. Fechner RE, Mills SE. *Tumors of the bones and joints.* Washington, DC: Armed Forces Institute of Pathology, 1993;203–209.
186. *Gray's anatomy. The anatomical basis of medicine and surgery,* 38th ed. New York. Churchill Livingstone, 1995;452–468.
187. Hall RL, Shereff MJ. Anatomy of the calcaneus. *Clin Orthop Relat Res* 1993;290:27–35.
188. Hart JAL. Intraosseous lipoma. *J Bone Joint Surg* 1973;55B:624–632.
189. Junghanns H. Lipomas (fatty marrow areas) in the vertebral column. In: *Handbuch der Speziellen Pathologischen Anatomie und Histologie,* Tome IX/4. Berlin: Springer-Verlag, 1939;333–334.
190. Keats TE. *Atlas of normal Roentgen variants that may simulate disease,* 5th ed. St Louis: Mosby Year Book, 1992;637–648.
191. Keats TE, Harrison RB. The calcaneal nutrient foramen: a useful sign in the differentiation of true from simulated cysts. *Skeletal Radiol* 1979;3:239–240.
192. Kenan S, Lewis MM, Abdelwahab IF, Hermann G, Klein MJ. Case report 652. Primary intraosseous low grade myxoid sarcoma of the scapula (myxoid liposarcoma). *Skeletal Radiol* 1991;20:73–75.
193. Köhler A, Zimmer EA. *Borderlands of normal and early pathologic findings in skeletal radiography,* 13th ed. Revised by Schmidt H, Freyschmidt J. Stuttgart: Thieme Verlag, 1993;797–814.
194. Kricun ME. *Imaging of bone tumors.* Philadelphia: WB Saunders, 1993;236–237.
195. Lagier R. Case report 128. Intraosseous lipoma. *Skeletal Radiol* 1980;5:267–269.
196. Leeson MC, Kay D, Smith BS. Intraosseous lipoma. *Clin Orthop* 1983;181:186–190.
197. Levey DS, Sartoris DJ, Resnick D. Advanced diagnostic imaging techniques for pedal osseous neoplasms. *Clin Pod Med Surg* 1993;10:655–682.
198. Levin MF, Vellet AD, Munk PL, McLean CA. Intraosseous lipoma of the distal femur: MRI appearance. *Skeletal Radiol* 1996;25:82–84.
199. Milgram JW. Intraosseous lipoma: Radiologic and pathologic manifestations. *Radiology* 1988;167:155–160.
200. Mueller MC, Robbins JL. Intramedullary lipoma of bone. Report of a case. *J Bone Joint Surg* 1960;42A:517–520.
201. Norman A, Steiner GC. Radiographic and morphological features of cyst formation in idiopathic bone infarction. *Radiology* 1983;146:335–338.
202. Posteraro RH. Radiographic evaluation of pedal osseous tumors. *Clin Pod Med Surg* 1993;10:633–653.
203. Poussa M, Holmstrom T. Intraosseous lipoma of the calcaneus: report of a case and a short review of the literature. *Acta Orthop* Scand 1976;47:570–574.
204. Ramos A, Castello J, Sartoris DJ, Greenway GD, Resnick D, Haghighi P. Osseous lipoma: CT appearance. *Radiology* 1985;157: 615–619.
205. Remagen W. Pathologische Anatomie der Femurkopfnekrose. *Orthopäde* 1990;19:174–181.
206. Resnick D, Kyriakos M, Greenway GD. Tumors and tumor-like lesions of bone: imaging and pathology of specific lesions. In: Resnick D. ed. *Bone and Joint Imaging.* Philadelphia: WB Saunders, 1989;1154–1156.
207. Resnick D, Niwayama J. *Diagnosis of Bone and Joint Disorders.* WB Saunders, 1988;3782–3786.
208. Salzer M, Gotzmann H. Parostale Lipome. (Parosteal lipomas.) *Bruns Beitr Klin Chir* 1963;206:501–505.
209. Salzer M, Salzer-Kuntschik M. Zur Frage der sogenannten zentralen Knochenlipome. *Beitr Pathol Anat* 1965;132:365–375.
210. Sirry A. The pseudo-cystic triangle in the normal os calcis. *Acta Radiol* 1951;36:516–520.
211. Wilner D. *Radiology of bone tumors and allied disorders.* Philadelphia: WB Saunders, 1982;387.
212. Zorn DT, Cordray DR, Randels PH. Intraosseous lipoma of bone involving the sacrum. *J Bone Joint Surg* 1971;53A:1201–1204.

Fibrocartilaginous Mesenchymoma

213. Bhaduri A, Deshpande RB. Fibrocartilaginous mesenchymoma versus fibrocartilaginous dysplasia: are these a single entity? *Am J Surg Pathol* 1995;19:1447–1448.
214. Bulichova LV, Unni KK, Bertoni F, Beabout JW. Fibrocartilaginous mesenchymoma of bone. *Am J Surg Pathol* 1993;17:830–836.
215. Campanacci M. *Bone and soft tissue tumors.* New York: Springer-Verlag, 1986;345–348.
216. Dahlin DC, Bertoni F, Beabout JW. Campanacci M: Fibrocartilaginous mesenchymoma with low grade malignancy. *Skeletal Radiol* 1984;12:263–269.
217. Ishida T, Dorfman HD. Massive chondroid differentiation in fibrous dysplasia of bone (fibrocartilaginous dysplasia). *Am J Surg Pathol* 1993;17:924–930.
218. Mirra JM. Intramedullary cartilage- and chondroid-producing tumors. In: Mirra JM, Picci P, Gold RH, eds. *Bone tumors: clinical, radiologic, and pathologic correlations,* vol 1. Philadelphia: Lea and Febiger, 1989;439–690.

Adamantinoma of Long Bones

219. Adler C-P. Case report 587. Adamantinoma of the tibia mimicking osteofibrous dysplasia. *Skeletal Radiol* 1990;19:55–58.
220. Alquacil-Garcia A, Alonso A, Pettigrew NM. Osteofibrous dysplasia (ossifying fibroma) of the tibia and fibula and adamantinoma. *Am J Clin Pathol* 1984;82:470–474.
221. Baker PL, Dockerty MD, Coventry MB. Adamantinoma (so-called) of the long bones. *J Bone Joint Surg* 1954;36A:704–720.
222. Campanacci M. Osteofibrous dysplasia of long bones. A new clinical entity. *Ital J Orthop Traumatol* 1976;2:221–237.
223. Campanacci M, Laus M, Giunti A, Gitelis S, Bertoni F. Adamantinoma of the long bones. The experience at the Istituto Ortopedico Rizzoli. *Am J Surg Pathol* 1981;5:533–542.
224. Czerniak B, Rojas-Corona RR, Dorfman HD. Morphologic diversity of long bone adamantinoma. The concept of differentiated (regressing) adamantinoma and its relationship to osteofibrous dysplasia. *Cancer* 1989;64:2319–2334.
225. Eisenstein W, Pitcock JA. Adamantinoma of the tibia: an eccrine carcinoma. *Arch Pathol Lab Med* 1984;108:246–250.
226. Fischer B. Über ein primäres Adamantinom der Tibia. *Frankfurter Z Pathol* 1913;12:422–441.
227. Huvos AG, Marcove RC. Adamantinoma of long bones: a clinicopathological study of fourteen cases with vascular origin suggested. *J Bone Joint Surg* 1975;57:148–154.
228. Ishida T, Iijima T, Kikuchi F, Kitagawa T, Tanida T, Imamura T, Machinami R. A clinicopathological and immunohistochemical study of osteofibrous dysplasia, differentiated adamantinoma, and adamantinoma of long bones. *Skeletal Radiol* 1992;21:493–502.
229. Jundt G, Remberger K, Roessner A, Schulz A, Bohndorf K. Adamantinoma of long bones. A histopathological and immunohistochemical study of 23 cases. *Pathol Res Pract* 1995;191:112–120.
230. Keeney GL, Unni KK, Beabout JW, Pritchard DJ. Adamantinoma of

long bones. A clinicopathologic study of 85 cases. *Cancer* 1989;64: 730–737.

231. Knapp RH, Wick MR, Scheithauer BW, Unni KK. Adamantinoma of bone. An electron microscopic and immunohistochemical study. *Virchows Arch (A)* 1982;398:75–86.

232. Llombart-Bosch A, Ortuno-Pacheco G. Ultrastructural findings supporting the angioblastic nature of the so-called adamantinoma of the tibia. *Histopathology* 1978;2:189–200.

233. Markel SF. Ossifying fibroma of long bone. Its distinction from fibrous dysplasia and its association with adamantinoma of long bone. *Am J Clin Pathol* 1978;69:91–97.

234. Moon NF. Adamantinoma of the appendicular skeleton. A statistical review of reported cases and inclusion of 10 new cases. *Clin Orthop* 1965;43:189–213.

235. Moon NF, Mori H. Adamantinoma of the appendicular skeleton —updated. *Clin Orthop* 1986;204:215–237.

236. Rock MG, Beabout JW, Unni KK, Sim FH. Adamantinoma. *Orthopedics* 1983;6:472–477.

237. Rosai J. Adamantinoma of the tibia: Electron microscopic evidence of its epithelial origin. *Am J Clin Pathol* 1969;51:786–792.

238. Rosai J, Pinkus GS. Immunohistochemical demonstration of epithelial differentiation in adamantinoma of the tibia. *Am J Surg Pathol* 1982; 6:427–434.

239. Schajowicz F, Santini-Araujo E. Adamantinoma of the tibia masked by fibrous dysplasia. Report of three cases. *Clin Orthop* 1989;238: 294–301.

240. Schajowicz F. *Tumors and tumorlike lesions of bone: pathology, radiology, and treatment,* 2nd ed. Berlin: Springer-Verlag, 1994; 468–481.

241. Springfield DS, Rosenberg AE, Mankin HJ, Mindell ER. Relationship between osteofibrous dysplasia and adamantinoma. *Clin Orthop* 1994;309:234–244.

242. Sweet DE, Vinh TN, Devaney K. Cortical osteofibrous dysplasia of long bone and its relationship to adamantinoma. A clinicopathologic study of 30 cases. *Am J Surg Pathol* 1992;16:282–290.

243. Tehranzadeh J, Fanney D, Ghandur-Mnaymneh L, Ganz W, Mnaymneh W. Case report 517. Ulcerating adamantinoma of the tibia. *Skeletal Radiol* 1989;17:614–619.

244. Ueda Y, Roessner A, Bosse A, Edel G, Bocker W, Wuisman P. Juvenile intracortical adamantinoma of the tibia with predominant osteofibrous dysplasia-like features. *Pathol Res Pract* 1991;187:1039–1043.

245. Unni KK, Dahlin DC, Beabout JW, Ivins JC. Adamantinoma of long bones. *Cancer* 1974;34:1796–1805.

246. Weiss SW, Dorfman HD. Adamantinoma of long bone. An analysis of nine new cases with emphasis on metastasizing lesions and fibrous dysplasia-like changes. *Hum Pathol* 1977;8:141–153.

247. Yoneyama T, Winter WG, Milsow L. Tibial adamantinoma: its histogenesis from ultrastructural studies. *Cancer* 1977;40:1138–1142.

248. Zehr RJ, Recht MP, Bauer TW. Adamantinoma. *Skeletal Radiol* 1995; 24:553–555.

Chordoma

249. Abenoza P, Sibley RK. Chordoma: an immunohistochemical study. *Hum Pathol* 1987;17:744–747.

250. Azzarelli A, Quagliuolo V, Cerasoli S, Zucali R, Bignami P, Mazzaferro V, Dossena G, Gennari L. Chordoma: natural history and treatment results in 33 cases. *J Surg Oncol* 1988;37:185–191.

251. Beaugié JM, Mann CV, Butler ECB. Sacrococcygeal chordoma. *Br J Surg* 1969;56:586–588.

252. Belza MG, Urich H. Chordoma and malignant fibrous histiocytoma. Evidence of transformation. *Cancer* 1986;589:1082–1087.

253. Byers PD. A study of histological features distinguishing chordoma from chondrosarcoma. *Br J Cancer* 1981;43:229–232.

254. Chu TA. Chondroid chordoma of the sacrococcygeal region. *Arch Pathol Lab Med* 1987;111:861–864.

255. Coindre JM, Rivel J, Trojan M, De Mascarel J, De Mascarel A. Immunohistological study in chordomas. *J Pathol* 1986;150:61–63.

256. Coombs RJ, Coiner L. Sacral chordoma with unusual posterior radiographic presentation. *Skeletal Radiol* 1996;25:679–681.

257. Crawford T. The staining reactions of chordoma. *J Clin Pathol* 1958; 11:110–113.

258. Dabska M. Parachordoma. A new clinicopathologic entity. *Cancer* 1977;40:1586–1592.

259. Dahlin DC, MacCarty CS. Chordoma. A study of fifty-nine cases. *Cancer* 1952;5:1170–1178.

260. Dahlin DC, Unni KK. *Bone tumors: general aspects and data on 8,542 cases.* Springfield, IL: Charles C Thomas, 1986;379–393.

261. deBruine FT, Kroon HM. Spinal chordoma: radiologic features of 14 cases. *Am J Roentgenol* 1988;150:861–863.

262. Falconer MA, Bailey IC, Duchen LW. Surgical treatment of chordoma and chondroma of the skull base. *J Neurosurg* 1968;29: 261–275.

263. Fechner RE, Mills SE. *Tumors of the bones and joints.* Washington, DC: Armed Forces Institute of Pathology, 1993;239–244.

264. Firooznia H, Printo RS, Lin JP, Baruch HH, Zausner J. Chordoma: radiologic evaluation of 20 cases. *Am J Roentgenol* 1976;127:797–805.

265. Fisher H-P, Alles JU, Stambolis C. Skeletal chordoma. Clinico-pathological and differential diagnostic aspects. *Pathologe* 1983; 4:307–312.

266. Friedman I, Harrison DFN, Bird ES. The fine structure of chordoma with particular reference to the physaliphorous cell. *J Clin Pathol* 1962;15:116–125.

267. Healey JH, Lane JM. Chordoma: a critical review of diagnosis and treatment. *Orthop Clin North Am* 1989;20:417–426.

268. Higginbotham NL, Phillips RF, Farr HW, Hustu HO. Chordoma. Thirty-five-year study at Memorial Hospital. *Cancer* 1967;20: 1841–1850.

269. Hruban RH, Traganos F, Reuter VE, Huvos AG. Chordomas with malignant spindle cell components. *Am J Pathol* 1990;137:435–447.

270. Hudson TM. *Radiologic-pathologic correlation of musculoskeletal lesions.* Baltimore: Williams and Wilkins, 1987;287–303.

271. Huvos AG. *Bone tumors: diagnosis, treatment, and prognosis,* 2nd ed. Philadelphia. WB Saunders, 1991;599–624.

272. Kay S, Schatzki PF. Ultrastructural observations of a chordoma arising in the clivus. *Hum Pathol* 1972;3:403–413.

273. Krol G, Sundaresan N, Deck M. Computed tomography of axial chordomas. *J Computed Assist Tomogr* 1983;7:286–289.

274. Makek M, Leu HJ. Malignant fibrous histiocytoma arising in a recurrent chordoma. Case report and electron microscopic findings. *Virchows Arch (A)* 1982;397:241–250.

275. Martin RF, Melnick PJ, Warner NE, Terry R, Bullock WK, Schwinn CP. Chordoid sarcoma. *Am J Clin Pathol* 1973;59:623–635.

276. Meis JM, Giraldo AA. Chordoma. An immuno-histochemical study of 20 cases. *Arch Pathol Lab Med* 1988;112:553–556.

277. Meis JM, Raymond AK, Evans HL, Charles RE, Giraldo AA. Dedifferentiated chordoma. A clinico-pathogic and immunohistochemical study of three cases. *Am J Surg Pathol* 1987;11:516–525.

278. Meyer JE, Lepke RA, Lindfors KK, Pagani JJ, Hirschy JC, Hayman LA, Momose KJ, McGinnis B. Chordomas: their CT appearance in the cervical, thoracic and lumbar spine. *Radiology* 1984;153:693–696.

279. Miettinen M, Karaharju E, Järvinen H. Chordoma with a massive spindle-cell sarcomatous transformation. A light- and electron-microscopic and immunohistological study. *Am J Surg Pathol* 1987;11: 563–570.

280. Mulder JD, Kroon HM, Schütte HE, Taconis WK. *Radiologic Atlas of Bone Tumors.* Amsterdam: Elsevier, 1993;267–274.

281. Pardo-Min n FJ, Guillen FJ, Villas C, Vasquez JJ. A comparative ultrastructural study of chondrosarcoma, chordoid sarcoma, and chordoma. *Cancer* 1981;47:2611–2619.

282. Rich TA, Schiller A, Suit HD, Mankin HJ. Clinical and pathologic review of 48 cases of chordoma. *Cancer* 1985;56:182–187.

283. Risio M, Bagliani C, Leli R, Digirolamo P, Del Paro M, Coverliza S. Sacrococcygeal and vertebral chordomas. Report of three cases and review of the literature. *J Neurosurg Sci* 1985;29:211–227.

284. Rosenthal DI, Scott JA, Mankin HJ, Wismer GL, Brady TJ. Sacrococcygeal chordoma: magnetic resonance imaging and computed tomography. *Am J Roentgenol* 1985;145:143–147.

285. Smith J, Ludwig RL, Marcove RC. Sacrococcygeal chordoma. A clinicoradiological study of 60 patients. *Skeletal Radiol* 1987;16: 37–44.

286. Smith J, Reuter V, Demas B. Case report 576. Anaplastic sacrococcygeal chordoma (dedifferentiated chordoma). *Skeletal Radiol* 1989; 18:561–564.

287. Sze G, Uichanco LS III, Brant-Zawadzki MN, Davis RL, Gutin PH, Wilson CG, Norman D, Newton TH. Chordomas: MR imaging. *Radiology* 1988;166:187–191.

288. Taylor JR. Persistence of the notochordal canal in vertebrae. *J Anat* 1982;11:211–217.

289. Thiery JP, Mazabraud A, Mignot J, Durigon M. Electron microscopic

study of a sacral chordoma. Characterization of various evolutive stages of the tumoral cells. *Ann Anat Pathol* 1977;22:193–204.

290. Turner ML, Mulhern CB, Dalinka MK. Lesions of the sacrum. Differential diagnosis and radiological evaluation. *JAMA* 1981;245: 275–277.

291. Uhrenholt L, Stimpel H. Histochemistry of sacrococcygeal chordoma. *Acta Pathol Microbiol Scand (A)* 1985;93:203–204.

292. Weiss SW. Ultrastructure of the so-called chordoid sarcoma. Evidence supporting cartilaginous differentiation. *Cancer* 1976;37: 300–306.

293. Yuh WT, Flickinger FW, Barloon TJ, Montgomery WJ. MR imaging of unusual chordomas. *J Comput Assist Tomogr* 1988;12:30–35.

Leiomyosarcoma of Bone

294. Abdelwahab IF, Hermann G, Kenan S, Klein MJ, Lewis MM. Case report 794. Primary leiomyosarcoma of the right femur. *Skeletal Radiol* 1993;22:379–381.

295. Abdelwahab IF, Kenan S, Hermann G, Klein MJ, Lewis MM. Radiation-induced leiomyosarcoma. *Skeletal Radiol* 1995;24:81–83.

296. Angervall L, Berlin O, Kindblom LG, Stener B. Primary leiomyosarcoma of bone. A study of five cases. *Cancer* 1980;46:1270–1279.

297. Berlin O, Angervall L, Kindblom LG, Berlin IC, Stener B. Primary leiomyosarcoma of bone. A clinical, radiographic, pathologic-anatomic, and prognostic study of 16 cases. *Skeletal Radiol* 1987;16: 364–376.

298. Eady JL, McKinney JD, McDonald EC. Primary leiomyosarcoma of bone. *J Bone Joint Surg* 1987;69A:287–289.

299. Fornasier VL, Paley D. Leiomyosarcoma in bone: primary or secondary? A case report and review of the literature. *Skeletal Radiol* 1983;10:147–153.

300. Jundt G, Moll C, Nidecker A, Schilt R, Remagen W. Primary leiomyosarcoma of bone: report of eight cases. *Hum Pathol* 1994;25: 1205–1212.

301. Kawai T, Suzuki M, Mukai M, Hiroshima K, Shinmei M. Primary leiomyosarcoma of bone. An immunohistochemical and ultrastructural study. *Arch Pathol Lab Med* 1983;107:433–437.

302. Meister P, Konrad E, Gokel JM, Remberger K. Case report 59. Leiomyosarcoma of the humerus. *Skeletal Radiol* 1978;2:265–267.

303. Myers JL, Arocho J, Bernreuter W, Dunham W, Mazur MT. Leiomyosarcoma of bone. A clinicopathologic, immunohistochemical, and ultrastructural study of five cases. *Cancer* 1991;67: 1051–1056.

304. Overgaard J, Frederiksen P, Helmig O, Jensen OM. Primary leiomyosarcoma of bone. *Cancer* 1977;39:1664–1671.

305. Sanerkin NG. Primary leiomyosarcoma of the bone and its comparison with fibrosarcoma. A cytological, histological, and ultrastructural study. *Cancer* 1979;44:1375–1387.

306. Shamsuddin AK, Reyes F, Harvey JW, Toker C. Primary leiomyosarcoma of bone. *Hum Pathol* 1980;11:581–583.

307. Von Hochstetter AR, Eberle H, Ruettner JR. Primary leiomyosarcoma of extragnathic bones. *Cancer* 1984;53:2194–2200.

308. Wang TY, Erlandson RA, Marcove RC, Huvos AG. Primary leiomyosarcoma of bone. *Arch Pathol Lab Med* 1980;104:100–104.

309. Young MPA, Freemont AJ. Primary leiomyosarcoma of bone. *Histopathology* 1991;19:257–262.

Metastases

INTRODUCTION

Skeletal metastases are the most common variety of bone tumors and should always be considered in the differential diagnosis, particularly in older patients (57). In a series of 1000 consecutive autopsies of patients who died of carcinoma, metastases to bone were found in 27% (2). Approximately 70% of all malignant bone tumors are metastatic in origin (109). The incidence varies according to the type of primary neoplasm and the duration of disease. Some malignant tumors demonstrate a far greater predilection for osseous involvement than others. Cancers of the breast, prostate, lung, and kidney account for 80% of all metastatic cancers to bone (58). In men, carcinoma of the prostate is reported to account for almost 60% and carcinoma of the lung for 25% of all bone metastases. In women, carcinoma of the breast is responsible for almost 70% of all metastatic lesions, the remaining 30% being mainly due to carcinomas of the thyroid, uterus, and kidney (1,76). Other primary tumors responsible for bone metastases include carcinomas of the stomach, colon, urinary bladder, melanoma, and some neurogenic tumors (105). Some sarcomas, such as osteosarcoma and Ewing sarcoma, may occasionally metastasize to bones. In children aged 5 years and younger, neuroblastoma is usually the primary tumor responsible for metastatic disease. Because of their frequency, cancers of the breast, lung, and prostate are responsible for the majority of bone metastases. The usual route of metastasis is via tumor emboli, mostly carried through the lymphatic system and the ductus thoracicus to the central blood circulation, and then by the arterial system into the periphery (11).

Clinical Presentation

Metastases are relatively rare in patients below the age of 40. Therefore, patient age is an important discriminating factor in the diagnosis (71). Unlike primary tumors, metastases usually involve the axial skeleton (skull, spine, and pelvis) and the most proximal segments of limb bones. Only in extremely rare cases do metastatic tumors occur distal to the elbows and the knees (72,85). Most metastatic lesions are found in the vertebrae, ribs, pelvis, skull, femur, and humerus (71) (Fig. 1).

The majority of skeletal metastases are silent. When metastases are symptomatic, pain is the main clinical feature, although rarely a pathologic fracture through the lesion may focus attention on the disease (86). Clinical and laboratory examinations frequently disclose other signs of malignancy, such as weight loss, anemia, fever, and an elevated erythrocyte sedimentation rate. In addition, serum calcium and alkaline phosphatase levels are usually elevated (107). In the spine, metastases are frequently associated with neurologic symptoms caused by compression of the cord or nerve roots or even by complete obstruction of the thecal sac.

Imaging

Detection of skeletal metastases is not always possible on routine radiography, because destruction of the bone may not be visible (6,99,108). It has been estimated that 30% to 50% of normal bone mineral must be lost before a bone metastasis becomes visible on a plain radiograph (9). Radionuclide bone scan, including both planar and single proton emission CT (SPECT) imaging (15), is the best screening method for early detection of metastatic tumors and can detect lytic and blastic lesions (Fig. 2). CT and MRI may also be helpful, the latter modality being the most sensitive (99). On radiography, a metastatic lesion may resemble any of the benign or malignant lesions. There are no radiographic characteristics of metastasis. The type of bone destruction may be geographic, moth-eaten, or permeative, and the margins may be well or poorly defined. A periosteal reaction and a soft tissue mass may or may not be present, although the latter situation is more common. Metastases can be solitary or multiple, and they can be further subdivided into purely lytic, purely blas-

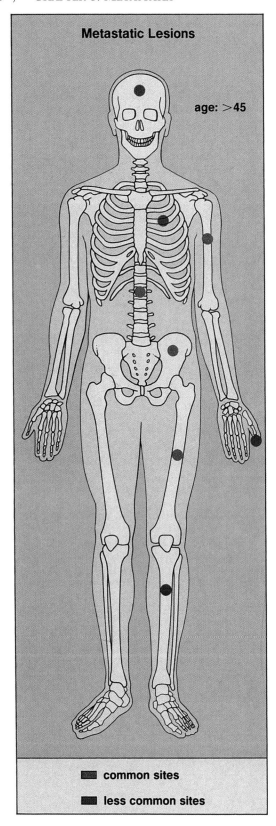

FIG. 1. Skeletal metastases:sites of predilection and peak age range.

tic, and mixed lesions. This distinction can be of considerable aid in analysis of the site of origin of the primary tumor (23). The primary sources of these lesions are as follows:

1. *Lytic lesions.* Osteolytic metastases are the most common, representing about 75% of all metastatic lesions. The primary source is usually a carcinoma of the kidney, lung, breast, GI tract, or thyroid (Figs. 3 and 4) (29).
2. *Sclerotic lesions.* Osteoblastic metastases represent approximately 15% of all metastatic lesions. In men they are caused mainly by a prostatic gland cancer and a seminoma (19) (Fig. 5A). In women the primary source is usually carcinoma of the breast, uterus (particularly cervix), or ovary (82) (Fig. 5B). In both genders, metastases may originate from carcinoid tumors (77,88,89), bladder (27), certain neurogenic tumors, including medulloblastoma (105), and osteosarcoma (34,63) (Fig. 6).
3. *Mixed lesions.* Mixed osteoblastic and osteolytic lesions represent approximately 10% of all metastatic lesions. Any primary tumor can give rise to mixed metastases, the most common primaries being breast and lung. Occasionally, some primary neoplasms may give both lytic and blastic metastases (Fig. 7).

Although metastases in the skeleton may appear similar, regardless of their primary source, in some instances their distribution, location, or morphologic appearance may suggest a site of origin (7,36,48,66,79,98,101). For example, 50% of skeletal metastases distal to the elbows and the knees, although unusual, originate from either bronchogenic or breast carcinoma (74) (Fig. 8). Although extremely rare, metastases to the hands and feet, particularly those affecting the distal phalanges (acrometastases), again indicate a primary tumor in the lung, less commonly in the breast or kidney (Fig. 9) (85). An extensive osteolysis of the distal phalanx, often accompanied by a soft tissue mass, is the usual presentation of this type of metastasis from bronchogenic carcinoma. Recently, characteristic cortical metastases were reported from bronchogenic carcinoma (23,24,41–43). These lesions produce a type of cortical destruction termed "cookie-bite" or "cookie-cutter" lesions (Fig. 10). The spread of malignant cells to involve the skeleton usually takes place via the hematogenous route. In such instances, the bulk of the tumor lodges in the marrow and spongy bone. Therefore, the initial radiography of metastatic lesions in the skeleton reveals the destruction of cancellous bone; only after further tumor growth is the cortex affected. An anastomosing vascular system in the cortex, originating in the overlying periosteum (103), probably serves as the pathway by which malignant cells from bronchogenic carcinoma reach the compact bone and initiate cortical destruction (32). Primary carcinomas of the kidney and bladder and melanoma may also give rise to cortical metastases (18,30,51). It is of interest that the majority of cortical metastases affect the femur (18,43).

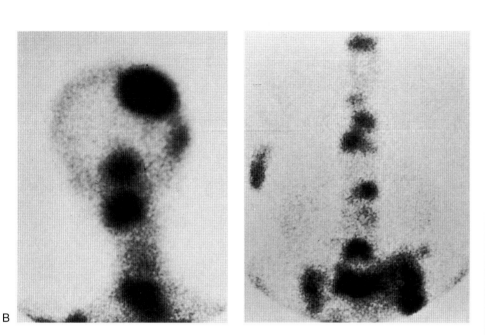

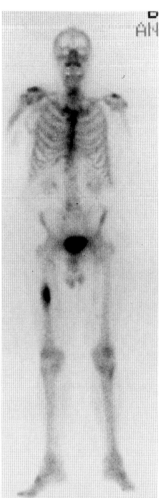

FIG. 2. Skeletal metastases:scintigraphy. A radionuclide bone scan was performed on a 68-year-old woman with breast carcinoma to determine the presence of metastases. After an intravenous injection of 15 mCi (555 MBq) of technetium-99m diphosphonate (MDP), an increased uptake of the radiopharmaceutical tracer is seen in the skull and cervical spine (**A**), and lumbar spine and pelvis (**B**), localizing the multiple metastases. (**C**) In another patient, a 55-year man with bronchogenic carcinoma, a radionuclide bone scan disclosed metastases to the thoracic spine, sternum, and right femur.

C

```
           Kidney            Breast

   Lung                            Thyroid


               OSTEOLYTIC
               METASTASES


         Stomach            Colon
```

FIG. 3. Origin of osteolytic metastases.

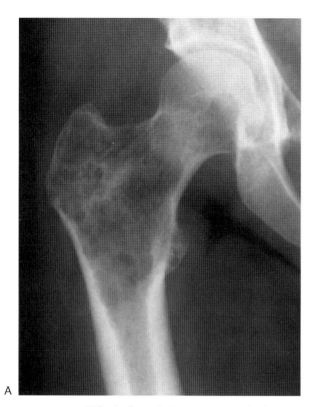

A

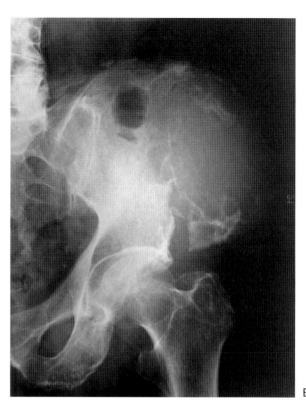

B

FIG. 4. Osteolytic metastases. **A:** An osteolytic metastasis to the proximal femur from carcinoma of the colon of a 52-year-old woman. **B:** An osteolytic metastasis to the left ilium from carcinoma of the thyroid of an 83-year-old man.

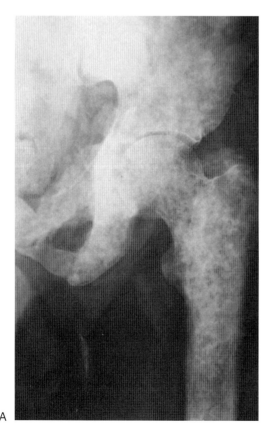

A

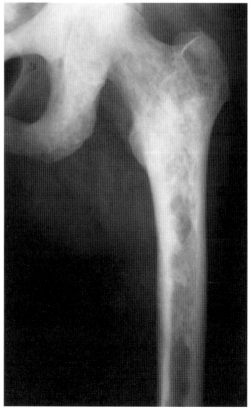

B

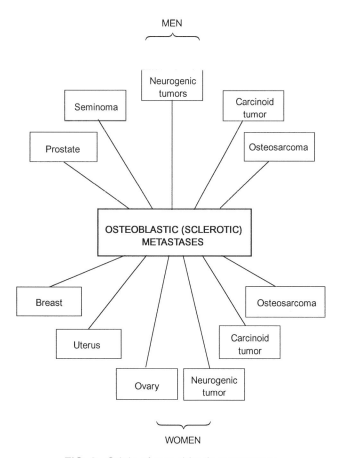

MEN

Neurogenic tumors

Seminoma

Carcinoid tumor

Prostate

Osteosarcoma

OSTEOBLASTIC (SCLEROTIC) METASTASES

Breast

Osteosarcoma

Uterus

Carcinoid tumor

Ovary

Neurogenic tumor

WOMEN

FIG. 6. Origin of osteoblastic metastases.

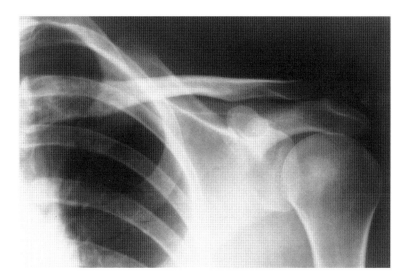

FIG. 7. Osteolytic and sclerotic metastases. Osteolytic metastasis in the medial end of the clavicle and sclerotic metastasis in the humeral head of a 27-year-old woman with a bronchial carcinoid tumor.

FIG. 5. Sclerotic metastases. **A:** Multiple sclerotic foci are scattered through the ilium, pubis, ischium, and proximal femur of a 55-year-old man with carcinoma of the prostate. **B:** Sclerotic metastases to the pubis, ischium, and proximal femur in a 57-year-old woman with breast carcinoma.

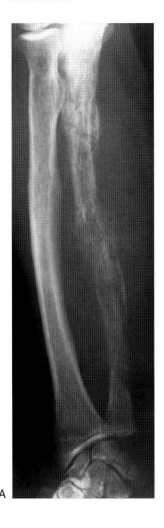

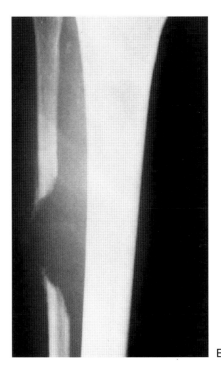

A

B

FIG. 8. Metastases distal to the elbows and the knees. **A:** Diffuse osteolytic metastases to the ulna in a
66-year-old woman with breast carcinoma. **B:** Osteolytic metastasis to the
midshaft of the right fibula of a 41-
year-old woman with hypernephroma.

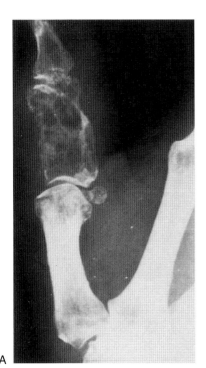

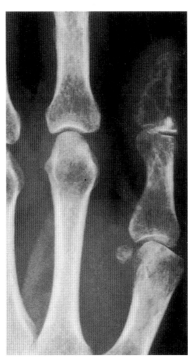

A

B

FIG. 9. Acrometastases. **A:** Osteolytic metastasis to the proximal phalanx of the left
thumb of a 63-year-old man with bronchogenic carcinoma. **B:** Osteolytic metastasis to
the distal phalanx of the right thumb of a 50-
year-old woman with breast carcinoma.

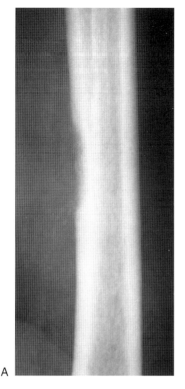

A

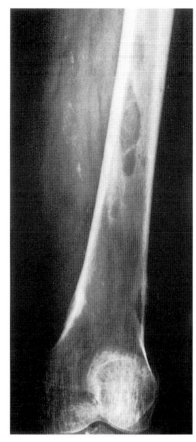

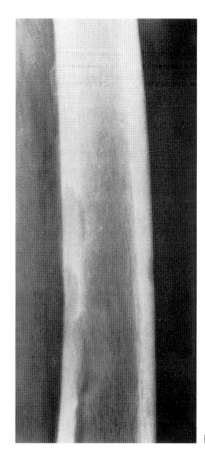

B, C

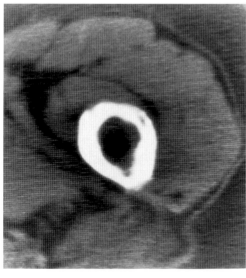

D

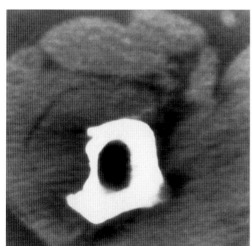

E

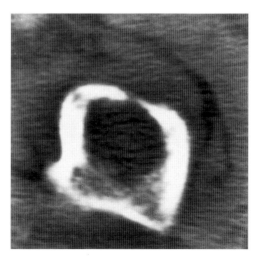

F

FIG. 10. Cortical metastases. **(A)** Osteolytic cortical metastasis to the femur in a 62-year-old man with bronchogenic carcinoma. **(B)** and **(C)** Osteolytic cortical metastases to the femur of an 82-year-old man with bronchogenic carcinoma. Note characteristic cookie-bite appearance of the lesion on the lateral radiograph. In three different patients, a 70-year-old man **(D)**, a 46-year-old woman **(E)**, and 72-year-old woman **(F)**, all with bronchogenic carcinoma, CT sections demonstrate cortical metastases in the femora.

373

In certain instances, the morphologic appearance of a metastasis may suggest a specific site of origin or may at least narrow the differential diagnostic possibilities (23). For example, bubbly, highly expansive, so-called blow-out metastatic lesions originate from a primary carcinoma of the kidney or thyroid (Fig. 11). Multiple round, dense foci or diffuse increases in bone density are often seen in metastatic carcinoma of the prostate (see Fig. 5A).

In general, metastatic bone disease is characterized by a combination of bone resorption and bone formation. Radiographic imaging of the lesions will reveal the predominant process (12,84). When osteolysis predominates, the lesions appear lytic, and when bone formation is dominant, they appear sclerotic (31,92). Multiple sclerotic metastases may present either in a focal pattern (multiple snowball appearance) or may have a diffuse pattern (generalized radiopacity of bones) (52). Bone formation in metastatic disease involves either a stromal or a reactive mechanism. Stromal new bone occurs only in lesions associated with the development of a surrounding fibrous stroma, as in carcinoma of the prostate, and reflects intramembranous ossification of areas within the stroma. In contrast, reactive bone represents an attempt to repair the injury caused by tumor cells. This type of formation occurs to some extent in all metastatic lesions, although it tends to be negligible in highly anaplastic or rapidly growing tumors (92). Bone destruction is always mediated by tumor-induced osteoclastic resorption. Primary tumors responsible for purely osteolytic metastases are usually located in the kidneys, lung, breast, thyroid, or gastrointestinal tract, whereas primaries responsible for osteoblastic metastases are usually located in the prostate gland. It must be pointed out, however, that after treatment (radiation ther-

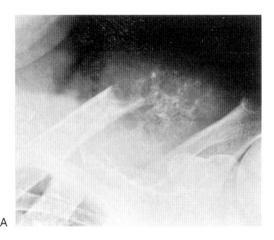

A

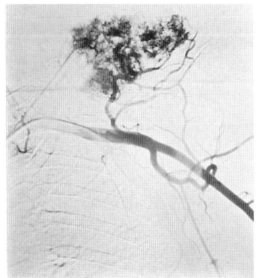

B

FIG. 11. Skeletal metastases. A 52-year-old man with renal cell carcinoma (hypernephroma) developed a solitary metastatic lesion in the acromial end of the left clavicle. **A:** Plain radiograph of the left shoulder shows an expansive blown-out lesion associated with a soft tissue mass destroying the acromial end of the clavicle. **B:** Subtraction study of a selective left subclavian arteriogram demonstrates hypervascularity of the tumor, a characteristic feature of metastatic hypernephroma. **C:** In another patient, a 59-year-old woman with hypernephroma, noted is a blown-out lesion associated with a soft tissue mass destroying the acromial end of the right clavicle, acromion, and glenoid.

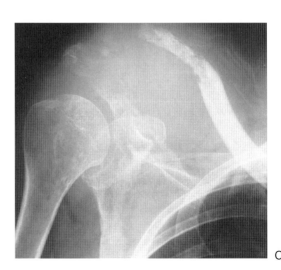

C

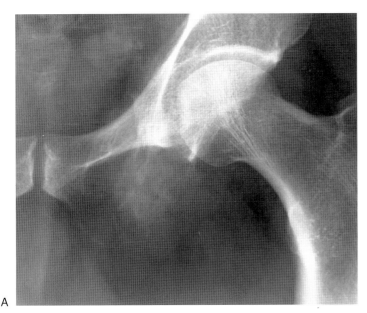

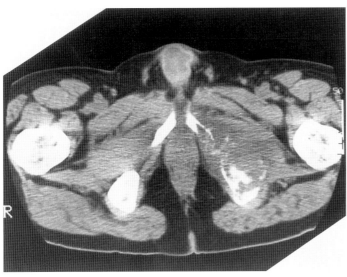

FIG. 12. Skeletal metastasis:computed tomography. **A:** An anteroposterior radiograph of the left hip of a 50-year-old man with hypernephroma shows an osteolytic lesion almost completely destroying the ischium. **B:** CT section demonstrates the extent of bone destruction and a soft tissue extension of metastasis.

apy, chemotherapy, or hormonal therapy), purely lytic lesions may become sclerotic.

Scintigraphy is almost invariably positive in bone metastases (80), and increased uptake is observed in both sclerotic and lytic lesions (see Fig. 2) (16,17,25,37,68,69, 83,87). This phenomenon is secondary to the increased bone turnover and reactive repair at the periphery of the lesion (3). Radionuclide bone scan is helpful for distinguishing metastatic disease from multiple myeloma because the latter usually presents with a normal uptake of a tracer (67). Only a few cases have been reported that exhibited negative bone scintigraphy in metastatic disease of the skeleton despite positive radiographic findings (14,59). This can be explained by the fact that bone density, as imaged by plain radiography, reflects net metabolic activity over an extended period of time and does not necessarily reflect current metabolic activity. Therefore, a radiographically blastic lesion with a low metabolic rate can produce a negative bone scan (21). Occasionally, very widespread metastatic disease produces a diffusely increased uptake throughout the skeleton rather than discrete hot spots. This so-called superscan appearance is identified by the abnormally intense bone uptake or by the absence of a normally visible activity in the kidneys, bladder, and soft tissues (10). Sometimes metastases cause cold spots (photopenic defects) when there is bone destruction but insignificant reactive bone formation; this may be observed in metastases from lung and breast carcinoma (10,49,53,61).

CT can contribute to the diagnosis of metastatic disease by frequently revealing a definite destructive lesion in bone in patients who have an abnormal radionuclide bone scan, a normal or inconclusive radiograph, or both (13,47,50,60, 62,70,90,91). This technique can also detect an associated soft tissue mass (Figs. 12 and 13).

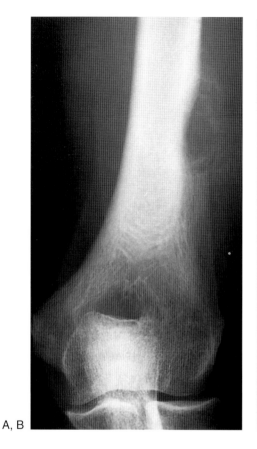
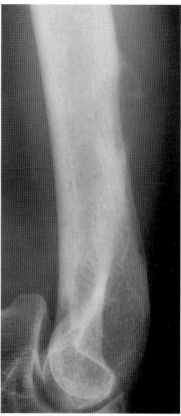
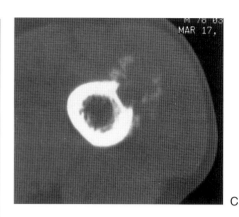

A, B

C

FIG. 13. Skeletal metastasis:computed tomography. **(A)** Anteroposterior and **(B)** lateral radiographs of the distal arm of a 78-year-old man with bronchogenic carcinoma show an osteolytic lesion in the posterolateral cortex of the distal humerus associated with periosteal reaction. **(C)** CT section shows cortical destruction, periosteal reaction, and a soft tissue mass.

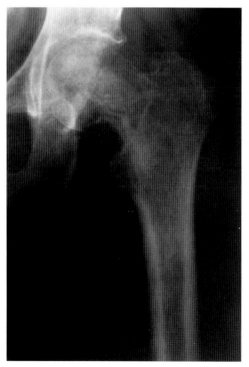
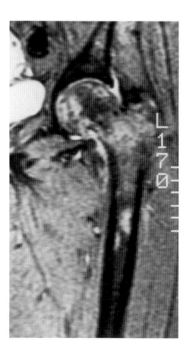

A, B

FIG. 14. Skeletal metastasis: magnetic resonance imaging. **A:** An anteroposterior radiograph of the left hip shows a diffuse osteolytic metastatic lesion in the proximal femur from breast carcinoma of a 60-year-old woman. **B:** Coronal T2*-weighted (MPGR, TR 550, TE 15, flip angle 15°) MRI demonstrates increased signal of the lesion. The uninvolved bone marrow remains of low signal intensity.

MRI is more sensitive than technetium scans for detection of metastatic disease (8,22,35,102). Focal, lytic metastases are characterized by a low signal on T1-weighted sequences, becoming bright on T2-weighting (4,20,104) (Fig. 14). Focal sclerotic metastases, such as those from a primary carcinoma in breast or prostate, induce an osteoblastic reaction with new bone formation. Therefore, both T1- and T2-weighted images reveal a low signal intensity.

Histopathology

On microscopic examination, two aspects must be considered. The first is that of the tumor tissue itself, which depends on the origin of the primary tumor. Metastatic tumor is often histologically identical or very similar to the primary, thus enabling accurate identification. In some cases, however, the tissue may be highly undifferentiated and its primary source therefore cannot be determined (58,100) (Fig. 15). The second histologic aspect is the effect of the metastasis on the bone, which constitutes a combination of reactive bone destruction and reactive proliferation (97). Some metastatic tumors are characterized primarily by bone destruction, others by bone proliferation, and still others exhibit a mixed reaction (Fig. 16). These effects appear on radiography as lytic, blastic, or mixed lesions, respectively (53).

A variety of osteoclast-stimulating factors are secreted by

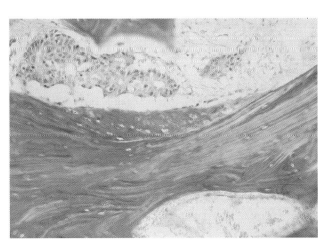

FIG. 16. Histopathology of metastasis. Trabecula of lamellar bone (*center left to right*) with attached cell-rich layer of new woven bone on upper surface and rim of osteoblasts on lower surface. Metastasis from grade 1 adenocarcinoma of prostate in upper marrow space (van Gieson, original magnification ×20.)

malignant cells. These include several growth factors, prostaglandins, cytokines, two transforming growth factors (α and β), and platelet-derived growth factor (27). Secretion of these substances by metastatic cells probably increases the number and activity of osteoclasts, and thus induces bone resorption. *In vitro* studies have demonstrated direct osteolysis at the contact point between tumor cells and bone in cultured human breast cancer cells (73). Nevertheless, it is widely believed at present that the bone resorption observed *in vivo* is due to osteoclastic activity rather than representing a direct effect of malignant cells, although malignant cells can occasionally be observed in resorption bays on bone surfaces (27).

The increased bone in osteoblastic metastases exhibits two patterns, which are usually observed in association with each other. New osteoid is produced on the surface of existing cancellous bone, resulting in trabeculae that are thicker than normal. Osteoblasts are also stimulated to form new trabeculae in marrow spaces that lie between preexisting medullary bone. Cultured prostate cancer cells have been demonstrated to secrete osteoblast-stimulating factor (27).

DIFFERENTIAL DIAGNOSIS

Radiology

There are no characteristic radiologic features of metastasis. A metastatic lesion may look like a primary benign or malignant tumor, like a focus of infection, like a metabolic disease, or even like a posttraumatic abnormality. The length of the lesion is often a helpful clue because long lesions (10 cm or greater) frequently represent a primary malignant tu-

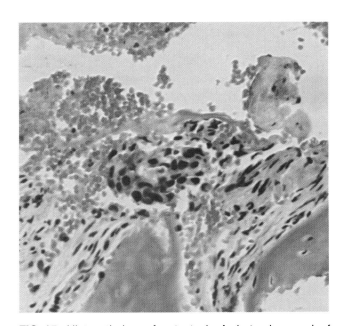

FIG. 15. Histopathology of metastasis. A photomicrograph of a needle biopsy obtained from a vertebral body with a sclerotic lesion suspected to be metastatic. There is evidence of reactive bone formation as well as fibrous scarring, and a conglomerate of atypical cells, strongly suggestive of a tumor, however, the definite diagnosis as to the origin of this lesion is difficult (hematoxylin and eosin, original magnification ×400). (Reprinted from Bullough PG. *Atlas of orthopedic pathology,* 2nd ed. New York:Gower, 1992;17.28.)

mor, whereas most metastatic lesions are smaller, between 2 and 4 cm in length. A recent study evaluated the usefulness of MRI in discriminating osseous metastases from benign lesions. The so-called bull's eye sign (a focus of high signal intensity in the center of an osseous lesion) proved to be a sign of a benign disease, whereas a halo sign (a rim of high signal intensity around an osseous lesion) proved to be a sign of metastasis (95).

From the practical point of view and to facilitate differential diagnosis, a division of metastatic lesions into those with a single focus or multiple foci, and further subdivision into lytic, blastic, or mixed, with further classification according to the particular site in the bone, should be attempted.

Solitary Metastasis

A single metastatic bone lesion must be distinguished from primary benign (and tumor-like) lesions and malignant tumors (64). In addition to the length of the lesion (see above), which can help in distinguishing a primary from a metastatic tumor, other helpful features are the presence (or absence) of a periosteal reaction and a soft tissue mass. A metastatic lesion usually presents without or with only a small soft tissue mass, although exceptions to this rule have been reported (Fig. 17, see also Figs. 11 and 12). A periosteal reaction is absent unless the mass breaks through the cortex. In some reported series, however, >30% of metastatic lesions demonstrated a periosteal response (106), particularly metastases from carcinoma of the prostate

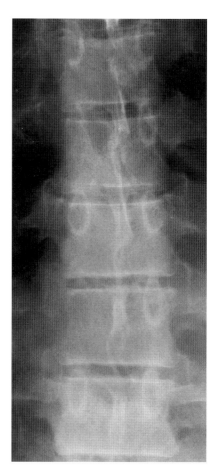

FIG. 18. Skeletal metastasis:differential diagnosis. Metastases from the bronchogenic carcinoma of a 45-year-old women destroyed the right pedicles of the vertebrae Th8 and Th10.

(5,65,78). In the spine, metastatic lesions usually destroy the pedicle (Fig. 18), a useful feature for distinguishing this lesion from myeloma or neurofibroma eroding the vertebral body (5,56).

Lytic Metastasis

Osteolytic metastasis, particularly at the articular end of a long bone or affecting apophyseal parts (such as the femoral trochanter or humeral tuberosity), must be differentiated from a *giant-cell tumor* and an *intraosseous ganglion*. The latter invariably exhibits a sclerotic border, a rare feature of metastatic lesions. At other sites, the differential diagnosis must include primary malignant bone tumors such as *fibrosarcoma, malignant fibrous histiocytoma, lymphoma, plasmacytoma,* and some benign conditions such as *hemangioma* and *brown tumor of hyperparathyroidism.* As mentioned above, differentiation solely on the basis of radiologic appearance is difficult, and clinical information is usually helpful.

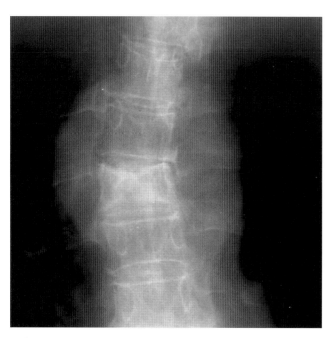

FIG. 17. Skeletal metastasis with soft tissue mass. A 70-year-old woman with breast carcinoma developed a skeletal metastasis to the thoracic vertebra. Note a large associated soft tissue mass.

Blastic Metastasis

A solitary osteoblastic metastasis should be differentiated from the *bone island*. On radiography, bone islands exhibit characteristic thorny radiations that blend imperceptibly with the normal trabeculae of the host bone, a feature not present in metastasis (81). Further confirmation is provided by the radionuclide bone scan, which is invariably positive in metastatic disease but is usually normal in bone islands (44). Occasionally, however, errors in diagnosis can be made, particularly if a bone island is very large (giant bone island) (46) or if it exhibits an increased uptake of the radiopharmaceutical tracer (45).

Occasionally, a sclerotic metastasis with exuberant sunburst periosteal reaction, such as metastasis from a prostatic carcinoma, can simulate the appearance of *osteosarcoma* (54).

A single sclerotic lesion at the medial (sternal) end of the clavicle, which often is mistaken for a metastasis, may in fact represent *condensing osteitis* of the clavicle. Clinically, this condition manifests with pain, and local swelling and tenderness. Radiography reveals a homogeneously dense sclerotic patch, usually limited to the inferior margin of the medial end of the clavicle (Fig. 19A, B). Although this part of the clavicle may be slightly expanded, periosteal reaction and a bone destruction are absent (39). CT reveals an obliteration

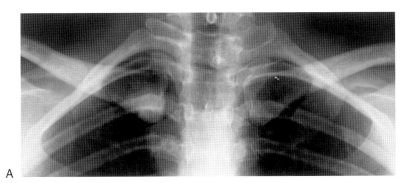

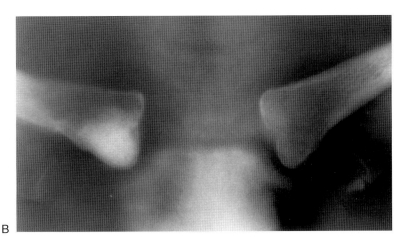

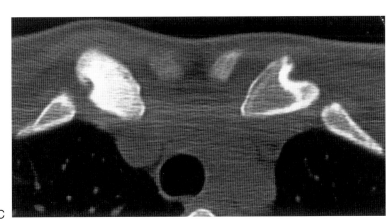

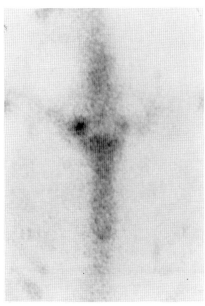

FIG. 19. Differential diagnosis of metastasis:condensing osteitis of the clavicle. **A:** Plain radiograph shows a sclerotic lesion in the inferior aspect of the right clavicle, originally thought to represent sclerotic metastasis. **B:** Trispiral tomography shows that the superior aspect of the clavicle is not affected. There is no evidence of periosteal reaction. **C:** CT section through the sternal ends of the clavicles shows homogeneous sclerosis of the right clavicular head and soft tissue swelling adjacent to it anteriorly. **D:** Radionuclide bone scan obtained after injection of 15 mCi (555 MBq) of 99m-methylene diphosphonate (MDP) shows increased uptake of the radiopharmaceutical tracer localized to the sternal end of the right clavicle. (Reprinted with permission from Greenspan A, *et al.* Condensing osteitis of the clavicle:a rare but frequently misdiagnosed condition. *Am J Roentgenol* 1991;156: 1011–1013.)

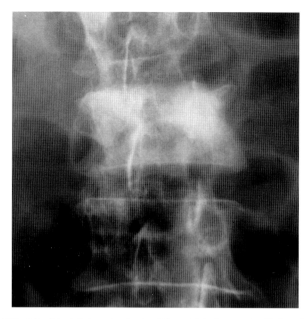

FIG. 20. Skeletal metastasis:differential diagnosis. Sclerotic metastasis to the lumbar vertebra of a 72-year-old man with prostatic carcinoma mimics Paget disease. Note, however, that the vertebral endplates are preserved and vertebral body is not enlarged.

of the marrow cavity, and radionuclide bone scan shows a significant focal increase in tracer uptake (Fig. 19C, D).

A sclerotic vertebra ("ivory vertebra") resulting from metastasis should be differentiated from *lymphoma, sclerosing hemangioma,* and *Paget disease* (28,94,96). Involvement by a lymphoma is usually indistinguishable from metastatic disease, although the clinical and laboratory data may be helpful. In Hodgkin lymphoma there is an occasional anterior scalloping of the vertebral body, which accentuates the anterior vertebral concavity and thus provides a useful differentiating feature. Hemangioma often presents with typical vertical striations or a honeycomb pattern. Paget disease characteristically enlarges affected vertebrae and causes disappearance or coarsening of the vertebral endplates. If a picture frame appearance is present typical for Paget disease, metastasis can be safely ruled out (**see Fig. 6-25**). Conversely, in metastatic lesions to the vertebrae the endplates remain preserved (Fig. 20).

Mixed Metastasis

A mixed (osteolytic and osteoblastic) solitary metastasis must be distinguished from a focus of **osteomyelitis, osteosarcoma**, and some primary round cell tumors, particularly **lymphoma**. Again, without additional clinical information it may be difficult to distinguish these lesions only on the basis of radiography.

Multiple Metastases

Multiple Lytic Metastases

Osteolytic metastases must be differentiated from *multiple myeloma* and *brown tumors of hyperparathyroidism*. In younger patients, *Langerhans cell granuloma* must be considered. Probably the best modality for distinguishing metastases from multiple myeloma is the radionuclide bone scan because, with only a few exceptions, metastatic lesions will exhibit an increased uptake of radiopharmaceutical tracer, whereas bone scan in multiple myeloma (except for the sclerotic variant) is usually normal. Helpful in distinguishing brown tumors of hyperparathyroidism are other hallmarks of this condition, such as diffuse osteopenia, loss of the lamina dura of the tooth sockets, subperiosteal bone resorption, and soft tissue calcifications. Laboratory data typical of hyperparathyroidism (particularly serum levels of calcium and phosphorus) will further enhance the difference.

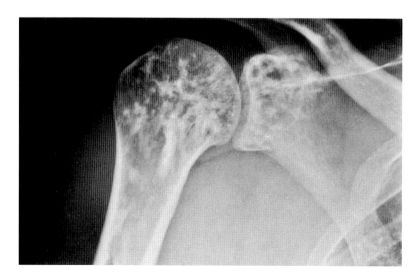

FIG. 21. Differential diagnosis of skeletal metastases:osteopoikilosis. Anteroposterior radiograph of the right shoulder of a 34-year-old man shows typical periarticular distribution of sclerotic foci of osteopoikilosis.

Because of their expansive nature, multiple metastases from kidney and thyroid should be differentiated from *pseudotumors of hemophilia*. In such cases the clinical information and laboratory data characteristic of the latter condition are extremely helpful.

Multiple Sclerotic Metastases

Sclerotic metastases should be differentiated from *osteopoikilosis* (33). Osteopoikilosis is classified among the sclerosing dysplasias of endochondral failure of bone formation and remodeling (38). Sclerotic foci in osteopoikilosis are typically distributed near the large joints, such as hips, knees, and shoulders (Fig. 21). An additional helpful radiologic feature is the scintigraphic appearance of the lesion: osteopoikilosis, unlike sclerotic metastases, exhibits a normal radionuclide bone scan (38). Other entities that may be confused with sclerotic metastatic disease include polyostotic **Paget disease** (Fig. 22), *mastocytosis,* and *secondary hyperparathyroidism*, in which sclerotic bone changes may predominate. A rare form of sclerosing myeloma (representing <1% of cases of multiple myeloma) (93) and *sclerosing hemangiomatosis* (55) may have a radiographic appearance similar to that of sclerotic metastases. In this situation, the

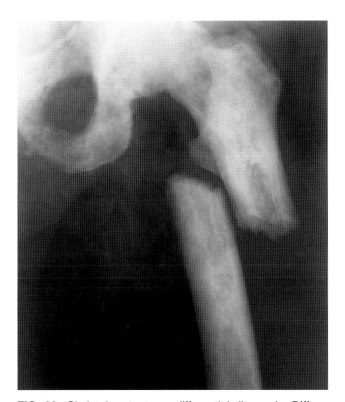

FIG. 22. Skeletal metastases:differential diagnosis. Diffuse sclerotic metastases to the pelvis and left femur causing a pathologic fracture of a 68-year-old man with prostate carcinoma mimic sclerotic changes of Paget disease.

clinical and laboratory data typical for myeloma, along with a good general physical condition and absence of abnormal laboratory data in hemangiomatosis, are helpful. Finally, *osteosarcomatosis* (synchronous or metachronous presentation of multifocal osteosarcoma) may also mimic metastatic disease (34). In such cases, a localization of the lesions in sites rarely affected by metastases, such as carpal and tarsal bones, metacarpals, epiphyses, and apophyses, as well as the radiographic morphology of the lesion consistent with osteosarcoma, lead to the correct diagnosis.

Cortical Metastasis

A solitary cortical metastasis should be differentiated, among other possibilities, from *osteoid osteoma, cortical bone abscess, plasmacytoma, hemangioma,* and *cortical osteosarcoma*. Cortical involvement associated with a soft tissue mass must be differentiated from an *aneurysmal bone cyst* and a primary soft tissue tumor invading the bone, including *synovial sarcoma*. Multiple cortical metastases should be differentiated from *hemangiomatosis* and any vascular lesion involving the cortex. The patient's age and clinical history, as well as the radiologic morphology of the lesion, are useful in differential diagnosis. A metastatic origin should always be considered in differential diagnosis of an osteolytic cortical lesion of a long bone in older patients and in patients with a known primary malignant condition (18).

Pathology

Histologically, metastatic tumors are easier to diagnose than many primary tumors because of their essentially epithelial pattern. Biopsies of suspected metastases are useful for the diagnosis in patients with known primary tumors, but only rarely are they helpful in identifying the exact site of an unknown primary tumor. A pathologist may be fortunate enough to identify an adenocarcinoma if gland formation is present and can make a list of differential diagnoses by comparing the morphologic features with the statistical likelihood of similarity in a primary tumor (40). Occasionally, the only identifying feature in the marrow spaces is a desmoplastic fibrotic reaction to tumor. If a bone biopsy reveals predominantly mature bone trabeculae with intertrabecular fibrosis, the differential diagnosis of metastatic carcinoma should be considered. Exceptionally, a metastatic lesion may exhibit a characteristic morphologic pattern that strongly suggests a primary tumor, such as the clear cells of renal carcinoma, follicular or giant cell carcinoma of the thyroid, or the pigment production of melanoma. A few neoplasms are associated with the production of enzymes or antigens that can be detected after the decalcification procedure. It is possible, for example, to perform a prostate-specific antigen

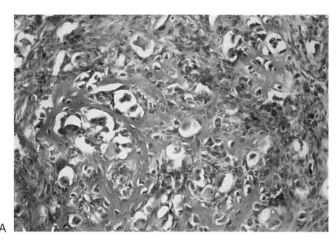
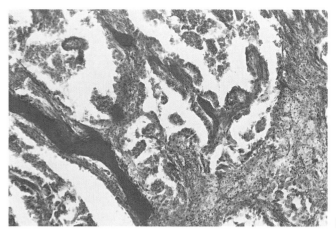

A
B

FIG. 23. Histopathology of skeletal metastases:differential diagnosis. **A:** Metastatic lesion from a well-differentiated papillary carcinoma of the thyroid exhibits formation of reactive bone that should not be mistaken for tumor bone of osteosarcoma (Giemsa, original magnification ×50). **B:** Metaplastic formation of narrow woven bone trabeculae is seen in the stroma of a well-differentiated papillary thyroid carcinoma. The bone is reactive and not produced by malignant cells (van Gieson, original magnification ×50).

study or a prostate-specific acid phosphatase by immunohistochemistry to identify a primary site in the prostate. At present, however, this method is used only rarely, and until specific antigens to other organ types become widely available it has limited practical value.

Osteoblastic metastases occasionally exhibit metastatic cells surrounded by rapidly proliferating osteoid, in a pattern that mimics *osteosarcoma* (Fig. 23). However, careful study of the reactive bone will reveal the regular distribution of the osteocytes, even if the bone has been formed by metaplasia. The immunohistochemical marker for cytokeratin or for other epithelial markers can distinguish neoplastic epithelial cells from the reactive osteoblasts and from the tumor cells of epithelioid osteosarcoma (27).

When osseous metastases are composed of spindle cells, with or without associated epithelioid-like neoplastic cells,

the diagnostic difficulties may be enormous. Differential diagnosis includes a number of primary osseous sarcomas, such as *malignant fibrous histiocytoma, leiomyosarcoma,* and *fibrosarcoma.* As a particular example, osseous metastases from spindle cell (sarcomatoid) renal cell carcinomas usually involve bone and may closely resemble malignant fibrous histiocytoma. Immunohistochemistry is extremely useful for distinguishing between these groups of lesions (27). However, some antigens are shared by both carcinomas and sarcomas. Vimentin, almost invariably present in sarcomas, may be synthesized by carcinoma cells and by those of malignant melanoma. Cytokeratin, present in most carcinomas, has been reported to occur in skeletal leiomyosarcoma (75) and other mesenchymal neoplasms (27). A useful immunohistochemical screening panel for the diagnosis of spindle cell lesions includes cytokeratin, epithelial mem-

TABLE 1. *Panel of immunohistochemical markers for spindle cell neoplasms*

	Antigens						
Tumor	Desmin	Vimentin	CK[a]	EMA[b]	S-100	MSA[c]	HMB-45[d]
Spindle cell carcinoma	−	+/−	+	+	+/−	−	−
Malignant melanoma	−	+	−	−	+	−	+
Malignant fibrous histiocytoma	−/+	+	−/+	−	−/+	−/+	−
Leiomyosarcoma	+	+/−	+/−	−	−	+	−
Fibrosarcoma	−	+	−	−	+	−	−

[a] Cytokeratin.
[b] Epithelial membrane antigen.
[c] Muscle specific actin.
[d] Melanocytic marker.
+/− = considerable number of positive, −/+ = very few positives.
Modified from Fechner RE, Mills SE. *Tumors of the bones and joints*, 3rd ed., Vol 8. Armed Forces Institute of Pathology, 1993 and from Brooks JSJ. Immunohistochemistry in the differential diagnosis of soft-tissue tumors, In Weiss SH, Brooks JSJ. eds. *Soft Tissue Tumors*, Baltimore, Williams and Wilkins, 1996, 65.

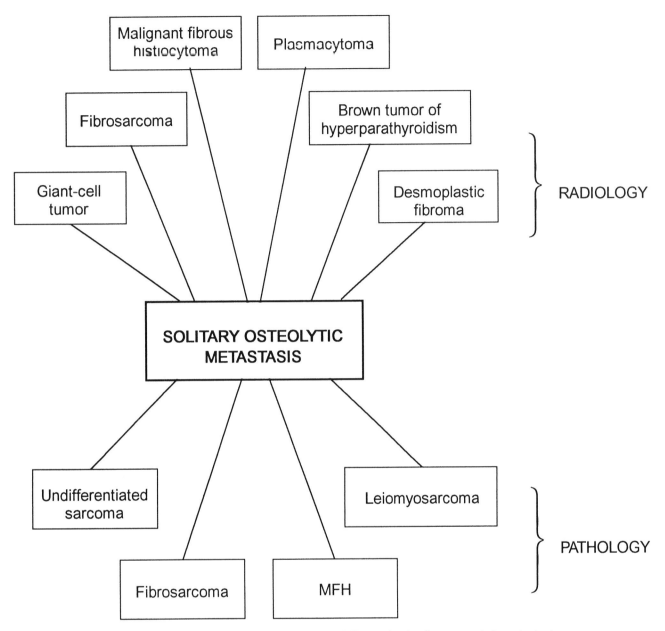

FIG. 24. Radiologic and pathologic differential diagnosis of solitary osteolytic metastasis.

brane antigen, S-100, vimentin, desmin, and muscle-specific actin. Positive findings for epithelial membrane antigen or keratin are strongly suggestive of metastatic carcinoma. Diffuse positivity for S-100 protein suggests a diagnosis of malignant melanoma, when the light microscopic appearance is appropriate. This can be confirmed by staining with the melanocyte marker HMB-45 (27).

If cytokeratin, epithelial membrane antigen, and S-100 markers are negative, the differential diagnosis must focus on primary sarcomas. In malignant fibrous histiocytoma, fibrosarcoma and leiomyosarcoma, some cells are vimentin-

positive. Furthermore, MFH and leiomyosarcoma may occasionally be positive for cytokeratin. However, the latter is strongly positive for muscle-specific actin, desmin, and smooth muscle actin (Table 1) (27).

The radiologic and pathologic differential diagnosis of solitary lytic metastasis is depicted in Fig. 24, of solitary blastic (sclerotic) metastasis in Fig. 25, whereas the differential diagnosis of multiple osteolytic and multiple osteoblastic metastases is depicted in Figs. 26 and 27, respectively. The radiologic and pathologic differential diagnosis of cortical metastases is depicted in Fig. 28.

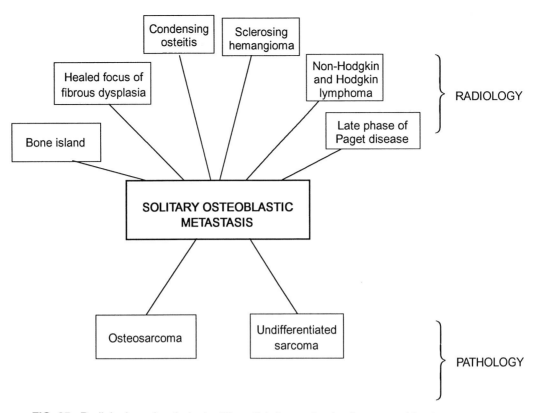

FIG. 25. Radiologic and pathologic differential diagnosis of solitary osteoblastic metastasis.

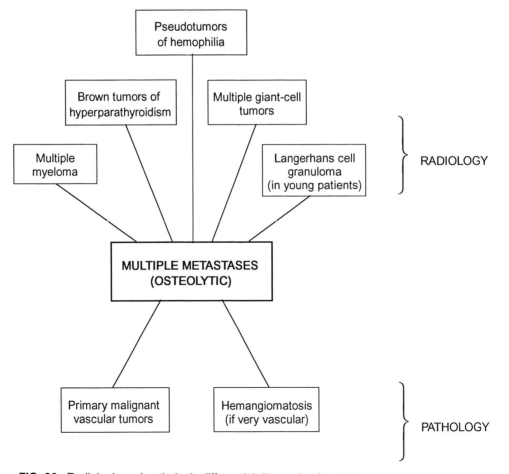

FIG. 26. Radiologic and pathologic differential diagnosis of multiple osteolytic metastases.

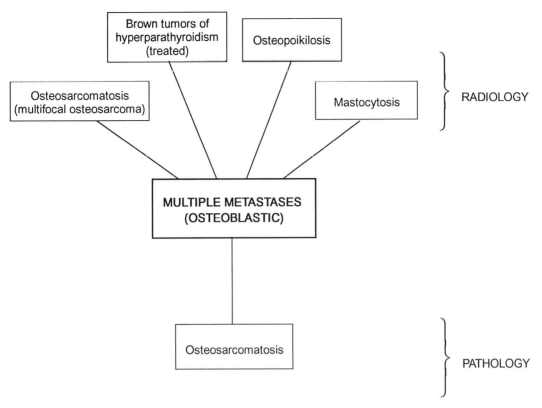

FIG. 27. Radiologic and pathologic differential diagnosis of multiple osteoblastic metastases.

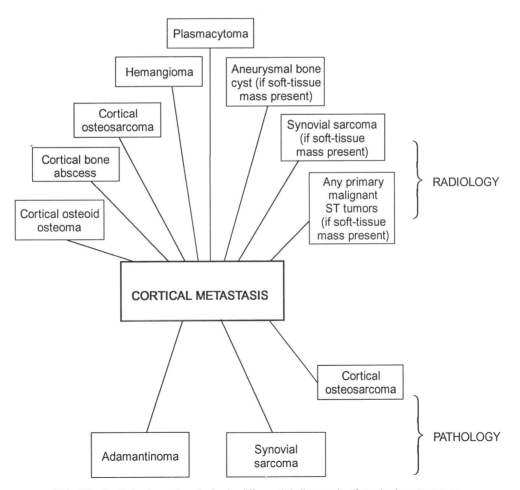

FIG. 28. Radiologic and pathologic differential diagnosis of cortical metastases.

REFERENCES

1. Abrams HL. Skeletal metastases in carcinoma. *Radiology* 1950;55: 534–538.
2. Abrams HL, Spiro R, Goldstein N. Metastases in carcinoma. Analysis of 1000 autopsied cases. *Cancer* 1950;3:74–85.
3. Alazraki N. Radionuclide techniques. In: Resnick D, ed. *Bone and joint imaging.* Philadelphia, WB Saunders, 1989;185–198.
4. Algra PR, Bloem JL. Magnetic resonance imaging of metastatic disease and multiple myeloma. In: Bloem JL, Sartoris DJ, eds. *MRI and CT of the musculoskeletal system.* Baltimore: Williams and Wilkins, 1992;218.
5. Algra PR, Heimans JJ, Valk J, Nauta JJ, Lachniet M, Van Kooten B. Do metastases in vertebrae begin in the body or the pedicles? Imaging study in 45 patients. *Am J Roentgenol* 1992;158:1275–1279.
6. Ardran GM. Bone destruction not demonstrable by radiography. *Br J Radiol* 1951; 24:107–109.
7. Asdourian PL, Weidenbaum M, Dewald RL, Hammerberg KW, Ramsey RG. The pattern of vertebral involvement in metastatic vertebral breast cancer. *Clin Orthop* 1991;250:164–170.
8. Avrahami E, Tadmor R, Dally O, Hadar H. Early MR demonstration of spinal metastases in patients with normal radiographs and CT and radionuclide bone scans. *J Comput Assist Tomogr* 1989;13:598–602.
9. Bachman AS, Sproul EE. Correlation of radiographic and autopsy findings in suspected metastases in the spine. *Bull NY Acad Med* 1940; 44:169–175.
10. Bassett LW, Steckel RJ. Imaging techniques in the detection of metastatic disease. *Semin Oncol* 1977;4:39–52.
11. Berrettoni B, Carter JR. Mechanisms of cancer metastasis to bone. *J Bone Joint Surg* 1986;68A:308–312.
12. Bloom RA, Libson E, Husband JE, Stoker DJ. The periosteal sunburst reaction to bone metastases. A literature review and report of 20 additional cases. *Skeletal Radiol* 1987;16:629–634.
13. Braunstein EM, Kuhns LR. Computed tomographic demonstration of spinal metastases. *Spine* 1983;8:912–915.
14. Brown B, Laorr A, Greenspan A, Stadalnik R. Negative bone scintigraphy with diffuse osteoblastic breast carcinoma metastases. *Clin Nucl Med* 1994;19:194–196.
15. Bushnell DL, Kahn D, Huston B, Bevering CG. Utility of SPECT imaging for determination of vertebral metastases in patients with known primary tumors. *Skeletal Radiol* 1995;24:13–16.
16. Caluser CI, Scott AM, Schnieder J, Macapinlac HA, Yeh SD, Larson SM. Value of lesion location and intensity of uptake in SPECT bone scintigraphy of the spine in patients with malignant tumors. *Radiology* 1992;185(S):315.
17. Citrin DL, Bessent RG, Greig WR. A comparison of the sensitivity and accuracy of the 99m Tc-phosphate bone scan and skeletal radiograph in the diagnosis of bone metastases. *Clin Radiol* 1977;28: 107–117.
18. Coerkamp EG, Kroon HM. Cortical bone metastases. *Radiology* 1988; 169:525 528.
19. Cumming J, Hacking N, Fairhurst J, Ackery D, Jenkins JD. Distribution of bony metastases in prostatic carcinoma. *Br J Urol* 1990;66: 411–414.
20. Daffner RA, Lupetin AR, Dash N, Deeb ZL, Sefczek RJ, Shapiro RL. MRI in the detection of malignancy infiltration of bone marrow. *Am J Roentgenol* 1986;1146:353–358.
21. Datz FL, Patch GG, Arias JM, Morton KA. *Nuclear medicine. A teaching file.* St. Louis: Mosby Year Book, 1992;28–29.
22. Delbeke D, Powers TA, Sandler MP. Negative scintigraphy with positive magnetic resonance imaging in bone metastases. *Skeletal Radiol* 1990;19:113–116.
23. Deutsch A, Resnick D. Eccentric cortical metastases to the skeleton from bronchogenic carcinoma. *Radiology* 1980;137:49–52.
24. Deutsch A, Resnick D, Niwayama G. Case report 145. Bilateral, almost symmetrical skeletal metastases (both femora) from bronchogenic carcinoma. *Skeletal Radiol* 1981;6:144–148.
25. Even-Sapir E, Martin RH, Barnes DC, Pringle CR, Iles SE, Mitchell MJ. Role of SPECT in differentiating malignant form benign lesions in the lower thoracic and lumbar vertebrae. *Radiology* 1993;187: 193–198.
26. Evison G, Pizey N, Roylance J. Bone formation associated with osseous metastases from bladder carcinoma. *Clin Radiol* 1981;32: 303–309.
27. Fechner RE, Mills SE. *Tumors of the bones and joints*, 3rd series, fascicle 8. Washington, DC: Armed Forces Institute of Pathology, 1993.
28. Fig LM, Gross MD. Metastatic prostate carcinoma mimicking Paget s disease on bone imaging. *Clin Nucl Med* 1989;14:777–778.
29. Forbes G. Radiographic manifestations of bone metastases from renal carcinoma. *Am J Roentgenol* 1977;129:61–66.
30. Foster D. Cortical skeletal metastasis in malignant melanoma. *Australas Radiol* 1982;20:545–560.
31. Galasko CSB. Mechanisms of lytic and blastic metastatic disease of bone. *Clin Orthop* 1982;69:20–27.
32. Galasko CSB. The anatomy and pathways of skeletal metastases. In: Weiss L, Gilbert H, eds. *Bone metastasis.* Boston: GK Hall, 1981; 49–63.
33. Ghandur-Mnaymneh L, Broder LE, Mnaymneh WA. Lobular carcinoma of the breast metastatic to bone with unusual clinical, radiologic, and pathologic features mimicking osteopoikilosis. *Cancer* 1984;53: 1801–1803.
34. Gherlinzoni F, Antoci B, Canale V. Multicentric osteosarcomata (osteosarcomatosis). *Skeletal Radiol* 1983;10:281–285.
35. Godersky JC, Smoker WR, Knutzon R. Use of magnetic resonance imaging in the evaluation of metastatic spinal disease. *Neurosurgery* 1987;21:676–680.
36. Gold RI, Seeger LL, Bassett LW, Steckel RJ. An integrated approach to the evaluation of metastatic bone disease. *Radiol Clin North Am* 1990;28:471–483.
37. Gosfield E, Alavi A, Kneeland B. Comparison of radionuclide bone scan and magnetic resonance imaging in detecting spinal metastases. *J Nucl Med* 1994;34:2191–2198.
38. Greenspan A. Sclerosing bone dysplasias—a tartet-site approach. *Skeletal Radiol* 1991;20:561–584.
39. Greenspan A, Gerscovich EO, Szabo RM, Matthews II JG. Condensing osteitis of the clavicle: a rare but frequently misdiagnosed condition. *Am J Roentgenol* 1991;156:1011–1015.
40. Greenspan A, Klein MJ. Radiology and pathology of bone tumors. In: Lewis MM, ed. *Musculoskeletal oncology: a multidisciplinary approach.* Philadelphia:WB Saunders, 1992;13–72.
41. Greenspan A, Klein MJ, Lewis MM. Case report 272. Skeletal cortical metastases in the left femur arising form bronchogenic carcinoma. *Skeletal Radiol* 1984;11:297–301.
42. Greenspan A, Klein MJ, Lewis MM. Case report 284. Osteolytic cortical metastasis in the femur from bronchogenic carcinoma. *Skeletal Radiol* 1984;12:146–150.
43. Greenspan A, Norman A. Osteolytic cortical destruction: an unusual pattern of skeletal metastases. *Skeletal Radiol* 1988;17:402–406.
44. Greenspan A, Stadalnik RC. Bone island: scintigraphic findings and their clinical application. *Can Assoc Radiol J* 1995;46:368–379.
45. Greenspan A, Steiner G, Knutzon R. Bone island (enostosis): clinical significance and radiologic and histologic correlations. *Skeletal Radiol* 1991;20:85–90.
46. Greenspan A, Klein MJ. Giant bone island. *Skeletal Radiol* 1996;25: 67–69.
47. Harbin WP. Metastatic disease and the nonspecific bone scan: value of spinal computed tomography. *Radiology* 1982;145:105–107.
48. Healey JH, Turnbull ADM, Miedema B, Lane JM. Acrometastases. A study of twenty-nine patients with osseous involvement of hand and feet. *J Bone Joint Surg* 1986;68:743–746.
49. Hellman RS, Wilson MA. Discordance of sclerosing skeletal secondaries between sequential scintigraphy and radiographs. *Clin Nucl Med* 1982;7:97–99.
50. Helms CA, Cann CE, Brunelle FO, Gilula LA, Chafetz N, Genant HK. Detection of bone-marrow metastases using quantitative computed tomography. *Radiology* 1981;140:745–750.
51. Hendrix RW, Rogers LF, Davis TM Jr. Cortical bone metastases. *Radiology* 1991;181:409–413.
52. Hove B, Gyldensted C. Spiculated vertebral metastases from prostatic carcinoma. *Neuroradiology* 1990;32:337–339.
53. Hudson TM. *Radiologic-pathologic correlation of musculoskeletal lesions.* Baltimore: Williams and Wilkins, 1987;421–440.
54. Igou D, Sundaram M, McDonald DJ, Janney C, Chalk DE. Appendicular metastatic prostate cancer simulating osteosarcoma, Paget's disease, and Paget's sarcoma. *Skeletal Radiol* 1995;24:447–449.
55. Ishida T, Dorfman HD, Steiner GC, Normatz A. Cystic angiomatosis of bone with sclerotic changes mimicking osteoblastic metastasis. *Skeletal Radiol* 1994;23:247–252.
56. Jacobson HG, Poppel MH, Shapiro JH, Grossberger S. The vertebral

pedicle sign: a Roentgen finding to differentiate metastatic carcinoma from multiple myeloma. *Am J Roentgenol* 1958;80:817–821.

57. Jaffe H. Tumors metastatic to the skeleton. In: *Tumors and tumorous conditions of the bones and joints.* Philadelphia: Lea and Febiger, 1958;594–595.

58. Johnston AD. Pathology of metastatic tumors in bone. *Clin Orthop* 1970;73:8–32.

59. Kattapuram SV, Khurana JS, Scott JA, el-Khoury GY. Negative scintigraphy with positive magnetic resonance imaging in bone metastases. *Skeletal Radiol* 1990;19:113–116.

60. Kido DK, Gould R, Taati F, Duncan A, Schnur J. Comparative sensitivity of CT scans, radiographs, and radionuclide bone scans in detecting metastatic calvarial lesions. *Radiology* 1978;128:371–375.

61. Kim EE, Deland FH, Maruyama Y. Decreased uptake in bone scans ("cold lesions") in metastatic carcinoma. *J Bone Joint Surg* 1978; 60A:844–846.

62. Kori SH. Computed tomographic evaluation of bone and soft tissue metastases. In: Weiss L, Gilbert H, eds. *Bone metastasis.* Boston: GK Hall, 1981;245–257.

63. Kumar N, David R, Madewell JE, Lindell MM Jr. Radiographic spectrum of osteogenic sarcoma. *Am J Roentgenol* 1987;148:767–772.

64. Legier JF, Tauber LN. Solitary metastases of occult prostatic carcinoma simulating osteogenic sarcoma. *Cancer* 1968;22:168–172.

65. Lehrer HZ, Maxfield WS, Nice CM. The periosteal sunburst pattern in metastatic bone tumors. *Am J Roentgenol* 1970;108:154–161.

66. Libson E, Bloom RA, Husband JE, Stocker DJ. Metastatic tumors of the bones of the hand and foot. A comparative review and report of 43 additional cases. *Skeletal Radiol* 1987;16:387–392.

67. Ludwig H, Kumpan W, Sinzinger H. Radiography and bone scintigraphy in multiple myeloma: a comparative analysis. *Br J Radiol* 1982; 55:173–181.

68. Mall JC, Beckerman C, Hoffer PB, Gottschalk H. A unified radiological approach to the detection of skeletal metastases. *Radiology* 1976: 118:323–328.

69. McDougall IR, Kriss JP. Screening for bone metastases. Are only scans necessary? *JAMA* 1975;231:46–50.

70. Muindi J, Coombes RC, Golding S, Powles TJ, Khan O, Husband J. The role of computed tomography in the detection of bone metastases in breast cancer patients. *Br J Radiol* 1983;56:233–236.

71. Mulder JD, Schütte HE, Kroon HM, Taconis WK. *Radiologic atlas of bone tumors.* Amsterdam: Elsevier, 1993.

72. Mulvey RB. Peripheral bone metastases. *Am J Roentgenol* 1964;91: 155–160.

73. Mundy GR, Spiro TP. The mechanisms of bone metastasis and bone destruction by tumor cells. In: Weiss L, Gilbert HA, eds. *Bone metastasis.* Boston: GK Hall, 1981;64–82.

74. Murray RO, Jacobson HG. *The radiology of skeletal disorders,* 2nd ed. New York: Churchill-Livingstone, 1977;585.

75. Myers JL, Arocho J, Bernreuter W, Dunham W, Mazur MT. Leiomyosarcoma of bone. A clinicopathologic, immunohistochemical, and ultrastructural study of five cases. *Cancer* 1991;67: 1051–1056.

76. Napoli LD, Hansen HH, Muggia FM, *et al.* The incidence of osseous involvement in lung cancer, with special reference to the development of osteoblastic changes. *Radiology* 1973;108:17–21.

77. Norman A, Greenspan A, Steiner G. Case report 173. Metastases from a bronchial carcinoid tumor. *Skeletal Radiol* 1981;7:155–157.

78. Norman A, Ulin R. A comparative study of periosteal new-bone responsc in metastatic bone tumors (solitary) and primary bone sarcomas. *Radiology* 1969;92:705–708.

79. Nystrom JS, Weiner JM, Wolf RM, Bateman JR, Viola MV. Identifying the primary site in metastatic cancer of unknown origin. *JAMA* 1979;241:381–383.

80. O Mara RE. Bone scanning in osseous metastatic disease. *JAMA* 1974;229:1915–1917.

81. Onitsuka H. Roentgenologic aspects of bone islands. *Radiology* 1977; 123:607–612.

82. Ontell FK, Greenspan A. Blastic osseous metastases in ovarian carcinoma. *Can Assoc Radiol J* 1995;46:231–234.

83. Osmond TD III, Pendergrass HP, Potsaid MS. Accuracy of 99M Tc-diphosphonate bone scans and roentgenograms in the detection of prostate, breast, and lung carcinoma metastases. *Am J Roentgenol* 1975;124:972–975.

84. Pagani JJ, Libshitz HI. Imaging bone metastases. *Radiol Clin North Am* 1982;20:545–560.

85. Panebianco AC, Kaupp HA. Bilateral thumb metastatis from breast carcinoma. *Arch Surg* 1968;96:216–218.

86. Papac RJ. Bone marrow metastases: a review. *Cancer* 1994;74: 2403–2413.

87. Parthasarathy KL, Landsberg R, Bakshi SP, Donoghue G, Merrin C. Detection of bone metastases in urogenital malignancies utilizing 99m Tc-labeled phosphate compounds. *Urology* 1978;11:99–102.

88. Peavy PW, Rogers JV Jr, Clements JL Jr, Burns JB. Unusual osteoblastic metastases from carcinoid tumors. *Radiology* 1973; 107:327–330.

89. Powell JM. Metastatic carcinoid of bone. Report of two cases and review of the literature. *Clin Orthop* 1988;230:266–272.

90. Rafii M, Firooznia H, Golimbu C, Beranbaum E. CT of skeletal metastasis. *Semin Ultrasound Comput Tomogr Magn Reson Imag* 1986;7:371–379.

91. Rafii M, Firooznia H, Kramer E, Golimbu C, Sanger J. The role of computed tomography in evaluation of skeletal metastases. *J Comput Tomogr* 1988;12:19–24.

92. Resnick D, Niwayama G. Skeletal metastases. In: Resnick D, ed. *Diagnosis of bone and joint disorders,* 3rd ed. Philadelphia: WB Suanders, 1995;3991–4064.

93. Sartoris DJ, Pate D, Haghighi P, Greenway G, Resnick D. Plasma cell sclerosis of bone: a spectrum of disease. *Can Assoc Radiol J* 1986;37: 25–34.

94. Schajowicz F, Velan O, Santini Araujo E, Plantalech L, Fongi E, Ottolenghi E, Fromm GA. Metastases of carcinoma in pagetic bone. *Clin Orthop* 1988;228:290–296.

95. Schweitzer ME, Levine C, Mitchell DG, Gannon FH, Gomella LG. Bull's-eyes and halos:useful MR discriminators of osseous metastases. *Radiology* 1993;188:249–252.

96. Shih WJ, Riley C, Magoun S, Ryo UY. Paget's disease mimicking skeletal metastases in a patient with coexisting prostatic carcinoma. *Eur J Nucl Med* 1988;15:422–423.

97. Sim FH, Frassica FJ. Metastatic bone disease. In: Unni KK, ed. *Bone tumors.* New York: Churchill-Livingstone, 1988;226.

98. Simon MA, Bartucci EJ. The search for the primary tumor in patients with skeletal metastases of unknown origin. *Cancer* 1986;58: 1088–1095.

99. Söderlund V. Radiological diagnosis of skeletal metastases. *Eur Radiol* 1996;6:587–595.

100. Spjut HJ, Dorfman HD, Fechner RE, Ackerman LV. *Tumors of bone and cartilage,* 2nd series, fascicle 5. Washington, DC: Armed Forces Institute of Pathology, 1971;347–390.

101. Thrall JH, Ellis BI. Skeletal metastases. *Radiol Clin North Am* 1987; 25:1155–1170.

102. Traill Z, Richards MA, Moore NR. Magnetic resonance imaging of metastatic bone disease. *Clin Orthop Relat Res* 1995;312:76–88.

103. Trias A, Fery A. Cortical circulation of long bones. *J Bone Joint Surg* 1979;61A:1052–1059.

104. Trillet V, Revel D, Combaret V. Bone marrow metastases in small cell lung cancer: detection with magnetic resonance imaging and monoclonal antibodies. *Br J Cancer* 1989;60:83–88.

105. Vieco PT, Azouz EM, Hoeffel J-C. Metastases to bone in medulloblastoma. A rcport of five cases. *Skeletal Radiol* 1989;18:445–449.

106. Vilar JL, Lezena AH, Pedrosa CS. Spiculated periosteal reaction in metastatic lesions in bone. *Skeletal Radiol* 1979;3:230–233.

107. Wilner D. Cancer metastasis to bone. In: *Radiology of bone tumors and allied disorders.* Philadelphia: WB Saunders, 1982;3641–3908.

108. Yamaguchi T, Tamai K, Yamato M, Honma K, Ueda Y, Saotome K. Intertrabecular pattern of tumors metastatic to bone. *Cancer* 1996;78: 1388–1394.

109. Yochum TR, Rowe LJ. Tumor and tumor-like processes. In: Yochum TR, Rowe LJ, eds. *Essentials of skeletal radiology,* vol 2. Baltimore: Williams and Wilkins, 1987;699–919.

CHAPTER 9

Tumors and Tumor-like Lesions of the Joints

BENIGN LESIONS
  Synovial (Osteo)chondromatosis
  Pigmented Villonodular Synovitis
  Localized (Pigmented) Nodular Tenosynovitis
      (Pigmented Giant-cell Tumor of the Synovium
      or the Tendon Sheath)

Synovial Hemangioma
MALIGNANT LESIONS
  Synovial Sarcoma
  Synovial Chondrosarcoma

BENIGN LESIONS

Synovial (Osteo)chondromatosis

Synovial osteochondromatosis (also known as synovial chondromatosis or synovial chondrometaplasia) is an uncommon benign disorder marked by the metaplastic proliferation of multiple cartilaginous nodules in the synovial membrane of the joints, bursae, or tendon sheaths (16,18). It is almost invariably monoarticular; rarely, multiple joints may be affected (24–26).

Clinical Presentation

The disorder is twice as common in men as in women and is usually discovered in the third to the fifth decade (16). The knee is a preferential site of involvement, with the hip, shoulder, and elbow accounting for most of the remaining cases (4,6) (Fig. 1). Patients usually report pain and swelling. Joint effusion, tenderness, limited motion in the joint, and a soft tissue mass are common clinical findings (5).

Imaging

The radiographic findings depend on the degree of calcification within the cartilaginous bodies, ranging from mere joint effusion to visualization of many radiopaque joint bodies, usually small and uniform in size (19,20) (Fig. 2). The best proof that the bodies are indeed intraarticular is achieved by arthrography or computed tomography (CT) (2) (Fig. 3). These modalities can visualize even noncalcified bodies (7). MRI may also be helpful: calcifications can be seen as signal void on T2-weighted images against the high-signal-intensity fluid and an inflamed hyperplastic synovium (11,26) (Figs. 4 and 5). In addition to revealing loose bodies in the joint, these modalities may demonstrate bony erosion (21).

Histopathology

By microscopy, many cartilaginous nodules are observed as they form beneath the thin layer of cells that line the surface of the synovial membrane (6,23) (Fig. 6). These nodules are highly cellular and the cells themselves may exhibit a moderate pleomorphism, with occasional plump and double nuclei (5). Although such cytologic atypia merely indicates an actively growing cartilaginous focus, an erroneous diagnosis of malignancy may sometimes be considered (Fig. 7). The cartilaginous nodules, which often are undergoing calcification and endochondral ossification, may detach and become loose bodies. The loose bodies continue to be viable and may increase in size as they receive nourishment from the synovial fluid (13) but they ossify no more.

Differential Diagnosis

Radiology

This condition should be differentiated from the secondary synovial osteochondromatosis caused by osteoarthritis, particularly in the knee and hip joints, and from synovial chondrosarcoma, either primary (arising *de novo* from the synovial membrane) or secondary (due to malignant transformation).

Distinguishing primary from *secondary synovial osteochondromatosis* usually presents no problems. In the latter condition there is invariably radiographic evidence of osteoarthritis with all of its typical features, such as narrowing of the radiographic joint space, subchondral sclerosis, and, occasionally, periarticular cysts or cyst-like lesions (Fig. 8). The loose bodies are fewer, larger, and invariably of different sizes. Conversely, in primary synovial chondromatosis the joint is not affected by any degenerative changes. In some cases, however, the bone may show erosions secondary to pressure of the calcified bodies on the

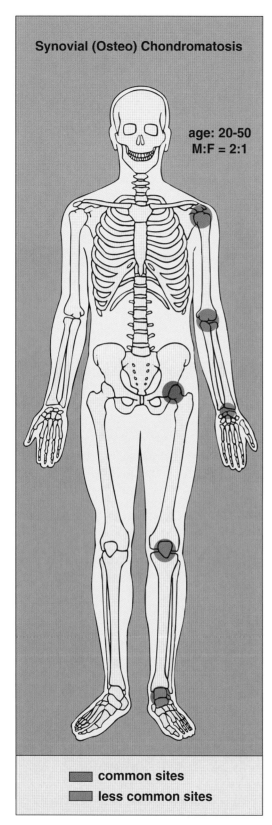

FIG. 1. Synovial (osteo)chondromatosis: skeletal sites of predilection, peak age range, and male-to-female ratio.

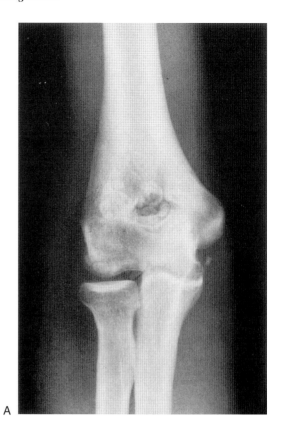

A

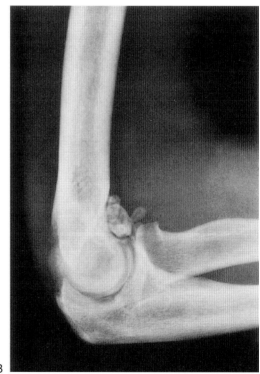

B

FIG. 2. Synovial (osteo)chondromatosis. (**A**) Anteroposterior and (**B**) lateral radiographs of the right elbow of a 23-year-old man who presented with pain and occasional locking in the elbow joint show numerous osteochondral bodies in the joint, which are regularly shaped and mostly uniform in size.

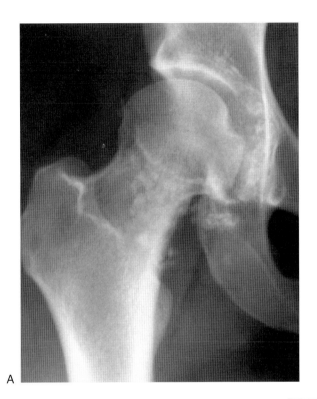

FIG. 3. Synovial (osteo)chondromatosis: computed tomography. (**A**) An anteroposterior radiograph of the right hip of a 27-year-old woman shows multiple osteochondral bodies around the femoral head and neck. Note preservation of the joint space. (**B**) and (**C**) Two CT sections, one through the femoral head, another through the femoral neck demonstrate unquestionably the intraarticular location of multiple osteochondral bodies.

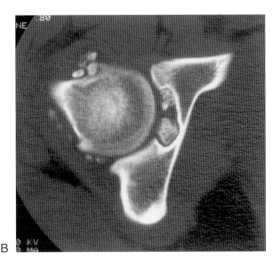

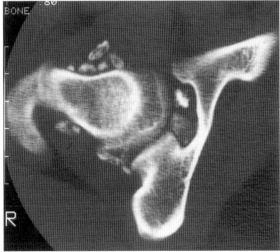

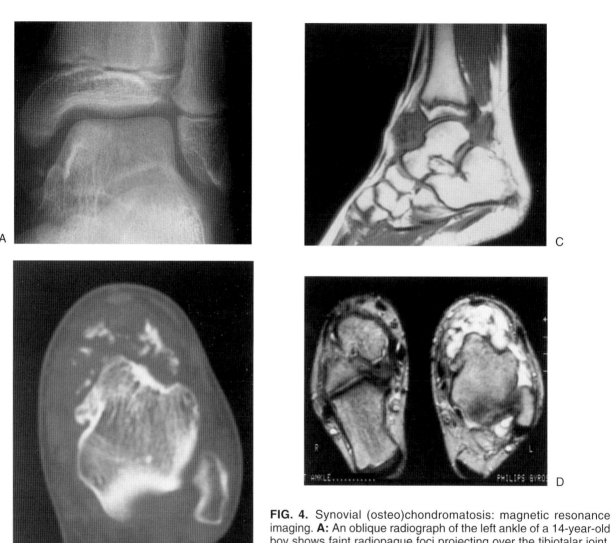

FIG. 4. Synovial (osteo)chondromatosis: magnetic resonance imaging. **A:** An oblique radiograph of the left ankle of a 14-year-old boy shows faint radiopaque foci projecting over the tibiotalar joint. **B:** CT section shows the location of calcified bodies in the anterior aspect of the joint. **C:** Sagittal T1-weighted (SE, TR 640, TE 20) MRI shows intermediate signal intensity of the fluid in the ankle joint and dispersed low-signal intensity osteochondral bodies. **D:** Coronal T2-weighted (SE, TR 2000, TE 80) MRI of the ankle joint clearly defines low-signal intensity osteochondral bodies within bright fluid.

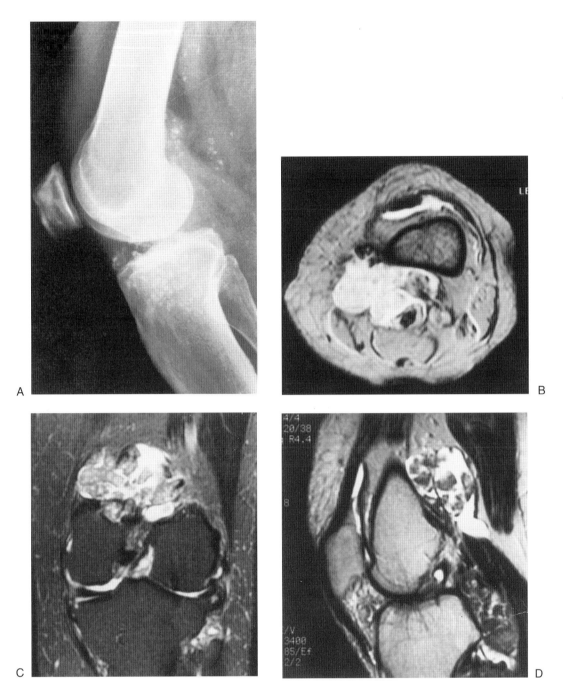

FIG. 5. Synovial (osteo)chondromatosis: magnetic resonance imaging. (**A**) Lateral radiograph of the left knee of a 50-year-old man shows multiple osteochondral bodies in and around the joint. (**B**) Axial T2*-weighted (MPGR, TR 500, TE 20, flip angle 30°) MRI demonstrates high signal joint effusion and multiple bodies of intermediate signal intensity, primarily located in a large popliteal cyst. (**C**) Coronal fast-spin echo (FSE, TR 2400, TE 85 Ef) and (**D**) sagittal fast spin echo (FSE, TR 3400, TE 85 Ef) MR images show to the better advantage the distribution of numerous osteochondral bodies.

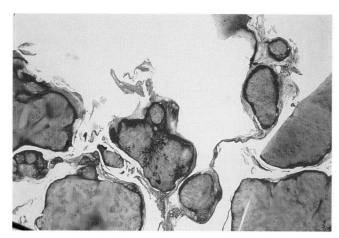

FIG. 6. Histopathology of synovial (osteo)chondromatosis. Photomicrograph of the synovium removed from the knee of a patient with primary synovial chondromatosis shows nodules of irregular cellular cartilage covered by a thin layer of synovium (hematoxylin and eosin, original magnification ×6).

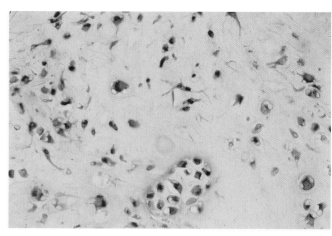

FIG. 7. Histopathology of synovial (osteo)chondromatosis. High-power photomicrograph shows pleomorphic cells with dark pleomorphic nuclei arranged in clusters (hematoxylin and eosin, original magnification ×100).

outer aspects of the cortex. The intraarticular bodies are numerous, small, and usually of uniform size (see Fig. 2).

More difficult is to distinguish *synovial chondromatosis* from synovial chondrosarcoma. The clinical and radiographic features have not been useful in this differentiation and are equally ineffective in distinguishing a secondary malignant lesion arising in synovial chondromatosis (1). In addition, both entities tend to have a protracted clinical course, and local re-

currence is common after synovectomy for synovial chondromatosis or local resection of synovial chondrosarcoma (12). The presence of frank bone destruction rather than merely erosions, and the association of a soft tissue mass, should always raise the concern about malignancy (8) (see Fig. 38). Although extension beyond the joint capsule should heighten the suspicion of malignancy, some cases of synovial chondromatosis have been reported to have an extraarticular extension (3,19).

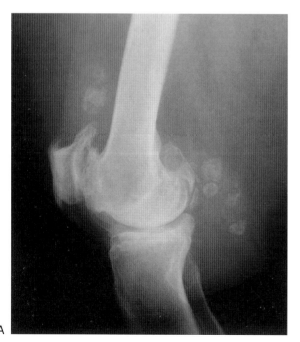
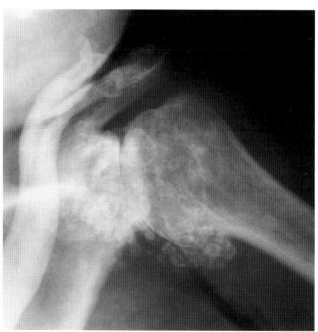

FIG. 8. Differential diagnosis of primary synovial (osteo)chondromatosis: secondary (osteo)chondromatosis due to osteoarthritis. **A:** A lateral radiograph of the knee in a 58-year-old man with advanced osteoarthritis of the femoropatellar joint compartment shows multiple osteochondral bodies in the suprapatellar bursa and within the popliteal cyst. **B:** A radiograph of the left shoulder in a 68-year-old woman with osteoarthritis of the glenohumeral joint shows multiple intraarticular osteochondral bodies.

The other conditions that can radiologically mimic synovial chondromatosis include pigmented villonodular synovitis, synovial hemangioma, and lipoma arborescens (9,10).

In *pigmented villonodular synovitis* the filling defects in the joint are more confluent and less distinct. Magnetic resonance imaging (MRI) may show foci of decreased intensity of the synovium in all sequences because of the paramagnetic effects of deposition of hemosiderin (13) (see Fig. 13). *Synovial hemangioma* usually presents as a single soft tissue mass. On MRI, T1-weighted images show that the lesion is either isointense or slightly higher (brighter) in signal intensity than surrounding muscles, but much lower in intensity than subcutaneous fat. On T2-weighted images the mass is invariably much brighter than fat (9) (see Fig. 25-26). Phleboliths and fibrofatty septa in the mass are common findings that show low signal characteristics.

Lipoma arborescens is a villous lipomatous proliferation of the synovial membrane (22). This rare condition usually affects the knee joint but has occasionally been reported in other joints, including the wrist and ankle (10). The disease has been variously reported to have a developmental, traumatic, inflammatory, or neoplastic origin, but its true etiology is still unknown. The clinical findings include slowly increasing but painless synovial thickening as well as joint effusion with sporadic exacerbation. Radiographic studies reveal a joint effusion accompanied by various degrees of osteoarthritis. Histologic examination demonstrates complete replacement of the subsynovial tissue by mature fat cells and the formation of proliferative villous projections.

Pathology

From the histopathologic standpoint it may be very difficult to distinguish *synovial chondrosarcoma* from synovial chondromatosis (14,15,17). The histopathologic distinction between primary and secondary malignant synovial lesions and synovial chondromatosis has been a matter of dispute. Occasional foci of increased cellularity showing hyperchromatic atypical cells, consistent with grade 1 chondrosarcoma, should not be considered sufficient evidence for a malignant change in synovial chondromatosis. However, evidence of aggressive growth (invasion) and lack of attachment of a lesion to the synovial lining support the diagnosis of malignancy.

The radiologic and pathologic differential diagnosis of synovial chondromatosis is depicted in Fig. 9.

Pigmented Villonodular Synovitis

Pigmented villonodular synovitis (PVNS) is a locally destructive fibrohistiocytic proliferation, characterized by many villous and nodular synovial protrusions (5), which affects joints, bursae, and tendon sheaths (48). PVNS was first described by Jaffe, Lichtenstein, and Sutro in 1941, who used this name to identify the lesion because of its yellow-brown, villous, and nodular appearance (62). The yellow-brown pigmentation is due to excessive deposits of lipid and hemosiderin. This condition can be diffuse or localized. When the entire synovium of the joint is affected and there is a major villous component, the condition is referred to as *diffuse pigmented villonodular synovitis*. When a discrete intra-

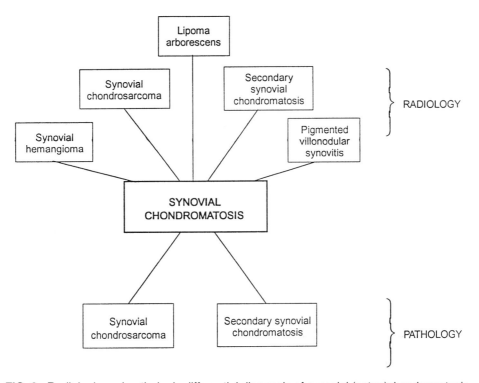

FIG. 9. Radiologic and pathologic differential diagnosis of synovial (osteo)chondromatosis.

articular mass is present, the condition is called *localized pigmented villonodular synovitis* (53,57) or (in the European literature) *pigmented giant-cell tumor of articulations*. When the process affects the tendon sheaths, it is called *localized giant-cell tumor of the tendon sheaths* (43,67,83). The diffuse form usually occurs in the knee, hip, elbow, or wrist and accounts for 23% of cases (70). The localized nodular form is often regarded as a separate entity. It consists of a single polypoid mass attached to the synovium. Nodular tenosynovitis is most often seen in the fingers and is the second most common soft tissue tumor of the hand, exceeded only by the ganglion (88).

Both the diffuse and the localized form of villonodular synovitis usually occur as a single lesion, mainly in young and middle-aged individuals of either sex (42,79). One of the most characteristic findings in PVNS is the ability of the hyperplastic synovium to invade the subchondral bone, producing cysts and erosions. Although the etiology is unknown (49) and is often controversial (55,56), some investigators have suggested an autoimmune pathogenesis (34). Trauma also is a suspected cause, since similar effects have been produced experimentally in animals by repeated injections of blood into the knee joint (88,99). Some investigators have suggested a disturbance in lipid metabolism as an etiologic factor (52,60). It has also been postulated by Jaffe and colleagues that these lesions may represent an inflammatory response to an unknown agent (62), and by Ray, Stout and Lattes et al. that they are true benign neoplasms (84,92). Although the latter theory was presumed to be supported by pathologic studies indicating that the histiocytes present in PVNS may function as facultative fibroblasts (77) and that foam cells may derive from histiocytes (45), relating PVNS to a benign neoplasm of fibrohistiocytic origin (55), these findings do not constitute definite proof that PVNS is a true neoplasm. Rather, they are indicative of a special form of a chronic proliferative inflammation process, as has already been postulated by Jaffe et al. (62).

Clinical Presentation

Clinically, PVNS is a slowly progressive process that manifests as mild pain and joint swelling with limitation of motion (27,49,91,97,100). Occasionally, increased skin temperature is noted over the affected joint (45). The knee joint is most commonly affected, and 66% of patients present with a bloody joint effusion (65). In fact, the presence of a serosanguinous synovial fluid in the absence of a history of recent trauma should strongly suggest the diagnosis of PVNS (55). The synovial fluid contains elevated levels of cholesterol (36,80), and fluid reaccumulates rapidly after aspiration (58). Other joints may be affected, including the hip, ankle, wrist, elbow, and shoulder (28,29,35,41,81,87). There is a 2:1 predilection for females. Patients range from 4 to 60 years of age, with a peak incidence in the third and fourth decade (5,76) (Fig. 10). The duration of symptoms can range from 6 months to as long as 25 years (30,44,71,72).

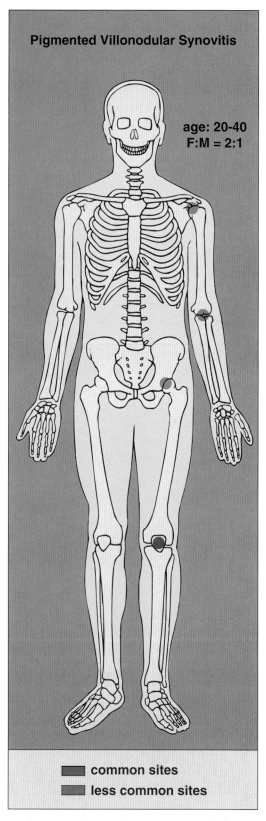

Pigmented Villonodular Synovitis

age: 20-40
F:M = 2:1

common sites
less common sites

FIG. 10. Pigmented villonodular synovitis: skeletal sites of predilection, peak age range, and male-to-female ratio.

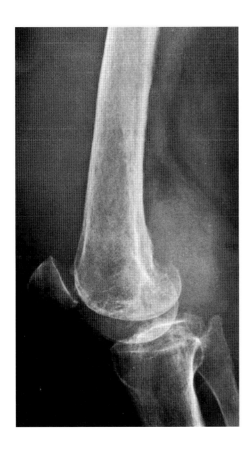

FIG. 11. Pigmented villonodular synovitis. Lateral radiograph of the knee of a 58-year-old man shows a large suprapatellar joint effusion and a dense, lumpy soft tissue mass eroding the posterior aspect of the lateral femoral condyle. Note that posteriorly the density is greater than that of a suprapatellar fluid.

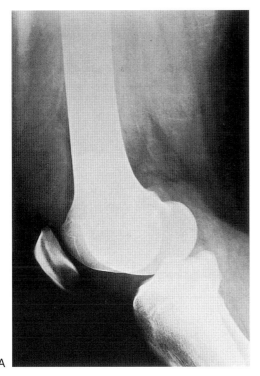
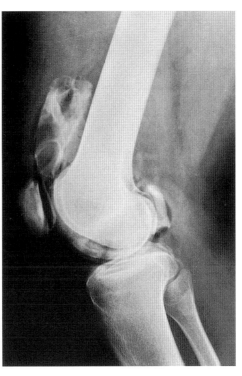

A   B

FIG. 12. Pigmented villonodular synovitis: arthrography. **A:** Lateral radiograph of the knee of a 25-year-old woman shows what appears to be a suprapatellar effusion. The density of the fluid , however, is increased, and there is some lobulation evident. **B:** Contrast arthrogram of the knee shows lobulated filling defects in the suprapatellar pouch, representing lumpy synovial masses. Joint aspiration yielded thick bloody fluid, which explains the increased density of the soft tissue mass seen on the plain film.

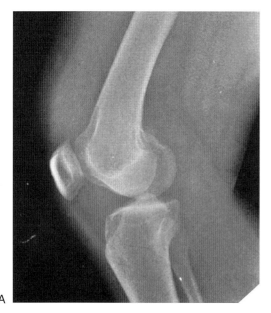

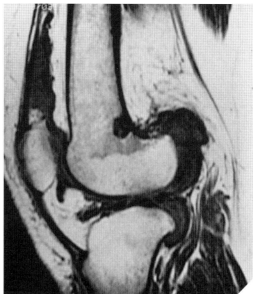

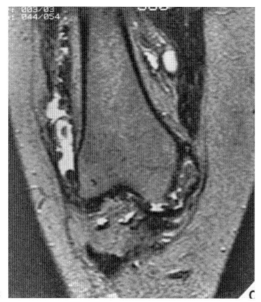

FIG. 13. Pigmented villonodular synovitis: magnetic resonance imaging. **A:** A lateral radiograph of the knee of a 22-year-old woman with several episodes of knee pain and swelling shows fullness in the suprapatellar bursa that was interpreted as joint effusion . Note also the increased density in the region of the popliteal fossa and subtle erosion of the posterior aspect of the distal femur. **B:** Sagittal T1-weighted (SE, TR 800, TE 20) MRI shows a lobulated mass in the suprapatellar bursa, extending into the knee joint and invading the infrapatellar fat. Note also the lobulated mass in the posterior aspect of the joint capsule, extending toward the posterior tibia. These masses exhibit an intermediate to low signal intensity. The erosion at the posterior aspect of the distal femur (supracondylar) is clearly demonstrated by an area of low signal intensity. **C:** Coronal T2-weighted (SE, TR 1800, TE 80) MRI demonstrates areas of high signal intensity that represent fluid and congested synovium, interspersed with areas of low signal intensity, characteristic of hemosiderin deposits.

Imaging

Plain radiography reveals a soft tissue density in the affected joint, frequently interpreted as joint effusion. However, the density is greater than that of a simple effusion, and it reflects not only a hemorrhagic fluid but also lobulated synovial masses (Fig. 11). A marginal, well-defined erosion of subchondral bone with a sclerotic margin may be present [incidence reported from 15% (38) to 50% (46)], usually on both sides of the affected articulation (101). Narrowing of the joint space has also been reported (55). In the hip, multiple cyst-like or erosive areas involving non-weight-bearing regions of the acetabulum, as well as the femoral head and neck, are characteristic (40). Calcifications are encountered only in exceptional cases (31).

Arthrography reveals multiple lobulated masses with villous projections, which appear as filling defects in the contrast-filled suprapatellar bursa (Fig. 12). Computed tomography effectively demonstrates the extent of the disease (37,68). The increase in iron content of the synovial fluid results in high Hounsfield values, a feature that can help in the differential diagnosis (85). MRI is extremely useful in making a diagnosis (32,33, 73,82,89,90,93,95,98) because on T2-weighted images the intraarticular masses demonstrate a combination of high-signal-intensity areas, representing fluid and congested synovium, interspersed with areas of intermediate to low signal intensity, secondary to random distribution of hemosiderin in the synovium (Fig. 13) (47,64). In general, MRI shows a low signal on both T1- and T2-weighted images because of hemosiderin deposition and thick fibrous tissue (11) (Fig. 14). In addition, within the mass signals consistent with fat can be noted, which are due

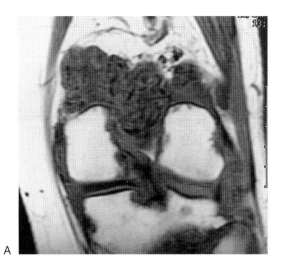

A

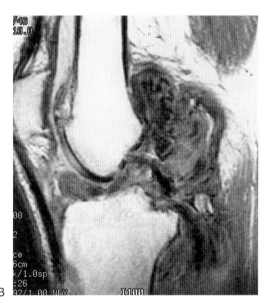

B

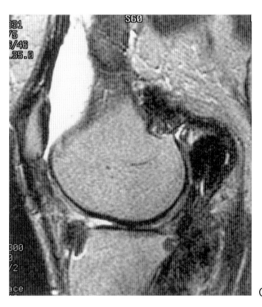

C

FIG. 14. Pigmented villonodular synovitis: magnetic resonance imaging. (**A**) Coronal and (**B**) sagittal T1-weighted (SE, TR 600, TE 12) MR images of the knee of a 40-year-old man show lobulated low-signal-intensity masses mainly localized to the popliteal fossa. (**C**) Sagittal T2-weighted (SE, TR 2300, TE 80) MRI shows high-intensity fluid in the suprapatellar bursa. The lobulated masses of pigmented villonodular synovitis remain of low signal intensity.

to clumps of lipid-laden macrophages (61). Other MRI findings include hyperplastic synovium and occasionally bone erosions. Administration of gadolinium in the form of Gd-DTPA leads to a notable increase in overall heterogeneity, which tends toward an overall increase in signal intensity of the capsule and septae (61). This enhancement of the synovium allows it to be differentiated from the fluid invariably present, which does not enhance. Apart from its diagnostic effectiveness, MRI also is useful in defining the extent of the disease (75).

Histopathology

On histologic examination, PVNS reveals a tumor-like proliferation of the synovial tissue. A dense infiltration of mononuclear histiocytes is observed, accompanied by plasma cells, lymphocytes, and variable numbers of resorptive giant cells (Fig. 15A, B). The villi are made up of a matrix that contains collagen and reticulin fibers, with a varied cell population. The villi are also covered by hyperplastic

and reactive-appearing synovial cells that may contain a large amount of hemosiderin (5). The synovial layer merges gradually with the underlying cell infiltrate that occupies the central core of the nodules (5). The stroma of the nodules contains variable amounts of collagen fibers and foci of large, epithelioid histiocytic cells that exhibit a macrophagic activity for hemosiderin and lipids (mainly cholesterol) (38,78) (Fig. 15C). Between these areas giant cells are present, some of which contain up to 50 nuclei (38,46). Dilatation of the blood vessels is often observed, and the histiocytic elements may contain variable amounts of hemosiderin or lipids (101). Mitotic figures are occasionally seen in the stromal and synovial cells (5). Electron microscopic studies have demonstrated that the histiocytic cell population of PVNS is not uniform but contains two basic cell types: (a) fibroblasts that produce collagen and proteoglycan and (b) macrophages that contain hemosiderin and lipids (54,55,86).

The pathologic spectrum of PVNS parallels the clinical features. Over time, the cellularity of the synovium diminishes and the degree of fibrosis increases (46). As the stroma

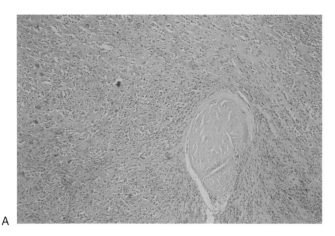

A

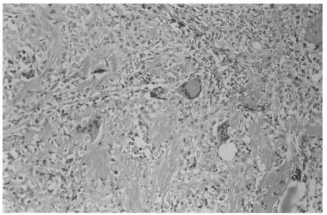

B

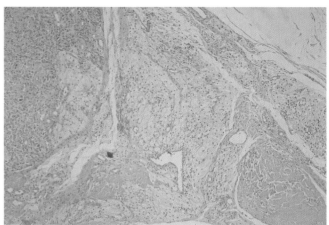

C

FIG. 15. Histopathology of pigmented villonodular synovitis. **A:** Extended strands of roundish histiocytic cells and scattered giant cells having formed bundles of condensed collagen (*center and upper right*). In other areas (*lower right*) the cells are more spindled (hematoxylin and eosin, original magnification ×25). **B:** At higher magnification noted is accumulation of mononuclear cells with interspersed giant cells, which have frequently peripherally arranged nuclei (*center*). Condensed collagen fibers sometimes resemble bone matrix (*bottom*) (hematoxylin and eosin, original magnification ×50). **C:** In another field of view noted are extended areas of lipid-laden macrophages and scattered hemosiderin-containing macrophages (hematoxylin and eosin, original magnification ×25).

becomes more fibrous, the numbers of foamy macrophages decrease and they may eventually disappear. Lesser numbers of lymphocytes and plasma cells remain, often in a perivascular distribution. Hemosiderin also persists, although much of it usually disappears (46).

Differential Diagnosis

Radiology

The most common diagnostic possibilities include hemophilia, synovial chondromatosis, synovial hemangioma, osteoarthritis, rheumatoid arthritis, and tuberculous arthritis (4,39,74). MRI is very effective in the differential diagnosis because it can reveal the presence of hemosiderin deposition in PVNS (47), whereas neither monoarticular *rheumatoid arthritis* nor *synovial hemangioma* clearly exhibits this feature. Some investigators, however, postulate that both hemophilia and synovial hemangioma may be associated with an intraarticular bleeding, and hence the hemosiderin deposition (79). Detection of diffuse hemosiderin clumps, synovial irregularity and thickening, and distention of the synovial sac usually suggest the diagnosis of PVNS (94).

Synovial chondromatosis may manifest with pressure erosions of the bone similar to those of PVNS, but it can be dis-

tinguished by the presence of multiple joint bodies, calcified or uncalcified (13). Synovial hemangioma is usually associated with the formation of phleboliths (9). *Synovial sarcoma* tends to have a shorter T1 and longer T2 on MRI compared with PVNS, and when calcifications are present the latter diagnosis can be excluded. *Lipoma aborescens* has a very characteristic appearance on MRI, with its signal compatible with fatty tissue and its typical frond-like synovial projections. In addition, there is very little or no enhancement of the mass after administration of gadolinium (10,59).

Hemophilia, unlike PVNS, usually affects multiple joints. The growth disturbances typical of this disorder are not a feature of PVNS. *Tuberculous arthritis,* like PVNS, favors the knee joint and the hip and tends to be monoarticular. On plain films, characteristic subchondral cysts and articular erosions are present, with relative preservation (at least in the early stages) of the joint space. However, the most consistent plain film finding of tuberculosis arthritis is severe juxtaarticular osteoporosis, which is not seen in PVNS.

Monoarticular *osteoarthritis* (degenerative joint disease) commonly occurs in an older population. Osteoarthritis affecting large joints, such as the knee and hip, may be characterized by cyst-like bony lesions that resemble those of PVNS. The presence of juxta-articular soft tissue masses is helpful in distinguishing PVNS from osteoarthritis and the former usually exhibits a lack of joint space narrowing. The formation of hypertrophic spurs that often occurs in degenerative joint disease is lacking in PVNS (46). Differentiation between *rheumatoid arthritis* and PVNS is sometimes more difficult because this arthropathy causes bony erosions secondary to the formation of a synovial pannus and to a chronic elevation of intraarticular pressure, which is a similar mechanism in both conditions (46). The lack of hypertrophic bone changes in rheumatoid arthritis constitutes another similarity to PVNS. Again, periarticular osteoporosis and the occasional formation of so-called rice bodies in rheumatoid arthritis serve as important differentiating points. Clinical information is also crucial in this situation.

Pathology

Rheumatoid arthritis may be characterized by synovial hypertrophy and proliferation of villi, which, however, are usually less prominent than in PVNS and during the acute phase contain an inflammatory infiltrate with many plasma cells. These villi also lack conspicuous hemosiderin deposits. *Hemophilia* is sometimes characterized by large hemosiderin deposits, but these are generally confined to the cells that line the synovium. The subsynovial tissue, also unlike the case with PVNS, almost completely lacks hemosiderin (5).

When PVNS invades the neighboring bone and radiologically appears like a primary epiphyseal bone tumor, the histologic presentation may mimic chondroblastoma, mainly because of the roundish appearance of histocytic elements (Remagen, unpublished observations) (Fig. 16).

Localized-pigmented Nodular Tenosynovitis [Pigmented Giant-Cell Tumor of the Synovium or the (Localized) Giant-Cell Tumor of the Tendon Sheath]

Clinical Presentation

This is the most common presentation of the localized nodular form of villonodular synovitis (96). It occurs predominantly in the tendon sheaths, mainly on the palmar aspect of the phalanges, and occasionally in the articular synovium. Unlike PVNS, there is a 2:1 male predominance (5), although some investigators report a slight female predominance (69). It is a well-circumscribed lesion that affects a small area of the synovium (61) or the tendon sheath (69). The main clinical symptom is pain, although the lesion is frequently asymptomatic (51,55).

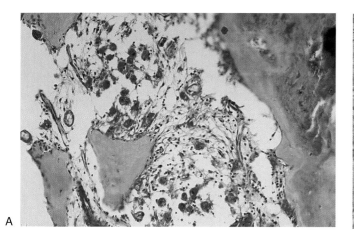

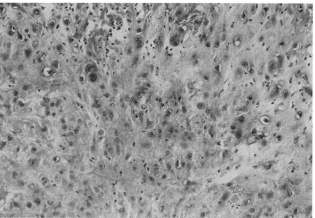

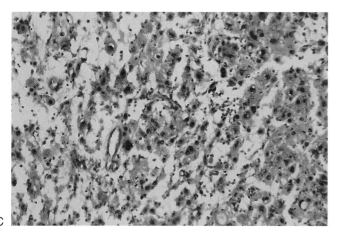

FIG. 16. Histopathology of pigmented villonodular synovitis: differential diagnosis. **A:** Cancellous bone from articular end of tibia shows infiltration by large roundish cells exhibiting some pleomorphism and nuclear hyperchromatism, originally mistaken for chondroblastoma (hematoxylin and eosin, original magnification ×100). **B:** With Giemsa stain the matrix even more resembles a chondroblastic tumor (Giemsa, original magnification ×100). **C:** The tissue obtained from the interior of the knee joint shows typical appearance of PVNS (hematoxylin and eosin, original magnification ×100).

Imaging

On radiography, localized nodular tenosynovitis is seen as a well-circumscribed, dense soft tissue mass, often in close approximation to a bony erosion (Fig. 17) (50). Pathologic fractures are exceedingly rare (102). Occasionally, the iron stored in histocytes may appear as fine dispersed densities within the soft tissue mass (Remagen, unpublished observations). MRI is rather characteristic. On T1- and T2-weighted images, lesions show predominantly low signal intensity equal to or slightly higher than skeletal muscle. On gadolinium-enhanced T1-weighted images, strong homogenous enhancement is seen (42). These findings reflect the underlying histologic composition of the lesion: hemosiderin deposition in xanthoma cells and abundant collagenous proliferation are responsible for low signal intensity on T1- and T2-weighted images. Strong homogenous enhancement reflects the presence of numerous proliferative capillaries in the collagenous stroma (42,63,66,69).

Histopathology

Pathologically, the tumor is firm, round, oval, or lobulated, and is usually contained within a dense fibrotic capsule. The size of the tumor varies from a few millimeters to several centimeters in diameter. Microscopic examination reveals collagenous connective tissue with a wide variation in the proportion of matrix to tumor cells (Fig. 18). The synovial cells are the basic component of this tumor. Although giant cells are a constant feature, they vary in number. Foam cells and hemosiderin-laden macrophages, although often identified, are not a constant feature. Xanthomatous cells often contain hemosiderin granules (42). The presence of hemosiderin results from the breakdown of erythrocytes that have extravasated into the tissue.

Differential Diagnosis

Radiology

The differential diagnosis includes synovial sarcoma, gout, amyloidosis, dermoid (dermal) inclusion cyst, glomus tumor, enchondroma, and periosteal chondroma.

Synovial sarcoma is more destructive, the soft tissue mass is usually larger than in giant-cell tumor of the tendon sheath, and, when true calcifications are present (imaging much coarser than the fine densities caused by hemosiderin deposits), the latter condition can safely be excluded. *A gouty tophus* may mimic nodular tenosynovitis, but it usually contains radiographically visible calcifications. The

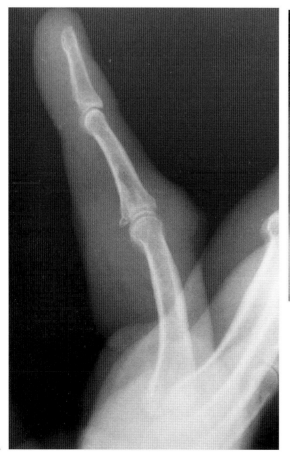

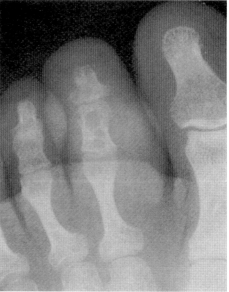

FIG. 17. Giant-cell tumor of the tendon sheath. **A:** A lateral radiograph of the index finger of a 58-year-old man shows a soft tissue mass at the site of the proximal interphalangeal joint. A small erosion is present at the base of the middle phalanx. **B:** In anteroposterior radiograph of the toes in a middle-aged man shows a soft tissue swelling of the second toe associated with several osteolytic defects in the middle phalanx. (Reprinted from Bullough PG. *Atlas of orthopedic pathology,* 2nd ed. New York: Gower, 1992;17.25.)

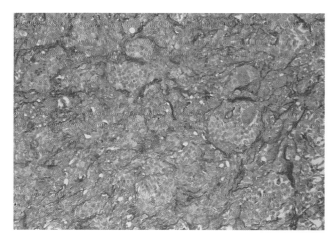

FIG. 18. Histopathology of giant cell tumor of the tendon sheath. The histiocytic character of the tumor tissue prevails. The collagen septae are less conspicuous (van Gieson, original magnification ×50).

bony erosion has a characteristic overhanging edge, and the affected joint is partially preserved.

Enchondroma exhibits a centric location and possesses lobulated borders, with frequent matrix calcifications. *Periosteal chondroma* may closely mimic giant-cell tumor of the tendon sheath but, again, almost invariably it displays visible soft tissue calcifications.

Pathology

The cleft-like structures in localized nodular tenosynovitis may suggest the glandular or biphasic form of *synovial sarcoma*. The large numbers of giant cells and the admixture of histiocytes help in the differential diagnosis to exclude the latter malignancy (5). In addition, the well-defined epithelioid cells characteristic of synovial sarcoma are not present. If the collagen produced appears very hyalinized and therefore resembles osteoid, the condition may at first glance be confused with *soft-tissue osteosarcoma* poor in matrix (Fig. 19). The monomorphism of the cells and the lack of other

malignant features in the nodular form of PVNS are then helpful in differentiation.

The radiologic and pathologic differential diagnosis of pigmented villonodular synovitis and a giant-cell tumor of the tendon sheath is depicted in Figs. 20 and 21, respectively.

Synovial Hemangioma

Clinical Presentation

Synovial hemangioma is a rare benign lesion that most commonly affects the knee joint, usually involving the anterior compartment (113,115). This lesion has also been found in the elbow (112), wrist, and ankle (108), as well as in tendon sheaths (121). Most cases affect children and adolescents. In one study, 75% of patients with synovial hemangioma of the knee joint presented before the age of 16 years, and 35% had a history of trauma at the site (117). A more recent study involving 20 patients places the average age at the time of presentation at 25 years (range 9 to 49 years) (108). Almost all patients with synovial hemangioma are symptomatic, frequently presenting with a swollen knee or with mild pain or limitation of movement in the joint (119). Sometimes patients report a history of recurrent episodes of joint swelling and various degrees of pain of several years duration. Synovial hemangioma is often associated with an adjacent cutaneous or deep soft tissue hemangioma. For this reason, some investigators classify knee joint lesions as intraarticular, juxtaarticular, or intermediate, depending on the extent of involvement (111). Synovial hemangioma is frequently misdiagnosed, and according to one estimate a correct preoperative diagnosis is made in only 22% of cases (108).

Imaging

Until recently, synovial hemangiomas were evaluated by a combination of plain radiography, arthrography, angiography, and contrast-enhanced CT. Although plain radiographs

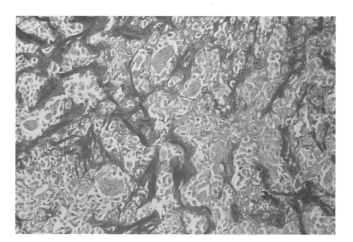

FIG. 19. Histopathology of giant-cell tumor of the tendon sheath. Sclerotic bundles of collagen fibers (*red structures*) resembling osteoid such as produced by malignant cells of osteosarcoma surround clusters of fairly large histiocytes with several giant cells (van Gieson, original magnification ×50).

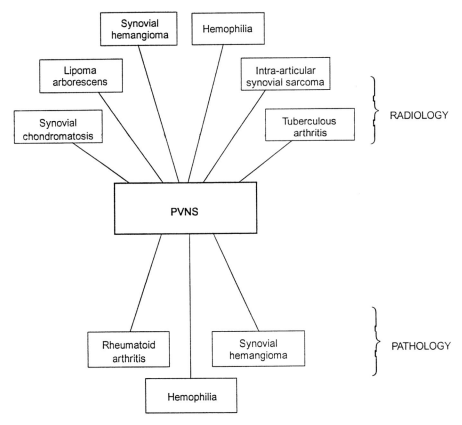

FIG. 20. Radiologic and pathologic differential diagnosis of pigmented villonodular synovitis.

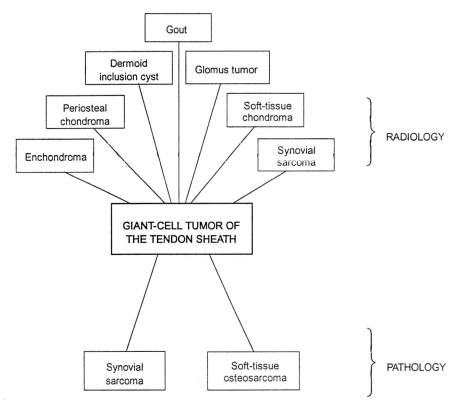

FIG. 21. Radiologic and pathologic differential diagnosis of giant-cell tumor of the tendon sheath.

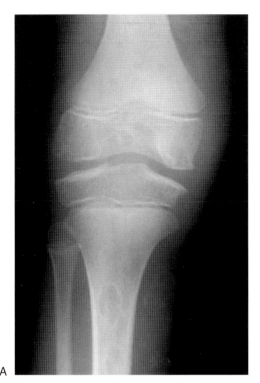
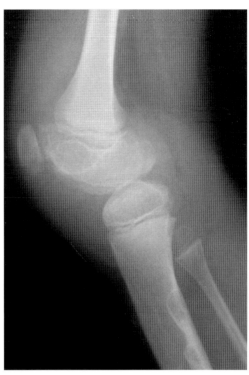

A

B

FIG. 22. Synovial hemangioma. (**A**) Anteroposterior and (**B**) lateral radiographs of the right knee of a 7-year-old boy show articular erosions at femoropatellar and femorotibial joint compartments. Soft tissue masses are seen anteriorly and posteriorly. An incidental finding is a nonossifying fibroma in the posterior tibia. (Reprinted with permission from Greenspan A, *et al.* Synovial hemangioma: imaging features in eight histologically proved cases, review of the literature, and differential diagnosis. *Skeletal Radiol* 1995;24:583–590.)

appear normal in at least half of the patients, they may reveal soft tissue swelling, a mass around the joint, joint effusion, or erosions (Fig. 22). Phleboliths, periosteal thickening, advanced maturation of the epiphysis, and arthritic changes are also occasionally noted on plain radiographs (117) (Fig. 23).

Arthrography usually shows nonspecific filling defects with a villous configuration. Angiograms yield much more specific information than plain films (116). They can often reveal a vascular lesion (114) and can demonstrate pathognomonic features of hemangioma, leading to a presumptive

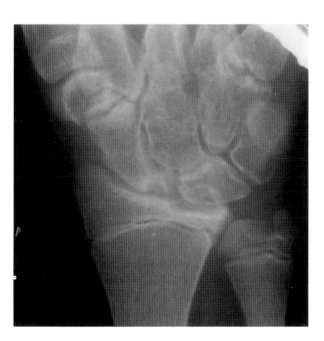

FIG. 23. Synovial hemangioma. Dorsovolar radiograph of the left wrist of a 15-year-old boy shows narrowing of the radiocarpal joint, and erosions of the scaphoid and lunate bones. Also noted are irregular articular surfaces of the trapezium-scaphoid and fifth carpometacarpal joints. (Reprinted with permission from Greenspan A, *et al.* Synovial hemangioma: imaging features in eight histologically proved cases, review of the literature, and differential diagnosis. *Skeletal Radiol* 1995;24:583–590.)

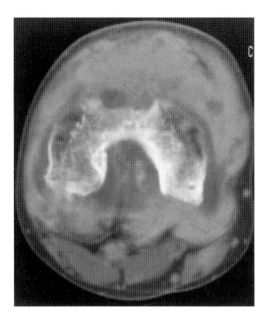

FIG. 24. Synovial hemangioma: computed tomography. CT axial section through the knee (same patient as illustrated in Fig. 9-22) shows marginal erosions of the femoral condyles. Heterogeneous masses are seen anteriorly and posteriorly with hypodense areas representing fat. (Reprinted with permission from Greenspan A, *et al.* Synovial hemangioma: imaging features in eight histologically proved cases, review of the literature, and differential diagnosis. *Skeletal Radiol* 1995;24:583–590.)

diagnosis. Contrast-enhanced CT of the joint typically reveals a heterogeneous-appearing soft tissue mass that displays tissue attenuation approximating that of skeletal muscle and contains areas of decreased attenuation, some approaching that of fat (106) (Fig. 24). CT is effective for demonstrating phleboliths and revealing patchy enhancement around them, as well as enhancement of tubular areas and contrast pooling within the lesion. In some cases CT reveals enlarged vessels feeding and draining the mass, as well as enlarged adjacent subcutaneous veins (110).

Recently, MRI has become the modality of choice for evaluation of hemangiomas because with this modality a presumptive diagnosis can be made. The soft tissue mass typically exhibits an intermediate signal intensity on T1-weighted sequences, appearing isointense with or slightly brighter than muscle but much less bright than fat. The mass is usually much brighter than subcutaneous fat on T2-weighted images and on fat suppression sequences (Fig. 25), and shows thin, often serpentine low-intensity septa within it (9,107,120) (Fig. 26). In general, the signal intensity characteristics of hemangiomas appear to be related to a number of factors, including slow flow, thrombosis, vessel occlusion, and increased free water in stagnant blood that pools in larger vessels and dilated sinuses, as well as to the variable amounts of adipose tissue in the lesion (106). After intravenous injection of gadolinium, there is evidence of enhancement of the hemangioma (107). In patients with a cav-

ernous hemangioma of the knee, fluid-fluid levels are also observed (**see Fig. 25B**), a finding recently reported also in soft tissue hemangiomas of this type (109).

Histopathology

Originating in the subsynovial layer mesenchyme of the synovial membrane, synovial hemangioma is a vascular lesion that contains variable amounts of adipose, fibrous, and muscle tissue, as well as thrombi in the vessels. When the lesion is completely intraarticular, it is usually well-circumscribed and apparently encapsulated, attached to the synovial membrane by a pedicle of variable size and adherent to the synovium on one or more surfaces by separable adhesions (105). Grossly, the tumor is a lobulated soft, brown, doughy mass with overlying villous synovium that is often stained mahogany-brown by hemosiderin. On microscopic examination, the lesion exhibits arborizing vascular channels of different sizes and a hyperplastic overlying synovium, which may show abundant iron deposition in chronic cases with repeated hemarthrosis (104) (Fig. 27).

Differential Diagnosis

Radiology

The differential diagnosis of synovial hemangioma includes *pigmented villonodular synovitis* (PVNS) and *synovial chondromatosis*. All proliferative chronic inflammatory processes, such as *rheumatoid arthritis, tuberculous arthritis*, and *hemophilic arthropathy*, should also be considered in the differential, but these conditions when involving the knee can usually be distinguished clinically. Because it is extremely uncommon, lipoma arborescens is rarely included in the differential diagnosis. MRI is diagnostic for this condition, showing typical frond-like projections of the lesion and fat characteristics (bright on T1- and intermediate on T2-weighted images). In PVNS, plain radiographs commonly reveal findings similar to those of synovial hemangioma, such as joint effusion and a mass in the suprapatellar bursa or popliteal fossa region. Radiographs may also demonstrate bone erosions on both sides of the joint, which in one study were reported in 26% of 81 patients (46). As in synovial hemangioma, arthrography in PVNS may demonstrate the synovial mass as a nonspecific filling defect (123). Without contrast enhancement, CT cannot identify decreased attenuation associated with fat within the tumor; contrast-enhanced CT, however, is diagnostic (37). The synovium in PVNS exhibits nodular thickening and masses of heterogeneous signal intensity. The majority of the lesion will display a higher signal intensity than muscle on both T1- and T2-weighted sequences, with other portions exhibiting a low signal intensity on all sequences, reflecting the hemosiderin content of the tumor (89). Synovial chondromatosis can often be diagnosed by plain radiography when nodules are calcified. Intraarticular osteochondral fragments

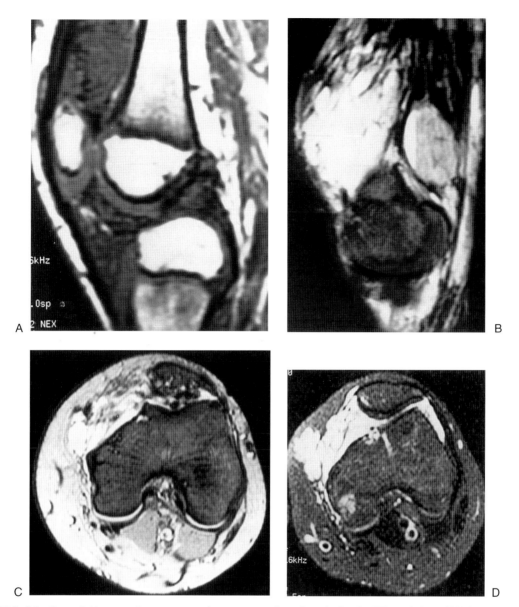

FIG. 25. Synovial hemangioma: magnetic resonance imaging. **A:** Sagittal T1-weighted (SE, TR 400, TE 11) MRI in a 9-year-old boy shows masses isointense with muscle involving the suprapatellar bursa and infrapatellar Hoffa fat. **B:** With fat-suppression technique the mass becomes very bright. The fluid-fluid level seen in the popliteal region is typical for cavernous type of synovial hemangioma.(**C**) In another patient, a 16-year-old girl, axial T2*-weighted (MPGR, TR 500, TE 15, flip angle 30°) MRI and (**D**) axial fast spin-echo (FSE, TR 5000, TE 85 Ef) image with fat suppression technique show the size and extent of the synovial hemangioma. (Reprinted with permission from Greenspan A, *et al.* Synovial hemangioma: imaging features in eight histologically proved cases, review of the literature, and differential diagnosis. *Skeletal Radiol* 1995;24:583–590.)

of uniform size are almost pathognomonic for this condition. CT may be helpful in demonstrating faint calcifications not otherwise seen, and MRI may be useful in delineating the extent of the disease. However, neither modality is of particular value in establishing the diagnosis of synovial chondromatosis (118).

Lipoma arborescens represents a villous lipomatous pro-

liferation of the synovial membrane (22). It is a very rare condition that affects men more commonly than women. It is a monoarticular disease, occurring primarily in the knee joint, but other joints, such as the wrists, ankle, and hips, are sometimes affected (10,59,103,122). Most patients report a long-standing, slowly progressive swelling of the joint, associated later with pain and limited motion. Plain radiogra-

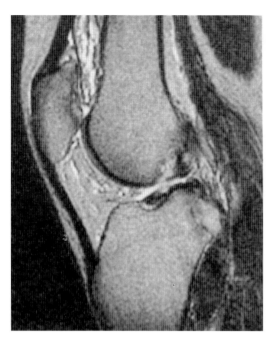

FIG. 26. Synovial hemangioma: magnetic resonance imaging. Sagittal T2-weighted (SE, TR 2000, TE 80) MRI of a 47-year-old woman demonstrates thin, low-intensity fibrofatty septa within the lesion. (Reprinted with permission from Greenspan A, *et al.* Synovial hemangioma: imaging features in eight histologically proved cases, review of the literature, and differential diagnosis. *Skeletal Radiology* 1995;24: 583–590.)

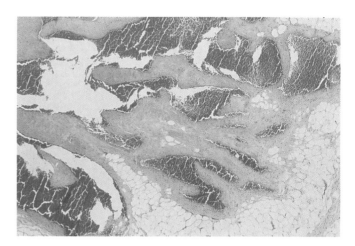

FIG. 27. Histopathology of synovial hemangioma. The vascular malformation consists of a network of connected blood-filled spaces within the loose connective tissue of the synovium (hematoxylin and eosin, original magnification ×12.5).

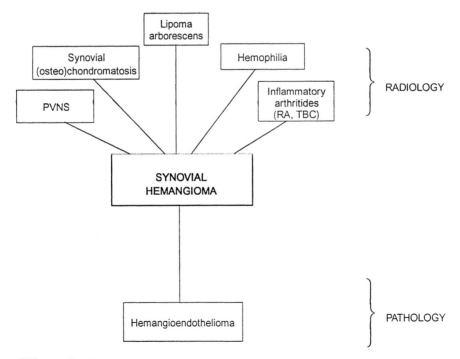

FIG. 28. Radiologic and pathologic differential diagnosis of synovial hemangioma.

phy shows only a soft tissue density within the joint, frequently interpreted as joint effusion. On CT, however, the synovial mass is obvious, and attenuation coefficient measurements are consistent with fat. There is very little or no enhancement of the mass after administration of intravenous contrast (59). The latter two features are useful in distinguishing this lesion from synovial hemangioma. The additional differential feature is the appearance of lipoma arborescens on MRI. The fatty areas of the synovial mass follow the signal intensity of subcutaneous fat on all pulse sequences (bright on T1 and intermediate on T2 weighting). In addition, MRI demonstrates typical frond-like synovial projections of the lesion.

Pathology

Synovial hemangioma in the great majority of cases can be diagnosed on a histopathologic basis with a high degree of confidence. Rarely, cases with atypical presentation may resemble *hemangioendothelioma.*

The radiologic and pathologic differential diagnosis of synovial hemangioma is depicted in Fig. 28.

MALIGNANT LESIONS

Synovial Sarcoma

Synovial sarcoma (synovioma) is an uncommon mesenchymal neoplasm, comprising about 8% to 10% of soft tissue sarcomas. Despite its name, it does not arise from synovium (149), although it may originate from any other structure, including joint capsules, bursae, and tendon sheaths (132).

Clinical Presentation

The tumor usually occurs before the age of 50 (132), most commonly between the ages of 16 and 36 years (131). There is no sex predilection. The extremities account for 83% of synovial sarcomas, but the most common sites are around the knee and foot (132) (Fig. 29). In exceptional instances the tumor may be intraarticular (5,130,147). Synovial sarcoma is usually slow growing with an indolent course, although in late stages it may demonstrate aggressiveness. Metastases to the lung by the hematogenous route and to the soft tissue have been reported (148). Schajowicz cites a local recurrence rate of >50% (155). The clinical symptoms usually include soft tissue swelling or a mass and progressive pain. On physical examination, a diffuse or a discrete soft tissue mass is present, usually tender on palpation.

Imaging

The radiographic features of synovial sarcoma include a soft tissue mass, usually in close proximity to a joint (Fig. 30) and occasionally associated with bone invasion

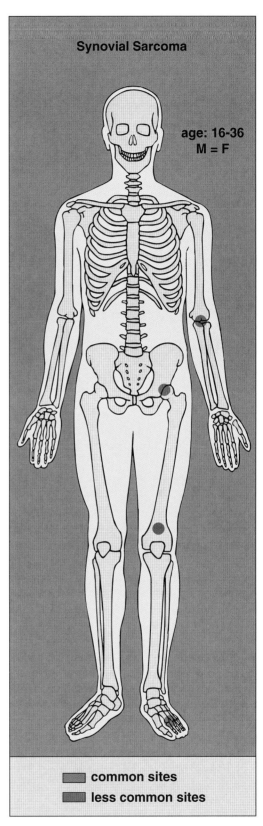

FIG. 29. Synovial sarcoma: skeletal sites of predilection, peak age range, and male-to-female ratio.

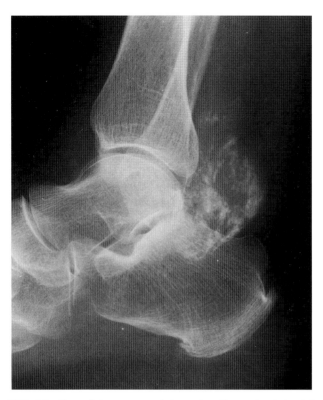

FIG. 30. Synovial sarcoma. A lateral radiograph of the left ankle of a 71-year-old woman shows a large calcified mass located in the soft tissues anteriorly to the Achilles tendon not affecting the adjacent bones.

(128,139). A periosteal reaction may also be observed (159). The soft tissue calcifications, usually amorphous in type, are present in about 25% to 30% of cases (132) (Fig. 31).

Computed tomography effectively demonstrates the extent of the soft-tissue mass, calcifications, and bone invasion (126). Magnetic resonance imaging shows the tumor to be an inhomogeneous, septated mass of low to intermediate intensity with infiltrative margins on T1-weighted sequences, displaying a high signal on T2 weighting (138,144, 145,152,160) (Figs. 32 and 33). The most extensive MRI study of this tumor in 34 patients showed that it tends to be deep, large (85% were >5 cm in diameter), and located in the extremities, with the epicenter close to a joint. The lesion was usually inhomogeneous on T2-weighted images and was clearly delineated from surrounding tissues. Forty-four percent of the cases had a high signal on both T1- and T2-weighted sequences, consistent with a hemorrhage within the tumor. Fluid-fluid levels, best visualized on T2-weighted images, were present in 18% of patients. The tumor frequently involved the adjacent bone, invading, eroding, or touching it in 71% of patients (141).

Histopathology

Synovial sarcoma, unlike the term implies, does not arise from synovial tissue (149,157). Most of the tumors occur in

extraarticular locations and bear no resemblance to synovium, neither ultrastructurally nor immunohistochemically (150). It has been suggested that synovial sarcoma originates from the pluripotential mesenchyme of the limb bud (162). Several studies have demonstrated a close relationship between cells that differentiate into osteoblasts and those that differentiate into synovioblasts (125,133,142). This factor may explain the formation of calcifications and ossifications in some synovial sarcomas.

Several subtypes of synovial sarcoma have been recognized (163). Among them are biphasic (fibrous and epithelial), monophasic, and poorly differentiated types (127). The classical biphasic type exhibits distinct spindle cell and epithelial components arranged in glandular or nest-like patterns (Fig. 34). The monophasic synovial sarcoma is composed of interdigitating fascicles and "ball-like" structures formed by the spindle cells (Fig. 35). Anastomosing vascular channels similar to those seen in hemangiopericytoma are occasionally present. Foci of calcification also may be observed usually localized in areas of hyalinization within the spindle cell elements of the tumor (132). At the ultrastructural level, abundant microvilli and many desmosomal attachments can be seen (127). The spindle cells are closely apposed to each other and appear polygonal or oval when viewed by electron microscopy. The cytoplasm demonstrates well-developed Golgi complexes, rough endoplasmic reticulum, polyribosomes, and glycogen particles (143). In the monophasic fibrous type, a spindle cell pattern predominates, with only a small number of epithelial cells. The

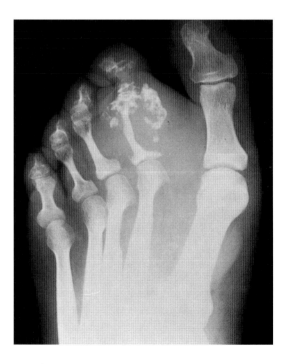

FIG. 31. Synovial sarcoma. A dorsoplantar radiograph of the right forefoot of a 55-year-old woman shows a large mass exhibiting coarse calcifications, eroding the proximal phalanx of the second toe. (Courtesy Dr. Harold Jacobson, Bronx, New York.)

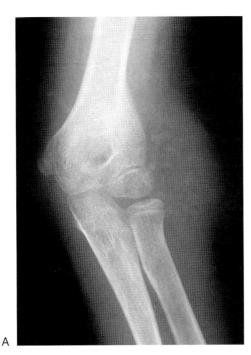

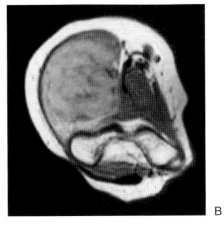

FIG. 32. Intraarticular synovial sarcoma. (**A**) An external oblique radiograph of the left elbow and (**B**) an axial T1-weighted (SE, TR 600, TE 20) MRI in an 8-year-old girl show a soft tissue mass arising from the elbow joint, displaying faint calcifications.

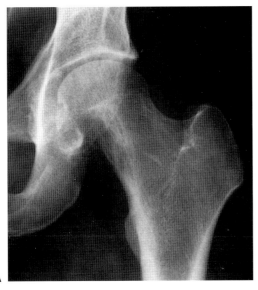

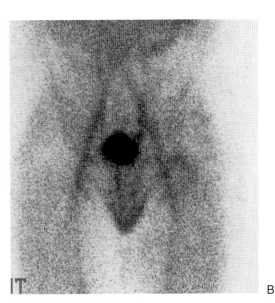

FIG. 33. Intraarticular synovial sarcoma. **A:** An anteroposterior radiograph of the left of a 37-year-old man shows an osteolytic lesion in the femoral neck bordered laterally by sclerotic margin. **B:** Scintigraphic (blood pool) examination demonstrates increased vascularity to the left hip joint.

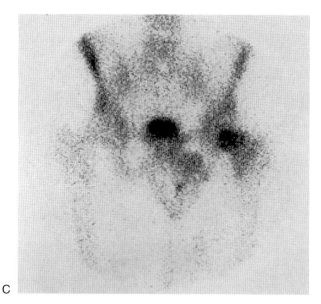

C

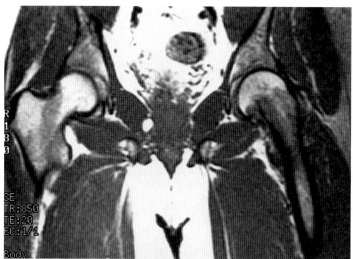

D

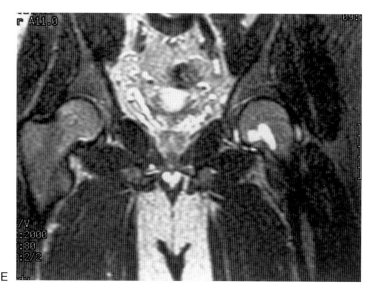

E

FIG. 33. *Continued.* **C:** Delayed radionuclide bone scan with 99m-technetium methylene diphosphonate (MDP) shows increased uptake of the radiopharmaceutical tracer in the femoral head and neck and around the hip joint. **D:** Coronal T1-weighted (SE, TR 850, TE 20) MRI shows a low-signal-intensity lesion affecting the medial aspect of the femoral neck. **E:** Coronal T2-weighted (SE, TR 2000, TE 80) MRI demonstrates increased signal in the femoral head and in the medial and lateral aspects of the hip joint.

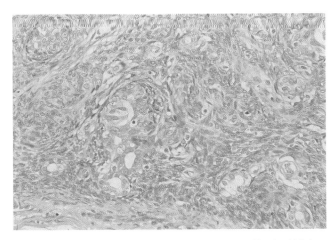

FIG. 34. Histopathology of synovial sarcoma. Typical biphasic appearance of synovial sarcoma with gland-like spaces (*left and below*) side-by-side with spindle-cell sarcomatous areas (hematoxylin and eosin, original magnification ×80).

monophasic epithelial type is rare and closely resembles metastatic carcinoma (127,135). This type exhibits glandular structures lined with epithelial cells. The poorly differentiated type contains cells resembling an intermediate form with characteristics of both epithelial and spindle cells (132). Immunohistochemical studies have shown a strong positivity for cytokeratin and epithelial membrane antigen in the epithelial areas, and a clear-cut positivity for the same markers, in addition to vimentin, in the spindle cell elements (5).

Differential Diagnosis

Radiology

The radiologic differential diagnosis should include soft-tissue chondroma, soft-tissue chondrosarcoma, soft-tissue

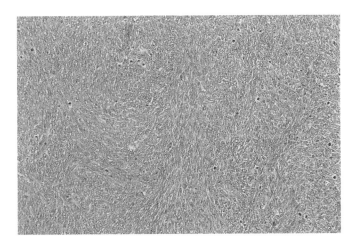

FIG. 35. Histopathology of synovial sarcoma. In rare cases, the tumor has a monophasic appearance without any gland-like patterns, resembling fibrosarcoma (hematoxylin and eosin, original magnification ×50).

osteosarcoma, soft-tissue fibrosarcoma or MFH, myositis ossificans, gout, and tumoral calcinosis. Except for fibrosarcoma and MFH, all of these entities exhibit calcifications. Therefore, if synovial sarcoma contains areas of mineralization, it may mimic the above-mentioned lesions (140,161).

Soft-tissue chondroma usually presents as a small and well-defined mass. Unlike synovial sarcoma, the lesion never invades bone. *Soft-tissue chondrosarcoma* is a rare tumor that usually arises in the proximal parts of the extremities and the buttocks (129). This neoplasm may display an aggressive behavior and hence may invade adjacent skeletal structures (156,165). *Soft-tissue osteosarcoma* is also much less common than synovial sarcoma. The preferred locations are the upper thighs and the buttocks. Like chondrosarcoma, this lesion may invade the bony structures. *Myositis ossificans* usually exhibits a distinctive zoning phenomenon, and juxtacortical lesions may evoke a well-organized periosteal reaction, although the cortex is not destroyed (124,137, 154). A *gouty tophus* usually occurs adjacent to the joint capsule, and calcifications are less sharply defined. The bony erosion usually exhibits a characteristic overhanging edge. *Tumoral calcinosis* is a rare metabolic disease characterized by the presence of single or multiple lobulated cystic masses containing chalky material (136). The condition can be idiopathic or associated with an abnormal phosphate metabolism with a high calcium-phosphate product, often due to secondary hyperparathyroidism (153). Radiographs reveal well-demarcated, well-lobulated heterogeneous calcific masses located around the joints (164). A consistent radiologic finding on conventional radiographs and CT is that of a dense calcified mass that is homogeneous except for a "chicken wire" pattern of lucencies within the mass, giving the calcifications a "cobblestone" appearance (158) that is not seen in synovial sarcoma. The adjacent bones are not invaded, although a pressure erosion of the cortex adjacent to the calcified mass may occasionally occur (158). The diagnosis of idiopathic tumoral calcinosis is one of exclusion. All other causes of soft tissue calcifications must be considered and excluded before this diagnosis is made.

Pathology

The histologic differential diagnosis includes soft-tissue osteosarcoma, parosteal osteosarcoma, periosteal fibrosarcoma, Ewing sarcoma, and metastatic carcinoma. Some synovial sarcomas are characterized by amorphous calcifications accompanied by extensive ossification, sometimes having a ribbon-like pattern, that simulates osteosarcoma (150). It is important to recognize this variant of synovial sarcoma with bone formation and to distinguish it from *extraskeletal* or *parosteal osteosarcoma*. The most important point in the recognition of synovial sarcoma is its biphasic pattern and the uniform appearance of the nuclei of the epithelial and spindle cells. Another factor that assists in the diagnosis of synovial sarcoma is the finding of amorphous concretions arranged in sheets and of small calcospherites located within spaces that are surrounded by flat or conspicuous epithelial cells (150). The cells are immunoreactive for cytokeratin and epithelial membrane antigen. A synovial sarcoma with an extensive spindle cell component may be confused with *fibrosarcoma* (134). Poorly differentiated round cell areas may resemble *Ewing sarcoma* (132). Moreover, tumors with predominant epithelial glandular (146) or squamous (151) components are difficult to differentiate from *metastatic carcinoma* (150). In this situation, as mentioned above, immunohistochemical markers for epithelial cells are of little help because the tumor cells that resemble epithelia are also positive despite their mesenchymal origin.

The radiologic and pathologic differential diagnosis of synovial sarcoma is depicted in Fig. 36.

Synovial Chondrosarcoma

Synovial chondrosarcoma is a rare tumor that originates from the synovial membrane. It may arise as a primary synovial tumor or it may develop as a malignant transformation of synovial chondromatosis (1,166,167). The concept of malignant degeneration of synovial chondromatosis is still controversial and the entity is rare: only 20 well-documented cases are on record (12,15,168–173).

Clinical Presentation

Most synovial chondrosarcomas are located in the knee joint. Rarely other joints such as the hip, elbow, or ankle are affected. These malignancies show a slight predominance in men and the patients range in age from 25 to 70 years (Fig. 37). The symptoms include pain and swelling, with duration in most patients exceeding 12 months (5). In patients with primary synovial chondromatosis, malignant transformation to synovial chondrosarcoma should be clinically suspected if there is development of a soft tissue mass at the site of the affected joint.

Imaging

Radiologically the presence of chondroid calcifications within the joint, destruction of the adjacent bones, and a soft tissue mass are highly suggestive of a synovial chondrosarcoma. In patients with documented primary synovial (osteo) chondromatosis, a soft tissue mass and destructive changes in the joint should alert to the development of a secondary synovial chondrosarcoma (Fig. 38). It has to be pointed out, however, that frequently both uncomplicated synovial chondromatosis and synovial chondrosarcoma may exhibit similar features on plain radiography and MRI (171).

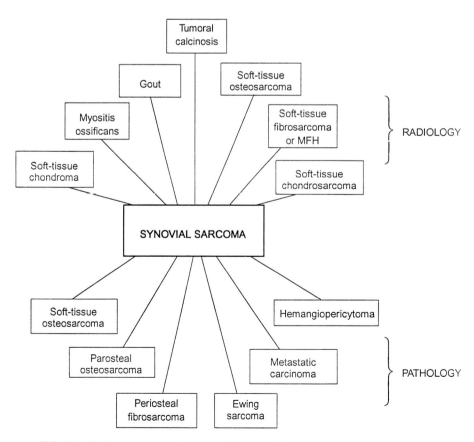

FIG. 36. Radiologic and pathologic differential diagnosis of synovial sarcoma.

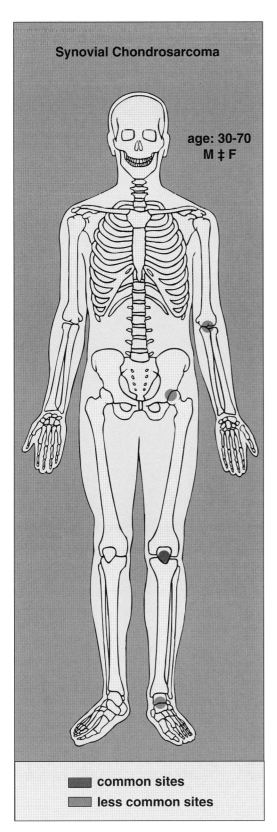

FIG. 37. Synovial chondrosarcoma: skeletal sites of predilection, peak age range, and male-to-female ratio.

Histopathology

The histopathologic distinction between primary synovial chondromatosis and secondary malignancy in synovial chondromatosis has been a matter of dispute. Manivel *et al.* (17) suggested that histologic features equivalent to those of grade 2 or 3 central chondrosarcoma must be present before chondrosarcoma arising in synovial chondromatosis can be diagnosed. Occasional foci of increased cellularity showing hyperchromatic atypical cells, consistent with grade 1 chondrosarcoma, should not be sufficient evidence for a malignant change in synovial chondromatosis (24). However, evidence of aggressive growth (invasion) and a lesion's lack of attachment to the synovial lining, combined with hypercellularity and pleomorphisms of the cells, should support the diagnosis of malignancy (Figs. 39 and 40).

Bertoni and co-workers have attempted to develop criteria for making this crucial distinction. They identified several microscopic features indicative of malignancy. The distinguishing features of synovial chondrosarcoma include the following: tumor cells arranged in sheets, myxoid changes in the matrix, hypercellularity with crowding and spindling of nuclei at the periphery, necrosis, and permeation of bone trabeculae. Remarking on the danger of misinterpreting synovial chondromatosis as chondrosarcoma on both radiographic and histopathologic examination, Bertoni and colleagues singled out pulmonary metastases as the only distinguishing feature (1).

Differential Diagnosis

Radiology

The main differential diagnosis is between synovial chondrosarcoma and *synovial (osteo)chondromatosis*. Frequently, the radiologic findings in both conditions are similar, although the development of destructive changes around the affected joint favors synovial chondrosarcoma. However, these destructive changes should be differentiated from periarticular erosions occasionally present in synovial chondromatosis (21). PVNS can usually be excluded without much difficulty because it does not exhibit calcifications and, in addition, shows somewhat characteristic MRI features.

Pathology

The difficulties in distinguishing secondary synovial chondrosarcoma from *synovial chondromatosis* have been discussed above.

The radiologic and pathologic differential diagnosis of synovial chondrosarcoma is depicted in Fig. 41.

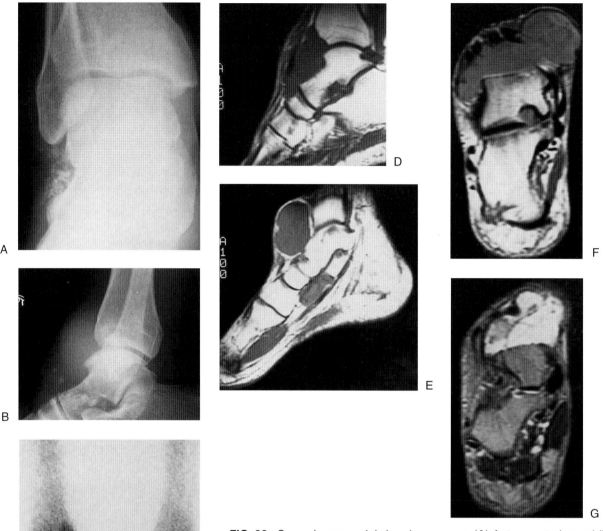

FIG. 38. Secondary synovial chondrosarcoma. (**A**) Anteroposterior and (**B**) lateral radiographs of the right ankle of a 64-year-old man with a long history of synovial chondromatosis show a large soft tissue mass on the dorsal aspect of the ankle joint, eroding the talus. Multiple calcifications, uniform in size and shape are noted laterally. (**C**) After injection of 15 mCi (555 MBq) of 99m-technetium-labeled methylene diphosphonate (MDP) there is increased uptake of radiopharmaceutical tracer in the right ankle. (**D**) Sagittal T1-weighted (SE, TR 400, TE 20) MRI shows the mass displaying intermediate signal intensity, isointense with the muscles. (**E**) Parasagittal T1-weighted (SE, TR 400, TE 20) image demonstrates the mass to be well encapsulated. (**F**) Coronal proton density (SE, TR 1800, TE 29) MRI shows that the mass is continuous with the ankle joint. (**G**) Coronal T2-weighted (SE, TR 2000, TE 80) image demonstrates the mass to be of high signal intensity. Punctate areas of low signal intensity within the mass represent calcifications. (Reprinted with permission from Ontell F, Greenspan A. Chondrosarcoma complicating synovial chondromatosis: findings with magnetic resonance imaging. *Can Assoc Radiol J* 1994;45:319–320.)

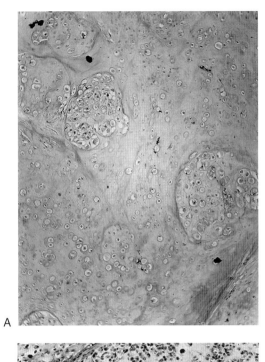

A

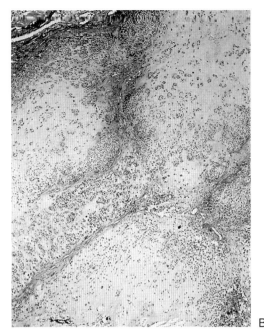

B

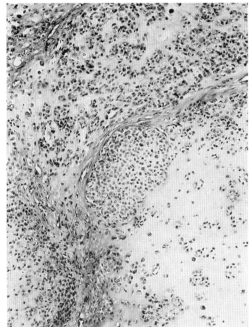

C

FIG. 39. Histopathology of secondary synovial chondrosarcoma. **A:** Clusters of chondrocytes exhibiting mild atypia are characteristic for synovial chondromatosis (hematoxylin and eosin, original magnification ×100). **B:** Marked hypercellularity is visible at the periphery of the cartilaginous lobules. These areas represent chondrosarcoma arising in synovial chondromatosis (hematoxylin and eosin, original magnification ×64). **C:** Higher power magnification shows chondrosarcomatous areas with marked hypercellularity and pleomorphism. Sheaths of cells are arranged without a pattern (hematoxylin and eosin, original magnification ×160). (Reprinted with permission from Ontell F, Greenspan A. Chondrosarcoma complicating synovial chondromatosis: findings with magnetic resonance imaging. *Can Assoc Radiol J* 1994;45:321.)

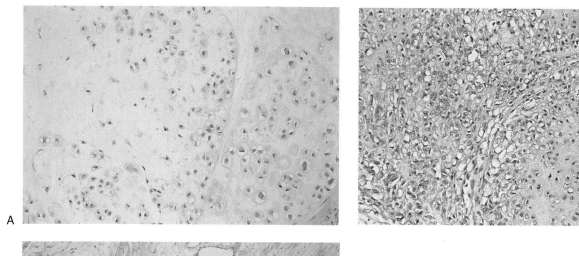

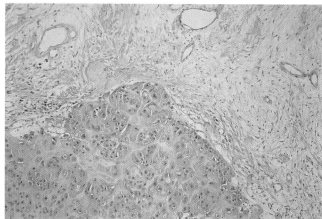

FIG. 40. Histopathology of secondary synovial chondrosarcoma. **A:** The chondrocytes with clearly pleomorphic, sometimes large blastic nuclei (*lower right corner*) are unevenly distributed. These differences in the nuclear size and structure, however, do not indicate malignancy, and may be features of uncomplicated synovial chondromatosis (hematoxylin and eosin, original magnification ×50). **B:** Smaller parts of the benign synovial lesion (*lower right*) border the cell-rich tissue of secondary chondrosarcoma of grade 2–3 (hematoxylin and eosin, original magnification ×50). **C:** At the proliferation line of the tumor against the fibrous connective tissue there is more matrix formation of the tumor, which here is a grade 2 sarcoma (hematoxylin and eosin, original magnification ×25).

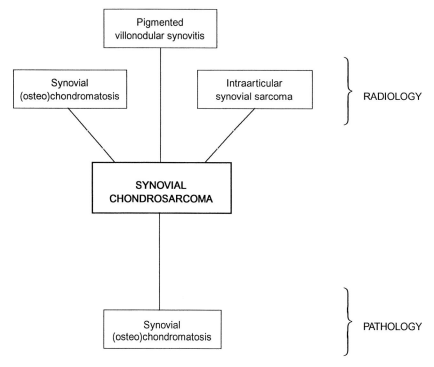

FIG. 41. Radiologic and pathologic differential diagnosis of synovial chondrosarcoma.

REFERENCES

Synovial Chondromatosis

1. Bertoni F, Unni KK, Beabout JW, Sim FH. Chondrosarcomas of the synovium. *Cancer* 1991;67:155–162.
2. Blacksin MF, Ghelman B, Freiberger RH, Salvata E. Synovial chondromatosis of the hip: evaluation with air computed arthrotomography. *Clin Imag* 1990;14:315–318.
3. Burnstein MI, Fisher DR, Yandow DR, Hafez GR, DeSmet AA. Case report 502. Intra-articular synovial chondromatosis of shoulder with extra-articular extension. *Skeletal Radiol* 1988;17:458–461.
4. Conway WF, Hayes CW. Miscellaneous lesions of bone. *Radiol Clin North Am* 1993;31:339–358.
5. Fechner RE, Mills SE. *Tumors of the bones and joint.* Washington, DC: Armed Forces Institute of Pathology, 1993.
6. Feldman F. Cartilaginous tumors and cartilage-forming tumor-like conditions of the bones and soft tissues. In: Ranniger K, ed. *Bone tumors.* Berlin: Springer-Verlag, 1977;83–242.
7. Ginaldi S. Computed tomography feature of synovial osteochondromatosis. *Skeletal Radiol* 1980;5:219–222.
8. Goldman RL, Lichtenstein L. Synovial chondrosarcoma. *Cancer* 1964;17:1233–1240.
9. Greenspan A, Azouz EM, Matthews J II, Décarie J-C. Synovial hemangioma: imaging features in eight histologically proved cases, review of the literature, and differential diagnosis. *Skeletal Radiol* 1995; 24:583–590.
10. Hallel T, Lew S, Bansal M. Villous lipomatous proliferation of the synovial membrane (lipoma arborescens). *J Bone Joint Surg* 1988; 70A:264–270.
11. Laorr A, Helms CA. *MRI of musculoskeletal masses: a practical text and atlas.* New York: Igaku-Shoin, 1997.
12. Hamilton A, Davis RI, Hayes D, Mollan RA. Chondrosarcoma developing in synovial chondromatosis. A case report. *J Bone Joint Surg* 1987;69B:137–140.
13. Hermann G, Abdelwahab IF, Klein MJ, Kenan S, Lewis M. Synovial chondromatosis. *Skeletal Radiol* 1995;24:298–300.
14. Kindblom L-G, Angervall L. Myxoid chondrosarcoma of the synovial tissue: a clinicopathologic, histochemical, and ultrastructural analysis. *Cancer* 1983;52:1886–1895.
15. King JW, Spjut HJ, Fechner RE, Vanderpool DW. Synovial chondromsarcoma of the knee joint. *J Bone Joint Surg* 1967; 49A:1389–1396.
16. Madewell JE, Sweet DE. Tumors and tumor-like lesions in or about joints. In: Resnick D, Niwayama M, eds. *Diagnosis of bone and joint disorders.* Philadelphia: WB Saunders, 1988.
17. Manivel JC, Dehner LP, Thompson R. Case report 460. Synovial chondrosarcoma of left knee. *Skeletal Radiol* 1988;17:66–71.
18. Maurice H, Crone M, Watt I. Synovial chondromatosis. *J Bone Joint Surg* 1988;70B:807–811.
19. Milgram JW. Synovial osteochondromatosis. A histopathological study of thirty cases. *J Bone Joint Surg* 1977;59A:792–801.
20. Murphy FP, Dahlin DC, Sullivan CR. Articular synovial chondromatosis. *J Bone Joint Surg* 1962;44A:77–86.
21. Norman A, Steiner GC. Bone erosion in synovial chondromatosis. *Radiology* 1986;161:749–752.
22. Ryu KN, Jaovisidha S, Schweitzer M, Motta AO, Resnick D. MR imaging of lipoma aborescens of the knee joint. *Am J Roentgenol* 1996;167:1229–1232.
23. Osburn AW, Bassett LW, Seeger LL, Mirra JM, Eckhardt JJ. Case report 609. Synovial (osteo)chondromatosis. *Skeletal Radiol* 1990;19: 237–241.
24. Schajowicz F. Synovial chondromatosis. In: *Tumors and tumorlike lesions of bones and joints.* New York: Springer-Verlag, 1981;541–545.
25. Trias A, Quintana O. Synovial chondrometaplasia: review of world literature and study of 18 Canadian cases. *Can J Surg* 1976;19: 151–158.
26. Tuckman G, Wirth CZ. Synovial osteochondromatosis of the shoulder: MR findings. *J Comput Assist Tomogr* 1989;13:360–361.

Pigmented Villonodular Synovitis

27. Abrahams TG, Pavlov H, Bansal M, Bullough P. Concentric joint space narrowing of the hip associated with hemosiderotic synovitis (HS) including pigmented villonodular synovitis (PVNS). *Skeletal Radiol* 1988;17:37–45.
28. Aghasi MK, Robinson D, Reif RM, Halperin N. Pigmented villonodular synovitis of the talus in a child. *Foot Ankle* 1988;9: 139–142.
29. Aglietti P, Di Muria GV, Salvati EA, Stringa G. Pigmented vollonodular synovitis of the hip joint (review of the literature and report of personal case material). *Ital J Orthop Traumatol* 1983;9: 487–496.
30. Atmore WG, Dahlin DC, Ghormley RK. Pigmented villonodular synovitis: a clinical and pathologic study. *Minn Med* 1956;39:196–202.
31. Baker ND, Klein JD, Weidner N, Weissman BN, Brick GW. Pigmented villonodular synovitis containing coarse calcifications. *Am J Roentgenol* 1989;153:1228–1230.
32. Balsara ZN, Staiken BF, Martinez AJ. MR image of localized giant cell tumor of the tendon sheath involving the knee. *J Comput Assist Tomogr* 1989;13:159–162.
33. Besette PR, Cooley PA, Johnson RP, Czarnecki DJ. Gadolinium-enhanced MRI of pigmented villonodular synovitis of the knee. *J Comput Assist Tomogr* 1992;16:992–994.
34. Bhawan J, Joris I, Cohen N, Majno G. Microcirculatory change in posttraumatic pigmented villonodular synovitis. *Arch Pathol Lab Med* 1980;104:328–332.
35. Boyd AD Jr, Sledge CB. Evaluation of the hip with pigmented villonodular synovitis. A case report. *Clin Orthop* 1992;275:180–186.
36. Breimer CW, Freiberger RH. Bone lesions associated with villonodular synovitis. *Am J Roentgenol* 1958;80:618–629.
37. Butt WP, Hardy G, Ostlere SJ. Pigmented villonodular synovitis of the knee: computed tomographic appearances. *Skeletal Radiol* 1990;19: 191–196.
38. Byers PD, Cotton RE, Deacon OW, Lowy M, Newman PH, Sissons HA, Thomson AD. The diagnosis and treatment of pigmented villonodular synovitis. *J Bone Joint Surg* 1968;50B:290–305.
39. Cavanagh R, Schwamm HA. RPC of the month from AFIP. *Radiology* 1971;100:409–414.
40. Cotten A, Flipo R-M, Chastanet P, Desvigne-Noulet M-C, Duquesnoy B, Delcambre B. Pigmented villonodular synovitis of the hip: review of radiographic features in 58 patients. *Skeletal Radiol* 1995;24:1–6.
41. Crawford GP, Offerman RJ. Pigmented villonodular synovitis in the hand. *Hand* 1980;12:282–287.
42. Crosby EB, Inglis A, Bullough PG. Multiple joint involvement with pigmented villonodular synovitis. *Radiology* 1977;122:671–672.
43. De Beuckeleer L, De Schepper A, De Belder F, Van Goethem J, Marques MCB, Broeckx J, Verstraete K, Vermaut F. Magnetic resonance imaging of localized giant cell tumour of the tendon sheath (MRI of localized GCTTS). *Eur Radiol* 1997;7:198–201.
44. Descamps F, Yasik E, Hardy D, Lafontaine M, Delince P. Pigmented villonodular synovitis of the hip. A case report and review of the literature. *Clin Rheumatol* 1991;10:184–190.
45. Docken WP. Pigmented villonodular synovitis: a review with illustrative case reports. *Semin Arthritis Rheum* 1979;9:1–22.
46. Dorwart RH, Genant HK, Johnston WH, Morris JM. Pigmented villonodular synovitis of synovial joints: clinical, pathologic, and radiologic features. *Am J Roentgenol* 1984;143:877–885.
47. Eustace SE, Harrison M, Srinivasen U, Stack J. Magnetic resonance imaging in pigmented villonodular synovitis. *Can Assoc Radiol J* 1994;45:283–286.
48. Enzinger FM, Weiss SW. Benign tumors and tumor-like lesions of synovial tissue. In: *Soft tissue tumors.* St. Louis, CV Mosby, 1988; 638–658.
49. Flandry F, Hughston JC. Pigmented villonodular synovitis. *J Bone Joint Surg* 1987;69A:942–949.
50. Fletcher AG Jr, Horn RC Jr. Giant-cell tumor of tendon sheath origin: a consideration of bone involvement and report of 2 cases with extensive bone destruction. *Ann Surg* 1951;133:374–385.
51. Fraire AE, Fechner RE. Intra-articular localized nodular synovitis of the knee. *Arch Pathol* 1972;93:473–476.
52. Galloway JDB, Broders AC, Ghormley RK. Xanthoma of tendon sheaths and synovial membranes. *Arch Surg* 1940;40:485–538.
53. Georgen TG, Resnick D, Niwayama G. Localized nodular synovitis of the knee: a report of two cases with abnormal arthrograms. *Am J Roentgenol* 1976;126:647–650.
54. Ghadially FN, Labonde JMA, Dick CE. Ultrastructure of pigmented villonodular synovitis. *J Pathol* 1979;127:19–26.
55. Goldman AB, DiCarlo EF. Pigmented villonodular synovitis. Diagnosis and differential diagnosis. *Radiol Clin North Am* 1988;26: 1327–1347.

56. Granowitz SP, D Antonio J, Mankin HL. The pathogenesis and long-term end results of pigmented villonodular synovitis. *Clin Orthop* 1976;114:335–351.
57. Granowitz SP, Mankin HJ. Localized pigmented villonodular synovitis of the knee. Report of five cases. *J Bone Joint Surg* 1967; 49A:122–128.
58. Greenfield MM, Wallace KM. Pigmented villonodular synovitis. *Radiology* 1950;54:350–356.
59. Grieten M, Buckwalter KA, Cardinal E, Rougraff B. Case report 873. Lipoma arborescens (villous lipomatous proliferation of the synovial membrane). *Skeletal Radiol* 1994;23:652–655.
60. Hirohata K. Light microscopic and electron microscopic studies of individual cells in pigmented villonodular synovitis and bursitis. *Kobe J Med Sci* 1968;14:251–279.
61. Hughes TH, Sartoris DJ, Schweitzer ME, Resnick DL. Pigmented villonodular synovitis: MRI characteristics. *Skeletal Radiol* 1995;24: 7–12.
62. Jaffe HL, Lichtenstein L, Sutro CJ. Pigmented villonodular synovitis, bursitis and tenosynovitis. *Arch Pathol Lab Med* 1941;31: 731–765.
63. Jelinek JS, Kransdorf MJ, Shmookler BM, Aboulafia AA, Malawer MM. Giant cell tumor of the tendon sheath: MR findings in nine cases. *Am J Roentgenol* 1994;162:919–922.
64. Jelinek JS, Kransdorf MJ, Utz JA, Hudson-Berry B Jr, Thompson JD, Heekin RD, Radowich MS. Imaging of pigmented villonodular synovitis with emphasis on MR imaging. *Am J Roentgenol* 1989;152: 337–342.
65. Jergesen HE, Mankin HJ, Schiller AL. Diffuse pigmented villonodular synovitis of the knee mimicking primary bone neoplasms. A report of two cases. *J Bone Joint Surg* 1978;60A:825–829.
66. Karasick D, Karasick S. Giant cell tumor of tendon sheath: spectrum of radiologic findings. *Skeletal Radiol* 1992;21:219–224.
67. Jones FE, Soule EM, Coventry MB. Fibrous xanthoma of synovium (giant-cell tumor of tendon sheath, pigmented nodular synovitis). A study of 118 cases. *J Bone Joint Surg* 1969;51A:76–86.
68. Keenan MG. Computed tomography in pigmented villonodular synovitis of the hip. *J Rheumatol* 1987;14:1181–1183.
69. Khan S, Neumann CH, Steinbach LS, Harrington KD. MRI of giant cell tumor of tendon sheath of the hand: a report of three cases. *Eur Radiol* 1995;5:467–470.
70. Kerr R. Diffuse pigmented villonodular synovitis. *Orthopedics* 1989; 12:1008–1012.
71. Kindblom LG, Gunterberg B. Pigmented villonodular synovitis involving bone. Case report. *J Bone Joint Surg* 1978;60A:830–832.
72. Klompmaker J, Veth RPH, Robinson PH, Molenaar WM, Nielsen HKL. Pigmented villonodular synovitis. *Arch Orthop Trauma Surg* 1990;109:205–210.
73. Kottal AR, Vogler JB, Matamoros A, Alexander AH, Cookson JL. Pigmented villonodular synovitis: a report of MR imaging in two cases. *Radiology* 1987;163:551–553.
74. Kursunoglu-Brahme S, Riccio T, Weisman MH, Resnick D, Zvaifler N, Sanders ME, Fix C. Rheumatoid knee: role of gadopentetate-enhanced MR imaging. *Radiology* 1990;176: 831–835.
75. Mandelbaum BR, Grant TT, Hartzman S, Reicher MA, Flannigan B, Bassett LW, Mirra J, Finerman AM. The use of MRI to assist in the diagnosis of pigmented villonodular synovitis of the knee. *Clin Orthop* 1988;231:135–139.
76. McMaster PE. Pigmented villonodular synovitis with invasion of bone. Report of six cases. *J Bone Joint Surg* 1960;42A:1170–1183.
77. Miller WE. Villonodular synovitis: pigmented and nonpigmented variations. *South Med J* 1982;75:1084–1086.
78. Mulder JD, Kroon HM, Schütte HE, Taconis WK. *Radiologic atlas of bone tumors.* Amsterdam: Elsevier, 1993.
79. Myers BW, Masi AT. Pigmented villonodular synovitis and tenosynovitis, a clinical epidemiologic study of 166 cases and literature review. *Medicine* 1980;59:224–238.
80. Nilsonne U, Moberger G. Pigmented villonodular synovitis of joints: histological and clinical problems in diagnosis. *Acta Orthop Scand* 1983;24:67–70.
81. Patel MR, Zinberg EM. Pigmented villonodular synovitis of the wrist invading bone; report of a case. *J Hand Surg* 1984;9:854–858.
82. Poletti SC, Gates HS III, Martinez SM, Richardson WJ. The use of magnetic resonance imaging in the diagnosis of pigmented villonodular synovitis. *Orthopedics* 1990;13:185–190.
83. Rao AS, Vigorita VJ. Pigmented villonodular synovitis (giant-cell tumor of the tendon sheath and synovial membrane). A review of eighty-one cases. *J Bone Joint Surg* 1984;66A:76–94.
84. Ray RA, Morton CC, Lipinski KK, Corson JM, Fletcher JA. Cytogenetic evidence of clonality in a case of pigmented villonodular synovitis. *Cancer* 1991;67:121–125.
85. Rosenthal DI, Aronow S, Murray WT. Iron content of pigmented villonodular synovitis detected by computed tomography. *Radiology* 1979;133:409–411.
86. Schumacher HR, Lotke P, Athreya B, Rothfuss S. Pigmented villonodular synovitis: light and electron microscopic studies. *Semin Arthritis Rheum* 1982;12:32–43.
87. Schwartz GB, Coleman DA. Pigmented villonodular synovitis of the wrist and adjacent bone. *Orthop Rev* 1986;15:526–530.
88. Sherry JB, Anderson W. The natural history of pigmented villonodular synovitis of tendon sheath. *J Bone Joint Surg* 1956;37A: 1005–1011.
89. Spritzer CE, Dalinka MK, Kressel HY. Magnetic resonance imaging of pigmented villonodular synovitis: a report of two cases. *Skeletal Radiol* 1987;16:316–319.
90. Steinbach LS, Neumann CH, Stoller DW, Mills CM, Crues JV 3d, Lipman JK, Helms CA, Genant HK. MRI of the knee in diffuse pigmented villonodular synovitis. *Clin Imag* 1989;13:305–316.
91. Stiehl JB, Hackbarth DA. Recurrent pigmented villonodular synovitis of the hip joint, case report and review of the literature. *J Arthroplasty* 1991;6:S85–S90.
92. Stout AP, Lattes R. Tumors of the soft tissue. In: *Atlas of tumor pathology,* 2nd series, fascicle 1. Washington DC: Armed Forces Institute of Pathology, 1967.
93. Suh J, Griffith HJ, Galloway HR, Everson LI. MRI in the diagnosis of synovial disease. *Orthopedics* 1992;15:778–781.
94. Sundaram M, Chalk D, Merenda J, Verde JM, Salinas-Madrigal L. Case report 563. Pigmented villonodular synovitis (PVNS) of knee. *Skeletal Radiol* 1989;18:463–465.
95. Sundaram M, McGuire MH, Fletcher J, Wolverson MK, Heiberg E, Shields JB. Magnetic resonance imaging of lesions of synovial origin. *Skeletal Radiol* 1986;15:110–116.
96. Ushijima M, Hashimoto H, Tsuneyoshi M, Enjoji M. Giant cell tumor of the tendon sheath (nodular tenosynovitis). A study of 207 cases to compare the large joint group with the common digit group. *Cancer* 1986;57:875–884.
97. Wagner ML, Spjut HJ, Dutton RV, Glassman AL, Askew JB. Polyarticular pigmented villonodular synovitis. *Am J Roentgenol* 1981; 136:821–823.
98. Weisz GM, Gal A, Kitchener PN. Magnetic resonance imaging in the diagnosis of aggressive villonodular synovitis. *Clin Orthop* 1988;236: 303–306.
99. Young JM, Hudacek AG. Experimental production of pigmented villonodular synovitis in dogs. *Am J Pathol* 1981;19:379–392.
100. Yudd AP, Velchik MG. Pigmented villonodular synovitis of the hip. *Clin Nucl Med* 1985;10:441–442.
101. Zwass A, Abdelwahab IF, Klein MJ. Case report 463. Pigmented villonodular synovitis (PVNS) of the knee. *Skeletal Radiol* 1988;17: 81–84.
102. Zwass A, Greenspan A, Green SM. Giant cell tumor of the tendon sheath with a pathologic phalangeal fracture: a rare association. *Bull Hosp Joint Dis Orthop Inst* 1985;45:87–93.

Synovial Hemangioma

103. Armstrong SJ, Watt I. Lipoma arborescens of the knee. *Br J Radiol* 1989;62:178–180.
104. Bullough PG. *Atlas of orthopaedic pathology with clinical and radiologic correlations,* 2nd ed. New York: Gower, 1992.
105. Brodsky AE. Synovial hemangioma of the knee joint. *Bull Hosp Joint Dis* 1956;17:58–69.
106. Buetow PC, Kransdorf MJ, Moser RP Jr, Jelinek JS, Berrey BH. Radiologic appearance of intramuscular hemangioma with emphasis on MR imaging. *Am J Roentgenol* 1990;154:563–567.
107. Cotten A, Flipo RM, Herbaux B, Gougeon F, Lecomte-Houcke M, Chastanet P. Synovial haemangioma of the knee: a frequently misdiagnosed lesion. *Skeletal Radiol* 1995;24:257–261.
108. Devaney K, Vinh TN, Sweet DE. Synovial hemangioma: report of 20 cases with differential diagnostic considerations. *Hum Pathol* 1993; 24:737–745.

109. Ehara S, Son M, Tamakawa Y, Nishida J, Abe M, Hachiya J. Fluid-fluid levels in cavernous hemangioma of soft tissue. *Skeletal Radiol* 1994;23:107–109.

110. Hawnaur JM, Whitehouse RW, Jenkins JP, Isherwood I. Musculoskeletal haemangiomas: comparison of MRI with CT. *Skeletal Radiol* 1990;19:251–258.

111. Jacobs JE, Lee FW. Hemangioma of the knee joint. *J Bone Joint Surg* 1949;31A:831–836.

112. Larson IJ, Landry RN. Hemangioma of the synovial membrane. *J Bone Joint Surg* 1969;51A: 1210–1215.

113. Lenchik L, Poznanski AK, Donaldson JS, Sarwark JF. Case report 681. Synovial hemangioma of the knee. *Skeletal Radiol* 1991;20: 387–389.

114. Levin DC, Gordon DH, McSweeney J. Arteriography of peripheral hemangiomas. *Radiology* 1976;121:625–630.

115. Llauger J, Monill JM, Palmer J, Clotet M. Synovial hemangioma of the knee: MRI findings in two cases. *Skeletal Radiol* 1995;24: 579–581.

116. Madewell JE, Sweet DE. Tumors and tumor-like lesions in or about joints. In: Resnick D, ed. *Bone and joint imaging.* Philadelphia: WB Saunders, 1989;1184.

117. Moon NF. Synovial hemangioma of the knee joint. A review of previously reported cases and inclusion of two new cases. *Clin Orthop* 1973;90:183–190.

118. Osburn AW, Bassett LW, Seeger LL, Mirra JM, Eckardt JJ. Case report 609. Synovial (osteo)chondromatosis. *Skeletal Radiol* 1990;19: 237–241.

119. Resnick D, Oliphant M. Hemophilia-like arthropathy of the knee associated with cutaneous and synovial hemangiomas. *Radiology* 1975; 114:323–326.

120. Suh J-S, Hwang G, Hahn S-B. Soft tissue hemangiomas: MR manifestations in 23 patients. *Skeletal Radiol* 1994;23:621–625.

121. Waddell GF. A haemangioma involving tendons. *J Bone Joint Surg* 1967;49B:138–141.

122. Weitzman G. Lipoma arborescens of the knee. *J Bone Joint Surg* 1965;47A:1030–1033.

123. Wolfe RD, Giuliano VJ. Double-contrast arthrography in the diagnosis of pigmented villonodular synovitis of the knee. *Am J Roentgenol* 1970;110:793–799.

Synovial Sarcoma

124. Ackerman LV. Extra-osseous localized non-neoplastic bone and cartilage formation (so-called myositis ossificans). Clinical and pathological confusion with malignant neoplasms. *J Bone Joint Surg (Am)* 1958;40:279–298.

125. Ashton BA, Eagleson CC, Bab I, Owen ME. Distribution of fibroblastic colony-forming cells in rabbit bone marrow and assay of their osteogenic potential by an in vitro diffusion chamber method calcification. *Tissue Int* 1984;36:83–86.

126. Azouz EM, Vicker DB, Brown KLB. Computed tomography of synovial sarcoma of the foot. *J Can Assoc Radiol* 1984;35:85–87.

127. Blacksin M, Adesokan A, Benevenia J. Case report 871. Synovial sarcoma, monophasic type. *Skeletal Radiol* 1994;23:589–591.

128. Cadman NL, Soule EH, Kelly PJ. Synovial sarcoma: an analysis of 134 tumors. *Cancer* 1965;18:613–627.

129. Chung EB, Enzinger FM. Extraskeletal osteosarcoma. *Cancer* 1987; 60:1132–1142.

130. Campanacci M. *Bone and soft-tissue tumors.* New York: Springer-Verlag, 1990;998–1012.

131. Enterline HT. Histopathology of sarcomas. *Semin Oncol* 1981; 8:133–155.

132. Enzinger FM, Weiss SW. *Soft tissue tumors,* 3rd ed. St. Louis: CV Mosby, 1995;757–786.

133. Ernst M, Froesch ER. Growth hormone dependent stimulation of osteoblast-like cells in serum-free cultures via local synthesis of insulin-like growth factor 1. *Biochem Biophys Res Commun* 1988;151: 142–147.

134. Evans HL. Synovial sarcoma: a study of 23 biphasic and 17 probably monophasic examples. *Pathol Annu* 1980;15:309–313.

135. Farris KB, Reed RJ. Monophasic, glandular, synovial sarcomas and carcinomas of the soft tissues. *Arch Pathol Lab Med* 1982;106: 129–132.

136. Geirnaerdt MJA, Kroon HM, van der Heul RO, Hertkens III. Tumoral calcinosis. *Skeletal Radiol* 1995;24:148–151.

137. Goldman AB: Myositis ossificans circumscripta: a benign lesion with a malignant differential diagnosis. *Am J Roentgenol* 1976;126: 32–40.

138. Greenfield GB, Arrington JA, Kudryk BT. MRI of soft tissue tumors. *Skeletal Radiol* 1993;22:77–84.

139. Horowitz AL, Resnick D, Watson RC. The roentgen features of synovial sarcomas. *Clin Radiol* 1973;24:481–484.

140. Ishida T, Iijima T, Moriyama S, Nakamura C, Kitagawa T, Machinami R. Intra-articular calcifying synovial sarcoma mimicking synovial chondromatosis. *Skeletal Radiol* 1996;25:766–769.

141. Jones BC, Sundaram M, Kransdorf MJ. Synovial sarcoma: MR imaging findings in 34 patients. *Am J Roentgenol* 1993;161:827–830.

142. Jotereau FW, LeDouarin NM. The developmental relationship between osteocytes and osteoclasts: a study using the quail-chick nucleus marker in endochondral ossification. *Dev Biol* 1978;63: 253–265.

143. Krall RA, Kostinovsky M, Patchefsky AS. Synovial sarcoma: a clinical, pathological, and ultrastructural study of 26 cases supporting the recognition of monophasic variant. *Am J Surg Pathol* 1981; 5:137–151.

144. Kransdorf MJ, Jelinek JS, Moser RP, Utz JA, Brower AC, Hudson TM, Berrey BH. Soft-tissue masses: diagnosis using MR imaging. *Am J Roentgenol* 1989;153:541–547.

145. Mahajan H, Lorigan JG, Shirkhoda A. Synovial sarcoma: MR imaging. *Magn Reson Imag* 1989;7:211–216.

146. Majeste RM, Beckman EN. Synovial sarcoma with an overwhelming epithelial component. *Cancer* 1988;61:2527–2531.

147. McKinney CD, Mills SE, Fechner RE. Intraarticular synovial sarcoma. *Am J Surg Pathol* 1992;16:1017–1020.

148. Meyer CA, Kransdorf MJ, Moser PP Jr, Jelinek JS. Case report 716. Soft-tissue metastasis in synovial sarcoma. *Skeletal Radiol* 1992;21: 128–131.

149. Miettinen M, Virtanen I. Synovial sarcoma—a misnomer. *Am J Pathol* 1984;117:18–25.

150. Milchgrub S, Ghandur-Mnaymneh L, Dorfman HD, Albores-Saavedra J. Synovial sarcoma with extensive osteoid and bone formation. *Am J Surg Pathol* 1993;17:357–363.

151. Mirra JM, Wang S, Bhuta S. Synovial sarcoma with squamous differentiation of its mesenchymal glandular elements. *Am J Surg Pathol* 1984;8:791–796.

152. Morton MJ, Berquist TH, McLeod RA, Unni KK, Sim FH. MR imaging of synovial sarcoma. *Am J Roentgenol* 1991;156:337–340.

153. Murphey MD, Sartoris DJ, Quale JL, Pathria MN, Martin NL. Musculoskeletal manifestations of chronic renal insufficiency. *RadioGraphics* 1993;13:357–379.

154. Nuovo MA, Norman A, Chumas J, Ackerman LV. Myositis ossificans with atypical clinical, radiographic, or pathologic fingings: a review of 23 cases. *Skeletal Radiol* 1992;21:87–101.

155. Schajowicz F. *Tumors and tumorlike lesions of bone: pathology, radiology, and treatment,* 2nd ed. New York: Springer-Verlag, 1994.

156. Shapeero LG, Vanel D, Couanet D, Contesso G, Ackerman LV. Extraskeletal mesenchymal chondrosarcoma. *Radiology* 1993;186: 819–826.

157. Soule EH. Synovial sarcoma. *Am J Surg Pathol* 1986;10:78–82.

158. Steinbach LS, Johnston JO, Tepper EF, Honda GD, Martel W. Tumoral calcinosis: radiologic-pathologic correlation. *Skeletal Radiol* 1995;24:573–578.

159. Strickland B, Mackenzie DH. Bone involvement in synovial sarcoma. *J Faculty Radiol* 1959;10:64–72.

160. Sundaram M, McLeod RA. MR imaging of tumor and tumorlike lesions of bone and soft tissue. *Am J Roentgenol* 1990;155:817–824.

161. Varela-Duran J, Enzinger FM. Calcifying synovial sarcoma. *Cancer* 1982;50:345–352.

162. Witkin GB, Miettinen M, Rosai J. A biphasic tumor of the mediastinum with features of synovial sarcoma. *Am J Surg Pathol* 1989;13: 490–499.

163. Wright PH, Sim FH, Soule EH, Taylor WF. Synovial sarcoma. *J Bone Joint Surg* 1982;64A:112–122.

164. Wilbur JF, Slatopolsky E. Hyperphosphatemia and tumoral calcinosis. *Ann Intern Med* 1968;68:1044–1049.

165. Wu KK, Collon DJ, Guise ER. Extraosseous chondrosarcoma. *J Bone Joint Surg* 1980;62A:189–194.

Synovial Chondrosarcoma

166. Dahlin DC, Unni KK. Chondrosarcoma. In: *Bone tumors. General Aspects and Data on 8542 Cases,* 4th ed. Springfield, IL: Charles C Thomas, 1986;227–259.
167. Dunn EJ, McGavran MH, Nelson P, Greer RB III. Synovial chondrosarcoma. Report of a case. *J Bone Joint Surg* 1974;56A:811–813.
168. Hermann G, Klein MJ, Abdelwahab IF, Kenan S. Synovial chondrosarcoma arising in synovial chondromatosis of the right hip. *Skeletal Radiol* 1997:26:366-369.
169. Kaiser TE, Ivins JC, Unni KK. Malignant transformation of extra-articular synovial chondromatosis: report of a case. *Skeletal Radiol* 1980;5:223–226.
170. Milgram JW, Addison RG. Synovial osteochondromatosis of the knee. Chondromatous recurrence with possible chondrosarcomatous degeneration. *J Bone Joint Surg* 1976;58A:264–266.
171. Mullins F, Berard CW, Eisenberg SH. Chondrosarcoma following synovial chondromatosis. A case study. *Cancer* 1965;18:1180–1188.
172. Ontell F, Greenspan A. Chondrosarcoma complicating synovial chondromatosis: findings with magnetic resonance imaging. *Can Assoc Radiol J* 1994;45:318–323.
173. Perry BE, McQueen DA, Lin JJ. Synovial chondromatosis with malignant degeneration to chondrosarcoma. Report of a case. *J Bone Joint Surg* 1988;70A:1259–1261.

Subject Index